... a... and ... ...lon

... \D

Geriatric
Otolaryngology

Geriatric Otolaryngology

edited by

Karen H. Calhoun, M.D.
University of Missouri
Columbia, Missouri, U.S.A.

David E. Eibling, M.D.
University of Pittsburgh
Pittsburgh, Pennsylvania, U.S.A.

Associate Editors

Mark K. Wax, M.D.
Oregon Health and Science University
Portland, Oregon, U.S.A.

Karen M. Kost, M.D.
McGill University
Montreal, Quebec, Canada

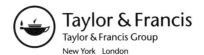
Taylor & Francis
Taylor & Francis Group
New York   London

Published in 2006 by
Taylor & Francis Group
270 Madison Avenue
New York, NY 10016

International Standard Book Number-10: 0-8247-2850-5 (Hardcover)
International Standard Book Number-13: 978-0-8247-2850-2 (Hardcover)

Library of Congress Cataloging-in-Publication Data

Catalog record is available from the Library of Congress

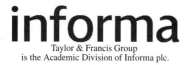

Taylor & Francis Group
is the Academic Division of Informa plc.

**Visit the Taylor & Francis Web site at
http://www.taylorandfrancis.com**

To all senior otolaryngologists who, like Sid Busis,
continue to practice into their 70s and 80s.

Preface

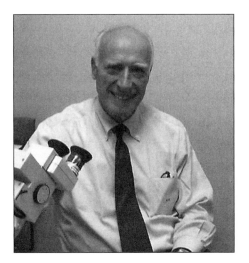

Sidney Busis

The goal of health care is to prolong life and relieve suffering. Each of us hopes to someday achieve elderly status, since the alternative is a life shortened by illness or other misfortune. Yet, simply achieving an advanced age is an imperfect goal for both our patients and ourselves. Our real aim, and that of our patients as well, is to live a rewarding and useful life for as long as is possible. This text is a guide for practitioners in our specialty to assist them in helping their elderly patients achieve their goal of health and the associated high levels of function for as long as possible. By doing so, our patients, and hopefully we as well, will continue to enjoy life and contribute in a meaningful manner to their (and our) professions, families, and communities. Each of us personally knows individuals who are role models in this regard and have been able to contribute much even in their advanced years.

This theme of long-term contribution to a community, even into advanced age, is perhaps demonstrated no better than by Sidney Busis, the author of Chapter 6 "Presbycusis" in this book. "Sid" was a solo private practitioner of otolaryngology for 54 years in Pittsburgh prior to his retirement at the end of 2004. At the age of 84 he continues to be an active contributor to his community, and to this book.

Sid Busis was born September 2, 1921, grew up in Pittsburgh, and attended the University of Pittsburgh for both undergraduate and medical school. During medical school he was an active-duty private in the army, and upon graduation in 1945 he was promoted to first lieutenant and assigned to Randolph Air Force Base where he trained to be a flight surgeon. In 1948, after discharge from the Army Air Corps, he began his training in otolaryngology at the University of Pittsburgh. During his residency he also found time for additional specialty training at the University of Pennsylvania and spent a summer with Chevalier Jackson, who was at Temple University.

Following his residency Sid entered practice and became a solo practitioner of general otolaryngology, later focusing his practice on diseases of the ear. He was a busy surgeon, often performing more than 700 procedures yearly. Although he was in private practice, he actively taught residents both in the operating room and in his office, directed many courses in Pittsburgh, and gave invited lectures. He contributed to the otolaryngology literature and presented instruction courses at the annual meeting of the American Academy of Otolaryngology yearly for 29 years. He also served as president of the medical staff of the Eye and Ear Hospital of Pittsburgh and as president of the American Neurotology Society.

In 1972 Sid recruited Eugene Myers to the University of Pittsburgh as chairman and the first full-time faculty member in the department. Over the next 33 years Dr. Myers served as department chair, and he and Sid remain close friends to this day.

Sid did much more for his community than practice otolaryngology and teach. He was, and remains, active in his local temple and community, serving as president of the United Jewish Federation of Pittsburgh and president of his congregation. He has donated both time and money through his leadership of local fund raising campaigns as well as several national nonprofit organizations. Sid has been a lifelong optimist. When he says "Do the math" he is not referring to the funds he has collected or to his years in practice, but rather to how lucky we all are to be alive at this time. "Do the math" means "Count your blessings," a message for all of us, regardless of age.

The significance of Sid's long career cannot be underestimated. Not only did he contribute in a meaningful way to his patients, his residents, and his community, but he continued to do so until into his eighties. His professional activities have spanned nearly 60 years, 54 years in solo private practice. When asked to author a chapter for this book when already 20 years past the age when most individuals are considering retirement, he eagerly accepted and in a short time produced a scholarly work. As you read his chapter, recall that Sid finished medical school at the end of World War II and that he has been in practice since before many or most of us were born.

The lifelong continuing contributions of Sidney Busis have served as an inspiration to the editors of this text. We hope that we, too, will be able to contribute over the years as he has shown to be possible.

As you read Sid's chapter, be reminded that many of our geriatric patients are capable and willing to contribute to their professions, families, and communities. Assisting them in achieving this goal through appropriate management of diseases and disorders of the ear, nose, and throat is, in fact, our responsibility as practitioners of our specialty.

Sid reminds us of what is possible for our patients, and ourselves, if we only believe it to be so.

Karen H. Calhoun M.D.
David E. Eibling M.D.
Karen M. Kost M.D.
Mark K. Wax M.D.

Contents

Contributors

Gopal Allada   Division of Pulmonary and Critical Care and Sleep Medicine, Department of Pulmonary and Critical Care, Oregon Health and Science University, Portland, Oregon, U.S.A.

Sonia Ancoli-Israel   Department of Psychiatry, University of California–San Diego and VA San Diego Healthcare System, San Diego, California, U.S.A.

Jonathan E. Aviv   Voice and Swallowing Center, Department of Otolaryngology—Head and Neck Surgery, College of Physicians and Surgeons, Columbia University, Columbia University Medical Center, New York–Presbyterian Hospital, New York, New York, U.S.A.

Vance D. Bachelder   Department of Biomedical Engineering, University of Minnesota Graduate School, Medical Instrumentation and Device (MIND) Laboratory/Bakken Institute, Minneapolis, Minnesota, U.S.A.

Steven Barczi   Section of Geriatrics, Department of Medicine, University of Wisconsin–Madison, and Geriatric Research Education and Clinical Center, William S. Middleton Veterans Hospital, Madison, Wisconsin, U.S.A.

Paul Bascom   Palliative Medicine and Comfort Care Team, Division of General Internal Medicine, Oregon Health and Science University, Portland, Oregon, U.S.A.

Amy R. Blanchard   Section of Pulmonary/Critical Care Medicine, Medical College of Georgia, Augusta, Georgia, U.S.A.

Michel A. Cramer Bornemann   Departments of Neurology and Pulmonary/Critical Care Medicine, Minnesota Regional Sleep Disorders Center, Hennepin County Medical Center, Minneapolis, Minnesota, U.S.A.

Sidney N. Busis   Department of Otolaryngology, University of Pittsburgh, Pittsburgh, Pennsylvania, U.S.A.

Stephen J. Chadwick   Department of Otolaryngology, Southern Illinois School of Medicine, Springfield, and ENTA Allergy Head and Neck Institute, Decatur, Illinois, U.S.A.

Ara A. Chalian Geriatric Committee AAO-HNS, Department of Otolaryngology—Head and Neck Surgery, University of Pennsylvania, Philadelphia, Pennsylvania, U.S.A.

Marshall Chasin Musicians' Clinics of Canada, Toronto, Ontario, Canada

Margaret A. Chen Division of Otolaryngology—Head and Neck Surgery, VA San Diego Healthcare System, and Department of Surgery, UCSD Medical Center, San Diego, California, U.S.A.

Daniel H. Coelho Section of Otolaryngology, Yale University School of Medicine, New Haven, Connecticut, U.S.A.

Bobby M. Collins Oral Medicine and Pathology, University of Pittsburgh School of Dental Medicine, Pittsburgh, Pennsylvania, U.S.A.

Nadine Connor Division of Otolaryngology, Department of Surgery, University of Wisconsin–Madison, Madison, Wisconsin, U.S.A.

Ted A. Cook Department of Otolaryngology—Head and Neck Surgery, Oregon Health and Science University, Portland, Oregon, U.S.A.

Robert L. Cross Jr. Department of Anesthesiology and Perioperative Medicine, Oregon Health and Science University, Portland, Oregon, U.S.A.

Sam J. Daniel Saliva Management Clinic, McGill University Health Center, Montreal Children's Hospital, Montreal, Quebec, Canada

Stephanie K. Daniels Research Service, VA Medical Center, and Department of Psychiatry and Neurology, Tulane University Health Sciences Center, New Orleans, Louisiana, U.S.A.

Terence M. Davidson Division of Otolaryngology—Head and Neck Surgery, VA San Diego Healthcare System, and Department of Surgery, UCSD Medical Center, San Diego, California, U.S.A.

Myrdalis Díaz-Ramírez Department of Anesthesiology and Perioperative Medicine, Oregon Health and Science University, Portland, Oregon, U.S.A.

Joanne DeLuzio Graduate Department of Speech-Language Pathology, University of Toronto, Toronto, Ontario, Canada

Richard L. Doty Smell and Taste Center, University of Pennsylvania Medical Center, Philadelphia, Pennsylvania, U.S.A.

Umamaheswar Duvvuri Division of Sino-Nasal Disorders and Allergy, Department of Otolaryngology, University of Pittsburgh, Pittsburgh, Pennsylvania, U.S.A.

David E. Eibling Department of Otolaryngology—Head and Neck Surgery, University of Pittsburgh School of Medicine, Pittsburgh, Pennsylvania, U.S.A.

Michelina Fato Department of Medicine, Western Pennsylvania Hospital, Pittsburgh, Pennsylvania, U.S.A.

Berrylin J. Ferguson Division of Sino-Nasal Disorders and Allergy, Department of Otolaryngology, University of Pittsburgh, Pittsburgh, Pennsylvania, U.S.A.

Lavinia Fiorentino Doctoral Program in Clinical Psychology, San Diego State University and University of California–San Diego, San Diego, California, U.S.A.

Karen J. Fong Department of Otolaryngology—Head and Neck Surgery, Oregon Health and Science University, Portland, Oregon, U.S.A.

Anne L. Foundas Department of Psychiatry and Neurology, Tulane University Health Sciences Center, and Neurology Section, VA Medical Center, New Orleans, Louisiana, U.S.A.

Oren Friedman Division of Facial Plastic and Reconstructive Surgery, Department of Otolaryngology, Mayo Clinic, Rochester, Minnesota, U.S.A.

Gerry F. Funk Department of Otolaryngology—Head and Neck Surgery, University of Iowa College of Medicine, Iowa City, Iowa, U.S.A.

Joseph M. Furman Division of Balance Disorders, Department of Otolaryngology, University of Pittsburgh, Pittsburgh, Pennsylvania, U.S.A.

Serge Gauthier McGill Center for Studies in Aging, McGill University, Montreal, Quebec, Canada

Eric Genden Department of Otolaryngology, Mount Sinai Medical Center, New York, New York, U.S.A.

Jack L. Gluckman Department of Otolaryngology—Head and Neck Surgery, University of Cincinnati Medical Center, Cincinnati, Ohio, U.S.A.

James S. Goodwin Department of Internal Medicine, Sealy Center on Aging, University of Texas Medical Branch, Galveston, Texas, U.S.A.

Timothy C. Hain Departments of Physical Therapy, Neurology, and Otolaryngology, Northwestern University Medical School, Chicago, Illinois, U.S.A.

Emily R. Hajjar Philadelphia College of Pharmacy, University of the Sciences in Philadelphia, Philadelphia, Pennsylvania, U.S.A.

Joseph T. Hanlon Department of Medicine (Geriatrics), University of Pittsburgh, Pittsburgh, Pennsylvania, U.S.A.

Richard Hanson Department of Anesthesiology and Perioperative Medicine, Oregon Health and Science University, Portland, Oregon, U.S.A.

Allen R. Huang Geriatric Medicine, McGill University Health Centre, Royal Victoria Hospital, Montreal, Quebec, Canada

Jonas T. Johnson   Department of Otolaryngology and Radiation Oncology, University of Pittsburgh School of Medicine, Pittsburgh, Pennsylvania, U.S.A.

Eric J. Kezirian   Department of Otolaryngology—Head and Neck Surgery, University of California–San Francisco, San Francisco, California, U.S.A.

Horst R. Konrad   Division of Otolaryngology—Head and Neck Surgery, Southern Illinois University School of Medicine, Springfield, Illinois, U.S.A.

Karen M. Kost   Department of Otolaryngology, McGill University, Montreal General Hospital, Montreal, Quebec, Canada

Miriam N. Lango   Department of Surgical Oncology, Fox Chase Cancer Center, Philadelphia, Pennsylvania, U.S.A.

Sue Ellen Linville   Department of Speech Pathology and Audiology, Marquette University, Milwaukee, Wisconsin, U.S.A.

Lianqi Liu   Department of Psychiatry, University of California–San Diego and VA San Diego Healthcare System, San Diego, California, U.S.A.

Robert H. Maisel   Department of Otolaryngology—Head and Neck Surgery, Minnesota Regional Sleep Disorders Center, Hennepin County Medical Center, Minneapolis, Minnesota, U.S.A.

Donna J. Millay   Division of OtoHNS, Department of Surgery, University of Vermont, Burlington, Vermont, U.S.A.

Natasha Mirza   Department of Otolaryngology—Head and Neck Surgery, University of Pennsylvania Health System and Philadelphia VA Medical Center, Philadelphia, Pennsylvania, U.S.A.

Laura O. Morris   Balance and Vestibular Program, Eye and Ear Institute, Centers for Rehab Services, Pittsburgh, Pennsylvania, U.S.A.

Thomas Murry   Voice and Swallowing Center, Department of Otolaryngology—Head and Neck Surgery, College of Physicians and Surgeons, Columbia University, Columbia University Medical Center, New York–Presbyterian Hospital, New York, New York, U.S.A.

Meiho Nakayama   Department of Otolaryngology, Aichi Medical University, Aichigun Aichiken, Japan

Julian M. Nedzelski   Department of Otolaryngology and Head and Neck Surgery, Sunnybrook and Women's College Health Sciences Centre and University of Toronto, Toronto, Ontario, Canada

Christopher D. Newell   Department of Anesthesia and Perioperative Medicine, Oregon Health and Science University, Portland, Oregon, U.S.A.

Amanda Ortmann   Communication Science and Disorders, University of Pittsburgh, and Department of Audiology and Speech Language Pathology, VA Pittsburgh Health Care System, Pittsburgh, Pennsylvania, U.S.A.

David W. Oslin   Department of Psychiatry, University of Pennsylvania, and Philadelphia VA Medical Center, Philadelphia, Pennsylvania, U.S.A.

Catherine V. Palmer   Communication Science and Disorders, University of Pittsburgh, and Audiology and Hearing Aids, Department of Otolaryngology, University of Pittsburgh Medical Center, Pittsburgh, Pennsylvania, U.S.A.

Kenny P. Pang   Department of Otolaryngology, Tan Tock Seng Hospital, Tan Tock Seng, Singapore, and Department of Otolaryngology—Head and Neck Surgery, Medical College of Georgia, Augusta, Georgia, U.S.A.

Steven M. Parnes   Department of Otolaryngology, Albany Medical Center, Albany, New York, U.S.A.

Richard J. Payne   Department of Otolaryngology, McGill University, Montreal General Hospital, Montreal, Quebec, Canada

Ronen Perez   Department of Otolaryngology and Head and Neck Surgery, Sunnybrook and Women's College Health Sciences Centre and University of Toronto, Toronto, Ontario, Canada

Karen T. Pitman   Department of Otolaryngology and Communicative Sciences, University of Mississippi Medical School, Jackson, Mississippi, U.S.A.

Mukaila A. Raji   Department of Internal Medicine, Geriatrics Clinics, Sealy Center on Aging, University of Texas Medical Branch, Galveston, Texas, U.S.A.

JoAnne Robbins   Sections of Geriatrics and Gastroenterology, Departments of Medicine and Radiology, University of Wisconsin–Madison, and Geriatric Research Education and Clinical Center, William S. Middleton Veterans Hospital, Madison, Wisconsin, U.S.A.

Adam T. Ross   Division of Facial Plastic and Reconstructive Sugery, Department of Otolaryngology, Medical University of South Carolina, Charleston, South Carolina, U.S.A.

Douglas A. Ross   Section of Otolaryngology, Yale University School of Medicine, New Haven, Connecticut, U.S.A.

Vanessa Sakadakis   Social Services Department, McGill University Health Centre, Royal Victoria Hospital, Montreal, Quebec, Canada

Clarence T. Sasaki   Section of Otolaryngology, Yale University School of Medicine, New Haven, Connecticut, U.S.A.

Robert Thayer Sataloff   Department of Otolaryngology—Head and Neck Surgery, Thomas Jefferson University and Graduate Hospital, Philadelphia, Pennsylvania, U.S.A.

Maisie Shindo   Division of Otolaryngology—Head and Neck Surgery, Department of Surgery, State University of New York–Stony Brook, Stony Brook, New York, U.S.A.

David Sibell   Department of Anesthesiology and Perioperative Medicine, Oregon Health and Science University, Portland, Oregon, U.S.A.

Azfar A. Siddiqui   School of Dental Medicine, Department of Maxillofacial Prosthetics, University of Pittsburgh, Pittsburgh, Pennsylvania, U.S.A.

Dana S. Smith   Department of Otolaryngology/Head and Neck Surgery, Oregon Health and Science University, Portland, Oregon, U.S.A.

Jeffrey P. Staab   Departments of Psychiatry and Otorhinolaryngology—Head and Neck Surgery, The Balance Center, University of Pennsylvania Health System, Philadelphia, Pennsylvania, U.S.A.

Hinrich Staecker   Department of Otolaryngology—Head and Neck Surgery, University of Kansas School of Medicine, Kansas City, Kansas, U.S.A.

Frances Tanzella   Division of Otolaryngology—Head and Neck Surgery, Department of Surgery, State University of New York–Stony Brook, Stony Brook, New York, U.S.A.

David J. Terris   Department of Otolaryngology—Head and Neck Surgery, Medical College of Georgia, Augusta, Georgia, U.S.A.

Cyrus Torchinsky   Division of Otolaryngology—Head and Neck Surgery, VA San Diego Healthcare System, and Department of Surgery, UCSD Medical Center, San Diego, California, U.S.A.

Cheryl Ellis Vaiani   Institute for the Medical Humanities, University of Texas Medical Branch, Galveston, Texas, U.S.A.

Tom D. Wang   Department of Otolaryngology—Head and Neck Surgery, Oregon Health and Science University, Portland, Oregon, U.S.A.

Mark K. Wax   Department of Otolaryngology/Head and Neck Surgery, Oregon Health and Science University, Portland, Oregon, U.S.A.

Edward M. Weaver   Department of Otolaryngology—Head and Neck Surgery, University of Washington, Seattle, Washington, U.S.A.

Susan L. Whitney   Departments of Physical Therapy and Otolaryngology, University of Pittsburgh, Pittsburgh, Pennsylvania, U.S.A.

Catherine P. Winslow   Department of Otolaryngology/Head and Neck Surgery, Oregon Health and Science University, Portland, Oregon, U.S.A.

Michael Wolfe   Department of Otolaryngology—Head and Neck Surgery, University of Cincinnati Medical Center, Cincinnati, Ohio, U.S.A.

Dario A. Yacovino   Departments of Physical Therapy, Neurology, and Otolaryngology, Northwestern University Medical School, Chicago, Illinois, U.S.A.

Mark J. Yaffe   Department of Family Medicine, St. Mary's Hospital Center, McGill University, Montreal, Quebec, Canada

Mark A. Zacharek   Department of Otolaryngology—Head and Neck Surgery, Henry Ford Hospital, Detroit, Michigan, U.S.A.

Steven M. Zeitels   Department of Otology and Laryngology, Harvard Medical School, Boston, Massachusetts, U.S.A.

Steven C. Zweig   Department of Family and Community Medicine, University of Missouri–Columbia School of Medicine, Columbia, Missouri, U.S.A.

1

Clinical Approach to the Geriatric Patient

Michelina Fato
Department of Medicine, Western Pennsylvania Hospital, Pittsburgh, Pennsylvania, U.S.A.

That time of year thou may'st in me behold
When yellow leaves, or none, or few, do hang
Upon those boughs which shake against the cold—
Bare ruin'd choirs where late the sweet birds sang
In me thou see'st the twilight of such day
As after Sunset fadeth in the West'
Which by and by black night doth take away,
Death's second self, that seals up all in rest.
In me thou see'st the glowing of such fire
That on the ashes of his youth doth lie,
As the death-bed whereon it must expire,
Consumed with that which it was nourish'd by.

This thou perceiv'st, which makes they love more strong
To love that well which thou must leave ere long.

William Shakespeare
"Sonnet 73"

Shakespeare's beautiful sonnet describes an aging speaker using a series of metaphors such as autumn and twilight. The sonnet allows us to feel sadness for one's loss of youth and eventual death. The field of geriatrics arouses similar feelings in physicians who care for the elderly, this mind-set often making it difficult for some to work with the elderly. Caring for the aged may remind the practitioner of the inevitability of the practitioner's own aging and eventual death. The physician may adopt a sense of futility and believe that there is nothing for the physician to offer an elderly patient that will make any difference. Ageism, a form of discrimination, is rampant in our youth-centered culture, and some physicians may just not want to deal with the complex problems that some elderly patients bring with them. Under-graduate and graduate medical education that continues to be inpatient based, with student exposure primarily to severely debilitated and institutionalized elderly, contributes to physician reluctance in dealing with this population as well.

However, over the next 20 to 50 years, it will become virtually impossible for any physician in any field (with the obvious exception of pediatric specialties) to avoid contact with an elderly patient. This chapter presents a clinical approach to the geriatric patient. It will help the otolaryngologist—hcad and neck surgeon—to be less fearful and feel more comfortable with this challenging and complex population, and hopefully even truly enjoy and gain satisfaction from working with these individuals.

DEMOGRAPHICS OF AGING IN AMERICA

Throughout human history, the age distribution of the population has resembled a pyramid. Improved and healthier living circumstances have contributed to lower death rates at younger ages. With decreasing fertility rates and decreasing death rates among younger cohorts, it is expected that as these younger cohorts age there will be a "squaring of the pyramid," (Figs. 1, 2) and that this will be a permanent change in the population.

The U.S. population is currently 294 million. Of these, 35 million (nearly 12%) are 65 years and older. This number is expected to double over the next 30 years. This dramatic shift in population demographics over the next three decades will lead to profound social, political, and economic changes in this country and most certainly within our current health care system. The number of Americans aged 80

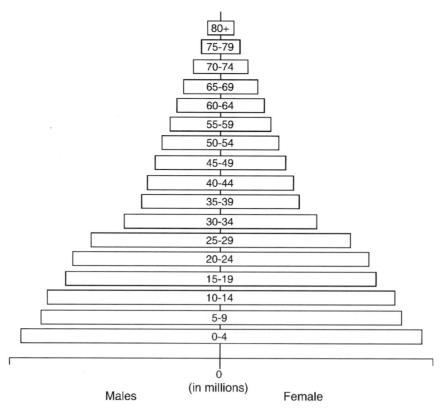

Figure 1   Age pyramid for humans prior to 1900.

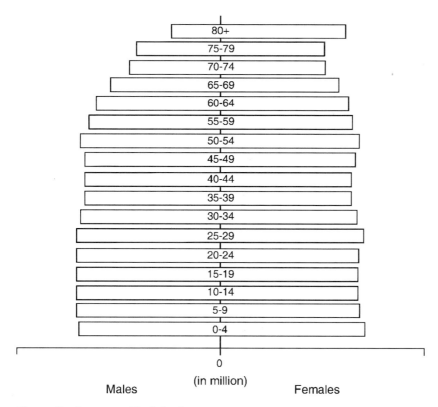

Figure 2 Age pyramid of the future.

and older is expected to rise to 32 million in 2050 and the number of centenarians will approach one million by then as well. Patients aged 65 and older accounted for 22% of all office visits to otolaryngologists in the year 2000; this number is projected to *double* in the next 30 years.

All physicians will be required to deal with the effects of this aging population. It is currently estimated that there is a shortage of more than 13,000 physicians needed to care for geriatric patients. It is projected that 35,000 geriatricians will be needed in the United States in 2030; we currently have about 9000. Without substantive changes in U.S. policies regarding medical education, it seems likely that current shortages will increase. Therefore, it is essential that *all* physicians, including subspecialists, develop a sound clinical approach that takes into account the special needs of this group.

Health Behavior

Studies show that older adults expect to be less healthy than younger adults. They also tend to view themselves as more healthy than they are (1). Overestimating their health may result in "explaining away" problems that in fact may be serious. In addition, health care professionals caring for elderly patients often tend to neglect signs and symptoms of disease, often, in fact, reassuring them that frailty and poor health are "normal" accompaniments of aging. Studies show that older persons tend to *underreport* symptoms and are more likely to minimize symptoms that are potentially serious (e.g., chest pain, bleeding, dyspnea, depression) (2,3). Reasons that elderly give for not reporting symptoms include "no big deal," "nobody cares," "nothing can be done about it," "don't want to bother people" (3). In addition, older persons most often attribute symptoms to aging and tend to adopt a wait and watch approach, accepting symptoms as inevitable and delaying seeking health care. To complicate matters, some physicians perceive that older patients have infinite numbers of complaints and may avoid obtaining a thorough history so as not to open "Pandora's box." There is no documented support for this and, in fact, younger patients tend to have more hypochondriacal symptoms than the elderly (4,5). Although the elderly underreport symptoms, it is important that physicians recognize that concurrence of disease is common in the elderly and that this multiplicity of problems poses serious risks to their health (6). Detecting treatable disease late in the course of illness results in functional decline and can result in catastrophic illness.

Functional decline is the end result for older people, especially for those over age 75, and may be the presenting sign of underlying disease. Elderly patients are less likely to be able to meet their own needs as time passes (7). The so-called geriatric syndromes (falls, confusion, incontinence, dizziness, failure to thrive) are defined as a set of specific functional capacities potentially lost due to a multiplicity of pathologies in multiple organ systems (8). A geriatric syndrome may be an unexpected initial presenting symptom or sign of a classic disease. For example, repeated falls may be the sole manifestation of pneumonia. Because functional loss in an elderly patient is usually a sign of disease, rapid assessment is crucial.

Disease in older patients may present in an atypical manner. The elderly may present with minimal or absent symptoms for many conditions associated with well-recognized symptoms in the younger population. Painless myocardial infarction has been documented in the elderly (9). Hypothyroidism may be more difficult to diagnose due to minimal clinical manifestations. It is important for the clinician to remember that common diseases may present in a nonspecific and atypical manner in the elderly, and that the older patient may underreport symptoms, even if present.

PRACTICAL APPROACH TO THE OFFICE VISIT

It must be recognized that the elderly have different needs than younger patients, and that these needs impact the entire spectrum of patient care. The actual environment in which the patient is evaluated may impact successful diagnosis and treatment. Although most commonly evaluation occurs within the physician's office, in the future it is likely that elderly patients will be evaluated in alternative settings such as the patient's home, nursing homes, assisted living facilities, rehabilitation centers, hospices, and acute care hospitals. Transportation needs will increasingly become an issue as the number of the elderly continues to rise. Older patients may depend on caregivers, government-funded modes of transportation, and paid drivers (jitney) to get to their appointments. This often leads to late arrivals or missed appointments. It is the physicians' responsibility to call older patients who miss an appointment if the visit is essential. There may be a multitude of reasons as to why the patient was unable to keep the appointment. In addition, there should be handicap access to parking and to the office. The length of the visit for a geriatric patient may need to be longer than for a younger patient; this will need to be individualized. It may take an older patient longer to get into the exam room, undress, sit on an exam table, and much longer to give a history. The physician may also need to review a long list of medications and a complex array of medical problems. In any setting, only about half as much light reaches the retina of elderly patients due to aging changes occurring in the ocular lens. Therefore, brighter lighting is required in both waiting rooms and exam rooms. In addition, any written forms that the patient is required to complete or any patient education materials need to be written in large print to accommodate for decreased vision in the elderly. Elderly patients should also be screened for health literacy (see appendix) as this may affect their ability to read medication labels, fill out forms, or read patient education materials (10). The temperature in the exam room should be between 70 and 80 degrees, since the elderly have increased vulnerability to temperature extremes. Greater than 50% of older patients have presbycusis, with resultant poor speech discrimination, particularly in the presence of background noise. Therefore, all distracting background noise in the examination room such as fans, music, etc., should be eliminated, and the setting should be quiet. The physician should speak in a lower pitched voice and face the patient directly to allow lip reading. Elderly patients often have difficulty arising from a sitting position; hence, chairs with a higher than standard seat, or even a mechanical lift to assist in arising, should be available. If an exam table is used, the office should ideally have a mechanical one that lowers and rises to assist the patient in getting on and off the table. If this is not available, a broad-based stool and handrail should be available for mounting and dismounting the exam table (8). A geriatric patient should never be left alone on the exam table to dismount after an exam. Assistance should be offered to reduce the risk of a fall. In addition, the office setting should be evaluated for fall hazards (loose rugs, exposed cords or wires, slippery floors, etc.) and appropriate remedies taken. Distracting and busy patterns on both walls and carpets should be avoided in both the waiting room and the exam room as this may increase the falls risk.

OBTAINING THE HISTORY

When obtaining the history from a geriatric patient, it is important to determine the patient's reliability as a historian as soon as possible. On the other hand, if a patient carries the diagnosis of dementia, one should not assume that the history is unreliable. Dementia includes a wide spectrum of disorders with differing cognitive ability. Patients may have minor cognitive deficits that would be noted only on extensive neuropsychiatric testing. One should begin the history with some simple questions and preface them by stating "these are a few questions that I ask of all of my patients." The physician or nurse should then proceed to ask time, place, date, and other orientation questions in addition to the reason for the visit. If the answers are not accurate and there is a concern of cognitive impairment, it is essential that a family member or caregiver accompany the patient to future visits. Regardless, it is still possible to get important information just by listening to the patient. If a family member is present, it is critical that the physician allow the patient to answer questions directly. If the patient is unable to do so, or if the physician needs clarification, only then should the family member be addressed. In addition, it is also important for the physician to be able to access old medical records and to speak with other providers that have cared for the patient.

Most elderly do not present with one chief complaint, but with multiple complaints that may or may not be inter-related. It is highly unlikely, in fact, that there will be one unifying disease, since most older patients have multiple disorders. This may be less of a problem in the otolaryngologist's office, since the physician is focusing on one system. However, it is important to keep in mind that all the complaints referable to the head and neck may not be attributable to one problem.

The importance of eliciting an adequate medication history cannot be overemphasized. Older patients tend to be on multiple prescribed medications and over-the-counter remedies. Some may be contraindicated and others may counteract each other. In all outpatient settings, it should be emphasized that every patient bring all their medication bottles to every visit. In addition to the prescribed medication bottles, the physician must specifically inquire about herbal and other remedies that are not prescribed. Elderly patients commonly use these, and often do not consider them to be "medications." If the patient is coming alone or if a family member is going to accompany the patient, they should be instructed to gather all medications in the home and bring them to their visit, including laxatives, vitamins, cold preparations, creams and lotions, herbs, etc. The physician can then review all the medications with the patient and ask about dosing.

SOCIAL HISTORY

The perception that the patient's social history is relevant only to the primary care provider can result in suboptimal specialty care in the elderly. Knowledge of the patient's living arrangements is essential and crucial to planning care for the patient. It is important to assess whether the patient lives alone, whether family members live nearby, whom they call in case of an emergency, and whether they see any one individual on a daily or regular basis. The availability of a caregiver will often impact on patient compliance with medications and any home care plan. Social isolation is a common problem in the elderly, and is addressed in a dedicated chapter in this text. It is known that individuals with extensive social networks do better in terms of function and have decreased mortality (11). The physician should also inquire about the home environment, particularly the presence of stairs in the home, loose rugs or other fall hazards, adequate heating and cooling, and neighborhood safety (the latter may be assessed by asking "do you feel safe in your home?"). It is extremely important to ask the patient about finances as many elderly in this country live at or below the federal poverty level. Questions such as "what is your monthly income and what is/are the source(s)" may be asked on an intake form. It is not unusual for an older person to be living on 400 dollars per month from Social Security. This directly affects both medication and visit compliance. Most insurers require co-payments per medication, which can quickly add up, making them unaffordable. In addition, patients on a very limited income may also not be able to afford the physician co-payment.

NUTRITION

Undernutrition increases in prevalence with age. However, with the increasing obesity rates in this country, we may see overnutrition as a growing problem among elderly patients in the future. Undernutrition is commonly a result of oral or gastro-intestinal disorders, medication side effects, psychiatric disease including dementia, inability to shop for or prepare food, lack of companionship, anorexia, poor dentition or ill-fitting dentures, and skipped meals. It is almost always multifactorial in the elderly. A low serum albumin is a good marker of poor nutritional status over the preceding months and correlates with mortality (12). Undernutrition contributes to sarcopenia and frailty in the old.

ALCOHOL, TOBACCO, AND DRUG USE DISORDERS

It is important to screen all elderly patients for drug, tobacco, and alcohol use disorders. Alcohol use disorders are not uncommon in the elderly and routine questions, such as in the CAGE questionnaire (see appendix), should be included in the history. Alcoholism may present as falls, depression, or dementia, and may be masked without careful questioning. Tobacco cessation is of benefit to health even beyond the age of 80 (13,14). The author has encountered several patients over the age of 60 who have heroin and/or cocaine addiction. Substance abuse disorders should be considered in all patients and appropriate screening, intervention, treatment, and referral should be done when necessary.

FUNCTIONAL STATUS

Patients should directly be asked about their ability to function at home. If there are any questions, screening with the BADL (basic activities of daily living) (see appendix) and IADL (instrumental activities of daily living) (see appendix) instruments should be performed (15,16). These tools may be administered by a registered nurse (RN), licensed practical nurse (LPN), or medical assistant (MA) prior to the physician visit. The BADL and IADL address such issues as mobility, bathing, transferring, continence, hygiene, shopping, cooking, managing money, using the telephone, etc., and are reliable indicators of performance. Loss of function, as measured by these instruments, contributes to a decline in health.

END OF LIFE

It is essential to determine individual preferences and values regarding end-of-life care prior to recommending or providing aggressive treatment measures. Often elderly patients are offered aggressive surgery or medical treatment and plans are made only to find out later that these are incongruent with the patient's goals. All patients should routinely be asked on their first visit, even to a subspecialist, whether they have executed a living will or have a proxy decision maker should they become unable to make health care decisions for themselves. These questions can be part of a routine intake questionnaire used by all patients. Neither of these advance directives requires a notary or an attorney, and standard forms are available through state medical societies. The patient and family can complete these forms together and then provide a copy to the physician. The physician should always respect the patient's wishes when they are voiced.

PHYSICAL EXAMINATION

Vital signs should always be obtained at every visit; this should include height, weight, BMI or waist circumference, blood pressure sitting and standing, pulse, and temperature. Orthostatic hypotension is common in the elderly and is often multifactorial in origin (e.g., medications, autonomic dysfunction). Screening with a handheld audiometer is also useful in the elderly and can easily be done by an MA.

General appearance should take note of dress (e.g., stains), hygiene (odor of urine or stool), youthful or aged appearance, frailty, and grooming. With the elderly patient, a picture is worth a thousand words!

Skin changes greatly with age. There is thinning and loss of elasticity. Wrinkling is more prominent in smokers and in individuals with a history of sun exposure. The head and neck area should be examined for actinic keratoses, basal cell carcinomas, and pigmented lesions that may indicate melanoma. Cherry angiomas and seborrheic keratoses, which are benign lesions, are commonly encountered.

Head and Neck Examination

This exam begins with careful observation of the skin for premalignant and malignant conditions. The temporal arteries should be palpated for pain, nodularity, and pulse. Visual acuity by a pocket Snellen chart held 10 inches from the eye is more practical than the wall chart. The whispered voice is as sensitive as an audioscope for detection of hearing loss (17). The ear canal and drum should be examined using an otoscope; cerumen impaction is a common cause of hearing loss. Oral examination should include palpation and inspection; if dentures are present they should be removed. It is important to examine for sores, oral cancers, and tooth and gum health. The neck examination should include the thyroid, the presence or absence of carotid bruits or other vascular sounds, and palpation for lymphadenopathy.

ELDER ABUSE AND NEGLECT

Elder abuse and neglect is a serious problem in the United States. It is widespread and affects thousands of vulnerable elderly. However, similar to child abuse and neglect, it is largely hidden under the shroud of family privacy. It is estimated that only about one out of 14 elder abuse cases are reported (18). Studies have indicated that abusers of elderly patients are most often caregivers, employees of facilities, or children of the abused. The most commonly abused are old-old females (mean age 84) in poor physical and mental health. Abuse of an elder person may be physical, psychological, or financial; it may also include neglect or a combination of these. Most states have mandatory reporting laws for elder abuse and neglect by health care providers. The physician should report any suspicions to Adult Protective Services within their local department on aging. All physician offices should screen on the intake questionnaire, asking such questions as "do you feel safe in your home?" It is important to interview an elderly patient alone in the exam room at some point during the history and physical exam. The presence of fresh and healing injuries or a history of repeated falls may suggest abuse; however, it is essential that the physician recognize that most types of abuse are not obvious, especially in the elderly. Dehydration and extensive decubitus ulcers may be evidence of neglect in institutionalized elderly. Neglect may also present in the office setting with poor hygiene, evidence of malnourishment, inappropriate dress, reports of being left in an unsafe situation, urine burns, and inability to obtain needed medications. Financial exploitation may manifest itself as unexplained loss of pension or social security checks or loss of personal belongings. Abandonment may present as being "dropped off" at the emergency room with no family available and no intention of a family member returning. It is important that such findings are documented in the medical record.

Elder abuse and neglect is a significant problem. Physicians have an extremely important role in assessing, detecting abuse and neglect, and notifying the appropriate authorities (19).

DEPRESSION AND SUICIDE

Depression is one of the most common treatable disorders in the elderly and continues to be treated mainly by primary care physicians. The etiology of depression in older patients is usually multifactorial; genetic, biologic, and psychosocial factors all play a role. Strong social support systems may offer protection from late-life depression and facilitate recovery. Physical health has a strong impact on the mental health of older adults. Epidemiologic studies have found that physical health is the strongest predictor of well-being and emotional health in the elderly (20). Therefore, in patients who may be given the diagnosis of advanced head and neck cancer, it is especially important to assess emotional well-being prior to and after the diagnosis has been given. The Geriatric Depression Scale (see appendix) is a screening instrument that can be included in an intake questionnaire and is highly sensitive (100%) (21). Even the simple question "Do you often feel sad or depressed?" has a sensitivity of 83%. Any patient with a positive screen should be referred for further evaluation. Suicide rates in late life are higher than at younger ages. Suicide is one of the top 10 causes of death in people over 65 (22,23). Older white men have the highest rate of any other age and sex group. The prevalence of alcohol use and dependence and poor health status are major risk factors for suicide in late life. All older patients should be screened for depression, especially prior to receiving bad news.

SUMMARY

When we "behold that time of year," to paraphrase Shakespeare, we need the proper skills. Elderly patients have unique health care needs. An approach to geriatric patients must be tailored appropriately to optimize the diagnosis and therapy for specific symptoms and disorders. As the numbers of elderly patients seeking medical care increases significantly over the next several decades, knowledge of the basic principles of geriatric medicine will become essential for all specialists. Optimal care of the geriatric patient will require that every otolaryngologist (with the exception of pediatric otolaryngologists) understand the unique health care needs and goals of the elderly. The author believes that this book will help meet these educational needs.

APPENDIX

INSTRUMENTAL ACTIVITIES OF DAILY LIVING
(SELF-RATED VERSION)

For each question, circle the points for the answer that best applies to your situation.

1. Can you use the telephone?
Without help   3
With some help   2
Completely unable to use the telephone   1
2. Can you get to places that are out of walking distance?
Without help   3
With some help   2
Completely unable to travel unless special arrangements are made   1
3. Can you go shopping for groceries?
Without help   3
With, some help   2
Completely unable to do any shopping   1
4. Can you prepare your own meals?
Without help   3
With some help   2
Completely unable to prepare any meals   1
5. Can yon do your own house work?
Without help   3
With some help   2
Completely unable to do any housework?   1
6. Can yon do your own handyman work?
Without help   3
Without some help   2
Completely unable to do any handyman work?   1
7. Can you do your own laundry?
Without help   3
Without some help   2
Completely unable to do any laundry at all?   1
8a. Do you take any medicines or use any medications?
Yes (If "yes," answer questions 8b.)
No (if "no," answer question Sc.)
8b. Do you take your own medicine?
Without help (in the right doses at the right time)   3
With some help (take medicine if someone prepares it for you and/or   2
    reminds you to take it)
Completely unable to take own medicine.   1
8c. If you had to take medicine, could you do it?
Without help (in the right doses at the right time)   3
With some help (take medicine if someone prepares it for you and/or   2
    reminds you to take it)
Completely unable to take own medicine.   1
9. Can you mange your own money?
Without help   3
With some help   2
Completely unable to handle money.   1

Scoring: The level of BADL dependence is graded via the score. Independent score 0–1. Dependence increases as the score approaches 6.
Source: From Ref. 24.

BASIC ACTIVITIES OF DAILY LIVING

Functional Abilities

1. Bathing–sponge bath, tub bath, or shower

   0 = no assistance (gets in and out of tub by self)
   1 = uses a device to got in or out of the-tub but able to bathe self
   2 = requires partial assistance with bathing
   3 = full bath, required (unable to bathe)

2. Dressing–includes getting clothes from closet and drawers (under and outer garments and able to use fasteners.

   0 = no assistance with getting clothes and dressing self
   1 = able to get clothes and get dressed, except for assistance with shoes
   2 = receives assistance with getting clothes or getting dressed
   3 = requires complete assistance or stays partly or completely undressed

3. Toileting–going to bathroom for bowel and urine elimation, self-cleaning and arranging clothes.

   0 = requires no assistance
   1 = requires no assistance but utilizes device (cane, walker, wheelchair, bedpan at night, but able to empty in sun.)
   2 = receives partial assistance with, going to the bathroom or in cleansing or arranging clothing
   3 = receives full assistance or does not go to the bathroom

4. Transfer

   0 = moves well in and out of bed and/or chair without assistance
   1 = moves well in and out of bed and/or chair with device
   2 = moves in and out of bed and/or chair with, assistance
   3 = requires full, assistance

5. Continence

   0 = controls urination and. bowel, movement completely by self
   1 = has occasional "accidents"
   2 = supervision helps keep bowel urine control or is incontinent
   3 = catheter is used

6. Feeding

   0 = able to prepare foods, serve and. feed self without assistance
   1 = requires .help in preparation of food but is able to feed self
   2 = requires help in preparation of food, cutting of meat, buttering
   3 = receives full assistance or is fed partly or completely by tubes.

Scoring: The level of BADL dependence is graded via the score. Independent score 0–1. Dependence increases as the score approaches 6.
Source: From Ref. 25.

CAGE QUESTIONNAIRE

- Have you ever felt you should **C**ut down on your drinking?
- Have people **A**nnoyed you by criticizing your drinking?
- Have you ever felt bad or **G**uilty about your drinking?
- Have you ever had a drink first thing in the morning to steady your nerves or to get rid of a hangover (**E**ye opener)?

Scoring: Two or more "Yes" answers are considered clinically significant.
Source: From Ref. 26.

GERIATRIC DEPRESSION SCALE

For each question, choose the best answer for how you felt over the past week.

1. Are you basically satisfied with your life?	Yes/NO
2. Have you, dropped many of your activities and interest?	YES/No
3. Do you feel that your life is empty?	YES/No
4. Do you often get bored?	YES/No
5. Are you in good spirits most of the time?	Yes/NO
6. Are you afraid that something bad is going to happen to you?	YES/No
7. Do you feel happy most of the time?	Yes/NO
8. Do you often feel helpless?	YES/No
9. Do you prefer to stay at home, rather than going out and doing new things?	YES/No
10. Do you feel you have more problems with memory than most?	YES/No
11. Do you think it is wonderful to be alive now?	Yes/NO
12. Do you feel pretty worthless the way you are now?	YES/No
13. Do you feel full of energy?	Yes/NO
14. Do you feel that your situation is hopeless?	YES/No
15. Do you think that most people are better off then you are?	YES/No

Scoring: The scale is scored as follows: 1 point for each response in capital letters. A score of 0 to 5 is normal; a score above 5 suggests depression.
Source: From Ref. 27.

RAPID ESTIMATE OF ADULT LITERACY IN MEDICINE (REALM) (30)

RAPID ESTIMATE OF ADULT LITERACY IN MEDICINE
(REALM)©

Terry Davis, PhD • Michael Crouch, MD • Sandy Long, PhD

Patient Name/
Subject # _____ Date of Birth _____

Reading
Level _____

Grade
Completed _____

Date _____ Clinic _____ Examiner _____

List 1		List 2		List 3	
fat	____	fatigue	____	allergic	____
flu	____	pelvic	____	menstrual	____
pill	____	jaundice	____	testicle	____
dose	____	infection	____	colitis	____
eye	____	exercise	____	emergen_	____
stress	____	behavior	____	me_	____
smear	____	prescription	____		
nerves	____	notify	____	_y	
germs	____	gallbladder	____	alcoholism	____
meals	____	calories	____	irritation	____
disease	____	de_	____	constipation	____
cancer	____			gonorrhea	____
caffeine	____	_nancy	____	inflammatory	____
attack	____	arthritis	____	diabetes	____
kidney	____	nutrition	____	hepatitis	____
hormone	____	menopause	____	antibiotics	____
herpes	____	appendix	____	diagnosis	____
seizure	____	abnormal	____	potassium	____
bowel	____	syphilis	____	anemia	____
asthma	____	hemorrhoids	____	obesity	____
rectal	____	nausea	____	osteoporosis	____
incest	____	directed	____	impetigo	____

SAMPLE COPY

SCORE	
List 1	_____
List 2	_____
List 3	_____
Raw Score	_____

Note: For copies of the REALM kit please contact:
Terry Davis, PhD
Prevention and Patient Education Project, Department of Medicine
LSU Health Sciences Center
1501 Kings Hwy., PO Box 33932
Shreveport, LA 71130-3932
Phone: (318) 675-4585
Source: From Refs. 28, 29.

REFERENCES

1. Ferraro K. Self-ratings of health among the old and the old-old. J Health Soc Behav 1980; 21:377.
2. Shanas E. The Health of Older People. Cambridge: Harvard University Press, 1961.
3. Brody EM. Tomorrow and tomorrow and tomorrow: toward squaring the suffering curve. In: Gaitz CM, et al., eds. Aging 2000: Our Healthcare Destiny. Vol. II. New York: Springer-Verlag, 1985.
4. Costa PT Jr, McCrae RR. Somatic complaints in males as a function of age and neuroticism: a longitudinal analysis. J Behav Med 1980; 3:245.
5. Stenback A, et al. Illness and health behavior in septuagenarians. Gerontologist 1978; 33:57.
6. Wilson LA, et al. Multiple disorders in the elderly. Lancet 1962; 2:841.
7. Bedsine RW. Geriatric medicine: an overview. Ann Rev Gerontol Geriatr 1980; 1:135.
8. Cassel, Christine K, et al. Geriatric Medicine, An Evidence-Based Approach. 4th ed. New York: Springer-Verlag, 2003.
9. Bayer AJ, et al. Changing presentation of myocardial infarction with increasing old age. J Am Geriatr Soc 1986; 34:263.
10. Wolf MS, Gazmararian JA, Baker DW. Health literacy and functional health status among older adults. Arch Int Med 2005; 165:1946–1952.
11. Berkman LF. Social networks, support, and health: taking the next step forward. Am J Epidemiol 1986; 123:559.
12. Corti M-C, et al. Serum albumin level and physical disability as predictors of mortality in older persons. JAMA 1994; 272:1036–1042.
13. LaCroix AZ, et al. Smoking and mortality among older men and women in three communities. N Engl J Med 1991; 324:1619–1625.
14. Kawachi I, et al. Smoking cessation and decreased risk of stroke in women. JAMA 1993; 269:232–236.
15. Katz S, Downs TD, Crash H, et al. Progress in development of the index of ADL. Gerontologist 1970; 10:20–30.
16. Lawton MP, Brody EM. Assessment of older people: self-maintaining and instrumental activities of daily living. Gerontologist 1969; 9:179–186.
17. Swan IRC, Browning GG. The whispered voice as a screening test for hearing impairment. J R Coll Gen Pract 1985; 35:197.
18. Pillemer K, Finkelhor D. The prevalence of elder abuse. Gerontologist 1988; 28(1):51–57.
19. AMA. Diagnostic and treatment guidelines on elder abuse and neglect. 1992; AA22:92698 20M 11/92.
20. Goldberg EL, Van Natta P, Comstock GW. Depressive symptoms, social networks and social support of elderly women. Am J Epidemiol 1985; 121:448–456.
21. Yasavage JA, Brink TL. Development and validation of a geriatric depression screening scale: a preliminary report. J Psychiatr Res 1983; 17:37–49.
22. Conwell Y. Suicide in elderly patients. In: Schneider LS, Reynolds CF, Lebowitz BD, Friedhoff AJ, eds. Diagnosis and Treatment of Depression in Late Life: Results of the NIH Consensus Development Conference. Washington, DC: American Psychiatric Press, 1994.
23. Murrell SA, Himmelfarb S, Wright K. Prevalence of depression and its correlates in older adults. Am J Epidemiol 1983; 117:173–185.
24. Lawton MP, Brody EM. Assessment of older people: self-maintaining and instrumental activities of daily living. Gerontologist 1969; 9(3):179–186.
25. Katz S, Ford AB, Moskowitz, RW, Jackson BA, Jaffe MW. Studies of illness in the aged. The index of ADL: A standardized measure of biological and psychological function.
26. Mayfield D, McLeod G, Hall P. The CAGE questionnaire: validation of new alcholism screening instrument. Am J Psychiatry 1974; 131(10):1121–1123.

27. Sheikh JI, Yesavage JA. Geriatric depression scale: recent evidence and development of a shorter version. Clin Gerontol 1986; 5:165–172.
28. Davis TC, Long SW, Jackson RH, et al. Rapid estimate of adult literacy in medicine: a shortened screening instrument. Fam Med 1993; 25:391–395.
29. Rapid estimate of adult literacy in medicine (REALM) http://www.ama.assn.org/ama/pub/category/9913.html.

2
Biology of Aging

Mukaila A. Raji
Department of Internal Medicine, Geriatrics Clinics, Sealy Center on Aging,
University of Texas Medical Branch, Galveston, Texas, U.S.A.

James S. Goodwin
Department of Internal Medicine, Sealy Center on Aging,
University of Texas Medical Branch, Galveston, Texas, U.S.A.

INTRODUCTION

As the U.S. population ages, a better understanding of the biological basis of development and aging is an important step towards reducing frailty and improving disability-free survival. There is a large body of research on what molecular and physiological changes occur with aging and senescence. Aging is characterized by decreased physiologic reserves and increasing prevalence of frailty and diseases (1–3). Prominent among the physiological changes are decline in immune, renal, neurological, and endocrine functions (Table 1) (4–6).

The differences in maximal lifespan between different species and in life expectancy in the same species raise a number of questions about the aging process. What are the mechanisms of aging? Are there ways to slow down the aging process? Can we live forever? The answers to these questions may lie in an in-depth understanding of the complex interaction of genetic programs and epigenetic factors that operate over the lifetime of an organism. In essence, nature (genes) and nurture (nongenetic factors such as environment, nutrition, and medical care) control aging phenotypes (1–3,7–9). Nature sets the limit and determines the responses of organisms to extrinsic factors (nurture). Nurture determines the extent to which the organism reaches the maximum of the genetic program. By modulating individuals' susceptibility to diseases and disability, these nurture–nature interactions determine health-related quality of life and life expectancy.

LIFE EXPECTANCY, LIFE QUALITY, AND LIFE SPAN

Life expectancy is defined as the age at which half of a specified population dies—the median lifespan for that species. In the Western world, the human life expectancy has increased from between 50 and 55 in the early 1900s to between 75 and 80 in the late 1990s (1,2,10,11). This increased life expectancy and better health-related quality of

Table 1 Physiology of Aging and Clinical Implications

Age-related decrease in enzymes (choline acetyl transferase) for acetylcholine synthesis in aging hippocampus	High risk of dementia and delirium
Impaired central processing of speech	Decreased word recognition
Decrease in olfactory and gustatory function	High risk for malnutrition
Decrease in muscle mass and increased fat mass	Decreased physical functioning
Impaired cellular and mucosal immunity, impaired immunosurveillance, and increased formation of autoantibodies	Susceptibility to infections and tumors
Thinning of epidermis, dermis, and subcutaneous fat	High risk of decubitus ulcers and poor wound healing post surgery
Decrease in total body water with an increase in body fat	Increased risk of drug toxicity
Decreased insulin sensitivity	Increased risk of diabetes
Decreased maximal heart rate and beta adrenergic sensitivity	Increased risk of orthostatic hypotension
Impaired diastolic function	Increased risk of heart failure and fluid overload
Decreased lung elasticity and increased V/Q mismatching	High risk for lung infections and postoperative atelectasis
Decrease in liver oxidative metabolism	High risk for drug toxicity
Decrease in renal blood flow, tubular function, and glomerular filtration rate	Increased risk for kidney failure and drug toxicity

life reflect major advances made in last century in hygiene, nutrition, vaccination, and discovery of antimicrobial agents (1,11,12). Additionally, better medical care for major diseases (especially heart attacks and cancers) and increasing adoption of healthier lifestyles (such as smoking cessation and exercise) play a major role in recent gains in life expectancy.

Yet, with all these advancements, there has been no change in the maximal life span of humans (1,11,12). The maximum life span refers to the ages of the oldest living members of the community, which in humans range from 90 to 125 (1,11,12). The maximum life span varies across species, a variation thought to reflect differences in metabolic rates and body size, among other factors (2,3). The interspecies life-span differences and the gains in human life expectancy have generated many theories regarding mechanisms of aging. These aging theories, in turn, have generated tremendous interest in the search for potential antiaging interventions.

THEORIES OF AGING

Theories of aging, summarized in Table 2, can be classified into two general categories: program (nature-determined and genetic) theories and error (nurture-determined and epigenetic) theories (1,2,7). This classification is convenient but artificial, as the molecular and cellular mechanisms of aging reflect multiple interactions of genetic and nongenetic factors. Genes modulate the ability of organisms to minimize the amount of error resulting from extrinsic and intrinsic stressors (such as free radicals and toxins). In turn, rates of error accumulation in response to stressors modulate the degree to which the organisms reach the maximal lifespan set by the genetic program.

Table 2 Theories of Aging

Program theories
Evolutionary theories
Disposable soma theory
Late-appearing lethal mutation theory
Antagonistic pleitropic gene theory
Cellular senescence theories
Replicative senescence theory
Telomere shortening theory
Longevity genes and accelerated aging theories
Programmed cell death and apoptosis theory
Hypothalamus–pituitary–adrenal–ovarian/testicular axis aging
Error theories
Free radical and mitochondrial dna damage theories
Caloric restriction and longevity
Mutation theories
DNA mutations
Advanced glycosylation end products formation
Lipid peroxidation and protein oxidation
Cross-linking of sugars and collagens

Source: From Refs. 1–3, 7–9.

Program Theories

Program theories are also known as intrinsic, developmental, or genetic theories of aging (1,2,7). These theories explain aging as largely a manifestation of a predetermined genetic program. According to these theories, there are predetermined periods for the onset of senescence in different cells, organs, and systems that ultimately lead to organismic deaths. These theories suggest the existence of tight control of development and senescence, in ways similar to fetal development, whereby genes are switched on and off at different phases of life. The switching on and off of genes is thought to determine risks of acquisition of diseases, disability, and death. Evidence for these theories is based on data from studies on evolution, cellular senescence and telomere shortening, programmed cell death, longevity-linked genes, and accelerated aging syndromes.

Evolutionary Theories

These theories posit that aging and senescence processes are set in motion once the organism undergoes stages of development, maturity, and reproduction—the main evolutionary purpose of "being" (1–3,7). In essence, the "program" optimizes reproduction (and child-rearing) at early life by keeping the body resistant to diseases and stemming the onset of frailty. As the reproductive role is accomplished and the body is no longer needed, genes that promote aging phenotypes progressively manifest— an idea aptly summarized in the disposable soma theories (3,13). Other theories based on this argument are:

1. *Late-appearing lethal mutation theory*—whereby genes whose protein products hasten organismic deaths manifest only after reproduction has been accomplished (3,14). An example is the Huntington's chorea gene, which

manifests after the carriers have had chance for procreation, after which—as evolutionary theory goes—the body is no longer needed (15,16).

2. *Antagonistic pleitropic gene theory*—states that genes (and their protein products) that facilitate survival and reproductive capability at earlier years may at later years heighten the risks of illnesses and death (3,17). For example, androgens are important for optimal male reproductive ability and muscle and bone functions; but at older age, the hormones increase the risks for prostate cancers and atherosclerotic cardiovascular diseases (2).

Cellular Senescence Theory

This theory states that the aging process reflects a predetermined age of each cell, an idea based on several observations and evidence for:

1. *Fixed division time for a given cell*—Hayflick and Moorhead's replicative senescence theory states that cells have a predetermined maximum number of population doublings (2,18). Several genes (such as retinoblastoma, p53, and p21 genes) have been identified as potential modulators of replicative senescence in various organisms (19–21). These genes suppress tumor formation and promote aging phenotypes by controlling the capacity of the cell to enter into the cell division cycle. For example, in cell cultures, fibroblasts have a fixed number of divisions before stopping, such that fibroblasts from the young undergo more divisions than those from the old before proliferative arrest (1,18). Additionally, cells from patients with accelerated aging such as Werner's syndrome manifest fewer divisions (as well as higher susceptibilities to genomic instability) compared with cells from normal controls of similar age (22,23).

2. *Telomere shortenings with cellular division*—Telomeres that cover the end of chromosomes protect genes from oxidative damage and fusion with other chromosomes (24). The telomeres shorten with each cell division. In germ cells and other cells that proliferate throughout life, the enzyme telomerase makes new telomeres and helps maintain a relatively constant telomere length (1,24). Further evidence for the role of telomeres comes from observations that some cancer cells exhibit excessive telomerase activity (1,25). Additional evidence also comes from the association of experimental lengthening of telomeres with an increase in the replicative life spans of those cells (26,27).

Longevity Genes and Accelerated Aging Syndromes

Evidence for longevity genes comes from several observations: aggregation of extended longevity in siblings of centenarians, clustering of certain genes in longest-living individuals, and the existence of patients with accelerated aging syndromes (8,9,28–30). These longevity genes appear to delay the onset of disease and age-related physiological decline. Thus, many centenarians remain active and independent, with delay of onset of diseases to the very last months of their life—a phenomenon referred to as compression of morbidity (31).

Examples of these longevity genes are possession of apolipoprotein E 2 alleles (as opposed to E 4 alleles) and polymorphisms of the angiotensin converting enzyme genes (Refs. 28, 29, 30 and others). Conversely, evidence for aging-promoting genes comes from the premature aging phenotypes found in patients with accelerated aging syndromes (Werner's and Hutchinson–Gilford syndromes—progeria).

These patients exhibit early onset of arteriosclerosis, wrinkled skin, and early menopause, among other features (1,23). The majority of these patients die before the age of 50.

Programmed Cell Death (Apoptosis) Theory

This theory states that cellular senescence and death reflect a "death" program that is triggered in response to some internal or external stimulus (1,7,32). This apoptotic program involves gradual disintegration of cells, condensation of both nuclear and cytoplasmic materials, fragmentation of these materials, and subsequent phagocytosis by nearby cells (1,33). Several genes are involved in programmed cell death including bcl-2 and bad genes, among others (1,7).

One way by which programmed cell death modulates aging phenotypes is through age-related apoptosis of cells subserving neuroimmunoendocrine functions. For example, with loss of hypothalamic neurons, there is progressive dysfunction in the hypothalamus–pituitary–adrenal–gonadal axis leading to aging phenotypes of osteoporosis, menopause, and sarcopenia. Similarly, programmed death of immune cells is associated with increased production of autoantibodies, decreased immunosurveillance, lower resistance to infections, and suboptimal free-radical scavenging and DNA repair capacity (1,2,7).

Error Theories

Error theories are also known as stochastic, extrinsic, or epigenetic theories (1,2,7). These theories explain the aging process and phenotypes as due to random accumulation of errors (such as mutations, damaged DNA, abnormally glycosylated proteins, and X-linked collagen, among others). These errors are thought to account for subsequent dysfunctions at molecular, cellular, and systemic levels. These dysfunctions ultimately lead to senescence and organismic deaths.

According to these theories, the errors can occur from exposure to internal and external factors such as infectious agents, ultraviolet radiation, toxins, and free radicals (1,2,7). Error formations by these factors are presumed to be random— stochastic—and outside of genetic control—epigenetic.

The main error theories are:

Free Radical/Mitochondrial DNA Damage Theories. They state that aging is in part due to progressive damage to vital structures (such as mitochondrial DNA) by reactive oxygen species (free radicals) (8,9,34–36). Free radicals are molecules with unpaired electrons and—by taking electrons from nearby molecules—they readily oxidize nearby cells and tissues. In particular, the oxidation of mitochondrial DNA leads to excessive generation of more free radicals in the respiratory chain cycle, causing more DNA oxidative damage, and the vicious cycle of continued free-radical generation continues. There are several free-radical scavengers (antioxidants) including super oxide dismutase, catalase, ascorbic acid, vitamin E, and glutathione S-transferase (GSTMI) (8,9,37).

Thus, these theories posit that aging starts with diminishing capacity of the organisms to remove free radicals and to repair damaged tissues. Evidence for the free-radical theories comes from mutations of antioxidant capacity experiments. In fruit flies and *C. elegans* worms, mutations that increase the superoxide dismutase activity (an antioxidant enzyme) extend the survival of these organisms (8,9,38,39). A study showed that having a specific genetic variant of the antioxidant enzyme was associated with better survival of cochlear cells in aged humans exposed to oxidative noise stress (37).

Other evidence supporting the free-radical theory comes from the salutary effect of caloric (dietary) restriction on longevity in insects, worms, and rats (40,41). Calorie restriction means having a 30% to 40% reduction of calories in diets that are otherwise balanced in proteins, carbohydrates, fats, and vitamins. Several mechanisms have been proposed to explain how lower caloric intake delays aging. These mechanisms include reduction of metabolic rates, decreased free-radical generation, and decreased oxidative damage to mitochondrial DNA and other organelles (1,2,7,34). The diet-restrictedorganisms exhibit delayed onset of several age-related physiological declines. The organisms show delayed decline in renal, cardiovascular, immune, and reproductive functions, delayed onset of cancers and osteoporosis, an increase in HDL, and a slow decline of dehydroepiandrosterone (1,2,7,41,42).

Mutation Theories. This theory attributes aging to random accumulations of genetic mutations (43–45). These mutations are thought to cause dysfunction in DNA transcription and RNA translation, and abnormal post-translational changes in proteins, lipids, and collagens.

Over time, damaged DNA is associated with higher risks of malignant transformation. As well, malformed and malfunctioning proteins accumulate, leading to tissue and system dysfunctions. One mechanism for dysfunctional proteins is through increased formation of advanced glycosylation end products, which have been implicated in cataract formation and loss of auditory hair cells (1,36,46). Onset and pace of the aging process depend on the capacity of organisms for DNA repair, for apoptosis of damaged cells to prevent neoplastic transformation, and for removal of altered proteins.

Lipid peroxidation, protein oxidation, and sugar and collagen cross-linking lead to compromised function in the neuroendocrine, immune and other systems. Thus, these physiological dysfunctions are thought to be important mechanisms for the aging process (1,2,7). The dysfunctions contribute to aging phenotypes in part by increasing the susceptibility of the aging animals to age-associated diseases: coronary arteriosclerosis, diabetes, Alzheimer's disease, cancers, and infections.

ANTIAGING INTERVENTIONS—INSIGHT AND POTENTIALS FROM AGING THEORIES

Approaches to slow down the development of aging phenotypes include diet restriction, use of antioxidants, and gene manipulations. To date, no data support extension of human lifespan by caloric restriction or usage of antioxidants, despite strong evidence in other species. On the other hand, better living conditions along with advances in nutrition, infection treatments, and medical care for major geriatric illnesses have contributed to the compression of morbidity to the very end of life, thus allowing for a longer lifetime of independent living.

SUMMARY AND CONCLUSION

The aging process is multifactorial, and no single theory can fully account for aging mechanisms. The aging process reflects the complexity of interactions between genes and the environment, and the adaptive capacity of organisms to respond to new challenges. Genetic programs set the limit of maximal life span for the organism. Reaching this limit depends on exposure to error-inducing intrinsic and extrinsic factors, and the organism's capacity to moderate these errors and to repair damaged cells.

REFERENCES

1. Troen BR. The biology of aging. Mount Sinai. J Med 2003; 70:3–22.
2. Weinert BT, Timiras PS. Physiology of aging. Invited review: theories of aging. J Appl Physiol 2003; 95:1706–1716.
3. Kirkwood TBL, Austad S. Why do we age? Nature 2000; 48:233–238.
4. Naranjo CA, Herrmann N, Mittmann N, Bremner KE. Recent advances in geriatric psychopharmacology. Drugs Aging 1995; 7:184–202.
5. Montamat SC, Cusack BJ, Vestal RE. Management of drug therapy in the elderly. NEJM 1989; 321:303–309.
6. Rochon PA, Gurwitz JH. Drug therapy. Lancet 1995; 346:32–36.
7. Semsei I. On the nature of aging. Mech Ageing Dev 2000; 117:93–108.
8. Robert L, Labat-Robert J. The mechanisms of aging. From genetic to epigenetic. Presse Med 2003; 32:605–614.
9. Knight JA. The biochemistry of aging. Adv Clin Chem 2000; 35:1–62.
10. Oeppen J, Vaupel JW. Broken limits to life expectancy. Science 2002; 296:1029–1031.
11. Olshansky SJ. The demography of aging. In: Cassel KC, Cohen HJ, Larson EB, et al., eds. Geriatric medicine. 3rd ed. New York: Springer-Verlag, 1997:29–36.
12. Hayflick L. The future of ageing. Nature 2000; 408:267–269.
13. Kirkwood TBL. Evolution of ageing. Nature 1977; 270:301–304.
14. Martin GM, Austad SN, Johnson TE. Genetic analysis of aging: role of oxidative damage and environmental stresses. Nat Genet 1996; 13:25–34.
15. Haldane JBS. New paths in genetics. London: Allen & Unwin, 1941.
16. Medawar PB. An unsolved problem of biology. London: Lewis, 1952.
17. Williams GC. Pleitropy, natural selection and the evolution of senescence. Evolution 1957; 11:398–411.
18. Hayflick L, Moorhead PS. The limited in vitro lifetime of human diploid cell strains. Exp Cell Res 1965; 37:614–636.
19. Atadja P, Wong H, Garkavtsev I, et al. Increased activity of p53 in senescing fibroblasts. Proc Natl Acad Sci USA 1995; 92:8348–8352.
20. Stein GH, Beeson M, Gordon L. Failure to phosphorylate the retinoblastoma gene product in senescent human fibroblasts. Science 1990; 249:666–699.
21. Shay JW, Pereira-Smith OM, Wright WE. A role for both RB and p53 in the regulation of human senescence. Exp Cell Res 1991; 196:33–39.
22. Brown WT. Genetic diseases of premature aging as models of senescence. Annu Rev Gerontol Geriatr 1990; 10:23–42.
23. Martin GM, Oshima J. Lessons from human progeroid syndromes. Nature 2000; 408: 262–266.
24. Harley CB, Futcher AB, Greider CW. Telomeres shorten during ageing of human fibroblasts. Nature 1990; 345:458–460.
25. Counter CM, Hirte HW, Baccheti S, Harley CB. Telomerase activity in human ovarian carcinoma. Proc Natl Acad Sci USA 1994; 91:2900–2904.
26. Bodnar AG, Oulette M, Frolkis M, et al. Extension of lifespan by introduction of telomerase into normal human cells. Science 1998; 279:349–352.

27. Wright WE, Brasiskyte D, Piatyszek MA, Shay JW. Experimental elongation of telomeres extends the lifespan of immortal x normal cell hybrids. EMBO J 1996; 15: 1734–1741.

28. Jazwinski SM. Longevity, genes, and aging. Science 1996; 273:54–59.

29. Schachter F, Faure-Delanef L, Guenot F, et al. Genetic associations with human longevity at the APOE and ACE loci. Nat Genet 1994; 6:29–32.

30. Perls T, Levenson R, Regan M, Puca A. What does it take to live to 100? Mech Ageing Dev 2002; 123:231–242.

31. Fries JF. Measuring and monitoring success in compressing morbidity. Ann Intern Med 2003; 139:455–459.

32. Lockshin RA, Zakeri ZF. Programmed cell death: new thoughts and relevance to aging. J Gerontol 1990; 45:B135–B140.

33. Ellis RE, Yuan JY, Horvitz HR. Mechanisms and functions of cell death. Annu Rev Cell Dev Biol 1991; 7:663–698.

34. Mandavilli BS, Santos JH, Van Houten B. Mitochondrial DNA repair and aging. Mutat Res 2002; 509:127–151.

35. Harman D. Aging: a theory based on free radical and radiation chemistry. J Gerontol 1957; 2:298–300.

36. Levine RL, Stadtman ER. Oxidative modification of proteins during aging. Exp Gerontol 2001; 36:1495–1502.

37. Rabinowitz PM, Pierce Wise J Sr, Hur Mobo B, Antonucci PG, Powell C, Slade M. Antioxidant status and hearing function in noise-exposed workers. Hear Res 2002; 173:164–171.

38. Tower J. Transgenic methods for increasing *Drosophila* lifespan. Mech Ageing Dev 2000; 118:1–14.

39. Melov S, Ravenscroft J, Malik S, et al. Extension of lifespan with superoxide dismutase/ catalase mimetics. Science 2000; 289:1567–1569.

40. Weindruch R, Walford RL. Dietary restriction in mice beginning at 1 year of age: effect on lifespan and spontaneous cancer incidence. Science 1982; 215:1415–1418.

41. Masoro EJ. Dietary restriction and aging. J Am Geriatr Soc 1993; 41:994–999.

42. Lane MA, Ingram DK, Ball SS, Roth GS. Dehydroepiandrosterone sulfate: a biomarker of primate aging slowed by calorie restriction. J Clin Endocrinol Metab 1997; 82:2093–2096.

43. Strehler BL, Freeman MR. Randomness, redundancy and repair: role and relevance to biological aging. Mech Ageing Dev 1980; 14:15–38.

44. Verzar F. The stages and consequences of aging of collagen. Gerontologia 1969; 15:233–239.

45. Cerami A. Hypothesis: glucose as a mediator of aging. J Am Geriatr Soc 1985; 33:626–634.

46. Ulrich P, Cerami A. Protein glycation, diabetes, and aging. Recent Prog Horm Res 2001; 56:1–21.

3

Introduction to Geriatric Otolaryngology

Hinrich Staecker

Department of Otolaryngology—Head and Neck Surgery, University of Kansas School of Medicine, Kansas City, Kansas, U.S.A.

INTRODUCTION

Otolaryngology as a specialty that deals with a wide variety of disorders that span from communication disorders to allergies and sinusitis to treatment of complex head and neck malignancies. Depending on the practice surveyed, up to one-third of patients seen by the average otolaryngologist are over the age of 65. With an aging population, health care of the elderly is becoming increasingly important. The importance of the older patient has been only partially recognized. Current otolaryngology texts do feature a section devoted to the care of the elderly patient. However, principles of geriatric medicine and issues of concern specific to geriatric patients in the realm of otolaryngology have not been widely applied. Furthermore, a significant portion of available literature dealing with geriatric issues in otolaryngology consists of case reports and case series. The purpose of this review is to assess the state-of-the-art knowledge for otolaryngologic care of the elderly and define important areas for future study in the care of the elderly.

THE AUDITORY SYSTEM

Epidemiology

The most common otolaryngologic disability affecting the elderly is hearing loss. Our understanding of age-related hearing degeneration has increased significantly through several large population-based studies. A wide variety of age-specific changes as well as the common otologic diseases occur in the elderly. Among the best-characterized populations that have been longitudinally studied is the Framingham cohort. A study of 1662 patients aged 60 to 90 showed an age-related increase in pure tone thresholds and a concurrent decrease in speech discrimination. The rate of hearing decline was found to be equal in men and women, but on average, men started with worse hearing. Interestingly, there was also a slight change in contralateral acoustic reflex thresholds. A further observation of the study was that only 10% of patients who were candidates for hearing aids used them (1). The rate of hearing decline has also been estimated by following a clinic population over a six-year period. Having the measurements taken by the same audiologist reduced variability in results. In a study of 1475 patients over this six-year period, an average decline in hearing of 1–8 dB was seen at 250 Hz, while a 10–15 dB decline in hearing was noted at 8 kHz. There appeared to be two main patterns of hearing degeneration. The low-frequency pattern of hearing loss appeared to be age dependent and women had worse thresholds than men. The high-frequency pattern of hearing loss had a different pattern of progression; the rate of threshold change decreased with age. This difference in pattern is interpreted as possibly representing a disorder of the stria vascularis (the organ that generates the endocochlear potential) for the low-frequency loss and a hair cell disorder for the high-frequency loss (2).

The Baltimore Longitudinal Study of Aging has examined 681 men and 416 women using standard pure tone auditometry from 1965 to present. The individuals were screened for prior otologic disease and noise exposure. This study demonstrated that the rate of loss in hearing sensitivity was greater in women than in men. In men, there was a decrease in hearing sensitivity that was detectable from age 30 on. In terms of gender differences, women tended to have better high-frequency hearing than men did and men had better low-frequency hearing. Overall, there was significant variation within the study group. A conclusion of this study was that there was an age-related decline in hearing (with the aforementioned gender factors) that was present in individuals without any history of noise exposure or evidence of noise exposure on their audiograms (3). This differs somewhat from the interpretation of the Framingham data, which suggested that the preponderance of male high-frequency hearing loss is related to occupational noise exposure. Epidemiological studies have consistently shown a 30% to 70% incidence of age-related hearing loss with widely variable assessment of the degree of impairment induced by the hearing loss. Overall, the degree of hearing loss increases with increasing age and is more prevalent in geriatric patients who are institutionalized (4,5).

Diseases of the Pinna and External Auditory Canal

Cerumen impaction can have a significant effect on the hearing of elderly patients. In a random sampling of hospitalized elderly patients over a one-year period, 30% were found to have cerumen impaction. Improved hearing was obtained in 75% of ears that underwent removal of cerumen (6).

Diseases of the Tympanic Membrane and Middle Ear

Tympanic Membrane Perforations

Numerous studies have examined the age-related risk of otologic surgery both in terms of complications and surgical outcome. Age over 65 has no impact on graft take rate in tympanoplasty (7). In a study of 42 elderly patients (age > 65) with otosclerosis, Vartiainen (8) determined that there was no significant increase in surgical complications and recovery of hearing was similar to that of 275 younger adult patients. Therefore, chronological age is not a contraindication to middle ear surgery either in terms of complications or in terms of outcomes of the surgery. No data comparing quality of life after surgery versus hearing aid placement are available. Also, there have been no controlled intervention trials to establish the best treatment of otosclerosis in older people.

Eustachian Tube Dysfunction (ETD)

ETD has been described in the elderly population but few studies have attempted to establish a clear etiology. When 36 temporal bones of younger adult and elderly patients were examined, calcifications of the eustachian tube cartilage and atrophy of the tensor veli palitini were found to increase in prevalence and severity with age (9). In another study, functional compliance was also found to change with aging, therefore affecting the overall function of the eustachian tube (10). No studies have examined the prevalence of serous otitis media in the elderly, and the contribution of ETD to hearing loss in older people has not been defined.

Presbycusis/Sensorineural Hearing Loss

The incidence and impact of age-related sensorineural hearing loss is well established. Recent studies are beginning to define deficits in addition to the previously described degeneration of the auditory hair cells, auditory neurons, and stria vascularis. Schuknecht and Gacek (11) classified presbycusis based on histologic criteria. In the authors' last review of the subject, they reported that the four diagnostic criteria of age-related hearing loss (sensory cell degeneration, neural degeneration, strial atrophy, and cochlear conductive loss) held up in a review of 21 cases that met the clinical diagnosis of presbycusis. Of note was the observation that most cases seemed to have a mixed pathological pattern. More recent analysis of temporal bone specimens has shown a high incidence of mutations of mitochondrial DNA within the peripheral auditory system (12).

Age-related changes in the central nervous system (central presbycusis) also play an important role in hearing deficits in older patients. There are clearly documented auditory brainstem response (ABR) changes that occur with aging. Standard ABR examines the auditory pathway from the cochlea to the inferior colliculus. In a study of 92 subjects aged 50 to 90, and 30 control subjects aged 20 to 29, there was a progressive delay in wave I, wave III, and wave V of the ABR. Interestingly, there was a lengthening in I–V and II–V interpeak intervals observed in the cohort of 70- to 79-year-olds that was not present in the oldest subjects (13). This may suggest that there is a cohort of the very aged that has better than average central (brainstem level) auditory processing. Auditory brainstem response and a central auditory test battery were used to study patients matched for peripheral hearing loss. Patients classified as having a retrocochlear loss (by ABR criteria) overall were poorer performers on the central auditory test battery (14).

A number of significant changes occur in the central processing of auditory information in elderly patients. In a study that compared a cohort of young (average age of 26) with a group of older (average age of 70) men, monaural and binaural temporal thresholds were measured. The elderly group showed poorer performance on both monaural and binaural processing tasks. These measurements were independent of peripheral system disease (15).

Stach et al. (16) investigated the prevalence of central presbycusis in a study of 700 patients aged 50 and older. One hundred consecutive patients from each five-year cohort with a complaint of hearing loss were enrolled and studied for the effects of central auditory processing on hearing. There was an age-related increase in central presbycusis that reached an incidence of 95% by the eighth decade of life. The results were controlled for absolute hearing threshold. This study also examined an age-matched "nonclinical" group (i.e., individuals without complaints of hearing loss). This population also demonstrated the presence of central auditory processing disorders, but at a lower rate. A study of 25 normal hearing, cognitively intact adults revealed that central auditory processing declined despite normal cognition, peripheral hearing sensitivity, and linguistic capability. The synthetic sentence identification–ipsilateral competing message test appeared to be the most sensitive measure of central auditory dysfunction (17). There are no clear data on the significance or the functional impact of these findings.

Impact of Presbycusis on Quality of Life

A number of studies have examined the impact of hearing loss on the elderly. A patient-based outcomes study was carried out on 2466 patients between the ages of 17 and 80. Patients were tested with standard audiologic measures as well as sentences in noise. There was an age-related decrease in performance of auditory tasks such as sentence identification that correlated with increasing hearing thresholds. There was also a matched increase in disability outcomes as measured by validated subjective outcome tools that identified features of communication disability that led to feelings of isolation and depression (13). In a study of over 1800 nursing home residents, sensory deprivation due to hearing loss was found to have a significant impact on social interaction. This was compounded when there was associated visual loss (18). Studies carried out on a cohort of 472 patients with mild to moderate hearing loss with disease-specific outcome measures revealed that even mild hearing losses had a significant impact on perceived emotional, social, and communication function. Sixty-six percent of individuals tested found that this represented a severe handicap for them despite hearing losses ranging from only 25–55 dB (19). In a follow-up study, 194 elderly patients were randomized into two groups, one receiving hearing aids immediately and one being placed on a waiting list. The effect of hearing aid use on quality of life was documented by a variety of outcome tools. There was a statistically significant effect on quality of life and cognitive function demonstrated in the patients that received treatment immediately (20).

A study on a population of over 1100 elderly found that hearing loss correlated with depression and decreased independence (21,22). A small ($n = 100$) case control study of normal subjects and patients with Alzheimer's disease did show an increase in the odds of having dementia with increasing hearing loss. Increasing degree of hearing loss, however, correlated with increased cognitive impairment in this population (23). There is some evidence to suggest that more accurate assessments of impairment can be derived from the patient's spouse and that discrepancies between hearing level and perceived deficit may be explained by the presence of central auditory processing deficits (24). Another interesting observation is that hearing loss in the elderly may be associated with depression. In a study of 43 geriatric patients with major depression, age of onset of depression correlated with decreased acuity of hearing. It was unclear from this study if the associated hearing loss could be purely related to increased age of the patient, but it does suggest that the association between hearing loss and depression in the elderly should be investigated (25).

Inheritance of Presbycusis

The inheritance patterns of presbycusis were studied in the Framingham cohort. Hearing levels in unrelated spouse pairs were compared to sibling pairs and parent–child pairs. Pure tone averages for low-, middle-, and high-frequency hearing were calculated to generate an audiometric pattern that was graded as normal, flat loss (consistent with strial atrophy), and high-frequency loss (consistent with sensory pathology). Hearing levels were correlated between the aforementioned groups. There was a grouping of hearing threshold changes within parent–child groups and within sibling groups. Sisters and mother–daughter and mother–son pairs showed an association of hearing threshold changes at all three frequency sets. The strial pattern of loss showed stronger aggregation and association among female relatives. The sensory pattern of hearing loss was found to aggregate in all related pairs except father–child pairs. This was interpreted as showing that there was a stronger heritable component to the strial pattern of sensory loss and that the inheritance of presbycusis had a genetic component in women and a mixed etiology in men (26). The Framingham study also suggested that patients with a history of noise exposure continue to be at greater risk of progression of hearing loss. This may offer an opportunity for intervention (27).

The Impact of Hearing Loss on Dementia

A number of studies have suggested that there is a link or at least an association between hearing loss and dementia (28). In a study of 30 patients with Alzheimer's disease and 22 patients with generalized cognitive impairment that presented to a memory disorders clinic, 98% of patients failed a pure tone hearing test (29). This indicates that certain selected populations may have extremely high rates of hearing loss. Gates et al. (30) examined hearing in a cohort of 82 elderly patients enrolled in a prospective Alzheimer's disease research program. Forty patients were judged to be non-demented based on the clinical dementia rating scale, and 42 were judged to have probable Alzheimer's disease based on clinical dementia rating scale scores. Pure tone testing showed no difference in the incidence of hearing loss in the two groups, but the probable Alzheimer's disease group had a much higher incidence of central auditory processing abnormalities. In a follow-up study, Gates et al. (30) examined patients from the Framingham study and found that hearing loss significantly lowered performance on the verbal portions of the mini mental state test. Patients were also tested with synthetic sentence identification with ipsilateral competing message (a test for central auditory dysfunction). A poor score in both ears was associated with a high relative risk of subsequent clinical dementia. This suggests that central auditory processing dysfunction may precede or be an early sign of some dementia.

Treatment of Presbycusis

It is well accepted that hearing aids are the treatment of choice for the moderately hearing impaired. The choice of hearing aids in the elderly needs to be carefully considered. In a study of in-the-canal (ITC) hearing aid use in 220 patients with an average age of 69, there was significant benefit from amplification. Yet elderly patients found ITC aids difficult to manipulate (31). It is important to take into account central processing as well as cognitive impairment in assessing the impact of these devices on the aging listener. Currently, no hearing aids provide clear transmission of sound in a noisy background, and furthermore, they do little to improve the function of persons with poor speech discrimination.

Despite the demonstrated impact of hearing loss on quality of life, only 14% of the elderly with hearing loss are fitted and use hearing aids. No clearly identifiable variable (i.e., age, degree of hearing loss, educational status, financial status) has been identified that consistently correlates with hearing aid use (19,20). Newer implantable hearing aids may help with problems of high-frequency gain and feedback, whereas cochlear implantation is beneficial to patients with very poor speech discrimination. Additional ways of improving the function of the hearing impaired is the use of assistive listening devices. Amplified doorbells and phones as well as personal amplification (headphones) for television viewing can improve the function of both the independent and non-independent elderly. For patients with profound hearing loss, cochlear implantation has become the treatment of choice. Shin et al. (32) examined the complication rates and outcomes in 27 patients older than 60 compared to a group of younger patients. This retrospective study as well as several more recent studies showed that there was no increased incidence in complications and that outcome in auditory function was not statistically different between the two groups (33,34). Some studies have also focused on quality-of-life and cost–benefit analysis after cochlear implantation in older patients and overall have concluded the procedure to be a cost-effective and beneficial intervention (35).

Neurotology

There are a limited number of papers devoted to neurotologic surgery in the elderly. Age was not found to be predictive of return to premorbid function in a series of Meniere's patients treated with labyrinthectomy (36). There are no large series of elderly patients treated with gentamicin for Meniere's disease that have been studied. Treatment of acoustic neuroma has been rapidly evolving over the last 10 years. Currently, age is not considered a contraindication for surgical management of the tumor. Some studies do, however, suggest that patient age may affect postoperative complications to some degree. Age >55 was found to be a statistically significant risk factor for the development of postoperative disequilibrium (7). A recent series of papers has examined the growth rate of acoustic neuroma. This has resulted in the observation that a selected group of patients may be candidates for observation rather than surgical excision or radiation. Current studies suggest that in growing tumors (30–40%), the average growth rate is 1 mm/yr, making no treatment other than observation with serial MRI possible in a selected patient population (37,38). De Cruiz et al. (39) examined the quality of life in postoperative acoustic neuroma patients. There was no statistically significant effect of age on patient-based outcome data.

Summary

Otologic disease, especially age-related hearing loss, is probably the most common otolaryngologic disorder afflicting the elderly. Treatment of presbycusis is currently limited to amplification. The overall low level of use and dissatisfaction with hearing aids is not thoroughly addressed in the literature.

Review of the current literature reveals that there are no age-related contraindications to middle ear surgery. There are no significant data available for neurotologic surgery. Recent developments in acoustic neuroma have shown that observation may be a reasonable choice in non-growing tumors in the elderly.

The last 10 years have shown that central auditory processing disorders, distinct from peripheral auditory degeneration, affect the hearing of the elderly. It is unclear at present what the impact of this disorder is on communication in the elderly. Advances are being made in the understanding of peripheral age-related auditory dysfunction with large cohort studies identifying both genetic and environmental factors. Thus far, even though there have been tremendous advances in molecular biology of presbycusis in animal models, no human "presbycusis" genes have been identified.

VESTIBULAR SYSTEM

Balance disorders, though probably as common as auditory problems in the elderly, are complex and have not been as fully studied. A large percentage of balance disorders in the elderly can be attributed to cardiovascular disease, neurologic disease, or medication effects. Most studies on patients with peripheral balance disorders have already had this population selected out.

Histological Studies

Recent archival temporal bone studies have shown that there is an age-related decline in both vestibular sensory and ganglion cells. Type I hair cells show a significant decline in the cristae, whereas type II hair cells are lost in both the cristae and the macular organs (40). There is also a decline of vestibular ganglion cells with age (41). In a histological study of human brainstems, Alvarez et al. (42) demonstrated that there was an age-related loss of neurons in the descending medial and lateral vestibular nuclei. The neurons of the superior vestibular nucleus were preserved (42).

Etiology of Dizziness

In a study by Davis (43), the etiology of dizziness in 117 consecutive patients (age > 50) was determined. The average duration of the complaint was 45 weeks. Seventy-one percent of patients had peripheral vestibular system dysfunction with benign paroxysmal positional vertigo (BPPV) being the cause of vertigo in one-third of these patients. Visual system disturbances were the primary diagnosis in 1% and proprioceptive disorders the primary diagnosis in 7%. Twenty-two percent were found to have metabolic or structural lesions of the brainstem. Psychiatric causes of dizziness were rare (43). In a study of 50 consecutive patients aged >60, symptoms of light-headedness and syncope were associated with a cardiovascular etiology of dizziness, whereas the symptom of vertigo was associated with peripheral vestibular disorders (44). Most patients in this study complained of their presenting symptoms for >1 year, suggesting that diagnosis and treatment of many of these types of complaints is ineffective. (The average duration was stated to be 45 weeks. That makes it unlikely that "most" patients had their symptoms for more than a year—that is what was cited in the study.)

Among the most common peripheral vestibular system pathologies is BPPV. In a cross-sectional study of patients complaining either of dizziness or balance disorders, unrecognized BPPV was found in 9% of patients. This diagnosis was associated with a history of falls, depression, and low activities of daily living scores (45). In a retrospective study of 1194 patients 70 years or older from a balance disorder clinic, 39% were found to have BPPV (46). This combination of findings suggests that all elderly patients complaining of dizziness, even when not complaining of the classic signs of BPPV, should be examined with a Dix-Hallpike maneuver.

BPPV is easily treatable with either an Epley maneuver or a variety of home exercises. The outcomes of Epley maneuver versus more conservative treatment have not been specifically examined in the elderly.

Developments in Vestibular Testing

Changes in vestibular test results with age have been well documented. This would be expected given the histologic data cited above. Posturography has recently been used to investigate functional balance in the elderly. Wolfson et al. (47) examined 234 elderly subjects (average age 76) and compared them to 34 young control subjects. There was a significantly poorer in response to conflicting balance information when comparing the elderly and the young individuals (47). Cohen et al. (48) specifically evaluated four age cohorts (<44, 45–69, 70–79, and 80–89); they found a continual age-related decline in sensory organization test scores that persisted into the ninth decade of life. These changes were not, however, directly associated with decrease in independence (48). Baloh et al. (49) prospectively examined 72 subjects (age 79–91) with normal neurological examinations and followed repeated posturography examinations on a yearly basis. They found that there was a significant increase in sway velocity and degree of sway with dynamic stimulation of balance over time. A standardized movement in the visual surround appears to increase sway and perturb balance to a greater degree in elderly subjects (50). Specific testing is needed to diagnose neurovestibular causes of dizziness and to determine fall risk.

Treatment of Age-Related Balance Problems

Few studies have rigorously looked at methodologies to improve balance in the elderly. Generally, balance disorders have been treated with physical therapy. The effect of Tai Chi was recently evaluated using posturography. Twenty-five test subjects who practiced Tai Chi were compared to 14 controls and were found to have statistically better outcomes on dynamic posturography (51). No long-term studies have correlated diagnosed peripheral vestibular system disease with treatment modality and outcome. There are also no prospective studies evaluating the pharmacologic treatment of vertigo.

Summary

Balance disorders are common and have a complex etiology. Even though balance disorders in the elderly can be related to a plethora of causes, histologic and epidemiological data suggest that a significant portion of balance disorders can be ascribed to disorders of the peripheral auditory system. No long-term prospective studies have combined the improvements in diagnostic techniques seen in the last 10 years with patient-based outcome measures. There are also little to no data available on the correlation between histological patterns of degeneration and changes in vestibular testing.

THE NOSE AND SINUSES

Smell

There has been little recent specific study of sinonasal disease in the elderly. Olfactory sensitivity has been found to decline with age. This may potentially be related to the degeneration of both peripheral and central olfactory pathways (52,53). One recent study has examined the smell sensitivity in normal elderly and patients with Alzheimer's disease (54). The 80 patients with Alzheimer's disease who were examined had awareness of olfactory sensitivity that was similar to that of chronic sinusitis patients (nine-fold less than normal elderly). Interestingly, 74% of the Alzheimer's disease patients and 77% of the normal elderly who were found to have abnormal smell sensitivity rated themselves as having normal smell sensitivity on a questionnaire.

Sinusitis/Nasal Discharge

A common symptom among elderly patients is postnasal drip that may be constant or induced by food (gustatory rhinitis). It is thought that this may be due to the loss of autonomic control, but it is more commonly a result of dehydration from reduced fluid intake or a side effect of medications (55). The allergy literature to some degree has addressed changes that occur during aging. Few studies have specifically examined the incidence or prevalence of sinusitis in the elderly. Knutson and Slavin (56) noted that sinusitis is common in the elderly and may have more subtle presenting signs. When sinusitis is properly treated, the management of asthma can be improved (57). The effect of sinus surgery for chronic sinusitis has been examined. In a study of 1112 patients who underwent endoscopic sinus surgery, patients aged older than 65 made up 15% of the patient population. This group had a higher incidence of minor complications, but final outcomes were similar to the other age groups (57).

TONGUE / ORAL CAVITY AND SWALLOWING

Swallowing

Normal Aging

In a study of normal volunteers ($n = 80$) divided into four age cohorts, liquid and semisolid swallows were studied with manometry and videofluoroscopy. Total swallowing time and time to initiation of oropharyngeal swallowing was prolonged in the advanced age. Upper esophageal sphincter pressure, peak pressure, and rate of bolus propagation did not appear to be affected by age greater than 65 (58). Other studies at least partially contradict these data, showing an overall slowing of pharyngeal swallowing time but also confirming an impairment in the opening of the upper esophageal sphincter (59). In a study of 53 asymptomatic individuals with an average age of 75, the repetitive oral suction test was applied to noninvasively evaluate swallowing function. Significant abnormalities in peak suction pressure, frequency of multiple swallows after one ingestion, frequency of polyphasic laryngeal movements, frequency of inspiration after swallowing, and frequency of coughing during or after swallowing were demonstrated. This suggested that a normal (non-dysphagic) population of patients has an increased incidence of a variety of physiologic abnormalities in the swallowing process and that concomitant disease may be more likely to result in pathologic dysphagia in the elderly who develop additional neurologic diseases (60–62). A series of elderly volunteers without symptoms of dysphagia were examined by endoscopy and fluoroscopy. Elderly subjects were found to require a much larger pharyngeal bolus to initiate swallowing (63). More recent studies have shown that with age there is an increase in pharyngeal swallow delay, a decrease in the duration of swallow, decreased cricopharyngeal opening, and decreased peristaltic amplitude and velocity (63,64). No studies have linked these changes or targeted treatment of these changes to improved nutritional status and quality of life in the elderly.

Despite swallowing pressure remaining constant across aging, the reserve capacity of pressure generation within the oral cavity is reduced. It was argued that concomitant illness might thus put elderly patients more at risk of dysphagia due to reduced reserves (65). Normal aging does not appear to result in problems with the coordination of swallowing and protective deglutitive vocal cord closure (66). However, pressure sensitivity in the supraglottis of normal aging volunteers appears to decrease with age (67). This loss of sensory function may contribute both to dysphagia and aspiration in the elderly. More recent studies have looked at healthy individuals between the ages of 80 and 94. Again, increases in pharyngeal delay as well as a decrease in muscular reserve were demonstrated. The authors concluded that there may be a role for exercise to improve reserve and possibly prevent later swallowing disorders (68).

Within the population aged greater than 65, 10% to 30% are estimated to have dysphagia, although this number is largely unsubstantiated (69). Some studies are beginning to address components of the swallowing system in a prospective fashion, allowing the establishment of measurement norms. Using four age cohorts (<50, 51–70, 71–85, and >85) with a sample of 30 in each, Jego et al. (70) studied by electromyogram (EMG) the activity of the mylohyoid muscle during swallowing. There were no significant differences among the groups. Rehabilitation of swallowing after head and neck cancer is vital for restoring the patient to a satisfactory functional state.

Xerostomia may significantly contribute to dysphagia and is common among the elderly. The incidence of this problem is estimated to be as high as one of five elderly noninstitutionalized adults. A study of 67 randomly selected elderly subjects (institutionalized and noninstitutionalized) showed that there was a statistically significant ($p < 0.001$) association between xerostomia (measured by sialometry and questionnaire) and inadequacy of nutritional intake (71). There is evidence in the literature that there is a normal degeneration in salivary gland function with age (72). However, several studies based on actual measurements of salivary flow suggest that despite this histologic evidence of loss of salivary acinar structure, flow rates do not decrease with age. Fisher and Ship (73) examined unstimulated and stimulated salivary flow rates in healthy (non-xerostomia) subjects aged 20 to 40 and 60 to 80 years old. No differences in unstimulated or stimulated parotid flow rates were seen between the two groups (73). Dehydration and recovery from dehydration does not have an age-related differential effect on salivary flow (74). The largest study completed examined 1493 subjects between ages 5 and 88 using the whole saliva test rather than just isolating parotid salivary flows. Resting salivary flow was demonstrated to decline in an age-related fashion, thus contradicting studies based on parotid salivary flow alone (75). Besides functioning in lubrication during mastication, saliva also produces substances that are important for protecting the mucosal and dental surfaces of the mouth from infection. A recent study of 45 non-hospitalized dentate elderly (aged 79–89) and 22 non-elderly (aged 21–51) demonstrated that there is an age-related decline in secretory leukocyte protease inhibitor and lysozyme (antimicrobial proteins found in saliva). Overall, protein levels and electrolytes in the saliva have been shown to not change with age (76). Astor et al. (77) observed that medication (particularly anticholinergics and antipsychotics) and systemic illness are probably the most common causes of xerostomia. In an analysis of 100 consecutive patients aged >60 presenting at a xerostomia clinic, 60% were found to have salivary gland hypofunction. Of these, two-thirds were found to suffer from Sjorgen's syndrome (78).

Summary

There are clear age-related changes in the physiology of swallowing. Yet, for the most part, this does not appear to result in clinically significant dysphagia.

LARYNX

Voice

Many studies have looked at the effect of aging on voice quality. A basic description of age-related voice changes include an alteration in voice pitch and increased variability in pitch. Fundamental frequency of the voice increased with age for males and decreased with age for females. Estimated subglottic pressure was increased with increasing age. Overall, for unclear reasons, women were found to have less age-related degeneration effects (79). In a longitudinal study of 20 patients, voice onset time and spectral features of the voice over 30 years were compared. The men tested showed a decrease in output in the 2–4 kHz part of the vocal spectrum. The voice onset time also became prolonged with age (80).

The histological changes in aging vocal cords have been studied. There is an increase in fatty degeneration of the laryngeal muscles and a decrease in fiber density and elastin fibers in the vocal folds (81). Increasing ossification of the larynx with age alters the elastic and biomechanical properties of the insertion points of the vocal cords. There is a concomitant loss of sulfated glycosaminoglycans in the vocal ligament tendon, resulting in stiffening of the insertion zones (82).

Several studies suggest that it is important to rule out a variety of disorders prior to making the diagnosis of "presbylarynges." Woo et al. (83) retrospectively reviewed 151 patients over the age of 60 presenting for evaluation at a voice clinic complaining of dysphonia. Only six patients were found to fit the diagnosis of presbylarynges with vocal fold bowing and breathiness. The remaining patients were found to have voice changes related to central nervous system dysfunction (i.e., stroke, Parkinson's disease), benign vocal cord lesions, inflammatory disorders, neoplasia, or vocal cord paralysis. In contrast, Hagen et al. (84) retrospectively reviewed 47 patients over the age of 60 presenting with dysphonia. This study found that up to 30% of these patients could be diagnosed with presbylarynges. Treatment for this disorder was speech therapy, with phonosurgery being reserved for failures of speech therapy.

Tucker reported the results of vocal fold medialization using a modification of the Isshiki technique in six patients with the diagnosis of presbylarynges. The report claims that there are significant short-term benefits in terms of voice improvement; however, progressive relaxation of laryngeal tissues makes the long-term results of this procedure unsatisfactory (85). Currently, no studies using more current concepts of laryngeal framework surgery have focused on the elderly voice.

Malignancies

Complications After Laryngectomy

In a retrospective study of 414 patients who underwent total laryngectomy, age greater than 65 or even age greater than 80 was not a variable contributing to medical or surgical complications (86). Pera et al. (87), as well as other retrospective studies, have confirmed these findings. In a study of 371 patients, Huygen et al. (88) also showed no increase in complications with age; however, age >70 was significantly predictive of death within three years after treatment. Patients older than 70 also have a higher incidence of developing a second primary after surgical or radiotherapeutic treatment of laryngeal cancer (89). Laryngectomy, though safe in the elderly, may have different long-term consequences. In a study of 58 patients post laryngectomy, a decrease in long-term expiratory function was found. This was more pronounced in patients over 65, even when age-related decrease in pulmonary function was considered. Treatment with bronchodilators reversed this trend (90).

Head and Neck Cancer

The effect of aging on head and neck cancer has been assessed in a number of retrospective studies. In these studies, the most common complications surveyed were mortality, myocardial infarction, pneumonia, pulmonary embolus, wound infection, post-op urinary tract infection, and postoperative bleeding. Change in mental status, percentage of patients who were converted from an independent to an institutionalized state, and incidence of decubitus ulcers were generally not examined. Management of cancers of the oral cavity is challenging from both an oncologic and a rehabilitative standpoint. A recent retrospective study in the British Journal of Cancer examined prognostic factors in the treatment of squamous cell carcinoma of the tongue. In stage I and II cancers, age > 65 was found to be a significant negative prognostic factor for survival. Age did not influence the prognosis of stage III and IV cancers (91). In a series of 187 poor-prognosis patients (recurrence of tongue cancer after radiotherapy), age at tumor presentation was found to be significant in determining outcome in men. Older men (age range 50–80) were statistically more likely to have shorter survival than age-matched women or younger individuals (92). Barzan et al. (93) examined prognostic factors in 438 patients with a variety of head and neck malignancies. Patients were divided into three groups by age. Age was not correlated with outcome. In a comparative study of major head and neck surgery, in 115 patients older than 70, Kowalski et al. (94) demonstrated that there was no age-related effect on surgical mortality. This was interpreted as an indication to treat elderly patients with standard oncologic protocols. McGuirt and Davis (95) found an increased incidence of complications in head and neck cancer patients aged over 80, but also found that this group had a similar prognosis for survival and function as younger patients. In a retrospective cohort study, age over 65 or over 80 was not found to be a risk factor for the development of distant metastasis after resection of stage III/IV head and neck cancer. Screening for distant metastasis in geriatric patients should therefore depend on disease-based risk factors rather than age (96,97). Janot et al. (98) prospectively compared the predictive effects of clinical and pathological information in 108 patients presenting with head and neck cancer. Multivariate analysis showed that age and nodal status were prognostic for survival. Age, tumor status, and histological differentiation were predictive of metastatic disease. In a retrospective study of 207 patients, Magnano et al. (99) found no effect of age on the incidence of metastatic disease. Age also does not appear to have an effect on the radiosensitivity of tumors (100). Recent attempts at curative radiotherapy for head and neck cancer have used an accelerated dosing schedule. Age >70 years as an independent variable was not found to have an increased incidence of radiotherapy complications such as mucositis and weight loss.

In terms of the defects and physical disabilities induced by aggressive resection of head and neck cancer, age does not appear to play a role. The development of microvascular techniques for reconstruction of defects of the oral cavity, pharynx, and hypopharynx has significantly improved the rehabilitation of these patients. Bridger et al. (101) retrospectively studied 26 patients older than 70 years and 91 patients younger than 70 years and found no differences in the postoperative complication rates for these two groups. Distribution of the type of cancer resected and the size of the defect were similar in the two groups. Shestak et al. (102) studied 92 patients in 10-year cohorts of age ranging from 50 to 80 years who underwent microvascular free flap reconstruction and found no statistically significant difference in complication rates in the patients ranging from age 70 to 79. Some older studies suggested that poor nutritional status may have more of an adverse effect on surgical outcome in older than in young patients. A retrospective study also demonstrated a significant difference in evaluation and preoperative treatment of malnutrition in elderly versus younger patients. Elderly patients had a higher complication rate when stratified by nutritional status, and younger patients were more likely to receive pre- and perioperative nutrition treatment (103).

Summary

From retrospective studies there appears to be no contraindication to standard oncologic treatment for head and neck cancer. Prospective studies are needed to confirm this. There is also little information on surgical decision making with regard to age.

CONCLUSIONS

Review of recent reports addressing various disorders encountered in elderly patients with otolaryngologic complaints demonstrates that some of these disorders behave differently in this population when compared with younger patient groups. Knowledge of these variations is necessary to optimize management of the geriatric patient. Opportunities exist for further investigation of the unique characteristics and response to therapy in this age group. Otolaryngologists who treat elderly patients are encouraged to actively seek and critically assess reports of disease characteristics and management in this population.

REFERENCES

1. Gates GA, Cooper JC, Kannel WB, Miller NJ. Hearing in the elderly: the Framingham cohort, 1983–1985. Patient basic audiometric test results. Ear Hear 1990; 11:247–256.
2. Gates GA, Cooper JC. Incidence of hearing decline in the elderly. Acta Otolaryngol 1991; 111:240–248.
3. Pearson JD, Morrell CH, Gordon-Salant S, et al. Gender differences in a longitudinal study of age-associated hearing loss. J Acoust Soc Am 1995; 97(2):1196–1205.

4. Parving A, Biering-Sorenson M, Bech B, Christensen B, Sorensen MS. Hearing in the elderly > or = 80 years of age. Prevalence of problems and sensitivity. Scand Audiol 1997; 26(2):99–106.

5. Stumer J, Hickson L, Worrall L. Hearing impairment, disability and handicap in elderly people living in residential care and in the community. Disabil Rehabil 1996; 18(2):76–82.

6. Lewis-Cullinan C, Janken JK. Effect of cerumen removal on the hearing ability of geriatric patients. J Adv Nurs 1997; 15:594–600.

7. Emmett JR. Age as a factor in the success of tympanoplasty: a comparison of outcomes in the young and old. Ear Nose Throat J 1999; 78(7):480–483.

8. Vartiainen E. Surgery in elderly patients with otosclerosis. Am J Otol 1995; 16:536–538.

9. Takasaki K, Sando I, Balaban CD, Haginomori S, Ishijima K, Kitagawa M. Histo-pathological changes of the eustachian tube cartilage and tensor veli palatini muscle with aging. Laryngoscope 1999; 109:1679–1683.

10. Kaneko A, Hosoda Y, Doi T, Tada N, Iwano T, Yamashita T. Tubal compliance-changes with age and in tubal malfunction. Auris Nasus Laryng 2001; 28:121–124.

11. Schuknecht HF, Gacek MR. Cochlear pathology in presbycusis. Ann Otol Rhinol Laryngol 1993; 102:16.

12. Fischel-Ghodsian N, Bykhovskaya Y, Taylor K, et al. Temporal bone analysis of patients with presbycusis reveals high frequency of mitochondrial mutations. Hear Res 1997; 110:147–154.

13. Lutman ME. Hearing disability in the elderly. Acta Otolaryngol Suppl 1990; 476: 239–248.

14. Rizzo SR Jr, Gutnick HN. Cochlear versus retrocochlear presbycusis: clinical correlates. Ear Hear 1991; 12:61–63.

15. Strouse A, Ashmead DH, Ohde RN, Grantham DW. Temporal processing in the aging auditory system. J Acoust Soc Am 1998; 104:2385–2399.

16. Stach BA, Spretnjak ML, Jerger J. The prevalence of central presbycusis in a clinical population. J Am Acad Audiol 1990; 1:109–115.

17. Rodriguez GP, DiSarno NJ, Hardiman CJ. Central auditory processing in normal-hearing elderly adults. Audiology 1990; 29(2):85–92.

18. Resnick HE, Fries BE, Verbrugge LM. Windows to their world: the effect of sensory impairments on social engagement and activity time in nursing home residents. J Gerontol B Psychol Sci Soc Sci 1997; 52(3):S135–S144.

19. Mulrow CD, Aguilar C, Endicott JE, et al. Association between hearing impairment and the quality of life of elderly individuals. J Am Geriatr Soc 1990; 38(1):45–50.

20. Mulrow CD, Aguilar C, Endicott JE, et al. Quality-of-life changes and hearing impairment. A randomized trial. Ann Intern Med 1990; 113(3):188–194.

21. Carabellese C, Appollonio I, Rozzini R, et al. Sensory impairment and quality of life in a community elderly population. J Am Geriatr Soc 1993; 41(4):401–407.

22. Ciurlia-Guy E, Cashman M, Lewsen B. Identifying hearing loss and hearing handicap among chronic care elderly people. Gerontologist 1993; 33(5):644–649.

23. Uhlmann RF, Larson EB, Rees TS, Koepsell TD, Duckert LG. Relationship of hearing impairment to dementia and cognitive dysfunction in older adults. JAMA 1989; 261(13):1916–1919.

24. Cnmiel R, Jerger J. Some factors affecting assessment of hearing handicap in the elderly. J Am Acad Audiol 1993; 4(4):249–257.

25. Kalayam B, Meyers BS, Kakuma T, et al. Age at onset of geriatric depression and sensorineural hearing deficits. Biol Psychiatry 1995; 38:649–658.

26. Gates GA, Couropmitree NN, Myers RH. Genetic associations in age-related hearing thresholds. Arch Otolaryngol Head Neck Surg 1999; 125:1285.

27. Gates GA, Schmid P, Kujawa SG, Nam B, D'Agostino R. Longitudinal threshold changes in older men with audiometric notches. Hear Res 2000; 141:220–228.

28. Strouse AL, Hall JW III, Burger MC. Central auditory processing in Alzheimer's disease. Ear Hear 1995; 16(2):230–238.

29. Gold M, Lightfoot LA, Hnath-Chisolm T. Hearing loss in a memory disorders clinic. A specially vulnerable population. Arch Neurol 1996; 53(9):922 928.
30. Gates GA, Karzon RK, Garcia P, et al. Auditory dysfunction in aging and senile dementia of the Alzheimer's type. Arch Neurol 1995; 52(6):626–634.
31. Parving A, Boisen G. In-the-canal hearing aids. Their use by and benefit for the young and elderly hearing-impaired. Scand Audiol 1990; 19:25–30.
32. Shin YJ, Fraysse B, Deguine O, et al. Benefits of cochlear implantation in elderly patients. Otolaryngol Head Neck Surg 2000; 122:602–606.
33. Kelsall DC, Shallop JK, Burnelli T. Cochlear implantation in the elderly. Am J Otol 1995; 16(5):609–615.
34. Sterkers O, Mosnier I, Ambert-Dahan E, Herelle-Dupuy E, Bozorg-Grayeli A, Bouccara D. Cochlear implants in elderly people; preliminary results. Acta Otolaryngol Suppl 2004; (552):64–67.
35. Francis HW, Chee N, Yeagle J, Cheng A, Niparko JK. Impact of cochlear implants on the functional health status of older adults. Laryngoscope 2002; 112(8 Pt 1):1482–1488.
36. Pereira KD, Kerr AG. Disability after labyrinthectomy. J Laryngol Otol 1996; (110): 216–218.
37. Bance ML, Walsh RM, Bath AP, Keller A, Tator CH, Rutka JA. The natural history of untreated vestibular schwannomas. Is there a role for conservative management? Rev Laryngol Otol Rhinol (Bord) 2000; 121(1):21–26.
38. Rosenberg SI. Natural history of acoustic neuromas. Laryngoscope 2000; 110:497–508.
39. DeCruiz MJ, Moffat DA, Hardy DG. Postoperative quality of life in vestibular schwannoma patients measured by the SF36 health questionnaire. Laryngoscope 2000; 110:151–155.
40. Merchant SN, Velazquez-Villasenor L, Tsuji K, Glynn RJ, Wall C III, Rauch SD. Temporal bone studies of the human peripheral vestibular system. Normative vestibular hair cell data. Ann Otol Rhinol Laryngol Suppl 2000; 181:3–13.
41. Velazquez-Villasenor L, Merchant SN, Tsuji K, Glynn RJ, Wall III, Rauch SD. Temporal bone studies of the human peripheral vestibular system. Normative Scarpa's ganglion cell data. Ann Otol Rhinol Laryngol 2000; 181:14–19.
42. Alvarez JC, Diaz C, Suarez C, et al. Aging and the human vestibular nuclei: morphometric analysis. Mech Aging Dev 2000; 114:149–172.
43. Davis LE. Dizziness in elderly men. J Am Geriatr Soc 1994; 42:1184–1188.
44. Lawson J, Fitzgerald J, Birchall J, Aldren CP, Kenny RA. Diagnosis of geriatric patients with severe dizziness. J Am Geriatr Soc 1999; 47:12–17.
45. Oghalai JS, Manolidis S, Barth JL, Stewart MG, Jenkins HA. Unrecognized benign paroxysmal positional vertigo in elderly patients. Otolaryngol Head Neck Surg 2000; 122:630–634.
46. Katsarkas A. Dizziness in aging: a retrospective study of 1,194 cases. Otolaryngol Head Neck Surg 1994; 110:296–301.
47. Wolfson L, Whipple R, Derby CA, et al. A dynamic posturography study of balance in healthy elderly. Neurology 1992; 42:2069–2075.
48. Cohen H, Heaton LG, Congdon SI, Jenkins HA. Changes in sensory organization test scores with age. Age Ageing 1996; 25:39–44.
49. Baloh RW, Corona S, Jacobson KM, Enrietta JA, Bell T. A prospective study of posturography in normal older people. J Am Geriatr Soc 1998; 46:438–443.
50. Borger LL, Whitney SL, Redfern MS, Furman JM. The influence of dynamic visual environments on postural sway in the elderly. J Vestib Res 1999; 9:197–205.
51. Wong AM, Lin YC, Chou SW, Tang FT, Wong PY. Coordination exercise and postural stability in elderly people: effect of Tai Chi Chuan. Arch Phys Med Rehabil 2001; 82:608–612.
52. Deems DA, Doty RL. Age-related changes in the phenyl ethyl alcohol odor detection threshold. Trans Pa Acad Ophthalmol Otolaryngol 1987; 39:646–650.

53. Schiffman SS. Taste and smell in disease (second of two parts). N Engl J Med 1983; 308(22):1337–1343.
54. Doty RL, Shaman P, Applebaum SL, Giberson R, Siksorski L, Rosenberg L. Smell identification ability: changes with age. Science 1984; 226:1441–1443.
55. Edelstein DR. Aging of the normal nose in adults. Laryngoscope 1996; 106:1–25.
56. Knutson JW, Slavin RG. Sinusitis in the aged: optimal management strategies. Drugs Aging 1995; 7:310–316.
57. Jiang RS, Hsu Cy. Endoscopic sinus surgery for the treatment of chronic sinusitis geriatric patients. Ear Nose Throat J 2001; 80:230–232.
58. Robbins J, Hamilton JW, Lof GL, Kempster GB. Oropharyngeal swallowing in normal adults of different ages. Gastroenterology 1992; 103:823–829.
59. McKee GJ, Johnston BT, McBride GB, Primrose WJ. Does age or sex affect pharyngeal swallowing? Clin Otolaryngol 1998; 23:100–106.
60. Nicosia MA, Hind JA, Roecker EB, et al. Age-effects on the temporal evolution of isometric and swallow pressure. J Gerontol A Biol Sci Med Sci 2000; 55:M634.
61. Nilsson H, Ekberg O, Olsson R, Hindfelt B. Quantitative assessment of oral and pharyngeal function in Parkinson's disease. Dysphagia 1996; 11(2):144–150.
62. Nilsson H, Ekberg O, Olsson R, Hindfelt B. Quantitative aspects of swallowing in an elderly nondysphagic population. Dysphagia 1996; 11(3):180–184.
63. Shaker R, Ren J, Zamir Z, Sarna A, Liu J, Sui Z. Effect of aging, position, and temperature on the threshold volume triggering pharyngeal swallows. Gastroenterology 1994; 107(2):396–402.
64. Tracey J, Logemann J, Kahrilas P, Jacob P, Kobara M, Krugler C. Preliminary observations on the effects of age on oropharyngeal deglutition. Dysphagia 1989; 4:90–94.
65. Robbins J, Levine R, Wood J, Roecker EB, Luschei E. Age effects on lingual pressure generation as a risk factor for dysphagia. J Gerontol A Biol Sci Med Sci 1995; 50:M257–262.
66. Zamir Z, Ren J, Hogan WJ, Shaker R. Coordination of deglutitive vocal cord closure and oral-pharynx swallowing events in the elderly. Eur J Gastroenterol Hepatol 1996; 8:425–429.
67. Aviv JE. Effects of aging on sensitivity of the pharyngeal and supraglottic areas. Am J Med 1997; 103(5A):76S.
68. Logemann JA, Pauloski BR, Rademaker AW, Colangelo LA, Kahrilas PJ, Smith CH. Temporal and biomechanical characteristics of oropharyngeal swallow in younger and older men. J Speech Lang Hear Res 2000; 43(5):1264–1274.
69. Barczi SR, Sullivan PA, Robbins J. How should dysphagia care of older adults differ? Establishing optimal practice patterns. Semin Speech Lang 2000; 21:347–361.
70. Jego A, Chassagne P, Landrin-Dutot I, et al. Does age play a role in mylohyoideus muscle function? Neurogastroenterol Motil 2001; 13:81–87.
71. Rhodus NL, Brown J. The association of xerostomia and inadequate intake in older adults. J Am Diet Assoc 1990; 90(12):1688–1692.
72. Scott J. A morphometric study of age changes in the histology of the ducts of human submandibular salivary glands. Arch Oral Biol 1977; 22(4):243–249.
73. Fischer D, Ship JA. Effect of age on variability of parotid salivary gland flow rates over time. Age Ageing 1999; 28(6):557–561.
74. Ship JA, Fischer DJ. The relationship between dehydration and parotid salivary gland function in young and older healthy adults. J Gerontol A Biol Sci Med Sci 1997; 52(5):M310–319.
75. Lopez-Jornet MP, Bermejo-Fenoll A. Is there an age-dependent decrease in resting secretion of saliva of healthy persons? A study of 1493 subjects. Braz Dent J 1994; 5(2): 93–98.
76. Wu AJ, Atkinson JC, Fox PC, Baum BJ, Ship JA. Cross-sectional and longitudinal analyses of stimulated parotid salivary constituents in healthy, different-aged subjects. J Gerontol 1993; 48(5):M219–224.

77. Astor FC, Hanft KL, Ciocon JO. Xerostomia: a prevalent condition in the elderly. Ear Nose Throat J 1999; 78:476–479.

78. Longman LP, Higham SM, Rai K, Edgar WM, Field EA. Salivary gland hypofunction in elderly patients attending a xerostomia clinic. Gerodontology 1995; 12(12):67–72.

79. Higgins MB, Saxman JH. A comparison of selected phonatory behaviors of health-aged young adults. J Speech Hear Res 1991; 34:1000–1010.

80. Decoster W, Debruyne F. Changes in spectral measures and voice-onset time with age: a cross-sectional and longitudinal study. Folia Phoniatr Logop 1997; 49:269–280.

81. Kahane JC. Histologic structure and properties of the human vocal folds. ENT J 1988; 67(5):324–325, 329–330.

82. Paulsen F, Kimpel M, Lockemann U, Tillmann B. Effects of ageing on the insertion zones of the human vocal folds. J Anat 2000; 196:41–54.

83. Woo P, Casper J, Colton R, Brewer D. Dysphonia in the aging: physiology versus disease. Laryngoscope 1992; 102:139–144.

84. Hagen P, Lyons GD, Nuss DW. Dysphonia in the elderly: diagnosis and management of age-related voice changes. South Med J 1996; 89:204–207.

85. Tucker HM. Laryngeal framework surgery in the management of the aged larynx. Ann Otol Rhinol Laryngol 1988; 97:534–536.

86. Arriaga MA, Kanel KT, Johnson JT, Myers EN. Medical complications in total laryngectomy: incidence and risk factors. Ann Otol Rhinol Laryngol 1990; 99(8):611–615.

87. Pera E, Moreno A, Galindo L. Prognostic factors in laryngeal carcinoma. A multifactorial study of 416 cases. Cancer 1986; 58:928–934.

88. Huygen PL, van den Broek P, Kazam I. Age and mortality in laryngeal cancer. Clin Otolaryngol 1980; 5:129–137.

89. Nikolaou AC, Markou CD, Petridis DG, Daniilidis IC. Second primary neoplasms in patients with laryngeal carcinomas. Laryngoscope 2000; 110(1):58–64.

90. Ackerstaff AH, Hilgers FJ, Van Zandwijk N. Long term pulmonary function after total laryngectomy. Clin Otolaryngol 1995; 20:547–551.

91. Kantola S, Parikka M, Jokinen K, Soini Y, Alho OP, Salo T. Prognostic factors in tongue cancer-relative importance of demographic, clinical and histopathological factors. Br J Cancer 2000; 83:614–619.

92. Llewelyn J, Mitchell R. Survival of patients who needed salvage surgery for recurrence after radiotherapy for oral carcinoma. Br J Oral Maxillofac Surg 1997; 35:424–428.

93. Barzan L, Veronesi A, Caruso G, et al. Head and neck cancer and ageing: a retrospective study in 438 patients. J Laryngol Otol 1990; 104:634–640.

94. Kowalski LP, Alcantara PS, Magrin J, Parise JO. A case-control study on complications and survival in elderly patients undergoing major head and neck surgery. Am J Surg 1994; 168:485–490.

95. McGuirt WF, Davis SP III. Demographic portrayal and outcome analysis of head and neck cancer surgery in the elderly. Arch Otolaryngol Head Neck Surg 1995; 121: 150–154.

96. Alvi A, Johnson JT. Development of distant metastasis after treatment of advanced-stage head and neck cancer. Head Neck 1997; 19(6):500–505.

97. Allal AS, Maire D, Becker M, Dulguerov P. Feasibility and early results of accelerated radiotherapy for head and neck carcinoma in the elderly. Cancer 2000; 88:648–652.

98. Janot F, Klijanienko J, Russo A, et al. Prognostic value of clinicopathological parameters in head and neck squamous cell carcinoma: a prospective analysis. Br J Surg 1996; 73:531–538.

99. Magnano M, Bongioannini G, Lerda W, et al. Lymphnode metastasis in head and neck squamous cell carcinoma: multivariate analysis of prognostic variables. J Exp Clin Cancer 1999; 18:79–83.

100. Stausbol-Gron B, Overgaard J. Relationship between tumour cell in vitro radiosensitivity and clinical outcome after curative radiotherapy for squamous cell carcinoma of the head and neck. Radiother Oncol 1999; 50(1):47–55.

101. Bridger AG, O'Brien CJ, Lee KK. Advanced patient age should not preclude the use of free-flap reconstruction for head and neck cancer. Am J Surg 1994; 168:425–428.
102. Shestak KC, Jones NF, Wu W, Johnson JT, Myers EN. Effect of advanced age and medical disease on the outcome of microvascular reconstruction for head and neck defects. Head Neck 1992; 28:14–18.
103. Lin BS, Robinson DS, Klimas NG. Effects of age and nutritional status on surgical outcomes in head and neck cancer. Ann Surg 1988; 207:267–273.

4

Cerumen Impaction

Cyrus Torchinsky and Terence M. Davidson
Division of Otolaryngology—Head and Neck Surgery, VA San Diego Healthcare System, and Department of Surgery, UCSD Medical Center, San Diego, California, U.S.A.

INTRODUCTION

Cerumen management is an integral and banal part of virtually every otolaryngologist's practice. While the management of earwax often provokes ribbing from our more "macho" surgical colleagues, it remains an important quality-of-life issue for our patients. Perhaps nowhere else is this more true than in the elderly population where impacted cerumen is a common problem that often leads to decreased functionality and cognition.

This chapter will be a compendium to assist practicing head and neck surgeons in managing cerumen in elderly patients and make suggestions for how to educate referring primary care physicians on how to manage cerumen in their office and when to refer for head and neck evaluation and assistance. To achieve this end, we will examine the anatomy and physiology of the external auditory canal as they relate to cerumen. This will include the recent biochemical efforts to determine the exact composition of cerumen so that a better ceruminolytic agent might be developed. Important in this discussion is the pathophysiology of cerumen impaction. The literature and current epidemiologic evidence examining the prevalence and impact of cerumen impaction in the elderly will be discussed. Then, after summarizing the limited clinical data on cerumen management, we will suggest our own practice algorithm for cerumen impaction. As a note, there is a semantic difference between cerumen, the product of specialized secretory glands and earwax, an amalgam of these secretions, and various other substances contained in the canal. Unless specified, we use these terms synonymously. After all, the offending substance we remove from our patients' ears is earwax.

ANATOMY AND PHYSIOLOGY OF CERUMEN

The external auditory canal is an approximately 2.5 cm long canal when measured from the external meatus to the tympanic membrane (TM). The lateral, cartilaginous part of the canal measures 8 mm. In the thick subcutaneous tissue in the outer or lateral third of the cartilaginous canal lie the numerous ceruminous and sebaceous glands that secrete what appears in the auditory canal as earwax (Fig. 1). Ceruminous glands are modified apocrine glands that have a coiled tubular structure resembling both sweat glands and secretory tissue in the breast (1). They lie deep to sebaceous glands, and in fact their ducts form a confluence with those emerging from the acini of sebaceous glands to empty adjacent to the hair follicles. Like all apocrine glands, the histology of ceruminous glands changes when glandular products are being secreted (2). While actively secreting cerumen, secretory cells have a columnar appearance. This changes to a cuboidal appearance when the glands are quiescent. Myoepithelial cells line the outer surface of the gland, aiding the propulsion of glandular products to the lumen of the external auditory canal (EAC).

Earwax is a mixture of the products of ceruminous and sebaceous glands, large sheets of desquamated keratinocytes, shed hair, and any other substances that may have made their way into the external auditory canal (i.e., personal hygiene products, dirt, or, commonly in our Southern California practice, sand). There is a wide range of colors for cerumen. Some earwax is dark brown or black while some is a golden-yellow to light brown hue. It is believed that all cerumen begins golden in color and the combination of dehydration, oxidation, and bacterial activity is what leads to the darker colors (3). While the exact source of the pigmentation is unknown, recent efforts at determining the chemical composition of cerumen by Burkhart et al. may have yielded an answer.

Not all cerumen is alike. Otolaryngologists working in communities with large Asian populations have long noted that these patients' wax differs from that of Caucasians. Asians have dry, also known as "rice bran," wax that is brittle, ash-like, and flaky appearing with a light grey to brownish grey color. This is opposed to the wet or sticky, gold to golden brown cerumen that is present in 98% of Caucasians

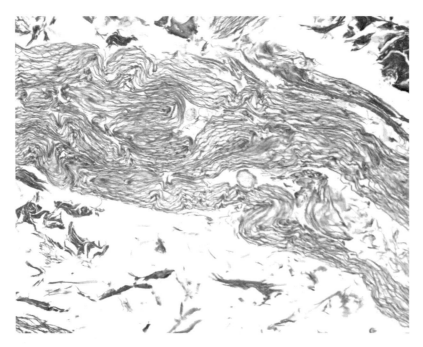

Figure 1 Low power (10X) paraffin-embedded section of an impacted cerumen plug demonstrating sheets of desquamated keratinocytes (*center of figure*).

and those of African and Latin descent (4). Rice bran wax also distinguishes itself by being odorless and less copious than wet cerumen. Asians produce significantly less cerumen than whites, Africans, or Latinos. Some investigators feel that this is the result of fewer ceruminous glands in the canal (5).

E. Matsunga in his 1962 paper "The Dimorphism in Human Normal Cerumen" described a simple Mendelian inheritance for cerumen phenotype. The exact locus of this gene was recently mapped by Tomita et al. (6) to the short arm of chromosome 16. This apparently inconsequential dichotomy of cerumen has yielded surprising avenues of research. Petrakis et al. (7) used cerumen phenotype to trace the migration across the Bering strait of native American peoples. This study was followed by work tracking the frequency and inheritance of cerumen phenotype in various tribes and led to the observation that the type of earwax is associated with breast secretions. Individuals with dry cerumen tend to produce fewer breast secretions. Given this correlation and the morphologic similarities between breast and ear tissue, Petrakis (8) extended this concept to the breast cancer finding that dry-type cerumen is associated with a reduced risk of this disease.

Wet and dry are not the only two subtypes of cerumen. Hawke (3) has further carried this classification to distinguish between soft and hard cerumen. Hard cerumen is more often found in adults and is characterized as having a dry, desiccated consistency while soft cerumen is wet and sticky and is typified by what we see in the pediatric population. Histologically, soft cerumen has small sheets of keratin squames, shed cells also known as corneocytes from the stratum corneum in external canal skin, while hard cerumen has larger, more tightly packed sheets of desquamated keratinocytes. Corneocytes are expanded in soft cerumen, and not in hard cerumen.

That earwax provides a protective function for the external auditory canal is undisputed. How it does this is a matter of some debate. It is certain that cerumen plays a role in lubricating and cleaning the external auditory canal. The chemical constituents of earwax are primarily hydrophobic compounds that help keep the otherwise damp, dark, and warm culture milieu [called the "greenhouse of the human body" by some (9)] of the external ear free of water. Cerumen is also very effective at trapping debris such as dirt, dust, shed hairs, and desquamated skin cells. The egress of this material is facilitated by the pattern of epithelial migration in the ear from the tympanic membrane outward. Jaw motion during mastication and speech further helps drive cerumen out of the canal. Cerumen has long been felt to act as protection against insects in the canal, although it is very difficult to scientifically verify this function (1).

Whether or not cerumen has intrinsic antimicrobial activity is controversial. Some evidence suggests that this is the case. Cerumen has a pH ranging from four to five and has both bacterio- and fungostatic properties, and it contains such bacteriocidal materials such as lysozyme, IgA, and fatty acids (10). However, in vitro work has been inconsistent. Stone and Fulghum (11) found that populations of some bacteria were reduced 17% to 99% by a 3% suspension of wet cerumen. They tested seven species of bacteria including *Staphylococcus aureus, Staphylococcus epidermis, Propionibacterium acnes, Corynebacterium* spp., *Eschericia coli*, and *Serratia marcescens*. Their results implied that more pathogenic species were more susceptible to the effects of cerumen as were bacteria in the logarithmic rather than stationary phase of growth. No difference was found between the wet and dry types of cerumen. Similar findings were also reported by Chai and Chai (12), who suspended dry cerumen in a 3% glycerol–sodium bicarbonate buffer, finding up to a 99% reduction in growth for

H. flu, *E. coli*, and *Serratia*, while growth rates were reduced by 30% to 80% for two *Pseudomonas*, one *Streptococcus*, and two *Staphylococcus* isolates. However, these results have been difficult to replicate. Campos et al. (13) found that cerumen suspensions more frequently increased rather than inhibited growth. A paper by Pata (14) showed reduction only in *S. epidermis* in cerumen from normal subjects. Intriguingly, the cerumen of patients with chronic otitis externa statistically inhibited growth of a pathogen, *E. coli*. Regardless of the end results of these studies, one thing that is clear is that at the very least cerumen acts a mechanical barrier to bacterial invasion of the very thin epidermis of the external auditory canal. Underproducers of cerumen are indeed predisposed to otitis externa, and the time-tested protocol of dry ear precautions for external otitis also gives hint that the drying properties provided by lipophilic compounds are important in preventing bacterial overgrowth of the external auditory canal.

The regulation of cerumen production has been well studied, albeit some years ago. Adrenergic agonists, smooth muscle stimulants, and the emotional states of anxiety and fear in addition to resulting in increased production of apocrine sweat result in increased cerumen. Also, the mechanical actions of cleaning or rubbing the canal wall have a milking action on the ceruminous glands, helping to extrude their contents. Cerumen secretion can also be stimulated by vigorous chewing (5). In addition to the amount of cerumen extruded into the canal, the quality of this secretion can change. Measured over an entire population, cerumen can change its chemical composition over the course of the seasons. The triglyceride content of earwax decreases significantly in the transition from winter to summer months (15). This is felt to be a consequence of changes in diet from these times.

The definitive studies of the biochemical composition of cerumen are the recent reports of Burkhart et al. (16,17). This group determined the constituent elements of wet hard cerumen in patients with obstructed ears. Their end goal is to use this information to discover a better ceruminolytic agent. Their first study determined the primary amino acid and simple sugar content of earwax. They found the major amino acid components to be glycine, glutamic acid, and serine. The most abundant carbohydrates in order of abundance were galactosamine, galactose, glucose, glucosamine, mannose, and fructose (16). This work was expanded one year later when the investigators used flash pyrolysis-gas chromatography/mass spectrometry to further elucidate the chemical composition of cerumen (17). The cerumen was first fractionated in a solution of deoxycholate, sodium chloride, and sodium phosphate. Then, the supernatant containing pure chemical constituents (i.e., the secretions of the ceruminous and sebaceous glands) and residue composed of squamous and proteinaceous debris were analyzed separately. This technique identified 152 principal compounds. These included aliphatic compounds, aromatics, nitrogen compounds, and possibly diterpenoids. This latter family of chemicals is quite interesting because among the diterpenoids are retinal and carotenoids. These compounds are abundant in plants and are major pigments in both fall foliage and carrots. The peak possibly representing diterpenoids was only found in the supernatant, indicating that Burkhart et al. (16,17) may have discovered the heretofore unknown pigment in earwax. The other peaks in their sample represented abundant squalene compounds and steroids. In addition to discovering the complexities of cerumen that yield its various physical properties [including some little known ones. For example, earwax was used as a binding agent for dyes in illuminated medieval manuscripts (18)], this study also yielded a potentially novel class of ceruminolytics: bile acids. Burkhart reported that primary and secondary bile acids in vitro were remarkably efficacious in dissolving the cerumen plug, perhaps due to the ability of the bile acids to form micelles with the cholesterol in cerumen. Although they suggest that they are developing clinical application of bile acids, no reports have emerged as of the time of this writing.

PATHOPHYSIOLOGY

Subjective complaints from patients with cerumen impaction include itching, pain, hearing loss, tinnitus, vertigo, and chronic otitis externa. Other reported symptoms include chronic cough, perhaps mediated through the auricular branch of the vagus (Arnold's nerve) that supplies the skin of the posterior and inferior wall of the canal (19).

Hearing loss has been quantified by pure tone audiometric testing in patients with cerumen impaction. These audiograms demonstrate gradually decreasing high-frequency threshold sensitivity as percent of canal occlusion increases (20). With an 80% to 90% occlusion, hearing loss only occurred at frequencies greater than 1000 Hz with threshold decreases from 15 dB to 20 dB. Increasing the occlusion to 95% resulted in an extra 5–10 dB of threshold loss in higher frequencies, but no changes in frequencies less than 1000 Hz. Only with complete blockage of the canal do we see hearing loss in the lower frequencies with an average pure tone loss of 40 dB across the spectrum. This explains the commonly encountered clinical phenomenon whereby patients do not complain of hearing loss until their canals are nearly or completely occluded. While there is high frequency loss prior to 100% occlusion of the EAC, patients do not perceive their deficit until impaction becomes severe enough to impact the frequencies used in speech. In their review, Roeser and Ballachanda make the point that any deficits from cerumen impaction may in fact be compounded by pre-existing sensorineural loss. This is especially true in elderly patients who have a high prevalence of presbycusis (9).

Another, perhaps often missed or misdiagnosed, consequence of cerumen impaction is decreased mental functioning. The association between cognitive impairment and hearing loss is inconsistently described. Peters et al. (21) found that hearing impaired individuals had a steeper decrease in their mental status scores over time compared with normal hearing individuals. Moreover, at least one study, Mulrow et al. (22), found that improvement of hearing was associated with improvement on the Folstein mini mental status exam, the Yesavage geriatric depression scale, and subjective surveys regarding emotional function and communication. Moore et al. studied how cleaning cerumen impaction influenced performance on the Folstein mini mental status exam (MMSE). In their cohort of 29 patients with cerumen impaction, this group found an average improvement of one point on the MMSE (23). Then, one must also consider the well-being of the elderly individual. A study examining quality of life and hearing impairment had 63% of respondents reporting severe emotional and social dysfunction as a result of their hearing loss. People with hearing loss also fare poorly on, and had "neurotic" or "borderline" profiles on, an anxiety questionnaire (24). The isolation caused by hearing impairment is difficult to quantify, but well understood by anyone regularly treating hearing impairment in a clinical practice.

Whether cerumen impaction is a disorder of overproduction or failure of migration is not certain. There is histological evidence that individuals with cerumen impaction have more distended ceruminous glands relative to nonimpacted controls (2). However, this distension could as easily be the result of obstruction at the exit point for cerumen as a symptom of overactivity of ceruminous glands.

The migration hypothesis as elucidated in a series of papers by Hawke's group is the more compelling. Robinson of Hawke's group examined impacted cerumen from 28 patients and found the combination of wet and hard cerumen to be the most associated with impaction (25). Robinson noted that these cerumen plugs contained more large sheets of keratin squames in them compared to earwax from non-impacted ears. Clinically, this type of cerumen plug often has a pearly white color and can lead to pressure and pain within the EAC, as the dead cells have a tendency to absorb water and expand. The presence of these sheets of keratinocytes could be explained by a failure of the inward to outward migration of epithelium within the external canal. This failure of migration is hypothesized to be a deficit in a protein that cleaves cell–cell connections allowing corneocytes (keratinocytes in the stratum corneum) to separate from each other and cells in the stratum lucidum below. This to date undiscovered protein has been named KADS (keratinocyte attachment destroying substance), and it may turn out to be a crucial component of the ear's self-cleaning mechanism. Without detachment, epithelial migration out of the canal is disrupted and the accumulating keratin ball serves to trap dirt, cerumen, and hair eventually forming a plug. To date, the only enzyme known to be involved in epithelial cell desquamation is steroid sulfatase. The target of steroid sulfatase is cholesterol sulfate, a known intracellular cement of sorts. In tissue from normal ear canals compared to those from patients with impacted cerumen, greater steroid sulfatase activity is seen in the deeper layers of the epithelium, supporting the hypothesis that this protein is involved with desquamation (dermatologists are well aware of disorders in keratinocyte detachment as they often treat patients with X-linked icthyosis). The desquamation hypothesis is also clinically relevant in the quest for the perfect ceruminolytic agent. In addition to addressing the chemical constituents of earwax, the ideal ceruminoltyic will be capable of disrupting the integrity of the keratin sheets in the ear canal (Fig. 1). This agent must be able to lyse the corneocytes' cell membrane, allowing them to expand and separate from each other and adjacent cells in the stratum lucidum of the epidermis (3).

The changes of normal aging also lead to a predisposition for cerumen impaction. As we age, the coarsening and lengthening of the hair within the external auditory canal acts as a physical impediment to self-cleaning of the ear. This is especially true in men. Additionally, there is a general decrease in the activity of cerumen glands in aging. This makes earwax drier and more difficult to clear from the canal. Another change of aging that can lead to cerumen impaction is the development of external ear canal exostoses. Finally, as the elderly are more frequent users of hearing aids, this cause of cerumen impaction must not be overlooked (26).

INCIDENCE

The geriatric population has the highest incidence of cerumen impaction of any age group with the exception of the mentally retarded and residents of institutions. There have been three studies by two investigators examining the prevalence of pathologic quantities of cerumen in the elderly. Mahoney examined the problem twice, first in 1987 and then again in 1993. In the first study, Mahoney (27) found that 34% of 133 elderly subjects had impacted cerumen and another 23% had "moderate to large" amounts of cerumen in their EACs. This matched up well with the follow-up study showing 25% to 42% of ears in nursing home residents aged 62–100 had "moderate to large" amounts of impacted cerumen (28). Perhaps the most concerning fact reported by Mahoney was that in spite of the identification of excessive cerumen, most ears were either inadequately treated or untreated. This was attributed to the unwillingness of physicians to perform ear irrigations and lack of training/knowledge in the nursing staff on the use of ceruminolytic agents, ear irrigation, or otoscopy. Janken and Lewis-Cullinan reported similar results, with 35% of 226 individuals 65 or over having impacted cerumen. Nineteen percent of this cohort had bilateral impaction (29).

TREATMENT

There are many safe and effective treatments for impacted cerumen. The challenge to the otolaryngologist is to determine which treatment to use with which patient. Before undertaking cerumen removal, a complete history should be taken. Has the patient had a history of this problem? Are there any signs suggesting tympanic membrane perforation? Were there complications of prior cerumen removals such as dizziness, bradycardia, etc.? This information is important because there have been reported cases of cardiac arrest arising from manipulation of the EAC, thought to be a response mediated by Arnold's nerve (30). Also one must know if this is an only hearing ear, for if so irrigation is contraindicated and the cerumen must be cleaned by direct visualization.

Before inserting an ear speculum, the external auditory meatus and canal should be inspected for signs of bleeding, erythema, swelling, or crusting to rule out a concomitant infection. The canal is best examined by pulling the pinna of the ear superiorly and posteriorly. If the speculum is inserted superiorly and anteriorly the drum should be visualized. In cases of impaction, one will see a plug of wax ranging from black to dark brown to white in color.

The treatment should proceed as follows. The majority of cases of cerumen impaction can be cleared by irrigation of the canal. Most otolaryngologic practices have a compressed air irrigation setup on hand, but a 20 cc syringe with a 14-gauge Angiocath can be used in lieu of more elaborate equipment. Commercial irrigators are also available, most often used in pediatrics. Typically, ears are irrigated with water, but some choose to add alcohol, hydrogen peroxide, or Burrow's solution. No one solution has a demonstrated clinical benefit over another solution. The irrigant must be warmed to body temperature to prevent stimulation of the vestibular system. When introducing the irrigant, care is taken to direct the stream laterally in the EAC. This prevents injury to the tympanic membrane as well as allowing the jet of water to pass behind the cerumen plug facilitating its egress from the canal. It is judicious to follow any irrigation procedure with a few drops of an antibiotic ear solution (31).

If irrigation fails, the next steps are the introduction of a ceruminolytic followed by removal under binocular otomicroscopy. Surprisingly, when one reviews all the literature involving the ideal ceruminolytic, no consensus arises to what is the best agent. Hydrogen peroxide, Burrow's solution, and acetic acid have been studied and proven to be of some benefit over no treatment, but no solution has consistently outperformed warmed tap water (32). Mineral oil is also used by many. Pediatricians have long been using docusate sodium as a ceruminolytic, and it remains the agent of choice in a handful of academic otolaryngology departments (33). The key to the use of any ceruminolytic is that it be warmed before introduction to the canal. Some authors claim this is especially true for Colace.

The ceruminolytic should be given five or so minutes to work on dissolving or loosening the plug before removal is attempted. How one proceeds from there is largely determined by what is seen in the canal. One preferred method is to use a five French otologic suction and roll the cerumen plug into a ball. (While suctioning the EAC be aware that many patients do not tolerate this procedure without discomfort. The noise is loud and it is possible to induce vertigo with this procedure, i.e., an air caloric stimulation.) The cerumen can in most instances be sucked out of the canal. If suction fails, with extreme care a Rosen hook may be introduced into the canal and either wedged behind or even into the cerumen plug to pull it out. Alternately, propitious use of a cerumen loop and cup forceps can be very effective. Any instrument used in the canal should have smoothed edges to avoid injury to canal skin. Given the high incidence of atelectatic drums in the elderly, extreme caution must be taken not to push the wax ball inwards. There are multiple documented cases of tympanic membrane perforation and even incostapedial dislocation that led to permanent sensorineural hearing loss (34). Caveats also include the thinned skin in the elderly. Even in young subjects there is no deep dermal tissue overlying the bony canal. With the thinning of skin that occurs with aging, interventions performed in the medial EAC can be extremely painful. It is also very easy to induce bleeding, which in addition to clouding the field of the microscope is of some distress to the patient and indicates a violation of EAC skin that may predispose to infection. If the wax plug is recalcitrant to the above interventions, it is best to stop, have the patient go home on a week-long regimen of your preferred ceruminolytic, and then follow up for removal.

COMPLICATIONS OF CERUMEN REMOVAL

Complications of cerumen removal can be protean and should be managed appropriately. As mentioned above, the already thin skin of the canal is further thinned by aging. Coupled with the fact that many elderly patients are on aspirin or other blood thinners, bleeding is a common complication. If bleeding arises, antibiotic otic drops can be administered. With a severely tender and edematous canal, oral antihistamines may be of some benefit to patient comfort and in fact speed healing.

Tympanic membrane perforation is another common complication. Small perforations usually heal on their own, but this can take from weeks to months in a geriatric patient. Also, tympanic membrane perforation can be associated with injury to the ossicles or even worse, perilymph fistula. The latter condition is especially suspected when nystagmus, tinnitus, and hearing loss follow treatment. Tinnitus without nystagmus may occur in absence of injury to the ossicles or even without a TM perforation. However, this form of tinnitus is usually self-limiting. If one is suspicious of perilymph fistula or ossicular injury, prompt referral to audiology for a fistula test and measurement of stapedial reflexes is indicated. Virtually all of the major complications of cerumen removal: TM perforation, ossicular disruption, and perilymph fistula are amenable to surgery. However, diagnosis must be made rapidly. If a fistula is indeed present per a fistula test by an audiologist, the patient should follow four to five days of bed rest and avoid Valsalva maneuvers. Use of stool softeners is encouraged if constipation is an issue. Perilymph fistulas typically present with a sensorineural hearing loss of 30–40 dB. This can be hard to parse out if there was preexisting sensorineural hearing loss (SNHL) in the patient. A 30 dB air bone gap usually indicates injury to the conductive component of the ear caused by the trauma of irrigation or too forceful removal with instruments (31).

Nausea and vomiting are common complications, which can be avoided by warming irrigation fluid and taking care to avoid suction in the context of a perforated tympanic membrane. Less common complications include cardiac arrest, visual changes, and otitis externa following cerumen removal.

There has been a large rise in the use of "alternative" medicines and therapies in the last 10 years. One such remedy is the ear candle, a homeopathic treatment that involves placing a hollow candle into the EAC and lighting the opposite end. This ostensibly creates a vacuum that sucks cerumen out. After the treatment, a substance resembling wax is left in the candle stub. This treatment has been touted in the popular press as being safe, effective, and cheap. While the cost of ear candling is indeed approximately one-fifth that of removal in a doctor's office, this practice is neither efficacious nor safe (35). None of the 20 candles tested generated negative pressure in a specially designed tympanometric setup. None of the impacted ears were cleared of cerumen, and in fact the investigators halted their study early due to injurious effects of the treatment. The wax-like substance in the candle stubs was examined with a mass spectrometer and found to have no earwax constituents, but it was rich in the alkanes that are commonly found in candle wax. A survey sent out by Seely's group found that burns to the auricle or EAC were common as were complete or partial occlusions of the EAC with candle wax and there was one report of a tympanic membrane perforation. Thus, otolaryngologists must be aware of this practice, counsel against its use, and be prepared to treat complications.

OUR PRACTICE ALGORITHM

Cerumen impaction in the elderly is a problem that should be primarily managed by primary care physicians. We suggest a simple algorithm that can be distributed to primary care physicians delineating management and referral guidelines (Fig. 2). Irrigation is the simplest and most readily available choice for impacted ears. Thus, this should be the first-line treatment using any of the base irrigants mentioned above (i.e., water warmed to body temperature with or without a combination of alcohol, hydrogen peroxide, vinegars, or Burrow's solution). Contraindications to irrigation include patients with chronic ear disease, a known tympanic membrane perforation, or an only hearing ear. These patients should have their cerumen removed under the binocular microscope and thus should be automatic referrals.

If the initial irrigation is not successful, a warmed ceruminolytic agent is instilled into the ear canal. After 15 minutes, the irrigation process is repeated. If the plug remains, the patient is sent home with a cerumen softener such as mineral oil. One week later the process is repeated. Failure to clear the plug necessitates referral to a specialist. When performing irrigations, physicians must know when to stop the procedure to avoid the aforementioned complications. To ensure that there is no reaccumulation of cerumen, patients can be instructed to use the otic preparation of Burrow's solution: Domeboro otic drops, two drops into each ear two to three times a week after showering. Burrow's solution, containing aluminum acetate, is an astringent which helps denature protein and by stimulating the EAC epithelium nurtures outwards epithelial migration.

Many patients will only suffer clinically apparent cerumen impaction every two or so years. Primary care physicians can easily manage these patients when they have problems. For those patients desiring more definitive management or in whom cerumen impaction is a chronic problem, we have two treatments. The first is the

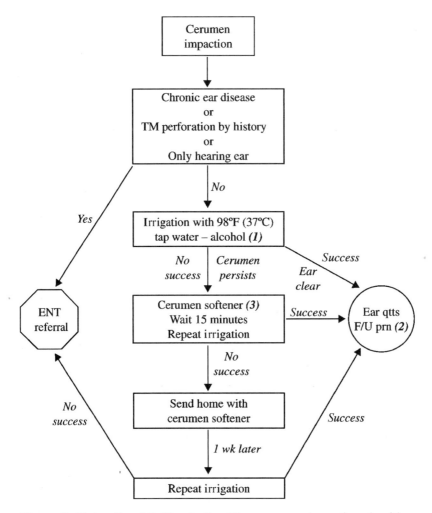

Figure 2   University of California–San Diego cerumen impaction algorithm.

abovementioned Domeboro otic prophylaxis. Alternatively, patients can instill two to three drops of mineral oil into each ear canal weekly. This can be followed by irrigation with a small bulb syringe.

HISTORICAL PRECEDENT AND CONCLUSIONS

> There is nothing new under the sun, but there are lots of old things we don't know.
>
> —Ambrose Bierce (1842–1914)

Ambrose Bierce's take on the famous quote from Ecclesiastes was made all too real in the final stages of preparing this chapter. A review of a textbook published in 1902 revealed that the otolaryngologists of that time had both a thorough understanding of the mechanisms of cerumen impaction as well as treatments that have been lost in the intervening century. We found this so interesting that the section on cerumen management is reproduced below for those who wish to read it.

Impacted Cerumen—Occlusion of the auditory canal by a mass of inspissated cerumen is the affection of the external ear which most frequently demands the attention of the aurist. Usually the patient is entirely unconscious of the presence of the mass until the canal is completely occluded by it. Then the hearing, which before had not been appreciably diminished, although the ceruminous plug may have all but filled the lumen of the canal, becomes at once greatly impaired, autophony manifests itself, and very frequently tinnitus makes its appearance to add to the discomfort and alarm of the patient. Although the mass develops very slowly, many months usually elapsing before it becomes inconveniently large, the symptoms just enumerated generally manifest themselves suddenly. The usual explanation of this is that water has run into the ear in washing or bathing, or in warm weather perspiration has found its way into it and has caused the plug, which previously had nearly filled the canal, to swell up sufficiently to make the occlusion complete. Occasionally it is a fluid which the individual has intentionally dropped into the ear or some manipulation on his part of the ceruminous mass, which brings about the sudden change. Exceptionally the same symptoms may result, accompanied, perhaps, by pain, from a smaller mass of wax (which left undisturbed might not have caused inconvenience for a long time) being dislodged and pushed down upon the drumhead by the efforts of the patient to remove it. Again, when the plug is very hard and occupies the outer portion of the meatus, it may, through the movements of the jaw, exert sufficient pressure upon the canal walls to cause pain, and perhaps inflammation, before it has become so large as to interfere with audition.

The plug varies greatly in consistency and in solubility, and frequently contains innumerable short, pale hairs (from the walls of the canal). Very often it is in part made up of pieces of exfoliated epidermis, and exceptionally it has as a nucleus some small foreign body which has found its way into the ear, or an old scab left by a former otitis. More frequently than not both ears are involved, so both should invariably be examined.

Among the rarer symptoms produced by the presence of impacted cerumen in the ear may be mentioned dizziness, reflex cough, perturbation of the mental faculties with inability to concentrate the mind in intellectual pursuits, disturbances of gait simulating those of locomotor ataxia (Risley), epileptiform convulsions, and, in a case reported by the writer (2), inability to swallow, accompanied by a feeling of oppression about the heart. The added danger which results in otitis media from a pre-existent occlusion of the meatus by impacted cerumen should also not be lost sight of.

With good illumination it is usually a very easy matter to detect the presence of a ceruminous plug in the auditory canal. It is seen as a dark brown mass filling the lumen of the canal, with its outer surface situated usually at about the line of juncture of the osseous and membranous portions of the meatus. Touched with a probe, it may appear quite hard, or may be soft and easily indented. Generally the inner extremity of the mass reaches to, and rests upon, the tympanic membrane.

The etiology of this affection has received considerable attention, and, while it cannot be claimed that it is as yet fully understood, there is a general agreement at least as to two points: in the first place, that, probably through reflex influence, the ceruminous glands are frequently abnormally active in the presence of chronic inflammatory affections of the nasopharynx; in the second place, that under such circumstances and often perhaps independently of such conditions, there is a disturbance of the normal outgrowth of the epidermis which covers the external surface of the drumhead and lines the walls of the meatus. This in health tends to transport the cerumen from the deeper portions of the canal to its external orifice, where it falls out or is removed in the ordinary daily ablutions. That catarrh of the nasopharynx is frequently present when there is a disposition to the formation of ceruminous plugs in the ears is a fact of daily observation, and there can be little doubt that it is an important factor in their causation. And the composition of many masses of impacted cerumen—made up, in great part, of layers of exfoliated epidermis, and sometimes enclosed in a thin pouch of epidermis which has been cast off entirely from the tympanic membrane and the walls of the meatus—would seem to show that under certain circumstances there is not only an arrest of the normal outgrowth of the epidermis, but an actual reversal in the direction of its growth, tending to a heaping up of epithelial débris in the deeper parts of the canal, as well as to an impaction of cerumen.

Treatment—It would seem that as to the manner of dealing with so simple a condition there could be but little room for difference of opinion, still less for contention. Such, however, is far from being the case, for one very high authority tells us in his excellent treatise upon diseases of the ear that the syringe should rarely be used for the removal of cerumen, and that with the curette and the angular forceps one may accomplish in ten or fifteen minutes what cannot be done with the syringe in an hour's time; while another excellent authority tells us in his book that in four or five years he has not met with a single instance in which by means of the syringe he has failed to remove impacted cerumen from the ear in one sitting of five minutes or less, and that as to the curetting method he feels that he cannot seriously argue the question. At the risk of seeming to be contentious himself, the writer cannot refrain from saying that this last expressed sentiment meets with his fullest endorsement. But still another very high authority, whose example in most things we are glad to follow, actually commends the introduction of a strong solution of caustic potash into the ear (of course with the exercise of extreme caution) in order to saponify quickly the ceruminous mass and so to facilitate its removal. As to this procedure, it may be remarked that in kindling, and especially in rekindling a fire, petroleum is a great saver of time; but, even so, it is not the part of wisdom to commend its general use in this way.

The method of dealing with impacted cerumen which the writer has found most convenient, and which he has employed for many years, is as follows: In the great majority of cases the syringe is chiefly relied upon. When, however, the ceruminous mass proves obdurate and does not easily undergo disintegration, the angular probe or the instrument for the removal of foreign bodies represented in Figure 490 is brought into requisition and the mass is partly broken up or separated from its attachment to the canal wall. After this the syringing is resumed, and usually with much better effect. Bicarbonate of soda is invariably added to the warm water (105–110°F) with which the syringing is done, as it unquestionably facilitates the removal of the wax and certainly does no harm to the syringe, as has been suggested. The quantity used is never accurately determined, but is approximately half an ounce to a quart. The ear is inspected from time to time to make sure that there is still cerumen in it, and that the syringing is not being kept up unnecessarily. As the mass diminishes in size and there is a likelihood that the stream of water may impinge upon the drumhead, the force with which it is thrown into the ear is lessened. The exact direction in which the stream strikes the impacted mass is not thought to be of especial moment, and no apprehension is felt that this may result in the plug being driven by the force of the water more deeply into the meatus, as some have imagined. When both ears are affected, unless the mass first attacked comes out very readily, the syringing is alternated from one ear to the other, as this saves time and appreciably diminishes the amount of syringing required. The intermittent stream of a piston syringe is employed, and is thought to be more efficacious than the continuous stream of a fountain syringe. The hard-rubber, kidney-shaped basin commonly employed by aurists has been long since discarded, because it is concave where it should be convex, and so does not fit well into the hollow beneath the ear, and because, moreover, it is so long and shallow that a very slight movement on the part of the patient is likely to cause its contents to slop over upon the clothing. Instead of this, a china bowl (one made of hard rubber or metal might be better, because less fragile) of the shape represented in Figure 489 is used, and has been found much better adapted to the purpose, since it is free from both of the faults mentioned. It is always held by the patient, over whose shoulder a napkin is spread, rather than by an assistant, unless the patient be a young child. When inspection with the speculum and mirror shows that all of the cerumen has been removed, two or three syringefuls of plain warm water are gently thrown into the ear to wash out the previously used soda solution. The ear is then dried with a spill of soft linen and closed with a bit of absorbent cotton, which in cold weather the patient is advised to wear until bedtime. If the plug proves to be exceptionally refractory or time be pressing, the patient is told to report the next day, and in the meantime to drop into the ear several times a little warm sweet oil, or, if it be inconvenient for him to do this, the ear is filled with a saturated solution of soda, and after perhaps a half-hour's wait the syringing is resumed. The cases in which the plug cannot be removed at one sitting are very exceptional, but the writer is compelled to admit that with the best skill he can command it is not unusual for him to spend many more than "five minutes" in accomplishing this result.

It occasionally happens that upon inspecting the ear it can be seen that the mass of cerumen does not extend into the deeper parts of the canal. Under such circumstances, if it is found to be of its usual firmness, it is often possible with the traction instrument (Fig. 490) to draw out the whole mass at a single effort, and so to save both time and trouble. If, however, even in such a case, the cerumen proves to be of such consistency that it can be removed only bit by bit, it is better to resort to the syringe without further ado.

The writer knows of no means by which the well-recognized disposition of impacted cerumen to recur after having been removed can be overcome, except in so far as the cure or amelioration of any accompanying inflammation of the nasopharynx tends to this result.

In summary, practicing otolaryngologists must have an understanding of the basic science of cerumen. Earwax is produced in the outer third of the cartilaginous canal and is composed of glandular products, desquamated skin, and whatever manages to get into the canal. There are ethnic morphological differences between dry, Asian cerumen, and the wet cerumen found in all other races. Whether or not cerumen has true antibiotic properties has been difficult to verify in vitro, but at the very least it helps keep the canal dry and protects the fragile EAC skin. Sophisticated biochemical techniques have been applied to determine the exact composition of cerumen and aid in the development of better ceruminolytics.

Earwax is cleared by the epithelial migration from the tympanic membrane to the auditory meatus as well as mechanical forces milking the canal during mastication. Recent work has rediscovered that cerumen impaction is more likely the result of a failure of the detachment of keratinocytes than overproduction. This disease process is likely genetic and exacerbated by the changes of aging. It is important that this easy to detect condition be diagnosed as the manifestations of disease are protean and treatments easy to administer.

Treatment of cerumen impaction is straightforward and most cases can be managed with a combination of irrigation and ceruminolytics. All agents work reasonably well, but there is still room for improvement. Early 20th century head and neck physicians used potash, a compound made by percolating water through a mixture of wood ash and lime (36). Perhaps not so ironically, potash is a saponifying agent like the bile acids recently suggested to be the optimal ceruminolytic. Referral to otolaryngologists should be made for patients with TM perforations, chronic ear disease, impacted only hearing ears, and impacted cerumen not easily cleaned by the primary care physician. Cerumen impaction prophylaxis can be obtained with Domeboro otic drops to encourage migration out of the EAC or with weekly application of mineral oil with or without self-irrigation.

REFERENCES

1. Kelly KE, Mohs DC. The external auditory canal. Anatomy and physiology. Otolaryngol Clin North Am 1996; 29(5):725–739.
2. Mandour MA, El-Ghazzawi EF, Toppozada HH, Malaty HA. Histological and histochemical study of the activity of ceruminous glands in normal and excessive wax accumulation. J Laryngol Otol 1974; 88(11):1075–1085.
3. Hawke M. Update on cerumen and ceruminolytics. Ear Nose Throat J 2002; 81(8 suppl 1): 23–24.
4. Matsunaga E. The dimorphism in human normal cerumen. Ann Hum Genet 1962; 25: 273–286.
5. Perry ET. The human ear canal. Springfield, IL: Charles C. Thomas, 1957.
6. Tomita H, Yamada K, Ghadami M, et al. Mapping of the wet/dry earwax locus to the pericentromeric region of chromosome 16. Lancet 2002; 359(9322):2000–2002.
7. Petrakis NL, Molohon KT, Tepper DJ. Cerumen in American Indians: genetic implications of sticky and dry types. Science 1967; 158(805):1192–1193.
8. Petrakis NL. Cerumen phenotype and epithelial dysplasia in nipple aspirates of breast fluid. Am J Phys Anthropol 1983; 62(1):115–118.
9. Roeser RJ, Ballachanda BB. Physiology, pathophysiology, and anthropology/epidemiology of human earcanal secretions. J Am Acad Audiol 1997; 8(6):391–400.
10. Osborne JE, Baty JD. Do patients with otitis externa produce biochemically different cerumen?. Clin Otolaryngol 1990; 15(1):59–61.
11. Stone M, Fulghum RS. Bactericidal activity of wet cerumen. Ann Otol Rhinol Laryngol 1984; 93(2 Pt 1):183–186.
12. Chai TJ, Chai TC. Bactericidal activity of cerumen. Antimicrob Agents Chemother 1980; 18(4):638–641.
13. Campos A, Betancor L, Arias A, et al. Influence of human wet cerumen on the growth of common and pathogenic bacteria of the ear. J Laryngol Otol 2000; 114(12):925–929.
14. Pata YS, Ozturk C, Akbas Y, Gorur K, Unal M, Ozcan C. Has cerumen a protective role in recurrent external otitis? Am J Otolaryngol 2003; 24(4):209–212.
15. Cipriani C, Taborelli G, Gaddia G, Melagrana A, Rebora A. Production rate and composition of cerumen: influence of sex and season. Laryngoscope 1990; 100(3):275–76.

16. Burkhart CN, Burkhart CG, Williams S, Andrews PC, Adappa V, Arbogast J. In pursuit of ceruminolytic agents: a study of earwax composition. Am J Otol 2000; 21(2):157–160.
17. Burkhart CN, Kruge MA, Burkhart CG, Black C. Cerumen composition by flash pyrolysis-gas chromatography/mass spectrometry. Otol Neurotol 2001; 22(6):715–722.
18. Petrakis NL. Earmarks of art history: cerumen and medieval art. Am J Otol 2000; 21(1):5–8.
19. Raman R. Impacted ear wax—a cause for unexplained cough? Arch Otolaryngol Head Neck Surg 1986; 112(6):679.
20. Chandler JR. Partial occlusion of the external auditory meatus: its effect upon air and bone conduction hearing acuity. Laryngoscope 1964; 74:22–54.
21. Peters CA, Potter JF, Scholer SG. Hearing impairment as a predictor of cognitive decline in dementia. J Am Geriatr Soc 1988; 36(11):981–986.
22. Mulrow CD, Aguilar C, Endicott JE, et al. Association between hearing impairment and the quality of life of elderly individuals. J Am Geriatr Soc 1990; 38(1):45–50.
23. Moore AM, Voytas J, Kowalski D, Maddens M. Cerumen, hearing, and cognition in the elderly. J Am Med Dir Assoc 2002; 3(3):136–139.
24. Mulrow CD, Aguilar C, Endicott JE, et al. Quality-of-life changes and hearing impairment. A randomized trial. Ann Intern Med 1990; 113(3):188–194.
25. Robinson AC, Hawke M, Naiberg J. Impacted cerumen: a disorder of keratinocyte separation in the superficial external ear canal? J Otolaryngol 1990; 19(2):86–90.
26. Naiberg JB, Robinson A, Kwok P, Hawke M. Swirls, wrinkles and the whole ball of wax (the source of keratin in cerumen). J Otolaryngol 1992; 21(2):142–148.
27. Mahoney DF. One simple solution to hearing impairment. Geriatr Nurs 1987; 8(5):242–245.
28. Mahoney DF. Cerumen impaction. Prevalence and detection in nursing homes. J Gerontol Nurs 1993; 19(4):23–30.
29. Lewis-Cullinan C, Janken JK. Effect of cerumen removal on the hearing ability of geriatric patients. J Adv Nurs 1990; 15(5):594–600.
30. Prasad KS. Cardiac depression on syringing the ear. A case report. J Laryngol Otol 1984; 98(10):1013.
31. Grossan M. Safe, effective techniques for cerumen removal. Geriatrics 2000; 55(1):80, 83–86.
32. Burton MJ, Doree CJ. Ear drops for the removal of ear wax. Cochrane Database Syst Rev 2003;(3):CD004400.
33. Chen DA, Caparosa RJ. A nonprescription cerumenolytic. Am J Otol 1991; 12(6):475–476.
34. Dinsdale RC, Roland PS, Manning SC, Meyerhoff WL. Catastrophic otologic injury from oral jet irrigation of the external auditory canal. Laryngoscope 1991; 101(1 Pt 1): 75–78.
35. Seely DR, Quigley SM, Langman AW. Ear candles—efficacy and safety. Laryngoscope 1996; 106(10):1226–1229.
36. Theobald S. Affections of the external ear. In: deScheintz GE, Randall BA, eds. An American Text-Book of Diseases of the Eye, Ear, Nose, and Throat. Philadelphia and London: WB Saunders and Co., 1901:699–703.

5

Amplification and the Geriatric Patient

Catherine V. Palmer
Communication Science and Disorders, University of Pittsburgh, and Audiology and Hearing Aids, Department of Otolaryngology, University of Pittsburgh Medical Center, Pittsburgh, Pennsylvania, U.S.A.

Amanda Ortmann
Communication Science and Disorders, University of Pittsburgh, and Department of Audiology and Speech Language Pathology, VA Pittsburgh Health Care System, Pittsburgh, Pennsylvania, U.S.A.

GENERAL DESCRIPTION OF THE CLINICAL PROBLEM

Improvements in technology and medicine over the past 50 years have resulted in significant increases in life expectancy. Twelve percent of the U.S. population was over the age of 65 in 2000; by 2050 that figure will nearly double (1). Along with the shifts in the demographics, there also will be a shift in the health status, with an increase in the number and severity of chronic health conditions affecting the population (2).

Hearing loss is the third most commonly reported chronic condition within the geriatric population (behind arthritis and hypertension) (2). According to the National Center on Deafness and Other Communication Disorders, 33% of the population over the age of 60 has hearing loss, increasing to 50% of those over 80 (3). Eight out of 10 residents of nursing homes suffer from hearing loss (4). Although hearing impairment is a prevalent problem among the elderly, only 20% of those affected actually use hearing aids (5). This is in remarkable contrast to visual impairment; 93% of the elderly population with visual problems wear glasses routinely (6). The sequellae of uncorrected hearing loss are very similar to those of visual impairment: decreased mobility, social isolation, and depression (7). Hearing aids and other assistive devices provide significant improvement of not only hearing function, but also of the overall quality of life of the elderly individual.

WHY IS HEARING LOSS PARTICULARLY IMPORTANT IN THE GERIATRIC POPULATION?

Currently, aging adults account for 43% of the hearing-impaired population (8). As the median age of Americans rise, an increase in the prevalence of hearing loss is to be expected. Health care professionals can assist with the needs of their

59

elderly patients by understanding the nature, repercussions, and remediation of hearing disorders.

Sensory impairments can limit the quality of life for both elderly individuals and their families. Uncorrected hearing loss leads to reduction of functional, psychological, and psychosocial well-being (9–11). Studies by Mulrow and colleagues (12) as well as Weinstein and Ventry (13) have found that even a mild to moderate hearing loss has a considerable effect on social and emotional handicaps (12,13). The elderly individuals judge the hearing handicap as being less severe than their spouse or partner (14). Thus, family members are often first to recognize the problem of the individual's hearing loss and encourage the use of amplification. Telephone communication often becomes an important link to family and safety as mobility is reduced with aging, with a concomitant requirement for amplification.

There is early evidence that uncorrected hearing loss may contribute to cognitive dysfunction (15). Uhlmann and colleagues (16) examined the relationship between hearing impairment and dementia and found that the prevalence of hearing impairment was higher in the demented adult sample than a comparable sample of adults free from dementia. Dementia and hearing loss interact to produce a more rapid cognitive decline in elderly individuals (17).

Management of hearing loss in the demented population is problematic (18). Although viewed by health care professionals as being hard to test and manage, these patients may often benefit from evaluation and amplification (19).

BASIC SCIENCE

Presbycusis disrupts both the peripheral and central portions of the auditory system (20). The peripheral loss of hair cells results in decreased audibility of the acoustic signal, particularly in the higher frequencies beyond 2000 Hz. The consonant properties of speech such as the "s," "sh," "f," "t," and "p" have acoustic energy within the range of 2000–8000 Hz and are therefore "dropped." Vowel properties of speech are preserved; hence, aging adults typically state that they hear conversations, but cannot understand what is being said.

The central component of presbycusis results in a degradation of the rapid processing of speech information, the ability to localize, and the ability to use binaural cues, and increases in severity with increasing age (21,22). Binaural cues are critical for separating speech from background noise. The elderly patient will often have difficulty understanding speech in the presence of background noise due to the central effects of aging, even in the presence of adequate amplification. An aural rehabilitation program should include not only amplification but also education regarding the use of various communication strategies, assistive listening devices (ALDs), and assertiveness.

HISTORY

Figure 1 displays a typical audiogram and word recognition results of an elderly individual. Hearing function is similar in both ears with normal or near-normal low-frequency hearing and decreased hearing sensitivity in the higher frequencies. This individual notes that this hearing loss has a negative effect on communication abilities and lifestyle. The audiogram suggests that the individual is a candidate for an aural

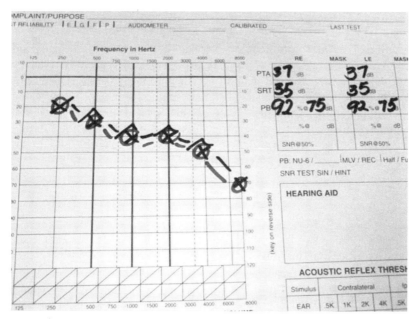

Figure 1 Audiogram of a typical aging hearing loss.

rehabilitation program. However, more information (history) about the individual is required in order to select the proper amplification device and counseling strategies.

Physical, psychosocial, or psychological changes associated with aging influence the auditory testing procedures and the aural rehabilitation design and outcome (10). Foremost among the physical changes that can interfere with the aural rehabilitation program are the individual's overall general health, visual deficits, and dexterity. Both advanced age and concomitant disease(s) may influence the individual's motivation and acceptance of the aural rehabilitation program. Manipulation of a hearing aid or other assistive listening device requires visual acuity and fine motor skills. Although not a contraindication, vision loss and decreased dexterity must be considered in the context of the aural rehabilitation program.

Cerumen production is a challenging physical change that impacts aural rehabilitation, as it can lead to malfunctioning of hearing aids by blocking the receiver opening in certain instruments. Some elderly hearing aid users require routine cerumen removal.

A major psychosocial change in aging adults that affects the aural rehabilitation program is the reduction of social activity. This reduction may or may not be the direct result of hearing loss. In order to be motivated to participate in a program designed to improve communication function, the aging individual must be involved in meaningful social interactions. Hearing-impaired adults experience some degree of social isolation and often require encouragement to seek increased social activities as part of their rehabilitation program.

Psychological changes such as cognitive decline and depression also can influence the diagnosis and treatment of hearing impairment in the elderly population. Hearing loss has been associated with a sense of helplessness, passivity, and negativism (23). These negative emotions will influence the aging patient's acceptance of the hearing aids. Aging individuals may need a longer timeframe to learn and retain new information (24).

PHYSICAL EXAMINATION

A case history is an integral component of every audiologic and/or hearing aid evaluation. It consists of specific questioning regarding hearing, tinnitus, balance function, situational performance, and general health. Otoscopy is performed with particular attention to ear texture and elasticity and checking for collapsing ear canal openings. These findings impact the choice of earphones for audiometric testing and later impact recommendations related to hearing aid selection and earmold material. The ear canal must be free from debris and the tympanic membrane visible and intact.

TESTING

Screening

The onset of presbycusis is subtle, and patients are frequently unaware of their hearing loss and do not seek evaluation of their hearing voluntarily. Routine screening of hearing loss by primary care physicians may be quite helpful in the detection of patients who would benefit from aural rehabilitation. Screening may be accomplished through a handheld device that functions as both an otoscope and an audiometer. For screening purposes, it performs a pure tone sweep across frequencies of 500, 1000, 2000, and 4000 Hz and the patient reports whether tones were heard. Background noise in the examination room must be kept to a minimum. There is some debate as to what intensities and frequencies should be used in the screening protocol to maximize the test's sensitivity and specificity (25).

The use of self-administered questionnaires regarding the patient's hearing handicap in certain situations is a simple and inexpensive approach to screening hearing. The hearing handicap inventory for the elderly-screening version is a 10-item, five-minute questionnaire that measures the degree of social and emotional hearing handicap (26). The American Academy of Otolaryngology devised the five minute hearing test, which is another self-administered questionnaire that can be used for screening purposes (27). These self-reported screening tests assess not only the patient's self-perceived hearing loss but also their motivation for hearing care.

Comprehensive Audiologic Examination

The routine audiologic test battery consists of pure tone and speech testing, static immittance, and acoustic reflexes. Word recognition scores, used for diagnostic purposes, also play a role in the aural rehabilitation program. If word recognition ability at audible levels is poor, then counseling must include realistic expectations of the results of amplification. Although such a patient will benefit from amplification, the patient usually must rely more heavily on visual cues and/or assistive listening devices.

A common challenge to rehabilitation in the hearing-impaired population is a reduced dynamic range, referring to the range between the thresholds of audibility and loudness discomfort. In age-related hearing loss, the elevated threshold of audibility contributes to the reduction of the dynamic range. The relationship between the change in audibility threshold and loudness discomfort level, however, is not linear due to recruitment. Recruitment is abnormal loudness gain for suprathreshold stimuli. In other words, sounds increase from very soft to uncomfortably loud rapidly with increasing stimuli. Determination of the elderly individual's loudness discomfort level when fitting a hearing aid or any other type of assistive listening device is important to ensure that the maximum output of the hearing aids does not exceed this level.

A salient characteristic of the elderly hearing-impaired listener is the decreased understanding of speech in the presence of background noise. In a study by Frisna and Frisna (28), a group of younger listeners and a group of elderly listeners with equivalent audiometric sensitivity completed a variety of speech recognition tasks in quiet and in background noise. It was found that although the elderly group's hearing sensitivity did not differ from the younger listeners, they performed significantly worse on speech recognition tasks in background noise than their younger counterparts. There are several speech recognition tests that quantify the difficulty the elderly patient is likely to experience with background noise, such as the hearing in noise test (HINT), and a shortened version of the speech in noise test (QUICKSIN). Performance on these tests may help guide the aural rehabilitation program.

TREATMENT OPTIONS

Testing is completed when the type, degree, and configuration of the hearing loss is defined for each ear separately; the individual's ability to understand words in quiet and in noise is documented; and the elderly individual's communication needs, challenges, and expectations are understood in the context of the individual's communication environment. All patients who exhibit a hearing loss, regardless of the severity, are candidates for an aural rehabilitation program and/or amplification. The aural rehabilitation program can be divided into four sections (Table 1): the selection of hearing aids or other listening devices (this session is called the hearing aid evaluation), the hearing aid fitting, orientation, and counseling.

During the hearing aid evaluation, many decisions regarding hearing aid features need to be made. Table 2 contains a list of all of the up front decisions that the elderly individuals, their family, and the audiologist need to consider. The following sections focus on five of the major considerations. These include style of hearing aid, hearing in noise, signal processing, use of the telephone, and safety.

Table 1 Four Components of an Aural Rehabilitation Program

Hearing aid selection and evaluation	Hearing aid fit	Hearing aid orientation	Counseling and training
Selection	Verification	Insertion and removal	Expectations
Monaural versus binaural	Validation	Care and maintenance	Communication strategies
Omnidirectional versus directional microphones		Use of volume control and/or memory push button	Understanding the hearing aid features
Hearing aid style		Use of hearing aid programs/memories	Listening practice
Telecoil			
Signal processing			
Use of other ALDs			

Abbreviation: ALDs, assistive listening devices.

Table 2   Up Front Considerations That Must be Made Prior to Ordering the Hearing Aid

Style of hearing aid
Monaural versus binaural amplification
Microphone type
Earmold type, earmold length, earmold venting
Sound channel characteristics
Bandwidth of the instrument
Receiver type
Output limiting
Volume control
Batteries (battery door locks)
Signal processing
Number of signal processing channels
Multimemory
Ability to fine tune (programmable)

The decisions are made based on empirical evidence, audiologist experience, and patient and family preference.

Hearing Aid Style

The common styles of hearing aids are behind the ear (BTE), in the ear (ITE), in the canal (ITC), and completely in the canal (CIC) (Fig. 2). In selecting the style (or the size) of the hearing aid, the audiologist must consider the individual's dexterity, ear canal size and texture, history of cerumen accumulation, and degree of hearing loss.

The BTE hearing aid has the most flexibility. BTE hearing aids have much more room for circuitry and options. The size and shape of the ear canal does not

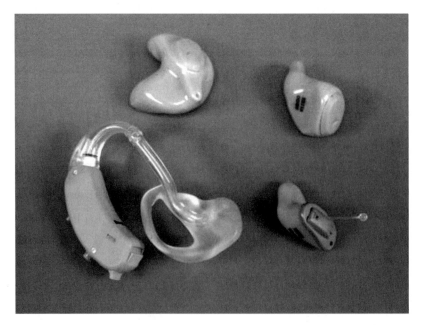

Figure 2   Four styles of hearing aids (*clockwise from bottom left*): behind the ear, in the ear, in the canal, completely in the canal.

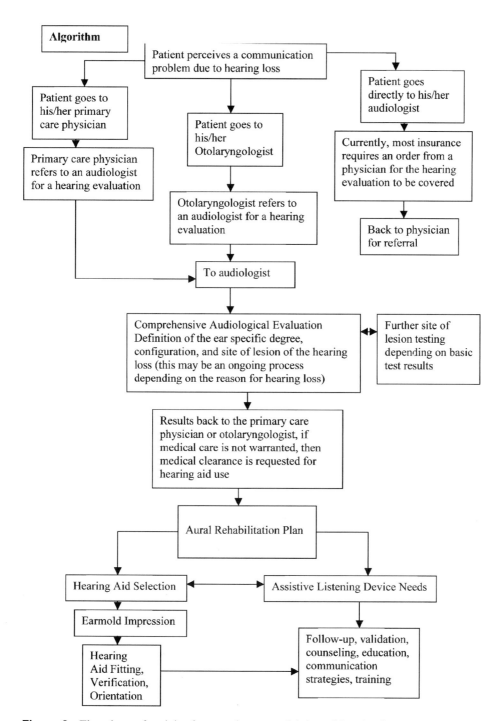

Figure 3 Flowchart of activity for a patient complaining of hearing loss.

interfere with the choices of hearing aid options for the patient using a BTE hearing aid. BTEs can provide the necessary gain to accommodate hearing losses ranging anywhere from mild to profound. BTE hearing aids are coupled to the ear with an earmold. By making specific changes to the earmold (length of tubing, belling of sound bore, vent sizes, etc.), a particular frequency/gain enhancement can be created. Patients usually report that these acoustic modifications sound more natural than electronic modifications accomplished through hearing aid circuitry. Other advantages of having a standard hearing aid coupled to a custom earmold include the ability to attach a loaner hearing aid to the user's earmold should the hearing aid need repair or service.

Another advantage of BTE hearing instruments is that care and maintenance is less problematic than with other types of hearing aids. With custom hearing aids that fit completely inside the ear canal and concha, the electronics, particularly the receiver, are vulnerable to cerumen blockage and damage from heat and moisture. Because the electronics of the BTE hearing aid are housed external to the ear canal, it is not vulnerable to these elements found in the ear canal. The earmold can accumulate cerumen blockage, but the patient simply brushes away the visible cerumen or disconnects the earmold from the hearing aid to soak the mold in a cup of warm water. If the elderly patient has a history of cerumen accumulation, a BTE hearing aid should be considered. Insertion, removal, and manipulation (changing the battery) of BTE instruments are relatively easy. Because it is bigger, it may be beneficial to an elderly individual who experiences problems with manual dexterity. Some patients find the bulkiness of this hearing aid a drawback to its use. However, with appropriate hair styling this aid can be very discreet. The earmold is made of a translucent plastic that blends in with the skin tone of the patient and the hearing aid portion is tucked neatly behind the ear.

ITE and ITC hearing aids are limited in their flexibility due to space limitations. A patient's ear canal may be too small to accommodate certain options such as a telecoil or directional microphones. These hearing aids typically fit a hearing loss range of mild to moderate. Due to the close proximity of the microphone and receiver, these hearing aids are more vulnerable to feedback, especially if the hearing loss is more severe. Feedback occurs when amplified sound "feeds" back into the microphone to be reamplified. Proper fit of these custom products is imperative.

Manipulation of these custom hearing aids may be more difficult for the elderly patient. The batteries in these hearing aids may be smaller in size and are not appropriate for someone with poor visual acuity and/or manual dexterity. However, several modifications can be made to reduce problems due to dexterity. A removal string can be added to ITE or ITC hearing aids for easier removal of the instrument from the ear. The volume control wheel can be stacked, making it more pronounced for easier manipulation. In some of the more advanced technology, the audiologist is able to enable and disable the volume control. This feature is very useful if you find an aging patient who is confused by the volume control. Rather than send the hearing aid back to have the volume control removed, it simply can be disabled.

There are individual differences in manipulation. For some older adults, insertion of one piece (the ITE) is easier than the two-piece BTE, which requires an extra step of looping the hearing aid behind the ear.

A CIC hearing aid may be the least visible of all the hearing instruments. A CIC hearing instrument fits deeply inside the patient's ear canal. The goal of a CIC is to take advantage of the acoustic properties of the external ear. However, it is not the best recommendation for an elderly individual for a number of reasons. It is the most limited in terms of flexibility and only can meet the needs of hearing loss in the mild-to-moderate range. There is no space for any additional options. Because of deep insertion, it is more prone to cerumen blockage, therefore requiring more cleaning and maintenance on the patient's part. For the elderly patient, extra visits into the clinic for repairs and frequent cerumen removal may be very difficult.

Table 3 Pros and Cons of Hearing Aid Styles

	BTE	ITE	ITC	CIC
Flexibility— hearing loss fitting range	Mild to profound	Mild to severe	Mild to severe	Mild to moderate
Flexibility— number of options	Very flexible	Dependent on size of ear canal	Dependent on size of ear canal	No options
Manipulation	Easy	Can be difficult	Can be difficult	Difficult
Care and maintenance	Minimal	Problems with earwax blockage	Problems with earwax blockage	A significant problem with earwax blockage
Cosmetic	Depends on hairstyle	Visible	Less visible	Least visible

Abbreviations: BTE, behind the ear; ITE, in the ear; ITC, in the canal; CIC, completely in the canal.

If a CIC is used, a wax guard system that the individual can replace on their own in order to avoid hearing aid repairs should be considered. The CIC is likely to be more difficult to insert for the elderly patient. The battery size is very small, so routine manipulations such as changing the battery are more difficult.

There also may be issues of occlusion effect with the CIC instruments. The occlusion effect is said to occur when patients state that their own voice sounds "hollow" or "in a barrel" due to the hearing aid occluding the ear canal. This effect is typically solved by venting the hearing aid or earmold so that the user does not feel so "plugged up" by the hearing aid. Due to the small size of a CIC hearing aid, adequate venting is not possible.

Selection of hearing aid style will be influenced by patient preference. Some patients will have a preconceived notion of what hearing aid style they want. It is important that the audiologist and patient compromise a few features and options in order to select an amplification device that the individual will wear. If the patient is forced to purchase an undesirable hearing aid style, then the hearing aid may not be used at all. The best hearing aids are the ones that the patient will wear. Table 3 is a comparison of hearing aid styles highlighting their pros and cons for the aging adult.

Hearing in Noise

An estimated 25% of hearing aid users are not wearing their hearing aids due to the negative effects of background noise (29). Due to the nature of age-related hearing loss, simple amplification is inadequate to provide maximum intelligibility in noise. Some of the solutions include binaural amplification, directional microphone technology, noise reduction circuitry, and the use of assistive listening devices.

Binaural Amplification

A significant advantage of binaural hearing is noise suppression since two ears are necessary to efficiently separate the speech signal from surrounding background noise (30). Binaural amplification provides the user with a 2–3 dB signal-to-noise ratio enhancement (31). It is critical to the success of the aural rehabilitation program to do everything possible to enhance the signal-to-noise ratio; hence, binaural amplification should be recommended and encouraged for most patients with presbycusis.

In 1980, Dirks and Wilson (32) noted that sounds presented binaurally are perceptually 3 dB louder than the actual level due to binaural summation. This is advantageous in that less gain is needed to achieve the same perception of loudness, resulting in less feedback. In addition to noise suppression and binaural summation, binaural hearing is critical to sound localization via comparison of the intensity and temporal cues from each ear individually. Binaural amplification aids the user's ability to localize sound, which may be important for the safety of the elderly individual in certain situations. Binaural interference is a phenomenon that occurs in some elderly patients who exhibit a large asymmetry in word recognition scores between the right and left ear and is a contraindication for binaural amplification (33). Word recognition scores should be tested individually and binaurally. If the binaural word recognition score is significantly poorer than that of the better ear, then binaural amplification may be inappropriate.

Directional Microphones

Directional microphones to improve performance in noise recently have been introduced and may benefit some individuals (34–37). All hearing aids dispensed have an omnidirectional microphone, which collects sounds from any directional source and passes them through to the amplifier without relative delay. A hearing aid with a directional microphone involves the use of an additional rear-facing microphone. Input from the additional rear microphone is delayed so that the signal from behind the person is cancelled. Thus, in a directional microphone hearing aid, sounds in front of the wearer are amplified, but the sounds behind them are attenuated. This type of technology provides significant improvement in the presence of background noise, provided that the noise is behind the patient and the signal is in front. The magnitude of the cancellation effect of the directional microphones increases as the listening environment becomes more unfavorable, even with the level of the noise being louder than the level of speech (34).

Hearing aids that have directional microphone technology are equipped with a push button or a switch so that the user can turn the directional program on and off. In quiet listening environments, the user should have the hearing aid switched to omnidirectional mode so that all sounds are amplified regardless of location. Once the listener enters a noisy situation, such as a restaurant, the user can either press the push button or a switch to change into the directional microphone program. For elderly patients with manual dexterity handicaps, a remote control can be ordered to change between the programs stored in the hearing aid.

Recently, automatic microphone technology has emerged. Automatic microphones switch back and forth between omnidirectional and directional modes automatically based on the sound environment. This technology is advantageous for the elderly population in that it is more hands free. However, the patient can override this automatic directional program by manipulating the push button or remote control. This may be important in situations such as crossing a busy street. The hearing aid will consider this "noisy" and switch into the directional setting, but for safety the individuals may want to hear all around them.

A proper and thorough hearing aid orientation is critical to the use and benefit of directional microphones. The elderly patient has to understand the use of the multiple programs stored in the hearing aid and how to manipulate or change them via the push-button or remote control. In addition, the aging patient needs to understand that they must orient themselves so that the noise is predominantly behind them and the speaker in front of them in order for the directional microphones to be of benefit.

Noise Reduction Circuitry

Noise, when analyzed spectrally and temporally, has a broad frequency band and is steady state or constant. In contrast, the acoustic properties of conversational speech are frequency specific and dynamic. Hearing aid engineers have used these contrasting properties to design noise reduction algorithms that will cancel or reduce steady-state sounds while maintaining the amplification of dynamic stimuli. For example, the sound of an air conditioner fan is a steady-state background noise—its intensity level and frequency band remain constant. A noise reduction circuit will cancel this noise so that it is not amplified by the hearing aid. Although noise reduction circuitry has not been shown to improve user understanding in noise, it may decrease the annoyance of the noise, which could lead to less effort expended in communication situations and/or less fatigue.

Assistive Listening Devices

Assistive listening devices (ALDs) are a family of instruments that can be either coupled to a hearing aid or used alone to assist the user in awareness and discrimination of speech and environmental sounds. Elderly patients with a profound hearing loss or very poor word recognition scores may need to rely on ALDs for not only maximum speech intelligibility in noise, but for safety concerns as well.

Some ALDs use a frequency-modulated radio signal (FM signal) that is coupled directly to the hearing aid via a "boot" (for a BTE hearing aid) or through an electromagnetic neckloop (for a BTE or ITE hearing aid). An FM system consists of an external microphone that is worn by the speaker and transmits the signal to the boot or neckloop. The hearing aid must be set to receive only the FM signal from the microphone or other assistive device such as those used in public places (e.g., churches, concert halls, and theaters). FM systems provide the greatest signal-to-noise ratio enhancement in that the hearing aid only receives what is transmitted from the microphone, which is inches away from the speaker's mouth since the microphone in the hearing aid is disconnected. Other ALDs include amplified telephones, infrared television amplifiers, and various alerting systems. These systems may be vital in ensuring the elderly individual's safety. Smoke detectors, doorbell ringers, and personal paging systems may alert an individual through a visual (flashing light), auditory (louder signal), or tactile (vibration) signal. ALDs may be somewhat cumbersome, so it is important that the most appropriate device be selected for the individual's needs and lifestyle.

Signal Processing

The basic components of a hearing aid are the microphone, amplifier, and the receiver. The analog electronic signal processing circuit within the amplifier divides the signal into different frequency bands (the number of these bands varies with the complexity of the circuit), which can be manipulated by changing the gain or the output characteristic of each band. These settings are done in the office by coupling the hearing aids to a computer and programming them with the appropriate software.

Within the past decade, there have been many significant changes in the electronic signal processing of the hearing aid with the advent of digital signal processing (DSP). Analog signals are converted to digital signals, which permits a nearly infinite number of possible signal alterations. While analog signal processing is limited to three bands or less for frequency shaping and compression, DSP technology can divide the signal into as many as 20 channels for processing. Thus, DSP technology has much more flexibility than analog technology (38).

As DSP technology continues to improve, more patients will benefit from the newer technology. Digital hearing aid sales comprised only 7% of the total number of hearing aid sales in 1998 whereas in 2002, 42.7% of hearing aid sales were digital technology (39). It is predicted that all hearing aids dispensed soon will be digital.

It is important to understand the relationship between DSP technology and hearing aid user performance. The primary predictor of speech recognition performance is audibility (40). Both analog and digital signal processing circuits have the capabilities to make the acoustic signal audible to the hearing aid user. Valente et al. (41) showed that performance on speech recognition tasks in noise were not significantly different when users were wearing either analog or digital hearing aids. Other research studies have supported this finding (42). Kochin (43) surveyed 500 individuals using DSP technology and 418 controls and found that DSP hearing aids receive an overall higher satisfaction rating. DSP technology also facilitates reduced feedback through feedback cancellation systems, expansion or gain reduction to reduce low-level noise, noise reduction algorithms, and automatic microphone technology.

Use of the Telephone

The telephone is an integral part of society and in many situations, the telephone may be the only connection between the elderly individual and family members or friends. Hearing aid users can use the telephone by either placing the receiver over the microphone or by activating a telecoil built into the hearing aid. A telecoil is a magnetic coil inside the hearing aid that picks up the electromagnetic field emitted from the receiver of the telephone (and from FM systems with neckloops) and amplifies the signal. Telecoils can be activated by a push button on the hearing aid, which, when pressed will turn off the microphone of the hearing aid and activate the telecoil. For elderly individuals with manual dexterity problems, the telecoil can be activated automatically by placing a telephone receiver directly on top of a hearing aid equipped with an automatic telecoil. The magnet in the telephone automatically switches the internal magnet in the hearing aid that engages the telecoil receiver. Once the phone is removed, the hearing aid will automatically change back to the regular microphone setting. The advantage of the telecoil is that since the microphone of the hearing aid is deactivated, feedback is eliminated when using the telephone. Some elderly individuals are unable to use the telephone with the hearing aid and often benefit from the use of amplified telephones. In order to use this option, however, the hearing aid must be removed and then replaced at the end of the telephone conversation.

Severe Unilateral Hearing Loss

An individual with a nonfunctioning ear along with a normal (or near-normal) hearing ear may experience difficulty localizing, hearing in noise, and hearing when communication is directed to the nonfunctioning side. Many individuals with this condition use a variety of communication strategies and environmental manipulations to accommodate this situation, but some patients will benefit from specific strategies. There are three potential solutions: (i) contralateral routing of signal (CROS) hearing aid, (ii) a bone-anchored hearing aid (BAHA) implanted on the nonfunctioning side, and (iii) a powerful conventional hearing aid in the nonfunctioning ear (transcranial CROS). Solution one is configured with a microphone pick up on the nonfunctioning side and the signal is transmitted via a cord or FM signal to a hearing aid case anchored on the normal ear. The signal is routed into the normal ear through an open ear canal fitting so the same ear can receive input normally from the "good" side. Solutions two (BAHA) and three (transcranial CROS) operate on the same principle. The signal is picked up on the nonfunctioning side and is delivered to the normal hearing cochlea via bone conduction.

Elderly patients with unilateral hearing loss may become aware of communication difficulty sooner than one would expect based on the reduced thresholds in the previously normal hearing ear. These individuals may be fully adapted to being a monaural listener and may only want improved performance in the mildly impaired ear rather than pursuing some type of CROS or transcranial solution. An alternative is a binaural contralateral routing of signal (BICROS) aid.

Middle Ear Implantable Hearing Aids

Several middle ear implantable hearing aids have been developed in the past several years. Some of these are partially implantable and others are designed to be fully implantable. The manufacturers of these instruments claim reduced feedback (high-pitched sound when amplified sound reaches the microphone and is reamplified) due to implantation, but the actual results have been varied. One would recommend a trial with traditional binaural amplification prior to recommending this type of instrument for the geriatric patient.

Cochlear Implant

An individual with severe to profound sensorineural hearing loss is a cochlear implant candidate. Candidacy for implantation is determined through a battery of performance tests and a hearing aid trial. The most common geriatric patient who would be a cochlear implant candidate would be an individual who suffered sudden, severe-to-profound, permanent sensorineural hearing loss as opposed to the individual who has functioned with this type of hearing loss over their lifetime.

Hearing Aid Fitting

During the hearing aid fitting, verification and validation of the hearing aid performance must be measured. This can be accomplished through a Real-Ear® measurement, which is a probe microphone system that measures the sound pressure level at the eardrum. Real-Ear verification is used to fine-tune the hearing aid until the hearing aid's output falls within this range so that soft sounds are audible and loud sounds are not uncomfortably loud.

Validation ensures that hearing aid performance meets the needs of the patient. This is obtained through the use of subjective questionnaires that look at handicap,

Table 4 Orientation Checklist

Battery insertion
On/off function
Volume control use
Hearing aid removal
Hearing aid insertion
Telephone use
Remote control/multimemory button (if applicable)
Cleaning and maintenance
What to do at night
Warranty explanation
Insurance information

disability, and satisfaction with hearing aids (44). The score tells the audiologist how much benefit the patient perceives from the hearing aids.

Hearing Aid Orientation

The elderly patients and their family members must understand how to use and take care of the hearing devices properly. The orientation session consists of instructions of insertion and removal, how and when to change the battery, how and when to change the hearing aid program designed for listening in background noise, a demonstration of telephone use, etc. (45). Documentation is given to the patient as well as the family or the caretaker. Table 4 provides a checklist of items that should be included in the orientation.

There are a number of helpful accessories for the aging patient such as "Fun Tak®" to hold the hearing aid and an extending magnet to capture batteries that may have fallen or to pick up the whole hearing aid if it has fallen and still has the battery in it. Moisture removal with a dehumidifier kit can add life to the hearing aid and greatly reduce repairs. Repairs may be a larger problem for the older patient who may find it difficult to travel to the clinic repeatedly. Other devices include a line to clip the aid to the shirt collar to reduce the possibility of loss and a battery tab to assist in battery insertion.

Counseling and Training

The new hearing aid wearer is adjusting to both how the hearing aids feel and how the world sounds and may not like the sound quality until there has been a period of adaptation. Often patients are aware of all sounds such as the sound of shoes on the floor, the refrigerator hum, etc., which creates an uncomfortable sensation. Several weeks are required to accommodate to this new sensation. Kochkin (46) reports that patients received greater satisfaction with their new hearing aids if they were provided with one to two hours of counseling regarding realistic expectations, and the use and care of the hearing aids. Abrahms et al. (47) reported that in a group of aging adults, hearing aid fittings plus aural rehabilitation (counseling) was more cost effective than hearing aid fittings alone.

REFERENCES

1. Pastor PN, Makuc DM, Reuben C, Xia H. Chartbook on Trends in the Health of Americans. Health, United States. Hyattsville, Maryland: National Center for Health Statistics, 2002.
2. National Center for Health Statistics. (www.cdc.gov/nchs/)
3. National Institute on Deafness and Other Communication Disorders. (www.nicdcd.nih.gov.)
4. Schow R, Nerbonne M. Hearing levels among elderly nursing home residence. J Speech Hear Res 1980; 45:124–132.
5. American Speech-Language-Hearing Association. (www.asha.org.)
6. Desai M, Pratt LA, Lentzner H, Robinson KN. Trends in vision and hearing among older Americans. Aging trends No. 2. Hyattsville, Md.: National Center for Health Statistics, 2001.
7. Keller BK, Morton JL, Thomas VS, Potter JF. The effect of visual and hearing impairments on functional status. J Am Geriatr Soc 1999; 47:1319–1325.
8. Jamieson JR. The impact of hearing impairment. In: Katz J, ed. Handbook of clinical audiology. 4th ed. Baltimore: Williams & Wilkins, 1994:596–615.
9. Carabellese C, Appollonio I, Rozzini R, et al. Sensory impairment and quality of life in a community elderly population. J Am Geriatr Soc 1993; 41:401–407.
10. Palmer CV. Improvement of hearing function. In: Huntley RA, Helfer KS, eds. Communication in later life. Boston: Butterworth-Heinemann, 1995:181–223.
11. Bess FH, Lichtenstein MJ, Logan SA, Burger MC, Nelson E. Hearing impairment as a determinant of function in the elderly. J Am Geriatr Soc 1989; 37:123–128.
12. Mulrow C, Aguilar C, Endicott J, et al. Association between hearing impairment and the quality of life of elderly individuals. J Am Geriatr Soc 1990; 38:45–50.
13. Weinstein B, Ventry I. Hearing impairment and social isolation in the elderly. J Speech Hear Res 1982; 32:593–599.
14. Chmiel R, Jerger J. Some factors affecting the assessment of hearing handicap in the elderly. J Am Acad Audiol 1993; 4:249–257.
15. Gates GA, Karzon RK, Garcia P, et al. Auditory dysfunction in aging and senile dementia of the Alzheimer's type. Arch Neurol 1995; 52:626–634.
16. Uhlmann R, Larson E, Rees T, Koepsell T, Duckert L. Relationship of hearing impairment to dementia and cognitive dysfunction in older adults. JAMA 1989; 261:1916–1919.
17. Peters CA, Potter JF, Scholer SG. Hearing impairment as a predictor of cognitive decline in dementia. J Am Geriatr Soc 1988; 36:981–986.
18. Durrant J, Gilmartin K, Holland A, Kamerer D, Newall P. Hearing disorders management in Alzheimer's disease patients. Hear Instrum 1991; 42:32–35.
19. Palmer CV, Adams SW, Bourgeois M, Durrant, JD, Rossi M. Reduction in caregiver-identified problem behaviors in patients with Alzheimer disease post-hearing-aid fitting. J Speech Lang Hear Disord 1999; 42:312–328.
20. Willott JF. Anatomic and physiologic aging: a behavioral neuroscience perspective. J Am Acad Audiol 1998; 7:141–151.
21. Stach B, Spretnjak M, Jerger J. The prevalence of central presbycusis in a clinical population. J Am Acad Audiol 1990; 1:109–115.
22. Jerger J, Chmial R, Wilson N, Luchi R. Hearing impairment in older adults: new concepts. J Am Geriatr Soc 1995; 43:928–935.
23. Herbst K, Humphrey C. Hearing impairment and mental state in the elderly living at home. Br Med J Clin Res 1980; 281:903–905.
24. Canestrari R. Paced and self-paced learning in young and elderly adults. J Gerontol 1963; 18:165–168.
25. Schow RL. Considerations in selecting and validating an adult/elderly hearing screening protocol. Ear Hear 1991; 12:337–348.

26. Ventry IM, Weinstein BE. Identification of elderly people with hearing problems. ASHA 1983; 7:37–42.
27. American Academy of Otolaryngology—Head & Neck Surgery. The five minute hearing test. AAO-HNS Bull 1990; 9:43.
28. Frisna DR, Frisna RD. Speech recognition in noise and presbycusis: relations to possible neural mechanisms. Hear Res 1997; 106:95–104.
29. Kochin S. MarkeTrak V. "Why my hearing aids end up in the drawer": the consumer's perspective. Hear J 2000; 53(2):34,36,39–42.
30. Valente M. Binaural amplification: part II. Audecibel 1984; 12:10–14.
31. Hawkins D, Yacullo W. Signal to noise ratio advantange of binaural hearing aids and directional microphones under different levels of reverberation. Speech Hear Disord 1984; 49:278–286.
32. Dirks D, Wilson R. Binaural hearing in sound field. In: Libby ER, ed. Binaural Hearing and Amplification, Vol. 1. Chicago: Zeneron, 1980:105–122.
33. Jerger J, Silman S, Lew H, Chimel R. Case studies in binaural interference: converging evidence from behavioral and electrophysiologic measures. J Am Acad Audiol 1993; 4:122–131.
34. Valente M, Sweetow R, Potts LG, Bingea B. Digital versus analog signal processing: effect of directional microphone. J Am Acad Audiol 1999; 10:133–150.
35. Agnew J, Block M. HINT thresholds for a dual-microphone BTE. Hear Rev 1997; 4(9):26, 29–30.
36. Ricketts T. Impact of noise source configuration on directional hearing aid benefit and performance. Ear Hear 2000; 21:194–205.
37. Ricketts T, Dhar S. Comparison of performance across three directional hearing aids. J Am Acad Audiol 1999; 10:180–189.
38. Agnew J. Amplifiers and circuit algorithms for contemporary hearing aids. In: Valente M, ed. Hearing Aids: Standards, Options, and Limitations. 2nd ed. New York: Thieme, 2002:101–142.
39. Kochkin S. MarkeTrak VI. Ten year customer satisfaction trends in the US hearing instrument market. Hear Rev 2002; 9(10):14–25,46.
40. Humes L, Roberts L. Speech-recognition difficulties of the hearing-impaired elderly: the contributions of audibility. J Speech Hear Res 1990; 33:726–735.
41. Valente M, Fabry DA, Potts LG, Sandlin RE. Comparing the performance of the widex senso digital hearing aid with analog hearing aids. J Am Acad Audiol 1998; 9:342–360.
42. Newman CW, Sandridge SA. Review of research on digital signal processing. In: Valente M, ed. Hearing Aids: Standards, Options, and Limitations. 2nd ed. New York: Thieme, 2002:347–381.
43. Kochin S. Customer satisfaction with single and multiple microphone digital hearing aids. Hear Rev 2000 November:24–34.
44. Cox RM, Alexander GC. The abbreviated profile of hearing aid benefit. Ear Hear 1995; 16:176–186.
45. Mormer E, Palmer C. A systematic program for hearing aid orientation and adjustment. In: Sweetow R, ed. Counseling for Hearing Aid Fittings. San Diego, CA: Singular Publishing, 1999.
46. Kochin S. Factors impacting consumer choice of dispenser and hearing aid brand; use of ALDs and Computers. Hear Rev 2002; 9(12):12–23.
47. Abrahms H, Chisolm T, McArdle R. J Rehabil Res Dev 2002; 39(5):549–558.

ANNOTATED BIBLIOGRAPHY

Bogardus ST, Yeuh B, Shekelle PG. Screening and management of adult hearing loss in primary care: clinical applications. JAMA 2003; 289(15):1986–1990.

This is an excellent, comprehensive, critical review of the subject of adult hearing screening.

Campbell K. Essential audiology for physicians. San Diego: Singular Publishing Group, 1997

This text is aimed at the practicing physician and provides good detail related to audiology while being easily read and well organized.

Palmer CV. Improvement of hearing function. In: Huntley RA, Helfer KS, eds. Communication in later life. Boston: Butterworth-Heinemann, 1995:181–223.

This chapter provides a great deal of detail regarding modifications to procedures in audiology appropriate for the older adult.

Yueh B, Shapiro N, MacLean CH, Shekelle PG. Screening and management of adult hearing loss in primary care: scientific review. JAMA 2003; 289(15):1976–1985.

This complements the Bogardus et al. (2003) article with scientific underpinnings.

6
Presbycusis

Sidney N. Busis
Department of Otolaryngology, University of Pittsburgh, Pittsburgh, Pennsylvania, U.S.A.

Aging is inevitable. In his classic text, "Pathology of the Ear," Harold Schuknecht (1) writes, "Literally, we start aging at the moment of conception and never stop until we die; in the more usual sense, aging starts when growth ceases." Presbycusis, derived from two Greek words—presbus, an old man, and acusis, hearing—is the natural hearing loss that occurs as the auditory system ages. It is the most common type of hearing impairment in humans and is the most common cause of sensorineural hearing loss in the United States (2,3). Presbycusis is the third most prominent chronic medical condition in older Americans after hypertension and arthritis (3,4). It is estimated that 25–40% of the population aged 65 years and older, 40–66% of patients older than 75 years and more than 80–90% of patients older than 85 years are hearing impaired (3–5). The hearing loss that accompanies aging might be called age-related hearing loss because it can be a combination of presbycusis, genetic predisposition to hearing impairment, and noise-induced hearing loss due to occupational or recreational noise exposure or to living for years in our noisy society (called sociocusis). Also age-related changes in other systems may adversely affect auditory function (6). Among others, these changes may include diminished efficiency of the immune system, a tendency to produce antibodies to the body's own proteins, and cardiovascular changes that can affect the ear and the brain (6,7).

INCIDENCE

Understanding and managing presbycusis is important because in the United States there is a large, growing older population. According to the Administration on Aging of the U.S. Department of Health and Human Services, the older population (age 65 or older) numbered 35.6 million in 2002 and is projected to reach 40.2 million in 2010 and 54.6 million in 2020 (8). These older adults have a high risk of developing hearing loss to a degree that can greatly affect their quality of life, and most older people experience further declines in hearing sensitivity over time (5). Loss of hearing is frequently compared to loss of vision. Helen Keller, the famous deaf–blind author and lecturer, when asked to compare the loss of hearing to the loss of vision, reflected that visual loss separates people from "things" and hearing loss separates

77

people from "people." This separation from people explains the feeling of isolation that leads to withdrawal from family and friends and can cause serious depression in some people with presbycusis (9). Tinnitus that frequently accompanies presbycusis can also be a cause of major depression (10). Depression associated with hearing loss has been found to be independent of age and socioeconomic status (3). In the elderly, depression is more likely to occur when the individual has distressing medical conditions, as frequently occurs in older people, or when the individual is grieving because of the loss of a loved one or is sad because of other personal or family problems. From the medical perspective, the treatment of hearing loss by the use of hearing aids and assistive listening devices can decrease the morbidity of late-life depression regardless of causation (10).

RECOGNITION

Despite the recognized deleterious effects of hearing loss on the quality of life, hearing loss is underdiagnosed; for example, only 9% of internists offer hearing tests to patients over 65 years of age (3). Hearing loss is also undertreated; only 10–25% of patients with aidable hearing loss receive hearing aids (3,6,11). Although the definitive measure of hearing is a complete audiometric examination, screening tests, which can be performed in the primary care physician's office, are useful for identifying patients who may have an unrecognized significant hearing problem that should be addressed. A subjective screening method for older patients relies on the patient's own perception of a hearing problem. For this evaluation, a Hearing Handicap Inventory for the Elderly (HHIE) has been developed and has been found to be useful for quantifying hearing handicap in elderly persons (12). A screening version of the Hearing Handicap Inventory for the Elderly, known as the Hearing Handicap Inventory for Elderly-Screening (HHIE-S), a self-administered, 10-item, five-minute questionnaire, has been shown to identify patients with handicapping hearing impairments (Table 1) (3). Scores of 10 and above provide reasonable sensitivity and specificity for significant hearing loss (3). However, Gates et al. (13) in a study of 546 older individuals who had audiometric testing reported that a single global

Table 1 Questions from HHIE-S

Does a hearing problem cause you to feel embarrassed when meeting new people?
Does a hearing problem cause you to feel frustrated when talking to members of your family?
Do you have difficulty hearing when someone speaks in a whisper?
Do you feel handicapped by a hearing problem?
Does a hearing problem cause you difficulty when visiting friends, relatives or neighbors?
Does a hearing problem cause you to attend religious services less often than you would like?
Does a hearing problem cause you to have arguments with family members?
Does a hearing problem cause you difficulty when listening to TV or radio?
Do you feel that any difficulty with your hearing limits or hampers your personal or
    social life?
Does a hearing problem cause you difficulty when in a restaurant with relatives or friends?

The HHIE-S scores are yes, 4 points; sometimes, 2 points; or no, 0 points, to each. Scores range from 0 (no handicap) to 40 (maximum handicap). Scores of 10 and above provide reasonable sensitivity and specificity for significant hearing loss.
Abbreviation: HHIE-S, hearing handicap inventory for the elderly-screening version.
Source: From Ref. 3.

question, "Do you have a hearing problem now?" was more effective than the HHIE-S in identifying older individuals with unrecognized handicapping hearing loss. Comparing these two screening methods to audiometric examinations in the same patients, Gates found that the HHIE-S had a sensitivity of 35% and a specificity of 94%, and the global question had greater sensitivity, 71%, but lower specificity, 71%. For office screening in the primary care physician's office, a relatively simple test of hearing is the use of the AudioScope (Welch Allyn) that offers a choice of three screening loudness levels of sound at four frequencies (3). Patients who are found, by any screening method, to have a hearing problem should be referred for an otologic examination and audiometry.

Presbycusis usually becomes apparent in the later years of life; however, it may begin to be manifested as early as the third or fourth decade of life. The American National Standards Institute Standard ANSI S3.44-1996 includes tables listing decibels of hearing loss due to age starting in the third decade (14). The International Organization for Standardization Standard ISO 7029 (15) notes that it is well known that sensitivity of the human ear usually falls progressively with age and that the impairment of hearing develops more rapidly for sounds at the high frequencies than at the low frequencies. The Standard notes that the magnitude of this effect varies considerably among individuals. It is further noted that when testing the hearing of persons over 18 years of age, part of any observed hearing loss will probably be associated with age. It cautions that the decrease in hearing may not necessarily be caused by aging alone but by other injurious influences. Hearing losses in decibels at frequencies from 125 to 8000 Hz for different ages, beginning at age 20 through age 70, are listed in the Standard in Annex C. In the table, at the higher frequencies males have greater hearing impairments than females. Schuknecht (1) noted that women have significantly better hearing than men at 2000 Hz and above and surveys have indicated that presbycusis is greater in men than it is in women. This may be attributed to the likelihood that men are generally exposed to more noise in their lifetime, but the reason for the difference is probably more complex.

Pathologically, presbycusis may involve three fundamental neural systems: the peripheral auditory system, the central auditory pathways, and the cortical cognitive level (16,17). There is also experimental evidence that the aging middle ear may contribute to age-related hearing loss (2).

PERIPHERAL PATHOLOGY

Schuknecht (1) described four types of peripheral auditory pathology that can account for presbycusis: sensory, neural, strial, and cochlear conductive presbycusis.

Sensory presbycusis is characterized by a loss of hair cells beginning in the basal turn of the cochlea and extending into the speech frequency area. The criterion for neural presbycusis is loss of 50% or more of the cochlear neurons compared to neonatal normal (1). Strial presbycusis, also called metabolic presbycusis, is associated with loss of 30% or more of the tissue in the stria vascularis (2). Schuknecht postulated that loss of strial tissue affects the quality of endolymph, a change in endolymph that has a detrimental effect on the physical and chemical processes by which energy is made available to the hair cells. There is recent evidence that strial atrophy is the primary cause of cochlear aging (18). The pathology in cochlear conductive presbycusis is thought to be stiffness of the basilar membrane.

AUDIOMETRIC PATTERNS

Audiometrically, sensory presbycusis is characterized by normal hearing or a mild hearing loss in the lower frequencies with a sharp drop beginning at 1000 Hz to a severe loss in the higher frequencies.

Clinically, neural presbycusis is characterized by progressive loss of word recognition ability in the presence of stable pure tone thresholds. Audiometrically, neural presbycusis is a high-frequency loss with a more gradual curve from low frequency to high frequency.

Audiometrically, strial presbycusis is characterized by a flatter curve with somewhat poorer hearing in the high frequencies and with excellent word recognition scores. It has been reported that poor low-frequency hearing, typical of strial or metabolic presbycusis, is associated with cardiovascular diseases (heart attacks, stroke, intermittent claudication) and that this effect is present in both men and women but is greater in women (7,19).

The audiogram of cochlear conductive presbycusis shows a gradually descending pure tone threshold over a range of at least five octaves with a difference of at least 50 dB between the best and worst thresholds and not more than 25 dB difference between any two adjacent frequencies. Schuknecht (1) notes that the diagnosis of a cochlear conductive presbycusis is "derived by histologic exclusion of any reasonable light microscopic explanation for the gradual descending pure tone threshold type of hearing loss" (Fig. 1).

Schuknecht and Gacek (20) reported a fifth and a sixth type of peripheral presbycusis, mixed, and indeterminate presbycusis. Based on a survey of the entire collection of 1500 serially sectioned temporal bones at the Massachusetts Eye and Ear Infirmary, they confirmed that the concept of four basic pathologic types of peripheral presbycusis was valid. However, they concluded that (i) sensory cell losses were the least important cause of hearing loss in the aged; these lesions in the basal end of the cochlea caused an abrupt high-frequency loss and often merged with acoustic trauma lesions and could not be differentiated from them; (ii) neuronal lesions are constant and predictable expressions of aging and degrade the capability of word recognition; (iii) atrophy of the stria vascularis occurs as a prominent lesion of aging and principally involves the apical and middle turns of the cochlea and characteristically shows a flat audiometric pattern; (iv) light microscopic studies failed to reveal a pathologic correlate to explain a gradual descending pure tone curve and a cochlear conductive disorder seemed to be the most logical explanation; (v) many aging ears showed a significant involvement of two or more of the four basic types of pathology, resulting in a wide spectrum of alterations in pure tone thresholds and word recognition scores; this was called mixed presbycusis; and (vi) there was an indeterminate group consisting of 25% of cases that did not meet the criteria for any of the four types of presbycusis. It was assumed that the cause was morphological and/or chemical changes that could not be identified on light microscopy study.

CENTRAL AUDITORY PATHWAYS

Processing abnormalities occur in the central pathways as the auditory system ages. Research data suggest that central presbycusis is associated with deficits in one or more inhibitory neurotransmitter circuits (6). Normal neural processing involves an interplay and balance between excitatory and inhibitory synapses. Inhibitory

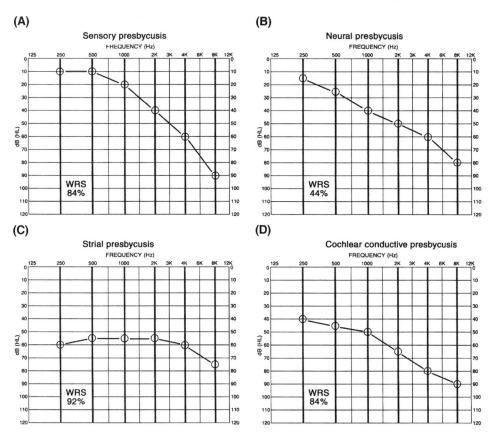

Figure 1 Examples of audiograms of the four basic types of peripheral pathology that account for presbycusis: (**A**) sensory, (**B**) neural, (**C**) strial, (**D**) cochlear conductive. *Abbreviation*: WRS, word recognition score. *Source*: From Ref. 1.

processes have been shown to play roles in auditory functions such as localization of sound and discrimination in noise (6). A study of central auditory aging supported the hypothesis that age-related changes in GABA (γ-aminobutyric acid) transmission in the inferior colliculus in the midbrain alter the balance between excitation and inhibition in the inferior colliculus (21). It was suggested that loss of the inhibitory function of GABA could affect hearing in the elderly (21). Glycine, another important inhibitory neurotransmitter, was found to be significantly decreased in the cochlear nucleus of old mice (6). Identification of specific neurotransmitter changes in parts of the nervous system important for speech processing could possibly lead to the development of pharmacotherapy for some types of age-related hearing loss (21).

Age-related changes in the central auditory pathways can result both from the effects of biological aging or from the loss or attenuation of neural input from ears that have peripheral pathology (22). From the behavioral neuroscience perspective, the central effects of biological aging are accompanied by the central effects of the cochlear pathology of aging. Age-related cochlear pathology causes changes in how frequency is "mapped" in the central auditory system and may impair neural inhibition (23). These effects of cochlear pathology on the central auditory system can impair binaural hearing and cause exaggerated "masking" of neural responses by noise. These changes in the central auditory system accelerate in the later years of life (23). Psychoacoustic research, on the other hand, has shown that high-level auditory skills such as temporal and binaural processing deteriorate with age irrespective of peripheral hearing loss and that the deterioration becomes more apparent as the complexity of the stimulus increases (6). This deterioration may lead to impaired ability to clearly understand speech, decreased ability to localize sound, and difficulty hearing in the presence of background noise. Auditory brainstem and auditory cortex temporal-resolution dysfunction have been implicated in age-related difficulty in speech processing and in speech recognition in noise (17,24).

It has been postulated experimentally that the auditory efferent system plays a role in enhancing signals in noise and, in particular, speech perception in noise (25). It has been shown in the mouse model that distortion product otoacoustic emissions (DPOAE) decrease with age (26). And, it was found that DPOAE were reduced in magnitude when white noise was presented to the opposite ear (25,26). This contralateral suppression of the DPOAE was attributed to activation of the medial olivocochlear system, which has an inhibitory effect on the outer hair cells. Contralateral suppression, measured by reduced DPOAE in the opposite ear, was less in older mice than in younger mice indicating a decline in the efferent system in older animals. This has also been shown in human subjects. Distortion product otoacoustic emissions were smaller in older individuals compared to younger individuals with the same normal hearing and normal middle ear function (25). The decline in the efferent system occurs before the decrease of the DPOAE due to age, and a functional decline in the olivocochlear system with age may explain one reason why the elderly have more difficulty hearing in background noise.

MOLECULAR MECHANISMS

The molecular mechanisms underlying aging and their relationship to presbycusis are being studied and an understanding of these mechanisms is emerging.

Mitochondria, organelles in the cytoplasm of cells, convert nutrients into energy. Mitochondria have been called the "power plants" in our cells that provide the energy needed to maintain body function and metabolism (27). They have a special type of DNA [mitochondrial DNA (mtDNA)] that may be more vulnerable to damage than the DNA in the chromosomes in the cell nucleus (6). In the respiratory mitochondrial chain, oxygen is reduced to water at the end of the chain. In this enzymatic, oxidative process, oxygen may be partially reduced. There is leakage of single electrons causing partial reduction of oxygen leading to the formation of superoxide. Superoxide is a chemical that is highly toxic to cells; it is one of a class of toxic chemicals called free radicals. Free radicals are chemical species with unpaired electrons; they are reactive because electrons like to pair up to form stable two-electron bonds and so are called "reactive oxygen species (ROS)" (27). Free radicals can also be produced elsewhere, e.g., endogenously by leukocytes to combat pathogens and exogenously by environmental pollutants such as cigarette smoke. Oxidative damage by ROS and other free radicals is neutralized by the human body's antioxidant defense systems; one important component of these systems is comprised of antioxidant enzymes including, among others, the antioxidant enzyme superoxide dismutase (27). In the elderly, there may be a significant increase in the production of ROS and/or a weakening of the antioxidant defenses; these are changes that can lead to presbycusis (6,28). This process may explain Schuknecht's postulate about strial presbycusis.

Among the several theories regarding the aging process, the "mitochondrial clock theory" has been considered the most engaging explanation for age-related hearing loss (28,29). According to this theory hypoperfusion of the cochlear tissue leads to ischemia and the formation of ROS (6) that are highly toxic to the auditory neuroepithelia. The ROS damage mtDNA, which, as noted, may be more vulnerable to damage than the DNA in chromosomes, resulting in specific mtDNA deletions and reduced mitochondrial membrane potential, eventually making the mitochondria bioenergetically inefficient (6,28). These specific mtDNA deletions are also known as the common aging deletion (28,29).

Continued research on the molecular mechanisms involved in aging is important because it may lead to effective treatment for presbycusis with antioxidants that neutralize free radicals, dietary supplements, and special diets (6,29). There has been evidence that some compounds slow down the "mitochondrial clock," and it has been shown that experimental animals fed caloric-restricted diets and antioxidant-treated animals had more acute hearing than controls (23,28,29).

GENETIC FACTORS

Although familial hearing loss in humans may be difficult to document in the laboratory because causes other than heredity may contribute to the hearing loss of an older person, epidemiologic study has shown a relatively strong heritability for presbycusis, especially for the strial type with sensitivity loss for low frequencies (6,30). Numerous genes are known to be expressed in the auditory system and some of these may contribute to presbycusis and may determine the severity and the time of onset of age-related hearing loss. But none have been proven to account for presbycusis (6,31). In a mouse model, a non-syndromic age-related hearing loss gene (Ahl) has been identified (6). There is no evidence that this gene or a similar gene is responsible for presbycusis in humans (E. W. Rubel, personal communication, 2004).

Gene mutations may account for non-syndromic hearing loss. In the mouse, the gene Cdh23 may predispose to early onset age-related hearing loss dependent on genetic factors including a mitochondrial mutation (32). Mutation in the homologous human gene, CDH23, may contribute to susceptibility to presbycusis (33).

EVALUATION

Clinically, age-related hearing loss is the foremost communication problem of the elderly. Presbycusis is characterized by the gradual, insidious onset of diminished hearing, of which the individual is frequently unaware. The hearing loss is often first apparent to family members and friends who urge the patient to seek medical attention. Presbycusis is bilaterally symmetrical and usually first affects the high frequencies, the sounds of consonants such as "s" and "t," sounds that enhance the intelligibility of speech (9). Many children have high-pitched voices and speak rapidly; although their speech may be easily heard, it is often difficult to understand. This explains the common cry of grandparents, "I can't understand my grandchildren!" Because of recruitment, people with cochlear hearing losses may have a narrow "dynamic range of hearing" in that when speech is soft they cannot hear it, yet when it is somewhat louder it sounds too loud and is unpleasant and annoying. People with presbycusis usually have trouble hearing in noisy places and they may also have trouble localizing sound and difficulty perceiving sudden, rapid changes in speech. Presbycusis is frequently accompanied by high-pitched tinnitus, which occasionally becomes a major problem in addition to the hearing impairment.

Although in many cases the diagnosis of presbycusis may seem apparent after a cursory history and physical examination and an audiologic test, there are other causes of sensorineural hearing loss simulating presbycusis so that a complete history and physical examination should be performed. The differential diagnosis for presbycusis includes hearing loss due to occupational or recreational noise exposure, acoustic or physical trauma, heredity and gene mutation, ototoxicity, acoustic tumor, and systemic disease. Conductive and mixed hearing losses due to external and middle ear disease also occur in older people.

The history encompasses all aspects of an otologic history including questions about: (i) whether the hearing loss is the same in both ears or greater in one ear; (ii) the onset and progression of the hearing loss; (iii) situations in which it is difficult to hear, such as more trouble hearing in quiet places or in noisy places; (iv) hearing the telephone ring and hearing on the telephone; (v) hearing in a one-to-one conversation; (vi) hearing women's and children's voices; (vii) fluctuations in hearing; (viii) the presence and the description of tinnitus, dizziness, balance disturbance, ear fullness, pain, or aural discharge; (ix) prior ear disease or ear operations and ear or head physical trauma; (x) occupational, recreational, or military noise exposure, with or without wearing hearing protection devices; (xi) immediate and extended family history of hearing loss; and (xii) the use of hearing aids. Responses to these questions will help quantify the hearing difficulty the patient is experiencing and may suggest etiologies other than, or in addition to, the aging process.

Review of the patient's social and general medical history is also important, since it may reveal activities, systemic diseases, injuries or medications that can contribute to hearing impairment.

The examination consists of examining the head and neck including: (i) the nose, nasopharynx, and pharynx; (ii) the areas about the external ear; (iii) the ear canal and tympanic membrane preferably using a microscope; (iv) the tympanic membrane for mobility with the pneumatic otoscope; (v) the tympanic membrane microscopically while the patient breathes through the mouth and nose to see if there is accompanying movement of the tympanic membrane indicating a patulous eustachian tube; (vi) evaluation of seventh nerve function; (vii) testing the corneal reflex for fifth nerve function; (viii) examining for nystagmus in all positions of the eyes; (ix) auscultation of the head and neck if the patient has objective or pulsatile tinnitus; and (x) office vestibular tests if there is a history of vertigo and a fistula test if there is anything to suggest a perilymph fistula. As with the history, abnormalities on physical examination may suggest etiologies other than, or in addition to, the aging process. For example, there are abnormalities of the ear canals and middle ears that can impair hearing. Dry, hard cerumen is frequently found impacted in the ear canals of older people and should be removed (34). Impacted cerumen can cause a conductive hearing loss and it often impairs the function of hearing aids. Middle ear effusion is not uncommon in the elderly.

Audiologic evaluation includes air and bone conduction pure tone threshold tests, speech reception thresholds, and word recognition scores (speech discrimination). Hearing is also tested in a sound field in quiet and in noise and, if the patient has hearing aids, with and without the aids in place. If on audiometric testing there is a question about the relationship between air and bone conduction thresholds, tuning fork tests (Rinné and Weber tests) can be useful in interpretation. Audiometry is an essential element for diagnosis, for measuring the extent of the patient's hearing loss, and for evaluating the effectiveness of hearing aids. Tympanometry, as another diagnostic tool, is performed to measure middle ear pressure and compliance and for testing acoustic reflexes.

Although special tests of auditory function, distortion product otoacoustic emissions, auditory brain stem responses, and electrocochleography have been shown experimentally and clinically to be abnormal in patients with presbycusis, these tests are not specific enough for the clinical diagnosis of presbycusis to warrant their routine use in the evaluation of patients for presbycusis (35–40). For patients with problematic diagnoses, these tests can be useful. In consideration of the possibility of systemic disease contributing to the sensorineural hearing loss, a battery of screening blood tests is indicated unless the patient's primary care physician has performed the tests recently, as is frequently the case (Table 2) (41). If there is significant asymmetry in the hearing thresholds of one ear compared to the other or if there has been the recent onset of unilateral tinnitus, the possibility of a acoustic tumor or other central nervous system lesion should be considered and a magnetic resonance image (MRI) of the brain with special attention to the internal auditory canals and cerebellopontine angles should be performed.

The vast majority of the elderly who have a hearing loss, have a sensorineural hearing loss. If the patient has a conductive or a mixed hearing loss, the external and middle ears are studied further including consideration of a computed tomography (CT) scan of the temporal bones.

MANAGEMENT

The basic principles of the management of presbycusis are education and amplification. An elderly person suspected of having a hearing problem should be encouraged to have a complete otologic examination, including audiometry, and a medical examination to determine if there are any systemic conditions that might affect hearing.

Counseling is most important. The persons with the hearing loss must understand what is happening in their auditory systems. They should be shown the

Table 2 Screening Blood Tests

Complete blood count and differential
Platelet count
Sedimentation rate
Cholesterol (HDL and LDL)
Triglycerides
TSH
Free T-4
HbA1c
RPR
ANA
Rheumatoid factor
Otoblot test if the patient has a rapidly progressing sensorineural hearing loss or there is other
    evidence of autoimmune disease

Abbreviations: HDL, high-density lipoprotein; LDL, low-density lipoprotein; TSH, thyroid stimulating hormone; ANA, antinuclear antibody; RPR, rapid plasma reagin.

Table 3   Guides to Better Hearing

Hearing is our most important means of communicating with each other. It is a combination of speaking and listening that can be a relaxed, pleasant exchange, or it can be a frustrating experience. Successful communication is equally dependent on the speaker and the listener. A normal-hearing person may sometimes misunderstand a sentence or a word. This is acceptable to all. However, when a person with a hearing impairment misunderstands a sentence or a word, it is immediately assumed that the listener is to blame for the misunderstanding. It may, in fact, have been due to the manner in which the sentence or words were spoken and so the fault of the speaker. Therefore, these are guides to help both the speaker and the listener.

For the speaker
When communicating with a person who has a hearing loss, you must be very aware of when and how you talk. If the suggestions listed below are followed carefully, the person to whom you are speaking will understand you better:
1. Always alert the person before you speak. For example, call the person by name first and then when the person looks at you begin to speak.
2. Speak a little more slowly and a little more distinctly, softly accenting important syllables
3. Speak a little louder than usual; however, do not shout.
4. If the person to whom you are speaking does not understand you, do not keep repeating the same words. Rephrase. Say it another way, using different words.
5. Never talk with your back turned to someone with a hearing loss.
6. Never call to or try to talk to a person from a distance that you know or suspect is too far for the person to hear you.
7. Avoid eating, chewing, or covering your mouth with your hands while speaking.
8. Remember that a person who has a hearing loss usually has more difficulty hearing when there is a lot of noise around. Therefore, when talking in a noisy place, try to be even more careful about how you speak. If possible, before speaking, try to reduce the noise level, for example by turning down the radio or television, or moving into a quieter place.
9. Be patient and understanding.

For the listener
The following suggestions will help you to hear and understand people better:
1. Don't be embarrassed to tell people that you have hearing problem. Most people will be considerate and be more careful with their speech.
2. Learn to look directly at the speaker's face. Watch the speaker's facial expressions and watch the speaker's lips. Be determined to master "speech reading," the ability to understand speech better by watching a speaker's facial expressions and the lip movements.
3. In any situation, especially when in a group, always place yourself so that you can hear best:
   (a) If you have one ear that is better than the other, always arrange to have your better ear facing the speaker or other source of sound.
   (b) If there is strong lighting in the room, always place yourself with your back facing the light so that the light falls on the speaker's face.
   (c) Try to be about 6 ft from the speaker. This is an ideal distance for watching facial expressions, lip movements, and gestures.
4. Ask a speaker whom you find particularly difficult to hear to speak a little more slowly and distinctly.
5. Make every effort to relax. Strain causes tension and makes it more difficult to hear and to read speech.
6. Maintain good general health and get plenty of rest.

audiogram and have an explanation of its meaning and what hearing problems might be expected. It is best to have this discussion in the presence of family members. Everyone in the family should be advised as to the best ways to cope with hearing loss and should be given a list of suggestions as to how the patient and the family can use the patient's hearing most effectively (Table 3). It is just as important

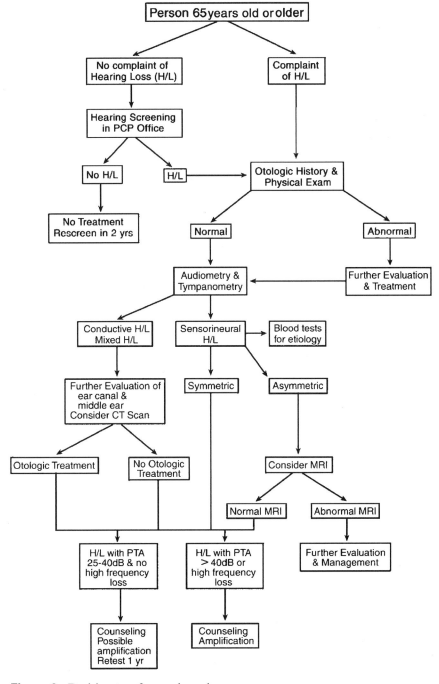

Figure 2 Decision tree for presbycusis.

for normal-hearing members of the family to know how to speak, as it is for the hearing impaired to know how to listen. Family members can be understanding and tolerant so that there is a harmonious family life or hearing loss can be used as a weapon causing continuous frustration and strife.

There is no proven medical or surgical treatment to stop or slow the aging of the auditory system. There are proprietary vitamin, mineral, and antioxidant preparations, and nutritional supplements marketed to help hearing. Although they may be helpful, there is no evidence-based medical treatment. As with many bodily dysfunctions, a healthy lifestyle—proper diet, maintaining a healthy body mass index, nonsmoking, regular exercise, avoidance of loud noise and ototoxic substances and other health risks, and periodic medical checkups—helps the person with presbycusis (6).

If the hearing loss is significantly affecting the patient's quality of life, the patient should be evaluated for a hearing aid and given information about assistive listening devices (41). Although rarely indicated for patients with presbycusis, if a severe-to-profound hearing loss develops, a cochlear implant might be considered (Fig. 2) (41).

In summary, age-related hearing loss is a major health problem in the United States, affecting the quality of life of millions of people. For now there is no evidence-based medical treatment; however, there is ongoing active research on the auditory system and in related fields so that hopefully effective medical treatment will be available in the future. In the meantime, early detection and evaluation of hearing loss in the elderly can be beneficial to them and their families leading to counseling and the provision of appropriate amplification by hearing aids and assistive listening devices.

REFERENCES

1. Schuknecht HF. Pathology of the Ear. 2nd ed. Philadelphia: Lea & Febiger, 1993.
2. Gratton MA, Vazquez AE. Age-related hearing loss: current research. Curr Opin Otolaryngol Head Neck Surg 2003; 11:367–371.
3. Yueh B, Shapiro N, MacLean CH, Shekelle PG. Screening and management of adult hearing loss in primary care. JAMA 2003; 289:1976–1984.
4. Bogardus ST Jr, Yueh B, Shekelle PG. Screening and management of adult hearing loss in primary care. JAMA 2003; 289:1986–1990.
5. Cruickshanks KJ, Tweed TS, Wiley TL, et al. The 5-year incidence and progression of hearing loss. Arch Otolaryngol Head Neck Surg 2003; 129:1041–1046.
6. Willott JF, Chisolm TH, Lister JJ. Modulation of presbycusis: current status and future directions. Audiol Neurootol 2001; 6:231–249.

   A comprehensive treatise on presbycusis including discussions of variables related to biologic aging, genetics, noise-induced hearing loss, moderately augmented acoustic environment, neural plasticity and the central auditory system, neural plasticity and hearing aids, socioeconomic and cultural barriers to hearing aid use, lifestyle, medical variables, pharmaceutical interventions for presbycusis, and cognitive variables.

7. Gates GA, Cobb JL, D'Agostino RB, Wolf PA. The relation of hearing in the elderly to the presence of cardiovascular disease and cardiovascular risk factors. Arch Otolaryngol Head Neck Surg 1993; 119:156–161.
8. Administration on Aging. A profile of older Americans. U.S. Department of Health and Human Services, Washington, DC 2003:1–16.
9. McCartney JH, Nadler G. How to help your patient cope with hearing loss. Geriatrics 1979; 34:69–71, 75–76.

10. Kalayam B, Meyers BS, Kakuma T, et al. Age at onset of geriatric depression and sensorineural hearing deficits. Biol Psychiatry 1995; 38:649–658.
11. Gates GA, Cooper JC Jr, Kannel WB, Miller NJ. Hearing in the elderly: the Framingham cohort, 1983–1985. Part I. Basic audiometric test results. Ear Hear 1990; 11:247–256.
12. Ventry IM, Weinstein BE. The hearing handicap inventory for the elderly: a new tool. Ear Hear 1982; 3:128–134.
13. Gates GA, Murphy M, Rees TS, Fraher A. Screening for handicapping hearing loss in the elderly. J Fam Pract 2003; 52:56–62.
14. The American National Standards Institute. Determination of occupational noise exposure and estimation of noise-induced hearing impairment. American National Standard ANSI S3.44, 1996.
15. International Organization for Standardization. Acoustics—statistical distribution of hearing thresholds as a function of age. 2nd ed. International Standard ISO 7029, 2000–05–01.
16. Cohn ES. Hearing loss with aging. Clin Geriatr Med 1999; 15:14.
17. Frisina DR, Frisina RD. Speech recognition in noise and presbycusis: relations to possible neural mechanisms. Hear Res 1997; 106:95–104.

One of the main complaints of people with presbycusis is the inability to understand speech in the presence of background noise. This paper clearly addresses the issue clinically and defines the central auditory dysfunction that may account for this common complaint.

18. Gates GA, Mills D, Nam BH, D'Agostino R, Rubel EW. Effects of age on the distortion product otoacoustic emission growth functions. Hear Res 2002; 163:53–60.
19. Gates GA, Rees TS. Hear ye? Hear ye! Successful auditory aging. West J Med 1997; 167:247–252.
20. Schuknecht HF, Gacek MR. Cochlear pathology in presbycusis. Ann Otol Rhinol Laryngol 1993; 102:1–16.

This is a thoughtful and authoritative extension of Schuknecht's classic work on cochlear pathology in presbycusis. Schuknecht's chapter on cochlear pathology in Ref. 1 should be reviewed in conjunction with this paper.

21. Caspary DM, Milbrandt JC, Helfert RH. Central auditory aging: GABA changes in the inferior colliculus. Exp Gerontol 1995; 30:349–360.
22. Chisolm TH, Willott JF, Lister JJ. The aging auditory system: anatomic and physiologic changes and implications for rehabilitation. Int J Audiol 2003; 42:2S3–10.
23. Willott JF. Anatomic and physiologic aging: a behavioral neuroscience perspective. J Am Acad Audiol 1996; 7:141–151.
24. Tremblay KL, Piskosz M, Souza P. Effects of age and age-related hearing loss on the neural representation of speech cues. Clin Neurophysiol 2003; 114:1332–1343.
25. Kim S, Frisina DR, Frisina RD. Effects of age on contralateral suppression of distortion product otoacoustic emissions in human listeners with normal hearing. Audiol Neurootol 2002; 7:348–357.
26. Jacobson M, Kim S, Romney J, Zhu X, Frisina RD. Contralateral suppression of distortion-product otoacoustic emissions declines with age: a comparison of findings in CBA mice with human listeners. Laryngoscope 2003; 113:1707–1713.
27. Frei B. Reactive oxygen species and antioxidant vitamins: mechanisms of action. Am J Med 1994; 97:3A-5S–13S.

This is a scholarly overview of the mechanisms of the production of reactive oxygen species in biologic systems and the various antioxidant defense systems that provide protection against oxidative damage to biologic macromolecules.

28. Seidman MD, Ahmad N, Bai U. Molecular mechanisms of age-related hearing loss. Ageing Res Rev 2002; 1:331–343.

     An excellent presentation of the various molecular mechanisms underlying age-related hearing loss and a discussion of potential ways to mitigate the effects of aging on hearing.

29. Seidman MD. Effects of dietary restriction and antioxidants on presbyacusis. Laryngoscope 2000; 110:727–738.
30. Gates GA, Couropmitree NN, Myers RH. Genetic associations in age-related hearing thresholds. Arch Otolaryngol Head Neck Surg 1999; 125:654–659.
31. Jennings CR, Jones NS. Review article presbyacusis. J Laryngol Otol 2001; 115:171–178.
32. Noben-Trauth K, Zheng QY, Johnson KR. Association of cadherin 23 with polygenic inheritance and genetic modification of sensorineural hearing loss. Nat Genet 2003; 35:21–23.
33. Siemens J, Lillo C, Dumont RA, et al. Nature Cadherin 23 is a component of the tip link in hair-cell stereocilia. Nature 2004; 428:950–955.
34. Busis SN, Gaca GJ. Removing cerumen: technique, risks, and informed consent. JAMA 1988; 260:99–100.
35. Parham K. Distortion product otoacoustic emissions in the C57BL/6J mouse model of age-related hearing loss. Hear Res 1997; 112:216–234.
36. Lonsbury-Martin BL, Cutler WM, Martin GK. Evidence for the influence of aging on distortion-product otoacoustic emissions in humans. J Acoust Soc Am 1991; 89: 1749–1759.
37. Cilento BW, Norton SJ, Gates GA. The effects of aging and hearing loss on distortion product otoacoustic emissions. Otolaryngol Head Neck Surg 2003; 129:382–389.
38. Rosenhall U, Pedersen K, Dotevall M. Effects of presbycusis and other types of hearing loss on auditory brainstem responses. Scand Audiol 1986; 15:179–185.
39. Boettcher FA. Presbyacusis and the auditory brainstem response. J Speech Lang Hear Res 2002; 45:1249–1261.
40. Oku T, Hasegewa M. The influence of aging on auditory brainstem response and electrocochleography in the elderly. ORL J Otorhinolaryngol Relat Spec 1997; 59:141–146.
41. Marcincuk MC, Roland PS. Geriatric hearing loss. Understanding the causes and providing appropriate treatment. Geriatrics 2002; 57:44–51.

7

Tinnitus in the Elderly Patient

Steven M. Parnes
Department of Otolaryngology, Albany Medical Center, Albany, New York, U.S.A.

TINNITUS

Tinnitus is an otologic symptom experienced by nearly every individual at some time. It is the perception of sound or noise, which originates in the head and not external to the individual. Tinnitus should be characterized not as a *disease*, but rather, a complex *symptom* that requires a thorough evaluation with appropriate diagnostic tests for successful management (1). Subjectively, patients may describe tinnitus as either a pure tone or multiple tones that can be high pitched or low pitched. It is often characterized as a ringing, buzzing, roaring, clicking, or hissing sound. Patients may describe tinnitus as pulsatile in nature. While it can be steady or intermittent, patients usually perceive tinnitus more often at night in a quiet environment.

Although tinnitus is poorly understood, it is very common. One of the first efforts to determine the prevalence of tinnitus was a national study conducted throughout England in 1978 (2). The study methodology was a questionnaire with 19,000 respondents. Approximately one in six (16–19%) of respondents over the age of 17 had experienced spontaneous tinnitus lasting more than five minutes. While 8% had a type of tinnitus that was bothersome and interfered with sleep or concentration, only 0.5% felt that it severely hampered their ability to have a normal life. In 1996, the National Center for Health Statistics (United States) conducted a survey to study the prevalence of tinnitus (3). With all ages considered, the prevalence was 3%; however, tinnitus was present in 1% of those surveyed under the age of 45, and 9% over the age of 65 (Fig. 1). These results, as well as others, confirm the clinical impression that an increasing incidence of tinnitus correlates with increasing age (1–3). An estimated 40–60 million people in the United States experience tinnitus, the symptom occurring most commonly between the ages of 40 and 70, more in men than in women, and rarely in children (4). In fact, one has stated that nearly the entire population will have this symptom at some time in their lives, with approximately 10 million people finding the symptom to be severe or troubling.

Tinnitus is closely correlated with hearing loss. As the population ages, hearing deteriorates and the symptom of tinnitus becomes not only more prevalent but also more bothersome (Fig. 2). A study comparing a tinnitus group to a cohort without tinnitus demonstrated an increasing incidence of hearing loss in the tinnitus group (5).

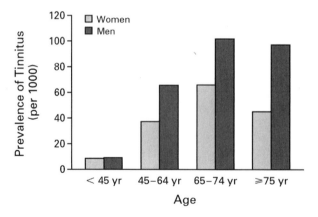

Figure 1 The prevalence of tinnitus in U.S. the population. *Source*: From Ref. 4.

The prevalence increases with the severity of hearing loss regardless of the frequency affected by the hearing loss, with tinnitus appearing to stabilize after age 75.

The characteristics—and etiologies—of tinnitus can be divided into two major categories, *objective* or *subjective*. Objective tinnitus refers to tinnitus that is audible to the physician or another person while subjective tinnitus is apparent only to the sufferer. This definition is rather arbitrary since it is dependent on the fastidiousness of the observer and not on the actual pathophysiology of the patient's tinnitus. The use of an amplifying stethoscope is more likely to lead to the identification of "objective" tinnitus then routine auscultation in the normal milieu. It is therefore more appropriate to delineate tinnitus into those generated by para-auditory structures versus *sensorineural tinnitus*, more likely to be encountered (6).

TINNITUS THAT ORIGINATES FROM PARA-AUDITORY STRUCTURES (OBJECTIVE TINNITUS)

Tinnitus that can be objectively heard can be further divided into vascular noises or "clicking." Vascular sounds may be due to venous hum, arterial turbulence, vascular neoplasm, arteriovenous fistulas, intracranial hypertension, or other vascular tumors,

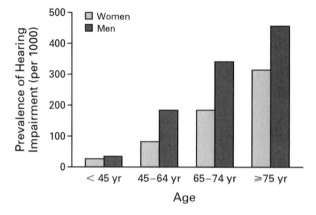

Figure 2 The prevalence of hearing loss in the U.S. population. *Source*: From Ref. 4.

and typically are synchronous with the heartbeat. Tinnitus described as clicking in nature is usually secondary to muscular myoclonus, usually from the palate. The astute clinician will differentiate between the patient's symptoms of random clicking or pulsatile nature of the tinnitus in an effort to elucidate the etiology.

Vascular Tinnitus

If the patient describes a pulsating type noise, this certainly suggests a vascular etiology even if the examiner is unable to appreciate it (6,7). The tinnitus can be described as a harsh, sharp sound, although if it is of venous origin it would be more like humming machinery with rhythmic accentuations since the sounds are vascular in origin. In addition to doing a careful head and neck exam with particular emphasis on the ear canal and eardrum, it is important to auscultate the patient in various positions. Auscultation should be done with a stethoscope near the eye, the preauricular area, parietal scalp, mastoid, and neck. An instrument likely to be found only in an otolaryngologist's office is a Toynbee stethoscope, which is a rubber tubing with ear inserts on both ends. This allows the examiner to appreciate the sound more easily. Furthermore, one should note during auscultation whether light neck compression obliterates the sound. Obliteration with light pressure suggests a venous etiology rather than an arterial cause in which greater pressure would be necessary. One should be particularly cautious in the elderly since significant carotid arthrosclerotic disease may be present and compression may trigger an embolic or occlusive event. Otoscopy of the tympanic membrane will rule out middle ear effusion, which can accentuate vascular sounds, and also identify any masses behind the eardrum. If a reddish vascular mass is noted, this could suggest a glomus tympanicum or glomus jugulare. A bluish mass in the hypotympanum suggests a dehiscent jugular bulb, where a reddish one in the anterior middle ear space suggests a dehiscent carotid artery. Employing magnification might be helpful to visualize the possible findings, and if increasing pressure in the ear canal results in blanching of the mass (Brown's sign), this provides additional confirmation of the presence of a vascular tumor. In addition to an audiogram, tympanometry can be useful in these patients since regular pulsations can be seen on the tracing.

Paragangliomas such as glomus jugulare tumors are highly vascular tumors composed of non-chromaffin paraganglioma cells that originate from chemoreceptors or baroreceptors. They are found along the carotid body, jugular bulb, and the middle ear. Patients may have more than one tumor; therefore, further investigation with magnetic resonance imaging as well as arteriography are required if a paraganglioma is suspected.

Arteriovenous malformations can also lead to a pulsatile-type tinnitus. In this case, examination of the patient is usually normal. Again, one must be dependent on imaging studies particularly magnetic resonance imaging (MRI), magnetic resonance angiographs (MRAs) and if necessary a four-vessel arteriograph. If this diagnosis is made, then these are usually treated with arterial embolization if possible.

Venous hum is another vascular sound that can be differentiated from sounds of arterial origin in that the venous sound is more low pitched and softer and can be obliterated by light pressure on the neck. Treatment is somewhat controversial. Ligation of the internal jugular vein has been performed, but many patients develop recurrent symptoms years later; hence, counseling and reassurance are appropriate for most patients, especially the elderly. In some instances, a magnetic resonance venograph (MRV) may be appropriate to define the abnormality. Pseudotumor cerebri can present in a similar fashion so that a fundoscopic examination to rule out papilledema should be performed (7). Pseudotumor cerebri usually occurs in young obese female patients (or in association with anemia or polycythemia) and is unlikely to be encountered in the geriatric population.

The exact etiology of pulsatile tinnitus remains unidentified in the majority of elderly patients who present with the complaint. Most will have normal findings on physical examination and unremarkable imaging studies. The internal carotid artery courses within 1–2 mm of the cochlea, so a plausible explanation is that sounds of turbulent blood flow coursing through the neck vessels is transmitted to the inner ear. An ongoing paradigm shift in the management of occlusive vascular disease of the extracranial cerebral circulation may reduce the threshold of intervention for future patients with vascular stenosis. Hence, evaluation of these patients with ultrasonography to rule out significant atherosclerotic disease or stenosis may be warranted.

Muscle Contraction Tinnitus

Synchronous contraction of the palatal muscles (palatal myoclonus) is a nonvascular cause of objective tinnitus. An involuntary series of rapid, repetitive contractions of the tensor and levator palatini muscles occurring at a frequency of from 60 to 200 times a minute results in an audible click. The click can be heard by both the patient and the examiner and it is synchronous with the movement of the palate. Occasionally, opening the mouth decreases or eliminates the contractions, making diagnosis challenging. Palatal myoclonus is occasionally associated with neurological diseases such as brainstem infarcts and multiple sclerosis, but usually there is no specific etiology identified. Imaging with MRI is necessary and is usually normal in these individuals. Medications that have been used include clonazepam, carbamazepine, and diazepam, all of which have side effects that may be more severe than the primary complaint, particularly in the elderly. Chemodenervation of the involved muscle(s) with botulinum toxin provides some benefit, but care must be taken to avoid palatal paralysis, which can lead to dysphagia. Surgery is rarely indicated and often ineffective (1,6).

Patulous Eustachian Tube

Patients who suffer sudden weight loss sometimes complain of an ocean roar in the ear that is synchronous with respiration. The sound is worse after the patient wakes up and is up and about during the day, and is not as severe when reclining. Often they will paradoxically complain of a "plugged" feeling, as well as an "echo" when they speak due to transmission of sound through the open eustachian tube. On examination of the ear, one may observe movement of the tympanic membrane during respiration. Tympanometry can also detect an abnormal motion of the eardrum. Fortunately, the symptoms are short lived for most patients, although an occasional patient will have persistent and troublesome symptoms. In these cases, partial or total obliteration of the eustachian tube can be performed; however, this will often lead to middle ear effusion, requiring placement of a patulous eustachian (PE) tube. Effective treatment for this disorder remains elusive (1).

SENSORINEURAL (SUBJECTIVE) TINNITUS

This is far and away the most common type of tinnitus encountered. Despite its high prevalence, little is known about the underlying physiologic mechanisms. It is known to occur in patients who have suffered insults to the ear such as noise exposure or administration of certain pharmacologic agents. It has also been associated with other otologic diseases such as Meniere's disease and otosclerosis. Most authorities believe that the illusion of sound is actually generated within the central nervous system (CNS). This is supported by the fact that tinnitus can persist in individuals in whom the auditory nerve has been severed (8). A number of theories exist. One is that deprivation of input to the auditory nervous system releases central neurons from inhibition. Another is that the sensation is due to spontaneous neural activity resulting from ephaptic excitation of one nerve fiber by adjacent fibers or synchronous hair cell discharges (9). Not all attribute the source to the CNS. One theory suggests that outer hair cell damage results in decoupling the stereocilia from the tectorial membrane, leading to an increased discharge rate that evolves from the damaged segment of the outer hair. The lack of a pure animal model has limited the possibility of studying the mechanisms of hearing loss-related tinnitus. None of the theories enumerated above have been substantiated or accepted by all otolaryngologists.

Causes and Evaluation

The etiology of tinnitus can be divided into the following potential causes: otologic, cardiovascular, metabolic, neurologic, pharmacologic, dental, and psychological factors. The greatest number will be due to otologic factors specifically noise exposure and presbycusis. Other disease processes involving the ear can result in tinnitus, such as Meniere's disease, otosclerosis, and labyrinthitis. Unilateral tinnitus presents a particular problem since one of the chief complaints of patients with an acoustic neuroma is unilateral tinnitus and hearing loss. An MRI is the diagnostic test of choice. Whether routine testing is warranted in the elderly population is a matter of some debate.

All patients should undergo a careful history and physical examination. In particular, the history should focus on the onset and duration of tinnitus and whether there is any history of noise exposure. A tinnitus handicap scale has been developed to document problems associated with tinnitus to determine the impact of the symptom on the patient's quality of life (QOL). It is apparent that many of these patients suffer from underlying psychiatric disorders and it is important that a clinician is cognizant of this fact (9,13). An audiogram should be obtained in all patients, as well as tympanometry depending on specific circumstances. The audiologist can also determine the loudness or pitch of the tinnitus using tinnitus-matching techniques. This is usually unnecessary unless one is considering a masking device for the treatment (14). Imaging studies may be occasionally warranted in specific cases such as unilateral nature, sudden onset, etc. Diagnosis and treatment of a specific otologic condition may or may not relieve the patient of tinnitus.

Cardiovascular problems should be considered, particularly hypertension and anemia, since there seems to be a higher incidence of tinnitus in this patient population. Thyroid dysfunction has been noted as well. Nine percent of patients who have head trauma have tinnitus, so asking about prior head injuries may assist in history taking (1). Postconcussive tinnitus usually occurs in a delayed fashion, beginning one to two weeks after the incident. One must be careful about making a causal association because of risk of secondary gain if litigation is possible.

Another common cause of tinnitus is as a side effect of certain drugs and medications. Aspirin and aspirin-like medications are the most common etiologic drugs. Tinnitus caused by these drugs is dose-dependent and is reversible, unlike that caused by the aminoglycosides. Tinnitus may be one of the first symptoms of irreversible otologic complications from aminoglycoside use. If unrecognized, patients may proceed to develop permanent hearing loss and loss of vestibular function. This risk has been reduced somewhat with the availability of aminoglycoside blood levels; nevertheless, the symptom of tinnitus mandates careful investigation in these patients. Caffeine may also be a culprit. Some authorities recommend that patients with tinnitus be asked to reduce or eliminate caffeine from their diet. Other drugs that have been implicated are nonsteroid inflammatory drugs and the heterocycline antidepressants (1).

A significant number of patients with temporal mandibular joint problems complain of tinnitus. Patients also note a sensation of fullness in the ear. Examination does not reveal any abnormality of the ear canal or eardrum, but palpation of the temporal mandibular joint may elicit pain, tenderness, and crepitus. A history of bruxism as well as joint malalignment are often associated with this complaint. Therapy is directed towards treating the temporomandibular joint (TMJ) abnormalities. Heat, analgesics, and a soft diet are important components of the treatment plan. A bite block may be necessary if significant bruxism is present.

It is important to recognize many patients whose QOL is severely affected by tinnitus have underlying psychological disorders. Psychological profiles of these patients demonstrate a pattern of difficulty in coping with the symptom as well as other associated psychological conditions (1,15,16). The question could be asked, "Does tinnitus cause depression?" It is apparent that most of these patients are not severely depressed and can be treated with appropriate counseling, thereby avoiding pharmacologic therapy. The converse question, "does depression cause tinnitus?" is also reasonable. However, there is no evidence to suggest that this is the case. In fact, despite the correlation between the *presence* of tinnitus and depression, there is no correlation between the *intensity* of the tinnitus and its effect on QOL (6,13).

Management

Therapy falls into several categories. First, there is treatment directed at the underlying condition. Specific otologic condition such as labyrinthitis, Meniere's disease, or otosclerosis can be addressed. Inciting factors such as noise exposure and drugs that can potentially produce tinnitus, such as aspirin and caffeine should be avoided. Other categories include medical therapy, surgical therapy, psychological approaches, and masking.

A number of pharmacological approaches have been tried over the years; however, no drug is presently approved by the Food and Drug Administration (FDA) with a specific indication for the treatment of tinnitus. Ginkgo biloba has become popular as a treatment strategy, but when subjected to double blind prospective studies it does not demonstrate effectiveness (6,14). No rigorous study has clearly determined that any medication will benefit patients with tinnitus, in that most studies have been anecdotal and poorly controlled (6,15,17). Patients who suffer from depression or significant anxiety with associated tinnitus may benefit from medical therapy of their depression and/or anxiety. Antidepressants represent the mainstay of this strategy, with specific medication choices, especially in the elderly, being beyond the intent of this chapter (13).

No surgical procedure is presently approved for tinnitus. Radical procedures, including trans-section of the cochlear nerve or labyrinthectomy have not been demonstrated to be efficacious (6,15). Surgical therapy directed at specific causes such as Meniere's disease or hearing loss (cochlear implantation) will occasionally result in reduction in tinnitus as an "extra added benefit" of the procedure. A number of studies have demonstrated some degree of tinnitus suppression after cochlear implantation and a modified cochlear implant intended for use in patients with severe tinnitus is under investigation (18,19). There is only a 25% chance of improving tinnitus with cochlear nerve resection, and the severity of tinnitus increased in some patients. Microvascular decompression of the eighth cranial nerve has also been performed by some for severe tinnitus, but this procedure remains controversial (20).

Avoidance of Silence

Perhaps the most effective therapy for tinnitus is *avoidance of silence*. In most instances, patients would have already discovered the effectiveness of background sound in reducing their awareness of tinnitus prior to their evaluation. The exact mechanism of action is unknown, but may be due to providing increased inhibition to central signal generators. Commercial devices are available, although many patients utilize a fan, radio, or some other mechanical or electronic device to assure a constant background sound. Discussion of this option with symptomatic patients is often all the "treatment" that they require.

Tinnitus Masker

Tinnitus maskers are devices similar to hearing aids that "avoid silence" by generating and transmitting a constant background sound into the ear(s). Maskers come in three broad categories, "pure" hearing aids, "pure maskers," and some combination of the two functions in one device. Patients with hearing loss who are fitted with hearing aids will often notice an improvement in their tinnitus. The aids act as "de facto maskers" by amplifying background environmental sounds. Masking devices are also specifically designed for patients with tinnitus. In the past, attempts were made to "frequency match" the masking device with the patient's tinnitus. However, more recently, "white noise" generators have been used instead, as they can be more easily fitted and have at least equal efficacy. Since most patients with tinnitus also have hearing loss, there is a hearing aid with an integral masking function specifically designed for these individuals (14). When used alone, these masking devices alone may be only transiently effective, with significant noncompliance. Therefore, these devices may be most effective when employed as a part of a "tinnitus retraining" (TRT) program.

Tinnitus Retraining

Jastreboff and Jastreboff (21) popularized a TRT program in the 1990s that utilizes white noise generators, patient education, and biofeedback. Tinnitus is not eliminated, but patients are taught coping strategies that improve their QOL. Most patients will gain some benefit, but it must be noted that this program is costly, time consuming, and not covered by insurance; hence, only the most highly motivated individuals complete it. In many instances, merely knowing that treatment is available will dramatically reduce the impact of the symptom and improve QOL. TRT (as well as other similar programs that employ patient education and biofeedback) should therefore be considered as part of the armamentarium for patients who are most distressed by the symptom (4,6,13,21).

CONCLUSIONS

Tinnitus is an extremely common symptom, particularly among the elderly. Telling the affected patient to "just live with it" is unhelpful and should be avoided. The elderly symptomatic patient will respond favorably to a concerned and sympathetic approach. A focused history and physical examination, along with audiometric investigation, will identify possible etiologies and facilitate directed therapy for some patients. Education, particularly the necessity to "avoid silence," and reassurance will benefit all patients to some degree. Fitting with a hearing aid, or masking device, may be beneficial. A few patients will suffer persistent significant reduction in QOL due to tinnitus and depression. Referral for treatment of depression is often necessary. TRT will be effective for most patients with the resources and insight to participate in the program. A considerable amount of information is available online. Excellent patient-centered resources can be found on the websites of the American Academy of Otolaryngology—Head and Neck Surgery Foundation and the American Tinnitus Association (22,23). The most critical point in this chapter is to remember that patients with tinnitus can be treated in a very satisfactory fashion.

REFERENCES

1. Schleuning AJ Jr, Martin WH. Tinnitus. 3rd ed. Head Neck Surg. Chapter 151, 1925–1933.
2. Coles RR. Epidemiology of tinnitus: (1) prevalance. J Laryngol Otol Suppl 1984; 9:7–15.
3. Adams PF, Hendershot GE, Marano MA. Current estimates from the National Health Interview survey, 1996. Hyattsville, Md.: National Center for Health Statistics, 1999.
4. Lockwood AH, Salvi RJ, Burkard RF. Tinnitus. N Engl J Med 2002; 347(9):904–910.
5. Coles RR. Epidemiology of tinnitus: (2) demographic and clinical features. J Laryngol Otol Suppl 1984; 23:441–452.
6. Jastreboff PJ, Gray WC, Mattox DE. Tinnitus and hyperacusis. In: Cummings CW, Fredrickson JM, Harker LA, et al., eds. Otolaryngol HNS, 3rd ed. St. Louis: Mosby, 1998:3198–3222.
7. Sismanis A. Pulsatile tinnitus. Otolaryngol Clin North Am 2003; 36(2):389–402.
8. Moller AR. Pathophysiology of tinnitus. Otolaryngol Clin North Am 2003; 36(2):249–266.
9. Eggermont JJ. Tinnitus: some thought about its origin. J Laryngol Otol Suppl 1984; 9:31.
10. Sweetow RW. Tinnitus reclassified: new oil and old lamp. Otolaryngol Head Neck Surg 1996; 114:582–585.
11. Tyler RS. Does tinnitus originate from hyperactive nerve fibers in the cochlea? J Neurophysiol 1984; 44:76–96.
12. Sewell WF. The relationship between the endocochlear potential and spontaneous activity in auditory nerve fibres of the cat. J Physiol 1984; 347:685–696.
13. Dobie RA. Depression and tinnitus. Otolaryngol Clin North Am 2003; 36(2):383–388.
14. Vernon JA, Meikle MB. Masking devices and alprazolam treatment for tinnitus. Otolaryngol Clin North Am 2003; 36(2):307–320.
15. Parnes SM. Current concepts in the clinical management of patients with tinnitus. Eur Arch Otorhinolaryngol 1997; 254:406–409.
16. Kirsch C, Blanchard E, Parnes S. Psychological characteristics of individuals high and low in their ability to cope with tinnitus. Psychom Med 1989; 51:209–217.
17. Seidman MD, Babu S. Alternative medications and other treatments for tinnitus: facts from fiction. Otolaryngol Clin North Am 2003; 36(2):359–381.
18. Miyamoto RT, Bichey BG. Cochlear implantation for tinnitus suppression. Otolaryngol Clin North Am 2003; 36(2):345–352.
19. House TW, Beackman DE. Tinnitus: surgical treatment. CIBA Fund Symp 1981; d5:xx.

20. Brookes GB. Vascular-decompression surgery for severe tinnitus. Am J Otol 1996; 17:569–576.
21. Jastreboff PJ, Jastreboff MM. Tinnitus retraining therapy for patients with tinnitus and decreased sound tolerance. Otolaryngol Clin North Am 2003; 36(2):321–336.
22. American Academy of Otolaryngology-HNS Foundation (www.entlink.org)
23. American Tinnitus Association (www.ata.org)

8

Hearing Protection for the Retired Adult

Marshall Chasin
Musicians' Clinics of Canada, Toronto, Ontario, Canada

Joanne DeLuzio
Graduate Department of Speech-Language Pathology, University of Toronto, Toronto, Ontario, Canada

INTRODUCTION

When one typically thinks of hearing protection, images of workers in a factory or on a construction site immediately come to mind. Depending on one's interest, an image of a rock star may also be conjured up. Research has shown that when it comes to causing hearing loss, music exposure is similar to noise exposure (1). Many issues arise when the topic of noise exposure is raised. Of these, the most common are:

1. Do I need to wear hearing protection when I mow my lawn?
2. I already have a hearing loss because of my age. Do I still need to protect my hearing?
3. What about the hearing of my teenage grandchildren?

Many common experiences such as lawnmower noise, listening to portable CD players while taking walks, and attending concerts—classical or otherwise—can subject the individual to potentially damaging levels of noise.

However, it is not just the level [measured in decibels A-weighted (dBA)], but also the duration of the exposure that can cause hearing loss. For example, there is nothing wrong with going to a concert on Friday evening, as long as one does not mow the lawn on Saturday morning. Various models of hearing loss [see, for example, Ref. (2)] indicate that 85 dBA exposure for 40 hours per week is identical to an exposure of 88 dBA for only 20 hours per week, a 91 dBA exposure for only 10 hours per week, and so on. That is, a 3-dB increase effectively halves the exposure time required to cause damage. While a senior citizen may not be exposed to 85 dBA of noise or music for 40 hours per week, they may be exposed for 5 to 10 hours per week at a deceptively high level. Maximum weekly "dosages" can be obtained by five hours of exposure to a portable music player at a volume of 4 out of 10. For those who like to listen to "portable music" while they walk, enjoy boating, and mow their own lawn, hearing protection is advised for the lawn work.

Does a previously existing hearing loss make a person more or less susceptible to further deterioration? Borg et al. (3), in reviewing a number of studies, concluded that just because a person already has a sensorineural hearing loss, they are no more and no less susceptible to future hearing loss from noise. The research indicates that it is just as important for a senior citizen to protect their hearing as it is for someone in their youth.

The third question suggests that senior citizens have an increasingly important role to play in advising their grandchildren about the maintenance of healthy hearing. Young people may not listen to mom and dad, but increasingly our senior citizens are being looked upon as being cool!

HEARING PROTECTION

Hearing protectors come in two forms—earplugs and earmuffs. As the name suggests, earplugs are inserted into the ear canal and earmuffs are worn over the ear and held to the head by a spring-loaded headband. Earplugs can be "one size fits all" or a custom fit where the individual has an impression taken of their ear.

Other than very specialized industrial applications, hearing protection does not cover or surround the entire head. Subsequently, there is a theoretical upper limit on the attenuation provided by any hearing protector. Many studies have examined the basis for the maximum attenuation levels from hearing protection (4–8). These factors pertain not only to the thickness and density of the material used in hearing protectors, but also to the level of bone-conducted sound transmission. For example, Berger (8) noted that at 2000 Hz, the bone conduction limit for hearing protection was only 40 dB. That is, hearing protection attenuations of greater than 40 dB in the 2000 Hz region are artifacts of the measuring system. Above this 40 dB range, sound is conducted through the temporal bone directly to the cochlea, by passing the air conduction route. Figure 1 shows the bone conduction limits across frequency for hearing protector attenuation.

Closely related to this is what is known as the occlusion effect. This is where there is an improvement of the lower frequency bone conduction thresholds upon occlusion of the ear canal. This results in the amplification of internal physiological noise (9). The essential characteristics of this phenomenon were first described by Josef Zwislocki in the 1950s (4,5). This occlusion effect is well known to hearing aid wearers. It typically results in an echo-like sensation being reported by hearing aid users. Extending the bore of the earplug into the inner or bony portion of the external ear canal can reduce the occlusion effect. This is one advantage of a custom earplug over a "one size fits all" type. The extent of the effect can be measured clinically in most audiology clinics.

Another feature of hearing protection is that the majority attenuate higher frequency sounds more than lower frequency sounds. Figure 2 shows the frequency-dependent characteristics of a typical industrial foam plug inserted deeply into the ear canal. If these plugs were not as deeply seated, low-frequency attenuations

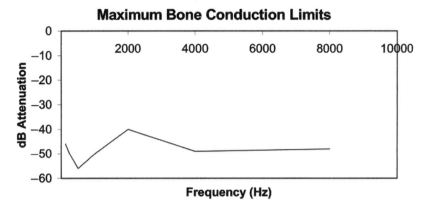

Figure 1 The maximum attenuations for bone conducted sound are shown, indicating that the maximum possible hearing protection attenuation in the 2000 Hz region is on the order of 40 dB. Maximum attenuations can exceed 40 dB at other frequencies however. *Source*: Adapted from Ref. 8.

of only 10–15 dB would be achieved. Two acoustic phenomena account for this frequency dependence:

1. Low-frequency sounds (i.e., long wavelengths) are acoustically "myopic" and do not see the obstruction well, while the higher-frequency (i.e., shorter wavelength) sounds acoustically "see" the obstruction. Thus, hearing protection will attenuate the higher-frequency consonants to a greater degree than the lower-frequency vowels and this creates "muffled" speech.
2. The human ear canal is a 25 mm (one inch) long tube that is closed at the tympanic membrane side and open at the other. It can be thought of as a quarter wavelength resonator with a frequency in the 2700 Hz region.

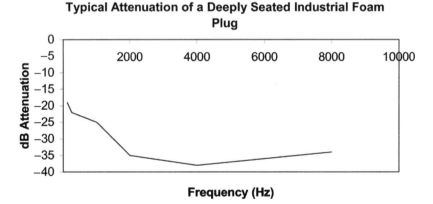

Figure 2 Typical attenuations for a deeply seated industrial foam earplug with maximum attenuations being less than 40 dB. A more shallow ear insertion would reduce the attenuation by 10–15 dB, especially for the lower frequencies.

Due to this configuration, the ear canal naturally amplifies consonants in the 2700 Hz region (the top octave of a piano keyboard) by about 17–20 dB.

Whenever the ear canal is occluded (with a hearing aid or an earplug), this naturally occurring resonance is lost. Plugging the ear canal is acoustically comparable to a musician inserting the hand into the bell of the French horn. With earplugs, high-frequency (insertion) loss is caused by the loss of the 2700 Hz resonance. The net effect from both of these physical phenomena is that high-frequency consonant sounds are attenuated more than lower-frequency ones.

In contrast, earmuffs do not modulate the natural ear resonance in the 2700 Hz region. This results in less relative high-frequency attenuation than if earplugs were used. Earmuffs do, however, yield greater attenuations in the 500–1000 Hz region. As an additional side effect, the level of the occlusion effect will be less with large volume earmuffs than with many earplug fittings. Even though many earmuffs provide a "more uniform" attenuation pattern than earplugs, one cannot state definitively that the use of earmuffs yield improved speech intelligibility in noise over that of the use of earplugs, since hearing loss configuration and large subject variability are confounding factors (10).

ACOUSTICALLY (AND ELECTRONICALLY) TUNED HEARING PROTECTION

Many people do not like to wear hearing protection. This is understandable given the nonuniform attenuation characteristics, the occlusion effect, and reduced speech intelligibility in noise. In order to resolve this problem, Killion et al. (11) devised a custom earplug with approximately 15 dB of attenuation over a wide range of frequencies. The earplug, named the ER-15^{TM} (manufactured by Etymotic Research, Inc.), has become widely accepted by musicians and music lovers, as well as some industrial workers who work in relatively quiet environments (<100 dBA). There is a noncustom form of this earplug called the ER-20. As the name suggests, this plug attenuates all sounds by about 20 dB (12). Figure 3 shows the attenuation characteristics of the ER-15 earplug and an industrial-type foam plug (from Fig. 2) for comparison purposes. Bilsom (another manufacturer of hearing protection) has come out with the NST^{TM} earplug. NST stands for "natural sound technology" and is a noncustom earplug giving a relatively flat attenuation characteristic.

Three benefits of a "flat attenuation" earplug are:

1. Hearing sounds (especially music) the way they were intended.
2. An improved ability to communicate in a noisy environment (over conventional hearing protection).
3. Improved localization for the direction of sound. Although it can be argued that this third point has relatively little importance for people not working in a noisy environment, the first two will certainly improve one's enjoyment of music.

It is a fallacy that more sound attenuation is better. As long as the earplug or earmuff is adequate, meaning that there is enough attenuation for the noise/music

Comparison of Industrial Foam plug to the ER-15

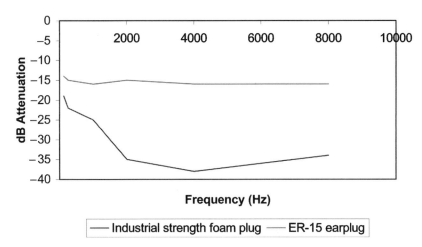

Figure 3 The attenuation characteristic of the custom ER-15 uniform attenuator earplug and for comparison purposes, the attenuation of a deeply seated industrial strength foam plug (Fig. 2).

environment—more is not better. More than the required attenuation can reduce speech intelligibility and reduce the overall ability to communicate. For many retired adults, their children, and grandchildren, 15–20 dB of attenuation is quite sufficient, while listening to music or attending a concert. Industrial strength (up to 40 dB) attenuation is not typically required for this type of recreational activity.

Hearing protection based on electronic characteristics rather than acoustic ones have recently been introduced. The first, active noise reduction (first reported on in 1933) is based on the principle that two identical signals when out of phase and added together will cancel each other out. While it is difficult to assess a quickly varying signal and generate another with the identical spectrum but 180° out of phase, it is a relatively easy task for steady-state signals, especially if they are low frequency (i.e., long wavelength). Active noise reduction hearing protection has not gained wide acceptance because of high cost, frequency limitation, and until recently a limitation to relatively steady-state signals. Recently, it has been gaining acceptance for certain uses such as long airplane flights. These earmuffs can cut out the constant drone of the airplane cabin. They can also be connected to a portable music player. The earmuffs, in cutting out some background noise, allow the listener to hear music at lower volumes, thus reducing the overall risk to hearing. By cutting out some lower frequency environmental noise, stress is also reduced.

In contrast, active sound transmission hearing protection has had its major use in hunting where optimal hearing of the movement of the prey has to be coupled with optimal hearing protection. A modified hearing aid circuit is typically utilized that allows for amplification at low input levels but attenuation or clipping at higher levels (such as the blast from a gun). An external monitoring microphone is used to assess the environmental noise/music level, and the amplification stages are reduced or disabled completely above a certain preselected level.

There are some reports in the literature regarding the use of compression or level-dependent hearing aid circuits such as the K-AMP, as well as the use of hearing aids that have been turned off (13,14). These have been shown to be quite useful, even for those with mild hearing losses, as long as there is no vent.

Many hearing aid manufacturers are offering a relatively new device—a combination of hearing aid and custom active hearing protector. In the hearing aid mode, such a device provides up to 40 dB of gain, but in the hearing protection mode becomes level dependent with peak gains of up to 15 dB. When the device is physically turned off, the shell provides attenuations of 25 dB in the lower frequencies and up to 35–40 dB in the higher frequencies.

Many senior citizens wear custom made hearing aids. Increasingly, these hearing aids use compression circuits that serve to not only amplify the softer sounds of speech but also attenuate or decrease the level of the louder environmental sounds. In this sense, many modern hearing aids are an example of electronic hearing protection. Not all hearing aids use the same circuitry, so it is important for the individual to contact their hearing health care professional to determine if their current amplification can be used as a hearing protector in noisy environments.

RATING HEARING PROTECTION

Many commercially available forms of hearing protection come with a noise reduction rating number on the package. This number can be misleading because a higher number is not necessarily better. Several single number rating schemes are in use throughout the world. The most commonly used scheme in the United States is the noise reduction rating (NRR). Most parts of Europe use an octave band method as well as the International Organization for Standardization (ISO) recommended single number rating (Berger, personal communication, 1995). Most provinces in Canada use the ABC scheme where hearing protectors are categorized according to a standard (Z94.2-94) into Class A, B, or C depending on their octave band attenuation values and the measured L_{eq}—a time-weighted average (15).

NRR has been in widespread use since 1979. However, Preves and Pehringer (16) have pointed out that the NRR calculation makes some simplifying assumptions and requires the use of various correction factors. The validity of these assumptions has led to some criticism of the NRR technique. For example, the National Institute for Occupational Safety and Health (NIOSH) felt that there should be a correction factor of 3 dB in the calculation of the NRR for reasons pertaining to spectral uncertainties. As this figure would be subtracted from the calculation, the NRR would be a worst-case scenario. NRR for each hearing protector is a measure based on the results of a number of subjects. Subsequently, a two standard deviation pad is also included as "a statistical adjustment so that the mean values are modified to reflect what some larger proportion of the population will actually achieve" (Berger, personal communication, 1995). This two standard deviation range covers approximately 95% of the population.

Although simplifying measures such as the NRR have made hearing protector characterization easier for the laboratories, the NRR tends to be affected by many artifacts when used for a different purpose than originally intended. It is, unfortunately, a widely held view that the higher the NRR, the better the hearing protector.

Depending on the noise or music level, the spectral shape, and the individual's communication or musical requirements, this is certainly not the case.

STRATEGIES FOR GRANDCHILDREN TO PROTECT THEIR HEARING

This section can be given as a handout to patients who have younger children or grandchildren. It is therefore written with the lay public in mind.

1. *Humming*: Most people with healthy ears have a natural sound attenuator in their middle ears called the stapedial reflex. This neurological reflex causes the stapedial muscle to contract upon loud sounds, thereby stiffening the middle ear bones or ossicles. This has the effect of reducing the transmission ability of the middle ear with the result that loud sounds do not get to the inner ear as effectively. All mammals have this reflex to varying degrees. From an evolutionary perspective, we have such a reflex to protect ourselves from our own voices. Depending on the study, this reflex has been shown to provide anywhere between 3 and 15 dB of hearing protection. Even if it is only 3 dB, this still cuts the damaging noise or music exposure in half so that a person can listen twice as long before the same damage occurs. A strategy to take advantage of this would be to elicit this natural reflex before a loud sounds such as a cymbal crash or when walking past a construction site. The stapedial reflex can be elicited simply by humming. This "fools" your ears into thinking that there is loud noise. Sustaining this hum throughout the loud sound will provide substantial hearing protection.
2. Hearing protection that attenuates sounds yet lets guitars still sound like guitars, drums like drums, and horns like horns is available. Such protection is widely available through most local hearing health care professionals. Many famous musicians and sound engineers wear this type of hearing protection and indeed forget that they are wearing anything in their ears.
3. Hearing loss is much like a dose of radiation. Small doses for short periods of time are not damaging, but even if relatively quiet noise or music exposure is heard for an extended period of time, hearing loss can ensue. As a rule of thumb, it takes the human ear about 16–18 hours to recover from loud noise. For the first 16–18 hours after a concert you may be suffering from a temporary hearing loss—usually noticed as a feeling of fullness or dullness, as if a piece of cotton is in your ear. Additional exposures within this critical 16–18-hour period would add significantly to the dose. However, additional doses of noise or music exposure separated by at least 16–18 hours do not contribute as significantly to the dose. Go ahead and enjoy the concert on Friday night, but do not mow your lawn until Sunday or better yet, get someone else to do it for you!

ACKNOWLEDGMENTS

Some of this information was derived from A. Behar, M. Chasin, and M. Cheesman, Noise Control—A Primer, San Diego: Singular Publishing Group, 2000.

REFERENCES

1. Chasin M. Musicians and the prevention of hearing loss. San Diego: Singular Publishing Group, 1996.
2. International Organization for Standardization (ISO). Acoustics—determination of occupational noise exposure and estimation of noise-induced hearing impairment. 2nd ed. International Standard ISO 1999. Geneva, Switzerland: Author, 1999.
3. Borg E, Canlon B, Engstrom B. Noise induced hearing loss: literature review and experiments in rabbits. Scand Audiol 1995; 24(suppl):40.
4. Zwislocki J. Acoustic attenuation between the ears. J Acoust Soc Am 1953; 25:752–759.
5. Zwislocki J. In search of the bone-conducted threshold in a sound field. J Acoust Soc Am 1957; 29:795–804.
6. Shaw EAG, Theissen GJ. Improved cushion for ear defenders. J Acoust Soc Am 1958; 30:24–36.
7. Shaw EAG, Theissen GJ. Acoustics of circumaural earphones. J Acoust Soc Am 1962; 34:1233–1243.
8. Berger EH. Methods for measuring the attenuation of hearing protection devices. J Acoust Soc Am 1986; 79:1655–1687.
9. Berger EH, Kerivan JE. Influence of physiological noise and the occlusion effect on the measurement of real-ear attenuation at threshold. J Acoust Soc Am 1983; 74:81–94.
10. Abel SM, Alberti PA, Haythornwaite C, Riko K. Speech intelligibility in noise with and without ear protectors. In: Alberti PW, ed. Personal Hearing Protection in Industry. New York: Raven Press, 1982:371–386.
11. Killion MC, DeVilbiss E, Stewart J. An earplug with uniform 15-dB attenuation. Hear J 1988; 41(5):14–16.
12. Killion MC, Stewart J, Falco R, Berger EH. Improved audibility earplug. U.S. Patent 5,113,967, 1992.
13. Killion MC. The parvum bonum, plus melius fallacy in earplug selection. In: Beilin L, Jensen GR, eds. Recent Developments in Hearing Aid Technology (15th Danavox Symposium). Kolding, Denmark: Scanticon, 1993:415–433.
14. Hétu R, Tran Quoc H, Tougas Y. Can an inactivated hearing aid act as a hearing protector? Canad Acoust 1992; 20(3):35–36.
15. Behar A, Desormeaux J. NRR, ABC, OR. Canad Acoust 1994; 22(1):27–30.
16. Preves DA, Pehringer JL. Calculating individual NRRs in situ using subminiature probe microphones. Hear Instrum 1983; 33(3):10–14.

9

Multisensory Impairment in Older Adults: Evaluation and Intervention

Susan L. Whitney
Departments of Physical Therapy and Otolaryngology, University of Pittsburgh, Pittsburgh, Pennsylvania, U.S.A.

Laura O. Morris
Balance and Vestibular Program, Eye and Ear Institute, Centers for Rehab Services, Pittsburgh, Pennsylvania, U.S.A.

INTRODUCTION

Multisensory deprivation disequilibrium is a condition that most commonly develops in the aging population. It occurs due to degradation of the three primary sensory systems used in balance: somatosensory, vestibular, and visual systems. These systems provide sensory information throughout the central nervous system regarding body position. The information is then coordinated and compared to memory of previous experiences and spatial maps. Areas of the cortex then develop a coordinated response from the neuromusculoskeletal system in order to maintain upright balance and perform such diverse activities as catching a ball or locomotion. This chapter addresses the clinical examination of the three primary sensory systems: somatosensory, vestibular, and visual.

No individual system provides all the sensory information required to determine position in space. Each system contributes its own unique and important information about body position and movement. As the normal older adult ages, some degradation of all three systems occur. In the healthy, active, aging adult, these changes are minimal and are inapparent. Decrement in the ability of the individual to perform balance-sensitive physical activities such as snow skiing or tennis is present, but inapparent. Peak performance may not be at the same level as someone younger; hence, older athletes characteristically compete within their own age group. A sedentary lifestyle with reduced levels of physical activity and stimulation can lead to decreased functional abilities purely due to deconditioning. Social factors such as a loss of a spouse, changing living environments, or retirement can lead to further inactivity, degrading a person's ability to maintain balance.

The risk for developing diseases that affect the sensory systems is greater in older adults. In isolation, a single impairment may not appear to have a significant effect on balance. However, defects in multiple systems can result in a devastating effect on an individual's ability to function. The relationship between incremental increase in sensory system decrement and functional loss is not linear as the systems are interconnected and interdependent. When multiple systems are involved, the term *multisensory impairment* is used.

Older adults experiencing multisensory impairment usually complain of imbalance, unsteadiness, dizziness, lightheadedness, and/or fear of falling when standing or walking. The symptoms usually subside with sitting or holding onto a stationary support. This improvement is due not to physical support, but due to increased proprioceptive input as to body position. A cane functions as much as a "feeler" as an extra supporting appendage. Typically, these symptoms do not develop acutely but gradually over a number of years. Patients may report a gradual onset of imbalance that has led to a decline in their ability to manage in dark environments or walk on uneven surfaces in their homes or community. Fear of falling may result in self-imposed limitations of activity. This reduction in activity further compromises function due to deconditioning and leads to complaints of fatigue and unsteadiness.

Many older persons report feeling "dizzy" when in actuality they feel a sense of imbalance. Terms such as lightheadedness may also be used for feeling unsteady or for presyncope. Those experiencing multisensory impairment may rarely report a sense of spinning or vertigo, which is a hallmark sign of vestibular impairment, but this is an uncommon description. Dizziness may also be due to systemic factors such as cardiovascular or metabolic abnormalities. It is often difficult to get an accurate description of symptoms, but it is worth the effort in order to accurately assess the etiology of symptoms.

The prevalence of dizziness in the elderly population is significant. Aggarwal et al. (1) reported an average prevalence of 9.6% in those over the age of 65, with those over the age of 85 reporting dizziness 18.4% of the time. The population worldwide is becoming older at a higher rate, which increases the importance of addressing multisensory impairment in older persons.

NORMAL AGE-RELATED CHANGES

Changes in sensory systems have been well documented in the literature. Baloh et al. (2) documented a decrease in gain of the vestibulo-ocular reflex in a longitudinal study of normal older adults. A loss of neurons in the vestibular nucleus between 40 and 90 years of age, occurring at a rate of approximately 3% per decade, has also been reported (3). Rauch et al. (4) documented a loss of hair cells, thereby decreasing the sensitivity of the peripheral system to high-frequency head movement that is often required for many activities of daily living. There are reductions in the gain of smooth pursuit and increases in saccade latencies with age.

Somatosensory changes in the older adult lead to a two- to tenfold decrease in the vibration threshold, indicating a reduced ability to feel the quality of contact between themselves and the surface below (5,6). A decrease in muscle spindle activity, sensitivity of skin receptors, and joint receptor activity also negatively influence postural control. Brocklehurst et al. (7) and Lord et al. (8) found that this age-related loss in somatosensation led to impaired control of postural sway and higher risk of falling.

The visual system degrades with age as well. Common age-related changes include a decrease in visual acuity, depth perception, and contrast sensitivity. The visual field narrows, reducing peripheral visual input. Behaviorally, these changes adversely affect the older adult's ability to accurately perceive their environment, including changes in surface conditions. Difficulty in avoiding obstacles, negotiating curbs and stairs, and efficiently moving in low light conditions may result. An increased risk for falling due to visual impairments is well documented and outlined later in the chapter.

PATHOLOGICAL SENSORY CHANGES IN THE OLDER ADULT

Although many older adults age successfully without documented pathology, the risk for developing many disease processes is higher. The labyrinthine system is vulnerable to vascular changes due to atherosclerosis, caused by cardiac disease or diabetes mellitus. Medications that impair balance may exert a greater effect on the older adult. The somatosensory system can be affected by peripheral neuropathy. According to Richardson and Ashton-Miller (9), the prevalence of peripheral neuropathy in developed countries may be as high as 20%. Diabetes mellitus accounts for many of these cases, but as many as 10% of adults have peripheral neuropathy from other causes. Richardson et al. (10,11) also found that older adults with identified peripheral neuropathy on electromyogram (EMG) had an increased risk of falling by a factor of 20 when compared to age- and sex-matched adults with normal peripheral nerves.

Changes to the visual system due to disease processes can also affect the older adult. Diabetes mellitus, multiple sclerosis, and myasthenia gravis can cause visual changes. Cataracts reduce visual acuity, although lens implants can now significantly reduce this visual deficit. Macular degeneration reduces foveal vision, while essentially maintaining the peripheral visual field. In contrast, glaucoma reduces peripheral vision, creating "tunnel vision." All of these diseases significantly impact an elderly adult from being able to accurately perceive their environment.

In addition to peripheral changes due to pathology, changes to the central nervous system (CNS) and its ability to integrate information are also more common in the older adult. Stroke and vascular changes in the CNS can affect integration and processing of information. Kerber et al. (12) found that higher ventricular-brain ratios, more frontal lobe atrophy, and more subcortical white matter lesions were found on magnetic resonance images (MRIs) in older adults with disequilibrium than with matched-age controls.

SOMATOSENSORY SCREENING

Several aspects of somatosensory function should be screened in order to determine the function of this system. A thorough screening should not take more than a few minutes and will be essentially painless for the patient. Because the primary focus is on balance function, these tests should be performed on the lower extremities, with the shoes and socks removed. Figure 1 illustrates a somatosensory screening test. As will be outlined in more detail later in the chapter, the use of a pain and sensation diagram may be helpful in gaining the patient's perception of sensory loss. Often the patient is unaware of the sensation loss or the extent of the impairment.

Vibration Sense

Vibration sense is tested by using a tuning fork. The vibrating fork is placed on a bony process, usually the first metatarsal head, the lateral malleolus, and/or the

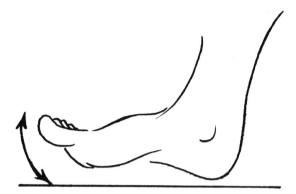

Figure 1 Proprioception should be tested by holding the lateral borders of the appendage and moving it up or down. The patient is asked to report whether their toe is "up" or "down" relative to the ground. Deficits in proprioception are never a normal finding in older adults.

fibular head or patella. The patient can be asked to vocalize the exact moment when the vibration stops, and the tester can stop the vibration with their fingers while maintaining contact of the fork with the skin. Another method, less objective, is to have the patient compare the tuning fork vibration on one extremity to the other. The difficulty with this comparison is that the vibration provided to the patient will vary depending on how hard one taps the tuning fork.

Proprioception

In order to test proprioception, one must hold both a proximal joint and the distal limb by its bony processes and move the distal limb up and down in small excursions (Fig. 1). It is important that one not touch too much of the toe or you will provide additional sensory input, making it easier for the subject to be accurate with the testing. The patient is asked to give the direction that the limb is moving while the eyes are closed. It is important to remember that the proprioceptive system is very sensitive and can sense movement in as little as 0.3°, so movement should be in very small excursions (9). Another gross test of proprioception, called *placing,* is to hold the limb in a similar manner and ask the patient to place the opposite limb in exactly the same position. Gross dysfunction can be ascertained quickly with this test. If deficits are noted, a neurologist should be contacted.

Cutaneous Sensation

Light touch is tested with the patient sitting with eyes closed, and the tester lightly touching the skin. Moving touch requires the patient to verbalize the direction that the tester moves on the limb. Taking two sharp objects, such as both ends of a protractor, tests two-point discrimination while randomly touching one or two points to the patient's skin. The patient must determine how many points are touching. The points can be varied in distance from one another to determine sensitivity. In sharp/dull testing, the tester randomly places a sharp or a dull object on the patient's skin, and the patient is asked to identify the object as either sharp or dull. All peripheral nerve and dermatome areas should be included in the testing.

Hot and Cold Sensation

Hot and cold sensation is impaired in many disease processes, and the patient may not be aware of the deficit. Loss or impaired hot/cold sensation can lead to significant safety risk. One way to test hot and cold is to use a metal object that has been heated or cooled, and place it on the patient's skin. Test tubes or similar containers of hot and cold water can also be used. As many patients have sensitive skin, one must ensure that the temperature is not too extreme.

Laboratory Tests of Sensory Loss

A nerve conduction velocity test can be performed by a physician or physical therapist and is used to assess sensory loss, tingling, pain, muscle cramping, or unexplained weakness distally. Typically, the test does not cause much pain as an electric shock is sent through the nerve. The test provides information about the speed of the nerve transmission. The nerve conduction velocity is most often accompanied by the more painful needle EMG test. A fine wire needle is inserted into the muscle to determine the speed of nerve transmission and also the examiner will "listen" to the sound of the muscle to make the diagnosis. The test takes approximately 25 minutes to 1.5 hours to perform.

VISUAL SCREENING

Directional E Test

Screening a person's visual acuity is important and can be performed in the physician's office. The easiest way to quickly assess vision is to use a directional E eye chart to determine the patient's acuity. Several studies have related falls to impairments in vision (13–16). Abdelhafiz and Austin (17) suggest that visual impairments are related to hip fracture in older persons. In addition to screening for visual acuity, depth perception and contrast sensitivity can be screened as both additional visual characteristics have been related to falls in older persons. Although the directional E test is the easiest to perform, testing contrast sensitivity will provide the clinician with greater insight into the patient's fall risk.

Contrast Sensitivity

An effective screening tool that has been directly related to falls is impaired contrast sensitivity (14). When testing contrast sensitivity, one has the patient read the letters until they can no longer see any (Fig. 2). The letters at the top of the chart are dark and then gradually become lighter. Poor contrast sensitivity has been related to falls risk. Having sharp contrast at the edge of objects such as curbs and the edge of steps can aid persons with impaired contrast sensitivity.

Macular Degeneration

Jack et al. (18) suggest that low vision is related to falling in older adults admitted to the hospital. A through eye history will help the physician better understand their patient's balance deficits when they present with multisensory disequilibrium. Referral to an ophthalmologist who specializes in low vision might be a consideration.

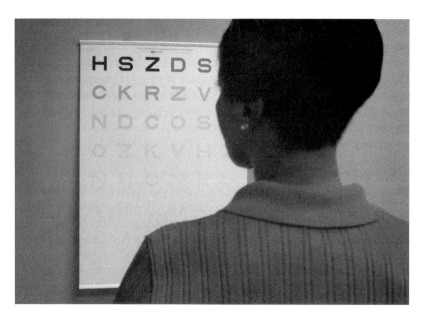

Figure 2 Testing for contrast sensitivity. A person stands in front of the chart and attempts to read as many letters as possible on the wall.

Cataracts

Brannan et al. (16) studied fall rates before and after cataract surgery. They demonstrated that after cataract surgery, person's fall rates decreased from 37% to 19% six months following surgery. As part of the history, it is important to determine if the person presently has cataracts.

Visual Field Testing

In order to determine if the patient has normal visual fields, the physician can sit in front of the patient or stand behind them. One should ask patients to look straight ahead and to tell you when they see your finger appear in their periphery. The physician is to move a finger from behind the patient's head towards the front on both the right and left sides and from over the top of their head. Looking for right/left symmetry in responses is important. Deficits in visual field testing could indicate either a peripheral or central disorder and if identified, would need further investigation to determine the location of the deficit.

Multifocal Lenses

Determining if the patient has multifocal lenses is important. Lord et al. (19) suggest that multifocal lenses impair both edge-contrast sensitivity and depth perception. These factors may predispose a person to greater risk of falling, especially on stairs. Asking about what type of lenses they have and when their last vision screen was is an important component of a through assessment of an older adult. If possible, having separate reading and distance lenses can help to solve the problem.

Cranial Nerves 3, 4, and 6

Assessing the motor performance of cranial nerves 3, 4, and 6 takes only a few seconds but can provide a wealth of information. The easiest method is to ask the patient to follow an H that you draw with your finger in front of the patient's face. When the eyes are following your finger, you are assessing all of the extraocular eye movements. For example, right and left horizontal eye movements assess the integrity of the lateral and medial rectus. If a deficit is identified, the patient should be referred to either an opthalmologist or a neurologist.

VESTIBULAR SCREENING FOR OLDER PEOPLE

There are several clinical tools that can be used to attempt to determine if the patient has a peripheral vestibular disorder. None are foolproof and the *best* way to test for vestibular dysfunction is through the use of a full vestibular test battery including calorics, an oculomotor screen, rotational chair testing, and computerized dynamic posturography. Sometimes circumstances do not permit the testing. The sensitivity and specificity of various clinical tools will be described.

Dix-Hallpike Test

The Dix-Hallpike test is crucial to assess in older adults as many patients have benign paroxysmal positional vertigo (BPPV), but it has not been diagnosed (20). It is suggested that the person start in long sitting with the head rotated 45° to either the right or the left. Then the person is brought to the head hanging position (approximately 30° over the edge of the bed). Excessive extension should be avoided in older persons as it might compromise their vertebrobasilar circulation. The speed of the Dix-Hallpike may need to be modified in older persons. If done too quickly, the person might experience a neck injury. With persons with a positive history of BPPV, sometimes a repeat Dix-Hallpike may be positive whereas the first maneuver was negative. If positive for a posterior canal disorder (the most common), the patient will exhibit a torsional upbeating nystagmus. The characteristic nystagmus is best visualized with Frenzel lenses or an infrared goggle system.

One must be careful to *not* perform the Dix-Hallpike test with persons with neck problems (cervical stenosis, cervical radiculopathies, significant vertebral artery disease, disc disease) and with persons with additional spinal deformities (Pagets disease, spinal cord injuries, low back dysfunction, and ankylosing spondylitis), depending on the severity of the disease. Persons with a history on examination of transient ischemic attacks and rheumatoid arthritis should also be carefully assessed. If there is a concern about performing the Dix-Hallpike test, one might consider using a tilt table to perform the maneuver. The head position changes in relation to gravity while on the tilt table but you will not be changing or stressing the neck and back of the older adult. Older adults feel more comfortable performing the test with their legs flexed in order to avoid low back pain. Having another person present can help to decrease their anxiety of having the test performed, as there is fear associated with placing the patient in the provocative position.

In addition, one can have the older adult with restricted neck motion move their entire body to the side if they do not have adequate neck range of motion prior to performing the Dix-Hallpike maneuver. If you decide that it is too difficult to assess the person in the office and send the patient to a physical therapist for the assessment and treatment of the BPPV, it is imperative that you provide details of the patient's laboratory testing, your concerns about doing the Dix-Hallpike, and your suspicion of BPPV. They will be able to manage the patient more successfully with greater knowledge of the patient's medical history and with lower risk of harm to the patient.

The Head Thrust

The head thrust test is a high acceleration movement of the head typically performed in the plane of the horizontal canal (21,22). It can also be performed in the other two planes of the semicircular canals. The patient tries to maintain fixation on a distant object during the test and one attempts to determine if the patient produces a catch up saccade. The second law of Ewald (Ewald, 1892, in Ref. 23) suggests that an asymmetric response occurs during the high-velocity movement. It must be performed passively, be unpredictable, and be of high acceleration to see the compensatory eye movement (22). The sensitivity of the test has been reported to be 54% and specificity was reported to be 100% (24).

Gaze Holding

It is important to determine if a patient can focus on an object without nystagmus. The patient is asked to focus on a nonmoving object. One can best visualize the nystagmus with an ophthalmoscope, as it is difficult with just one's vision to assess if there is movement. One should focus on the fundus to determine if there is movement. If there is movement, it could indicate that the person has an acute peripheral disorder or a brain disorder.

Questionnaires

In an older adult, in order to assess somatosensory impairments, one should have the patient complete a pain diagram (Fig. 3). On the diagram, which depicts the ventral and dorsal aspect of the body, the patient has an opportunity to describe any pain or sensory loss that they might be experiencing. The pain scale can be quantified and a comparison can be made in future visits to the clinic.

Another helpful paper and pencil tool that can provide additional information to the physician is the Activities-Specific Balance Confidence (ABC) Scale (25–27). It is a 16-item questionnaire that was developed to assess balance confidence in older persons that is rated on a 10-point scale from 0 to 100. Scores are added and then divided by 1600 for a percent score. The ABC has been used in persons with vestibular disorders. In older adults, scores of less than 80 indicate functional impairments and scores of less than 50 indicate that the person is often housebound (28). The ABC could be used as a screening tool to determine the patient's perceived functional impairment (29). The staff can supply and score the questionnaire prior to the patient's physician interview.

A third questionnaire particularly helpful to an otolaryngologist is the Dizziness Handicap Inventory (DHI) (30). The DHI consists of 25 items that assist the physician in determining the patient's extent of perceived dizziness. With DHI scores of >60, people had an increased chance of reporting a fall (Whitney et al., in press).

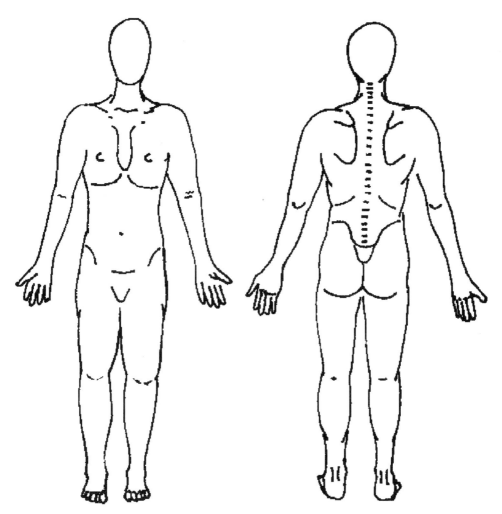

Figure 3 A pain diagram that can be used to determine if the patient has sensory loss or impairment.

Quick Screening Techniques to Assess Fall Risk

One of the easiest methods to assess fall risk and also help in the diagnosis of a vestibular disorder is to have the older adults stand on a piece of high-density temper foam (T-foam). Weber and Cass (31) suggested that the ability to stand on the T-foam correlated to computerized dynamic posturography. They reported a sensitivity of 95% and a specificity of 90% in persons with vestibular dysfunction on conditions 4 and 5 (standing on foam, eyes open and closed).

The foam pad must be placed on a nonslip surface and the patient must be carefully guarded to ensure that they do not fall. If the person falls off the foam with eyes open, it suggests that they have difficulty walking on uneven surfaces, even with good light. When falling off the T-foam with the eyes closed, it may suggest a vestibular disorder. These persons will report that they have difficulty walking in the dark. One must closely guard the patient as they attempt to stand on the high-density T-foam, as it is not uncommon for them to fall off the foam.

An easy way to assess overall strength is to ask the person to move from sit to stand without using their arms. If they have difficulty with this task, they are at risk for falling (32).

The Romberg test can help to provide an assessment of overall dorsal column function. It was designed as a test of lower extremity sensation. Persons with diabetes are unable to maintain the Romberg position and many community-living older adults also have difficulty performing the Romberg test. Not all older adults with vestibular dysfunction fall during the Romberg test. Guard the person closely, as it is not uncommon for the person to fall.

When assessing an older adult, it is recommended that all three tests be performed. If they fall during the Romberg test, it may or may not indicate significant pathology in the older person. A positive Romberg is seen in community-living older adults. If the patient falls during standing on the foam pad and/or cannot rise from the chair, a referral to physical therapy may be indicated.

INTERVENTION FOR MULTISENSORY DISEQUILIBRIUM

Once an assessment of sensory systems is complete and impairments identified, the next step involves appropriate medical and rehabilitative intervention. A review of medications is always advised in order to identify possible adverse effects. A careful review of the history may reveal an underlying etiology, as outlined in Table 1. If any of the sensory impairments can be treated medically, the appropriate physician should address this. Table 2 lists disorders and diseases that can cause sensory or gait dysfunction in older adults.

Rehabilitation for multisensory disequilibrium has been found to be effective in managing the balance deficit and functional impairment. A systematic approach of assessing both sensory and motor deficits, functional impairment, and disability is followed by treatment that addresses education and improving function. Fall risk reduction education is an integral part of the therapy process, as described in Chapter 14, "Balance Rehabilitation." If a sensory system has a partial or temporary impairment (visual, vestibular, or somatosensory), the therapist attempts to improve function of the impaired system by increasing the weighting or use of that system while decreasing the use of the other two sensory systems. For somatosensation, the therapist will encourage eyes closed activities on a firm surface in order to decrease the use of visual feedback. Also, Maki et al. (33) demonstrated that patients with cutaneous impairment improved in postural reactions with a raised boundary on the plantar surface of their feet. Older adults also demonstrated less postural sway when they wore vibrating insoles compared to young persons (34). Physical therapists may be able to provide avenues for patients to improve somatosensation and thereby improve overall stability. If damage to a sensory system is permanent or progressive, in the case of complete bilateral vestibular loss or severe visual impairment, rehabilitation focuses on compensation by improving the use of the "better" functioning sensory systems (35). In some cases, the best avenue for intervention is to improve strength and motor function, and to teach compensation for the sensory impairment(s). The use of a straight cane is a good compensatory tool for impaired visual and somatosensory systems (36). The upper extremity can assist in providing extra somatosensory feedback, while the cane helps in assessing depth and uneven surfaces that the visual system may not be able to perceive (36,37). Reversing the effects of deconditioning is essential in this population, as the lack

Table 1 What Older Adults Complain of, Possible Working Diagnoses, and Tests to Perform to Confirm the Diagnosis

Patient comments	Possible diagnosis	Tests to perform
I can't stand for a long time. If I stand for longer than a few minutes, my legs start to shake.	Orthostatic tremor Severe muscle weakness	Needle EMG Refer to a physical therapist
I get dizzy when I get out of bed or when I go from sitting to standing.	Orthostatic hypotension or BPPV	Supine, sitting, and standing BP (check for a drop in diastolic pressure of 10 μmmHg or more) Dix-Hallpike test Check for bruits Possible referral to a cardiologist
I am slowing down and falling. I lose my balance when I turn while walking. It is hard to roll over in bed.	Parkinson's disease or a basal ganglia disorder	Refer to a neurologist
I lose my balance. Sometimes I see double.	Stroke, head injury, chronic subdural hematoma	MRI
I feel like I spin when I roll over in bed.	BPPV	Dix-Hallpike test and either treat or refer to a physical therapist
I faint sometimes and have fallen.	Autonomic dysfunction, transient ischemic attack	Refer to a neurologist and/or cardiologist
I fall down but do not pass out.	Attack of Tumarkins or a true drop attack	Treat conservatively for Meinere's disease depending on their risk of fracture and send to a neurologist
I feel like my feet have lead in them—they are heavy.	Peripheral neuropathy, diabetes	Needle EMG, vibration, and distal sensory testing
I keep bumping into things and I can't see as well. I don't see people coming up next to me.	Visual impairment: cataracts, glaucoma, multifocal lenses, visual field deficit; stroke, head trauma	Visual screen, refer to ophthalmologist
I am losing confidence; I feel that I need a cane, I am afraid to leave the house.	Multisensory disequilibrium	Assess sensation, vision, and balance

Abbreviations: EMG, electromyogram; MRI, magentic resonance imaging; BPPV, benign paroxysmal positional vertigo.

Table 2 Disorders and Diseases That Can Cause Sensory Loss or Gait Disorders in Older Adults

Brain disorders
    Basal ganglia disorders (Parkinson's disease)
    Cerebellar degeneration
    Chronic subdural hematoma
    Dementia
    Depression
    Head trauma
    Normal pressure hydrocephalus
    Orthostatic tremor
    Stroke
    Transient ischemic attacks
Spinal disorders
    Cervical myelopathy
    Mononeuropathy
    Peripheral neuropathy
    Spinal stenosis
    Spinal tumors
Systemic disorders
    Alcoholism
    Diabetes Mellitus
    Neuropathy (HIV, Lyme disease)
Vascular disorders
    Baroreceptor dysfunction
    Postural hypotension
Visual disorders
    Macular degeneration
Medication
    Medication-induced
    Status post organ transplant
Anterior horn cell disorder
    Amytrophic lateral sclerosis
Musculoskeletal
    Foot deformities
    Weakness

of balance leads to less physical activity, which only exacerbates the deficits. By providing a safe environment to exercise in a rehabilitation setting, as well as sound recommendations for activities at home, patients can increase their activity level safely with greater confidence (38,39). Efficacy of such rehabilitation has been documented by Rose and Clark and Shumway-Cook et al. (39–44) in which multiple and specific dimensions of the postural control system demonstrated significant improvements in balance and mobility.

In summary, multisensory disequilibrium is a disorder that affects a significant number of older adults. It results in an overall sense of imbalance and instability while in an upright position. It involves degradation of the sensory systems responsible for balance function, both due to normal aging and pathological disease processes. The most effective way to manage the disorder is by a thorough assessment of the somatosensory, visual, and vestibular systems, and address intervention and rehabilitation according to the deficits identified. Improvement in overall functional mobility is sometimes possible with targeted intervention as long as appropriate causative factors are determined.

REFERENCES

1. Aggarwal NT, Bennett DA, et al. The prevalence of dizziness and its association with functional disability in a biracial community population. J Gerontol A Biol Sci Med Sci 2000; 55(5):M288–292.
2. Baloh RW, Enrietto J, et al. Age-related changes in vestibular function: a longitudinal study. Ann NY Acad Sci 2001; 942:210–219.
3. Lopez I, Honrubia V, et al. Aging and the human vestibular nucleus. J Vestib Res 1997; 7(1):77–85.
4. Rauch SD, Velazquez-Villasenor L, et al. Decreasing hair cell counts in aging humans. Ann NY Acad Sci 2001; 942:220–227.
5. Perret E, Regli F. Age and the perceptual threshold for vibratory stimuli. Eur Neurol 1970; 4(2):65–76.
6. Bergin PS, Bronstein AM, et al. Body sway and vibration perception thresholds in normal aging and in patients with polyneuropathy. J Neurol Neurosurg Psychiatry 1995; 58(3):335–340.
7. Brocklehurst JC, Robertson D, et al. Clinical correlates of sway in old age—sensory modalities. Age Ageing 1982; 11(1):1–10.
8. Lord SR, Ward JA, et al. Physiological factors associated with falls in older community-dwelling women. J Am Geriatr Soc 1994; 42(10):1110–1117.
9. Richardson JK, Ashton-Miller JA. Peripheral neuropathy: an often-overlooked cause of falls in the elderly. Postgrad Med 1996; 99(6):161–172.
10. Richardson JK, Ching C, et al. The relationship between electromyographically documented peripheral neuropathy and falls. J Am Geriatr Soc 1992; 40(10):1008–1012.
11. Richardson JK, Hurvitz EA. Peripheral neuropathy: a true risk factor for falls. J Gerontol A Biol Sci Med Sci 1995; 50(4):M211–215.
12. Kerber KA, Enrietto JA, et al. Disequilibrium in older people—a prospective study. Neurology 1998; 51(2):574–580.
13. Lord SR, Menz HB. Visual contributions to postural stability in older adults. Gerontology 2000; 46(6):306–310.
14. Lord SR, Dayhew J. Visual risk factors for falls in older people. J Am Geriatr Soc 2001; 49(5):508–515.
15. Tinetti ME. Where is the vision for fall prevention? J Am Geriatr Soc 2001; 49:676–677.
16. Brannan S, Dewar C, et al. A prospective study of the rate of falls before and after cataract surgery. Br J Ophthalmol 2003; 87(5):560–562.
17. Abdelhafiz AH, Austin CA. Visual factors should be assessed in older people presenting with falls or hip fracture. Age Ageing 2003; 32(1):26–30.
18. Jack CI, Smith T, et al. Prevalence of low vision in elderly patients admitted to an acute geriatric unit in Liverpool: elderly people who fall are more likely to have low vision. Gerontology 1995; 41(5):280–285.
19. Lord SR, Dayhew J, et al. Multifocal glasses impair edge-contrast sensitivity and depth perception and increase the risk of falls in older people. J Am Geriatr Soc 2002; 50(11):1760–1766.
20. Oghalai JS, Manolidis S, et al. Unrecognized benign paroxysmal positional vertigo in elderly patients. Otolaryngol Head Neck Surg 2000; 122(5):630–634.
21. Halmagyi GM, Curthoys IS, et al. The human horizontal vestibulo-ocular reflex in response to high-acceleration stimulation before and after unilateral vestibular neurectomy. Exp Brain Res 1990; 81(3):479–490.
22. Cremer PD, Halmagyi GM, et al. Semicircular canal plane head impulses detect absent function of individual semicircular canals. Brain 1998; 121(Pt 4):699–716.

23. Della Santina CC, Cremer PD, et al. Comparison of head thrust test with head autorotation test reveals that the vestibulo-ocular reflex is enhanced during voluntary head movements. Arch Otolaryngol Head Neck Surg 2002; 128(9):1044–1054.

24. Oliva M, Martin Garcia MA, et al. The head-thrust test (HTT): physiopathological considerations and its clinical use in daily practice. Acta Otorrinolaringol Esp 1998; 49(4):275–279.

25. Powell LE, Myers AM. The Activities-Specific Balance Confidence (ABC) Scale. J Gerontol Ser A Biol Sci Med Sci 1995; 50(1):M28–34.

26. Myers AM, Powell LE, et al. Psychological indicators of balance confidence: relationship to actual and perceived abilities. J Gerontol Ser A Biol Sci Med Sci 1996; 51(1):M37–43.

27. Myers RL, Laenger CJ. Virtual reality in rehabilitation. Disability Rehabil 1998; 20(3):111–112.

28. Myers AM, Fletcher P, et al. Discriminative and evaluative properties of the Activities-Specific Balance Confidence (ABC) Scale. J Gerontol 1998; 53A(4):M287–294.

29. Whitney SL, Hudak MT, et al. The activities-specific balance confidence scale and the dizziness handicap inventory: a comparison. J Vestib Res 1999; 9(4):253–259.

30. Jacobson GP, Newman CW. The development of the dizziness handicap inventory. Arch Otolaryngol Head Neck Surg 1990; 116(April):424–427.

31. Weber PC, Cass SP. Clinical assessment of postural stability. Am J Otol 1993; 14(6): 566–569.

32. Lord SR, Murray SM, et al. Sit-to-stand performance depends on sensation, speed, balance, and psychological status in addition to strength in older people. Gerontol A Biol Sci Med Sci 2002; 57(8):M539–543.

33. Maki BE, Perry SD, et al. Effect of facilitation of sensation from planter foot-surface boundaries on postural stabilization in young and older adults. J Gerontol Ser A Biol Sci Med Sci 1999; 54(6):M281–287.

34. Priplata AA, Niemi JB, et al. Vibrating insoles and balance control in elderly people. Lancet 2003; 362(9390):1123–1124.

35. Herdman SJ. Physical therapy management of vestibular disorders in older patients. Phys Ther Pract 1992; 1(1):77–87.

36. Nandapalan V, Smith CA, et al. Objective measurement of the benefit of walking sticks in peripheral vestibular balance disorders, using the sway weigh balance platform. J Laryngol Otol 1995; 109(9):836–840.

37. Jeka JJ. Light touch contact as a balance aid. Phys Ther 1997; 77(5):476–487.

38. Cohen HS, Kimball KT. Increased independence and decreased vertigo after vestibular rehabilitation. Otolaryngol Head Neck Surg 2003; 128(1):60–70.

39. Whitney SL, Wrisley DM, et al. The effect of age on vestibular rehabilitation outcomes. Laryngoscope 2002; 112(10):1785–1790.

40. Rose DJ, Clark S. Can the control of bodily orientation be significantly improved in a group of older adults with a history of falling? J Am Geriatric Soc 2000; 48: 275–282.

41. Shumway-Cook A, Gruber W, et al. The effect of multidimensional exercises on balance, mobility, and fall risk in community-dwelling older adults. Phys Ther 1997; 7(1):46–57.

42. Horak FB, Jonesrycewicz C, et al. Effects of vestibular rehabilitation on dizziness and imbalance. Otolaryngol Head Neck Surg 1992; 106(2):175–180.

43. Shepard NT, Telian SA. Programmatic vestibular rehabilitation. Head Neck Surg 1995; 112:173–182.

44. Strupp M, Arbusow V, et al. Vestibular exercises improve central vestibulospinal compensation after vestibular neuritis. Neurology 1998; 51(3):838–844.

ANNOTATED BIBLIOGRAPHY

Lord SR, Dayhew J. Visual risk factors for falls in older people. J Am Geriatr Soc 2001; 49(5):508–515.

This paper provides an excellent overview of the visual deficits that are commonly associated with falling in older persons.

Oghalai JS, Manolidis S, et al. Unrecognized benign paroxysmal positional vertigo in elderly patients. Otolaryngol Head Neck Surg 2000; 122(5):630–634.

The article describes a group of older adults who present to the clinic without complaints of dizziness or balance disorders. Nine percent had undiagnosed BPPV and 61% had dizziness when questioned.

10
Mal de Debarquement

Timothy C. Hain and Dario A. Yacovino
Departments of Physical Therapy, Neurology, and Otolaryngology, Northwestern University Medical School, Chicago, Illinois, U.S.A.

GENERAL DESCRIPTION OF THE CLINICAL PROBLEM

Mal de debarquement (MDD), literally "sickness of disembarkment," refers to inappropriate sensations of movement after exposure to motion. The syndrome typically follows a sea voyage, but similar sensations have been described following extended train travel, space flight, and after experience within a slowly rotating room (1,2). Symptoms usually include sensations of rocking and swaying accompanied by imbalance, but not rotational vertigo. MDD is distinguished from motion sickness, air sickness, simulator sickness, or seasickness (mal de mer) because subjects are predominantly symptom-free during the period of motion. MDD is distinguished from "landsickness" or post-motion vertigo by duration. Landsickness typically lasts less than 48 hours (3,4). We, like most other authors reporting on MDD, define it almost exclusively as a syndrome that persists for at least one month (4–7). It should be noted, however, that some authors refer to the very common short-lived, post-motion vertigo as MDD, and the longer duration form as "persistent MDD" (3).

As of 2003, only 46 subjects with mal de debarquement as defined above have been described in the literature (4–7). However, this syndrome is probably more common than the literature might lead us to believe, as the level of awareness in the general population as well as in health personnel is very low.

MDD occurs most commonly in middle-aged women (Fig. 1) but about 25% of reported cases of MDD have been in individuals over the age of 65. It has never been reported in children, and it is rarely encountered in persons in their 20s or 30s. The prevalence of vulnerability to MDD in the population is unknown.

BASIC SCIENCE

Literature describing persons with persistent MDD is sparse. Brown and Baloh (5) reported six cases of MDD in 1987. They noted that despite anecdotal reference to this syndrome, there had been no published definition or description. Five of their six subjects were females, ranging in age from 38 to 71 years. Five of the subjects

125

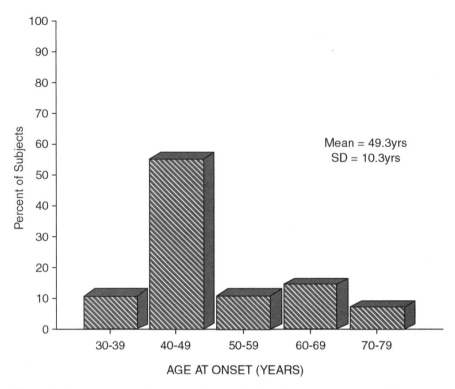

Figure 1 Age at onset of MDD syndrome, in decades. *Source*: From Ref. 7.

developed MDD after boat travel, with durations of exposure that varied from under five hours to 70 days. Subjects typically got little relief from antivertiginous medication. Three subjects exhibited a direction-changing positional nystagmus during electronystagmography. Caloric testing was normal in all. One patient had abnormally prolonged optokinetic afternystagmus, but the authors did not indicate whether this response was tested in all patients. Brown and Baloh suggested that MDD syndrome is caused by an abnormally persistent central nervous system (CNS) adaptation to the seagoing environment that causes a failure or delay of readaptation to the earth-stable environment.

Murphy (6) reported four cases of MDD. All of these were female, ranging between 36 and 48 years of age. The duration of motion exposure ranged from eight hours to seven days, and the duration of symptoms between four weeks and one year. Three subjects developed MDD after exposure to water travel, the remaining patient after sleeping on a water bed. One patient had direction-changing positional nystagmus. Amitriptyline was helpful in one patient and lorazepam in another. Murphy suggests that the sensations described by subjects are consistent with a perception of abnormal linear acceleration, and that because the utricle is known to be responsible for responding to linear acceleration, MDD syndrome may result from "utricular dysfunction." Murphy notes hormonal interaction with the vestibular system or brain, and/or inability of the brain to coordinate vestibular and ocular input as other possible causes.

Mair (4) reported 10 cases of MDD. Again, all subjects were female, with ages ranging from 15 to 66 years. Sea travel provoked symptoms in eight and air travel in the remainder. Onset followed exposure variously from two hours to two days, with all but one in less than 18 hours. While one patient had a symptom duration of only three days, all others had symptoms persisting for at least one month, ranging up to two years. Mair suggested that defective or delayed readaptation following cessation of motion might be an important causative factor. Mair also noted that gender differences have been previously shown to exist in susceptibility to motion sickness and in the degree to which visual cues are used for orientation.

Hain and associates (7) reported 27 cases of MDD. Nearly all were middle-aged females (26/27, mean age 49.3). Duration of symptoms ranged from six months to 10 years (mean 3.5, SD 2.5). Symptoms were constant in 85%. Neither meclizine nor transdermal scopolamine was helpful. Benzodiazepines were of the most benefit. Balance rehabilitation physical therapy was undertaken by 15 patients, who on average reported a small benefit.

Other authors have reported that a large percentage of persons disembarking from seagoing voyages experience a brief MDD syndrome, which by our definition would instead be termed "landsickness." Gordon et al. (8) surveyed 234 healthy crew members of seagoing vessels. They reported a high incidence of a short-lived MDD symptom complex (73%). Presumably, the majority of their subjects were male. As a follow-up to that study, Gordon et al. (3) studied 116 male crew members of seagoing vessels. The subjects ranged in age from 18 to 33 years and sailed once or twice a week. Seventy-two percent reported having experienced MDD. The duration of symptoms ranged from one minute to two days, lasting less than six hours in 88% of the men. They found a significant relationship between susceptibility to seasickness and the occurrence of MDD. A similar short-lived syndrome has been reported after flight-simulator training of pilots (9). None of the subjects in the Gordon et al. study would qualify as having MDD according to our criteria.

Similarly, Cohen (10) studied professional and amateur crew members participating in sailing on a 117-year-old sailing vessel. Cohen's sample included 36 men and 23 women. After the first sailing day, 37% reported landsickness symptoms, increasing to 41% after the second day, and then decreasing to 20% after further experience. Males and females did not differ significantly in the incidence, intensity, or duration of symptoms.

A number of other symptoms are reported by persons with MDD. Many suffer from migraine, ear pain, tinnitus, and ear fullness. A sensitivity to flashing lights and fluorescent lighting is commonly seen. Busy patterns can induce nausea. Also, symptoms of rocking may intensify while shopping in malls or grocery stores, or when walking in crowds. This probably reflects "visual dependence," which is often associated with vestibular disorders (11). Ataxia is commonly seen during periods of stress and as fatigue increases throughout the day. Family situations can change as well as employment as these are impacted by the illness. Anxiety and depression are common. Most individuals recover, but many have reoccurrences. Some have a recurrent variant with reactivation following a plane ride, another boat trip, or a long car ride.

POTENTIAL ETIOLOGIC FACTORS IN MDD

Given the consistency of the four studies on MDD, it would appear that, although landsickness may be common in both sexes following motion exposure, it is more likely to persist and become MDD in females. This has some implications regarding possible causes.

Migraine

The prevalence of migraine is estimated at 11% of the general population and about 20% in women during their reproductive years (12,13). Migraine has a similar female predominance at the age of 50 (3:1) when compared to MDD and occurs most commonly at the age of 35. Migraine has been strongly associated with motion sensitivity (14). From our data, almost one-fourth of the subjects fit the International Headache Society (IHS) criteria for migraine, with another almost 30% having recurring headaches (7). However, only one patient had a migraine on the MDD-provoking voyage, and in most of the subjects, the headaches have resolved. Studying a large group of migraine sufferers for MDD syndrome could help clarify the picture.

Hormones

There is a strong predominance of females in studies of MDD and also a relatively narrow age group. The predominance of females greatly exceeds that found in motion sickness among passengers at sea, where the ratio of females to males is about 5:3 (15). Anecdotal evidence suggests that MDD also lasts longer in women than in men. In our study, only about one-third were of postmenopausal ages and none were of premenarchal, suggesting that female hormones may facilitate this syndrome. Murphy (6) noted the age and female predominance in his subjects (4/4) and also postulated a hormonal effect. Based on this same evidence, one could also hypothesize that MDD is somehow related to factors biologically dependent on the presence of two copies of the X chromosome. On the other hand, landsickness clearly occurs in a large percentage of men after ocean voyages. These issues could be clarified by obtaining more data in this age group, studying males who are taking estrogen (e.g., for control of prostate cancer), and by further studies of MDD in large groups.

Inner Ear Pathology, in Particular, Meniere's Disease

The symptomatology of MDD subjects can overlap with Meniere's disease as many subjects complain of aural fullness, tinnitus, and hearing impairment (7). While no formal study has been done, it is possible that some patients with MDD actually have a variant of Meniere's disease, which coincidentally flared up following motion exposure.

Persistent CNS Adaptation to the Seagoing Environment

MDD syndrome does not have the features of a "pathologic" disease, in the sense that it does not appear to follow an injury. Rather, it is provoked by exposure to motion that does not trouble most individuals, at least not in a persistent manner. Movements such as that experienced in a boat expose a person to rhythmic upward and downward movements along with tilts to the left and right. During this time, the brain must adjust leg and body motion so that they counter the rhythmic pattern of shipboard motion. Adaptation to such movement is sometimes called "gaining sea legs."

While the appearance of a rocking sensation as a result of adaptation might seem implausible, as it implies the initiation of an oscillating pattern, experimentally a pendular nystagmus lasting up to 60 minutes can be induced in rabbits by 24 hours of exposure to torsional or parallel swing stimuli (16).

Psychogenic Etiology

MDD does not appear to have a psychogenic basis. Several studies have noted that the relatively late age of onset as well as the lack of other medical complaints is not supportive of a somatization disorder (5,7). The extreme female predominance also is not consistent with a psychogenic etiology, which is generally more evenly distributed according to gender.

History

A typical case history is as follows: A 50-year-old woman went on her first ocean cruise. She had some motion sickness on the cruise, which responded to transdermal scopolamine. After returning from the cruise she developed "landsickness," consisting of imbalance and a rocking sensation accompanied by fatigue and difficulty in concentrating. Her description was "imagine feeling like you are on rough seas 24 hours a day seven days a week."

The typical MDD patient presents with persistent landsickness after a seven-day ocean cruise. They complain of a constant rocking sensation that persists while awake. Frank vertigo (spinning) is unusual. Many patients with MDD report that they are able to drive, but that their symptoms return on getting out of the car. Normal persons may have landsickness for 48 hours, but MDD becomes likely with persistence beyond this time.

Physical Examination

The neurological and otological examination is usually normal, and the purpose of the physical examination is largely to exclude other entities. The tympanic membranes should be inspected for abnormality and hearing should be tested. The eye movements should be checked for nystagmus, impaired pursuit, and saccadic dysmetria or instability.

Neurologically, balance should be assessed with the eyes-closed tandem Romberg test. Most patients with MDD are able to stand for six seconds, in spite of complaints of rocking and unsteadiness. Reflexes and motor power are expected to be normal. Coordination of the limbs, speech, and head should be normal. There should be no tremor, rigidity, or upper motor neuron signs.

Diagnostic maneuvers for dizziness performed with the Frenzel goggles are often very helpful in differential diagnosis of vertigo (17). They should be performed in persons with MDD to exclude alternative diagnoses, particularly benign paroxysmal positional vertigo. There should be no spontaneous nystagmus. Positional testing is generally normal, but it may also sometimes reveal a low-amplitude direction changing positional nystagmus (5). Fistula testing should be performed in the clinic with Frenzel goggles if there is a history of SCUBA diving or onset of symptoms following an airplane flight.

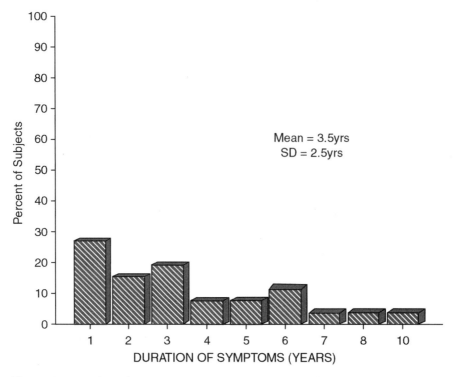

Figure 2 Duration of MDD symptoms. *Source*: From Ref. 7.

DIAGNOSIS OF MDD

The diagnosis is made by a combination of the history (rocking after prolonged exposure to a boat) and exclusion of reasonable alternatives. A typical patient is a woman of appropriate age who has gone on a cruise and who has been rocking for at least a month (Figs. 1, 2). Symptoms that would make MDD less likely would be rotational vertigo, double vision, or bouncing vision.

Table 1 outlines our recommendations for diagnostic testing. Because of the high prevalence of aural fullness, tinnitus, and subjective hearing loss in MDD, tests to exclude Meniere's disease should be done, and if there is a history of plane flight, perilymph fistula should also be considered (7). The electronystagmography (ENG) test result is usually normal, but occasionally it may find unusually strong or prolonged optokinetic afternystagmus or vestibular responses, and there is also

Table 1 Recommended Diagnostic Tests to Exclude Alternative Causes of Ataxia

Audiogram
ENG
ECOG if hearing is abnormal
MRI of brain if neurological examination is abnormal
Blood tests to exclude alternative causes (CBC, blood glucose, FTA, B12)

Abbreviations: ENG, electronystagmography; ECOG, electrocohleography; MRI, magnetic resonance imaging; FTA, fluorescent treponema antibody.

Table 2 Medications Probably Ineffective in MDD

Dramamine
Meclizine
Scopolamine

sometimes direction-changing positional nystagmus, as has been reported by Brown and Baloh (5).

Blood testing is normal in MDD. Nevertheless, blood testing for treatable causes of unsteadiness, such as B_{12} deficiency, syphilis, hypoglycemia, and anemia are recommended, to exclude other disorders. Magnetic resonance imaging (MRI) testing is nearly always normal in persons with MDD, but it is indicated in persons with central findings on neurological examination such as nystagmus or limb ataxia.

TREATMENT OF MDD

We will consider both treatments aimed at preventing MDD and treatments aimed at ameliorating the effects of MDD once it has occurred. If MDD is indeed related to inappropriate vestibular adaptation, medications that slow such adaptation (vestibular suppressants, benzodiazepines) might be tried. We know of no studies to date regarding the prevention of MDD through medication; patients with the recurrent variant of this condition have indicated that low doses of klonapin or lorazepam taken prior to the anticipated motion exposure are often effective. Anticholinergic medications such as scopolamine do not appear to be effective for prevention (7). Antihistamines such as meclizine are also ineffective (Table 2) (7). Certainly, for persons with a history of MDD, avoidance of further prolonged exposure to rocking motion seems prudent.

With respect to treatments of an ongoing MDD syndrome, there is evidence of a positive effect of benzodiazepines and amitriptyline (Table 3) (7). Meclizine and scopolamine were entirely ineffective. Occasionally patients have reported a good response to diverse medications such as gabapentin and carbamazepine. Finally, Brown and Baloh (5), Murphy (6), and Mair (4) all recommend vestibular rehabilitation or exercise for the MDD syndrome, although no results for this intervention were reported. Zimbelman and Walton reported a case of MDD that may have benefited from vestibular rehabilitation (18). However, no formal study has been done proving its efficacy.

In addition to vestibular rehabilitation therapy, medications that speed adaptation, for example, stimulants such as the amphetamine family, might be tried.

Table 3 Treatment of Ongoing Symptoms of MDD with Benzodiazepines

Drug	Dose (mg)	Interval	Adverse effects
Diazepam	2	BID	Sedation Pregnancy cat D
Klonapin	0.5	BID	Sedation Pregnancy cat D

Although there is anecdotal evidence that stimulants may be helpful, again, these medications have not been formally studied for MDD.

ALGORITHM

Figure 3 illustrates a decision tree regarding MDD. The diagnosis should be considered in a person who presents with a persistent rocking sensation following a prolonged movement exposure, such as a seven-day cruise. MDD is probable if the duration of symptoms is at least one month and alternative causes of dizziness have been excluded.

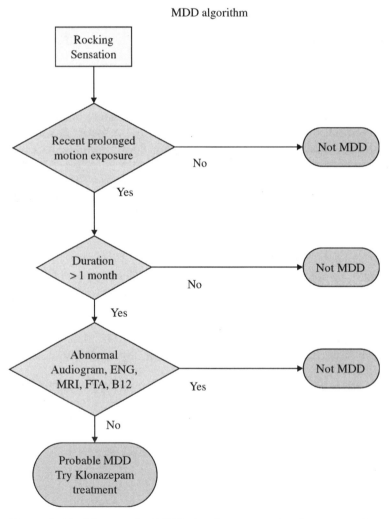

Figure 3 Decision tree for MDD showing progression from presenting symptoms through physical examination and testing to treatment. *Abbreviations*: MRI, magnetic resonance imaging; ENG, electronystagmography; FTA, fluorescent treponema antibody.

SUMMARY

In summary, persistent MDD is a prolonged sensation of rocking, swaying, imbalance, or other motion typically triggered by a seagoing voyage. The disorder appears to occur almost exclusively in females, with age of onset typically in the 40s. The cause is unclear. Symptoms usually diminish with time, but can last for years. Certainly, more work is required in order to obtain a greater understanding of this little-known disorder. An increased awareness among physicians may help lead to the clinical knowledge necessary to develop effective treatment strategies.

ACKNOWLEDGMENTS

We gratefully acknowledge the assistance of the MDD support group in writing this review article.

REFERENCES

1. Stott J. Adaptation to nauseogenic motion stimuli and its application in the treatment of airsickness. In: GH C, ed. Motion and Space Sickness. Boca Raton: CRC Press, 1990.
2. Graybiel A. Structural elements in the concept of motion sickness. Aerospace Med 1969; 40:351–367.
3. Gordon CR, Spitzer O, Doweck I, Melamed Y, Shupak A. Clinical features of mal de debarquement: adaptation and habituation to sea conditions. J Vestib Res 1995; 5(5):363–369.
4. Mair I. The mal de debarquement syndrome. J Audiol Med 1996; 5:21–25.
5. Brown JJ, Baloh RW. Persistent mal de debarquement syndrome: a motion-induced subjective disorder of balance. Am J Otolaryngol 1987; 8(4):219–222.
6. Murphy TP. Mal de debarquement syndrome: a forgotten entity? Otolaryngol Head Neck Surg 1993; 109(1):10–13.
7. Hain TC, Hanna PA, Rheinberger MA. Mal de debarquement. Arch Otolaryngol Head Neck Surg 1999; 125(6):615–620.
8. Gordon CR, Shupak A, Nachum Z. Mal de debarquement. Arch Otolaryngol Head Neck Surg 2000; 126(6):805–806.
9. Ungs TJ. Simulator induced syndrome: evidence for long-term after effects. Aviat Space Environ Med 1989; 60:252–255.
10. Cohen H. Mild mal de debarquement after sailing. Ann N Y Acad Sci 1996; 781:598–600.
11. Guerraz M, Yardley L, Bertholon P, et al. Visual vertigo: symptom assessment, spatial orientation and postural control. Brain 2001; 124:1646–1656.
12. Stewart WF, Lipton RB. Migraine headache: epidemiology and health care utilization. Cephalalgia 1993; 13(suppl 12):41–46.
13. Stewart WF, Shechter A, Rasmussen BK. Migraine prevalence. A review of population-based studies. Neurology 1994; 44(6 suppl 4):S17–S23.
14. Kayan A, Hood JD. Neuro-otological manifestations of migraine. Brain 1984; 107(Pt 4): 1123–1142.
15. Lawther A, Griffin MJ. A survey of the occurrence of motion sickness amongst passengers at sea. Aviat Space Environ Med 1988; 59:399–406.
16. Kleinschmidt HJ, Collewijn H. A search for habituation of vestibulo-ocular reactions to rotatory and linear sinusoidal accelerations in the rabbit. Exp Neurol 1975; 47(2):257–267.
17. Hain T. Approach to the Vertigo Patient. In: Biller J, ed. Practical Neurology. Philadelphia: Lippincott-Raven, 1997.
18. Zimbelman JL, Watson TM. Vestibular rehabilitation of a patient with persistent mal de debarquement. Physical Therapy Case Reports 1992; 2:129–133.

11

Meniere's Disease in the Elderly

Ronen Perez and Julian M. Nedzelski
Department of Otolaryngology and Head and Neck Surgery, Sunnybrook and Women's College Health Sciences Centre and University of Toronto, Toronto, Ontario, Canada

Meniere's disease is a disorder of the inner ear, which is characterized by vertiginous episodes, fluctuating hearing loss, and tinnitus. Although the disorder classically develops in middle age (peak 35–50 years), it is not uncommon in patients over 65 years old.

EPIDEMIOLOGY

The incidence and prevalence of Meniere's disease is reported to widely vary. While the incidence reported in the United Kingdom is 157 per 100,000, in France it is only eight per 100,000 (1). Since Meniere's disease is extremely rare in the pediatric population, the true incidence in the adult population is probably slightly higher (2). In a detailed thorough clinical study, Ballester et al. (3) reported that 15.3% of 432 active Meniere's patients were over 65. Sixty percent of these individuals had the initial presentation over the age of 65 and the remaining 40% presented with reactivation of long-standing disease. The authors of this chapter report approximately similar numbers with 9% of patients presenting with the disease over the age of 65 (4).

There are conflicting reports regarding sexual preponderance of the disease with respect to the full range of the population (5–8). While Ballester's study reported a clear female preponderance in the elderly population (46 women and 20 men), our data do not support this.

Published reports regarding the frequency of bilateral Meniere's disease vary from 2% to 78% of patients (9,10). The results of an ongoing study at the authors' institution seem to indicate that while the percentage of clinical Meniere's disease of the contralateral ear is relatively low, the percentage of patients with a contralateral low frequency hearing loss is higher. Kitahara et al. (11) reported that the percentage of bilateral involvement at the onset of the disease was higher in patients over 60.

Familial occurrence of the disease is also unclear but has been described in 14% of patients in a Swedish study and 5% of patients in a study conducted in the United Kingdom (12,13).

PATHOGENESIS

The widely accepted histopathologic changes associated with Meniere's disease relate to the membranous labyrinth. The hallmark of this disturbance is endolymphatic hydrops (14,15). Over-accumulation of endolymph is believed to cause anatomical distortion of the membranous labyrinth (16). Although it is widely known that hypertension is common among the elderly population, to the best of our knowledge there is no evidence in the literature to suggest a link between hypertension and the endolymphatic hydrops felt to be a feature of Meniere's.

Endolymph is produced by the stria vascularis in the cochlea and by dark cells scattered throughout the vestibular labyrinth. It is absorbed within the endolymphatic sac as well as the stria vascularis. Numerous mechanisms for the development of hydrops have been proposed. These include obstruction of the endolymphatic duct, dysfunction of the endolymphatic sac, overproduction of endolymph, infection, immune-mediated etiologies, and vascular disturbance (16–21).

A breakdown in the barrier between endolymph and perilymph is thought to be the significant event in the pathophysiology of the disease, especially in the acute attacks. The range of this barrier disturbance is thought to vary between a rupture to a small leakage (22–24). The rupture or leakage leads to potassium intoxication of the hair cells. This reversible hair cell depolarization transiently interferes with the mechanoelectrical transduction of these structures. This explains the sudden tinnitus increase, hearing loss, and vertigo (25). It has been shown that the membranous labyrinth easily heals restoring the normal potassium balance and consequently terminating the acute exacerbation (26). Repeated exposure of the hair cells to the high concentration of potassium is thought to cause the gradual deterioration in hearing and vestibular function (27). It has been shown histologically that the hair cells and the nerves remain unchanged in these patients. A decrease in the hair cell or neuronal population occurs rarely and only in the severe cases of the disease (11).

In the past decade, several studies have implicated an immune response as being responsible for endolymphatic hydrops (20,28–30). Known immune-mediated diseases such as Cogan's, and polyartheritis nodosa are known to cause inner ear disturbances (31,32). Circulating immune complexes were found in the serum of patients with Meniere's (30). C3 and C1q complement have been shown to be elevated in patients with the disease as have circulating serum antibodies to heat shock protein 70 (29,33). In addition, animal models of endolymphatic hydrops induced by a secondary immune response have been described (34).

The vascular etiology is of special interest with regard to the elderly population. The possibility of a common vascular mechanism for migraine headache and Meniere's syndrome has been proposed (6,35). Some studies suggest that altered microcirculation and venous drainage may be significant in the pathophysiology of Meniere's disease (21,36). Kimura et al. (37) postulated that endolymphatic hydrops may be a result of interference with the blood supply to the endolymphatic sac causing alteration in its function. The peak incidence of the disease in middle-aged patients does not support this theory.

DIAGNOSIS

History

A well-taken history is paramount for the diagnosis of Meniere's disease. Typically, Meniere's patients present with episodes of severe vertigo, tinnitus, and ipsilateral hearing loss (8). The duration of the episode is from minutes to hours, most commonly two to three hours. The vertiginous episodes may appear suddenly without warning although generally are preceded by increasing tinnitus and aural fullness (38). Approximately 60% of elderly patients diagnosed as having Meniere's have their initial episode at age 65 or older. The remaining 40% have an acute reactivation of long-standing disease (3).

Drop attacks are a rare occurrence in patients afflicted with Meniere's disease and consist of sudden falls without loss of consciousness or vertigo. They are thought to occur as a consequence of sudden alteration of proprioception by the extremity antigravity muscles. Patients often report a sensation of being "pushed to the ground by a giant hand." Tumarkin (39) described these attacks in 1936 and attributed them to acute otolithic dysfunction (40). Current thinking is that an inappropriate postural adjustment occurs as a result of an acute change in otolithic output (41). Less than 5% of Meniere's patients suffer from drop attacks during the course of their disease. Importantly, as many as 25% of patients, initially presenting with Meniere's symptoms over age 65, suffered from drop attacks (3). This is a significantly higher number than in the general Meniere's population. This observation is of importance for physicians treating the geriatric population for two main reasons: namely, the differential diagnosis with a possible vascular event often leads to an erroneous diagnosis. Secondly, the drop attacks may be associated with fractures, which have a tremendous impact on all aspects of life of the patients.

The sensorineural hearing loss associated with Meniere's typically fluctuates at onset of the disease. Additionally, in contrast to most other causes of sensorineural hearing loss (noise, age, ototoxicity), the hearing loss associated with Meniere's typically begins in the low frequencies (Fig. 1) (38). Meniere's disease in most cases is progressive, leading to a permanent hearing loss. Over time, the audiogram assumes a flat configuration.

It is well known that a majority of the elderly have varying degrees of hearing loss. The typical audiometric configuration associated with presbycusis is a symmetric downsloping sensorineural hearing loss (Fig. 2). The acute and chronic hearing loss associated with Meniere's in the elderly is superimposed on the presbycutic loss (Fig. 3). Because the low frequencies are most affected in early Meniere's disease and these are typically spared in presbycusis, afflicted elderly patients are especially handicapped in the involved ear early. Finally, because hearing loss, tinnitus, and balance-related complaints are commonly experienced by the elderly, the diagnosis of Meniere's is made difficult.

Physical Examination

As is the case in the general population, the physical examination in elderly Meniere's patients, apart from an asymmetric hearing loss, is normal. The diagnosis is primarily based on the history. A full and thorough ear, nose, and throat (ENT) and neuro-otologic exam should be performed. This by definition includes examination of all of the cranial nerves, and cerebellar as well as gait assessment. There are a

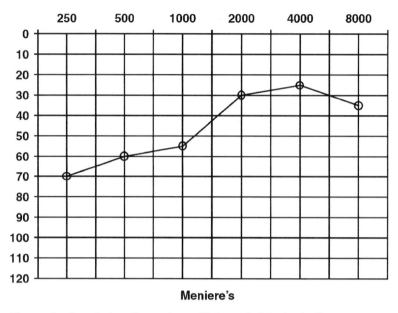

Figure 1 A typical audiometric profile in early Meniere's disease.

number of considerations in the geriatric population which need to be made. Special attention should be given to ruling out orthostatic hypotension. Orthostatic hypotension, a common finding in the elderly, may be described as a sensation of transient vertigo. The neck and skull should be carefully auscultated for bruits, which are barometers of vascular disease. The presence of nystagmus without vertigo is suspicious for central pathology and warrants further prompt investigation.

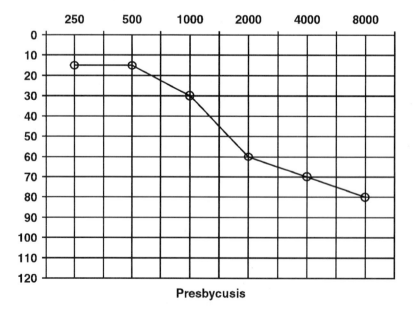

Figure 2 A typical audiometric profile for presbycusis.

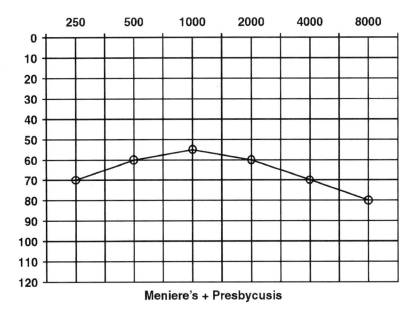

Meniere's + Presbycusis

Figure 3 An audiometric illustration of superimposed Meniere's disease and presbycusis-related hearing loss.

Investigations

As stated earlier, there is no diagnostic test for Meniere's disease. All tests should be viewed as corroborative.

Audiometric Evaluation

The typical sensorineural hearing loss associated with early onset Meniere's disease is primarily in the low frequencies and this finding contributes significantly to establishing the diagnosis. In the elderly, this is typically superimposed on the loss as a consequence of presbycusis. Both the hearing loss noted as a consequence of aging (presbycusis) and that of Meniere's disease can lead to a very poor quality of hearing, that is to say, the ability to discriminate especially conversations. The fact that this can dramatically fluctuate in the Meniere's afflicted ear makes it doubly frustrating for the elderly (42).

Electrocochleography

The summating potential in Meniere's patients is larger and with a higher negativity. This is a reflection of the distension of the basilar membrane into the scala vestibuli (43). The difficulty in obtaining reproducible recordings and the variability of the wave amplitude in different age groups limits the diagnostic use of this test in Meniere's patients.

Otoacoustic Emissions

Their value in the diagnosis of Meniere's is still questionable. Of special interest is the finding of smaller-amplitude emissions in the opposite ear. This may bear implications regarding impending disease in the contralateral ear.

Electronystagmography

The caloric test, one part in the battery of the electronystagmography tests, is useful in corroborating the affected ear. In 48–73% of patients with Meniere's disease a significant caloric response reduction is noted in the affected ear (44,45). An absent caloric response is reported in 6–11% of patients.

Differential Diagnosis

Meniere's disease in the elderly is relatively rare. However, given the higher incidence of drop spells in this patient population, it does pose as a consideration in the diagnosis of cerebrovascular disease. In Ballaster's study, five of the 39 patients with Meniere's initially diagnosed at age 65 or older (13%) were misdiagnosed as having a stroke because of the associated drop spells.

Another important differential diagnosis in the elderly patients is vertebro-basilar insufficiency (VBI). Sudden vertigo is the most common symptom of VBI in older patients. Approximately 50–60% of patients with VBI have spinning vertigo as their initial complaint (46). The vertigo usually lasts minutes and is often associated with nausea and vomiting. In all cases, it is associated with additional symptoms of brainstem involvement, thereby excluding the diagnosis of Meniere's.

Although benign paroxysmal positional vertigo (BPPV) is easily differentiated from Meniere's (especially by otolaryngologists), it is worth mentioning because it is the most common cause of peripheral vertigo and is common in the elderly. In BPPV, the vertigo typically lasts for seconds and always less than a minute. It occurs when assuming a certain head position typically with the involved ear undermost after rolling over in bed. In contrast to Meniere's disease, it is not associated with hearing loss or tinnitus. The nystagmus evoked in BPPV by the Dix-Hallpike maneuver has features, which are pathognomonic of the disease (47). That is to say, the nystagmus is rotatory, beating toward the undermost ear, delayed in onset, lasts for seconds, and is associated with marked symptoms of spinning and nausea.

The term "presbyvertigo" is not uncommonly used to describe an ill-defined sense of poor balance by elderly patients. They do not experience vertigo as such, do not realize any associated fluctuating aural symptoms nor do they experience any transient neurologic deficits. It is assumed that these symptoms are a consequence of combined vestibular hair cell loss, declining vision, and compromised proprioception.

TREATMENT

To date, there is no curative treatment for Meniere's disease. All treatment modalities are aimed at relieving the main symptoms, notably the debilitating vertigo with its associated nausea. Definitive treatment for vertigo and Meniere's associated drop attacks consist of vestibular ablation for the involved ear. It is our experience and Ballester's that the elderly show more tolerance to the vertigo attacks than the general population. Once the patients are reassured that the disease is not life threatening, they tolerate the vertigo quite well. This is not the case with regard to the drop attacks, which are extremely debilitating and potentially fatal. The hearing loss and tinnitus are also debilitating and as mentioned previously are superimposed on presbycusis causing significant hearing handicap.

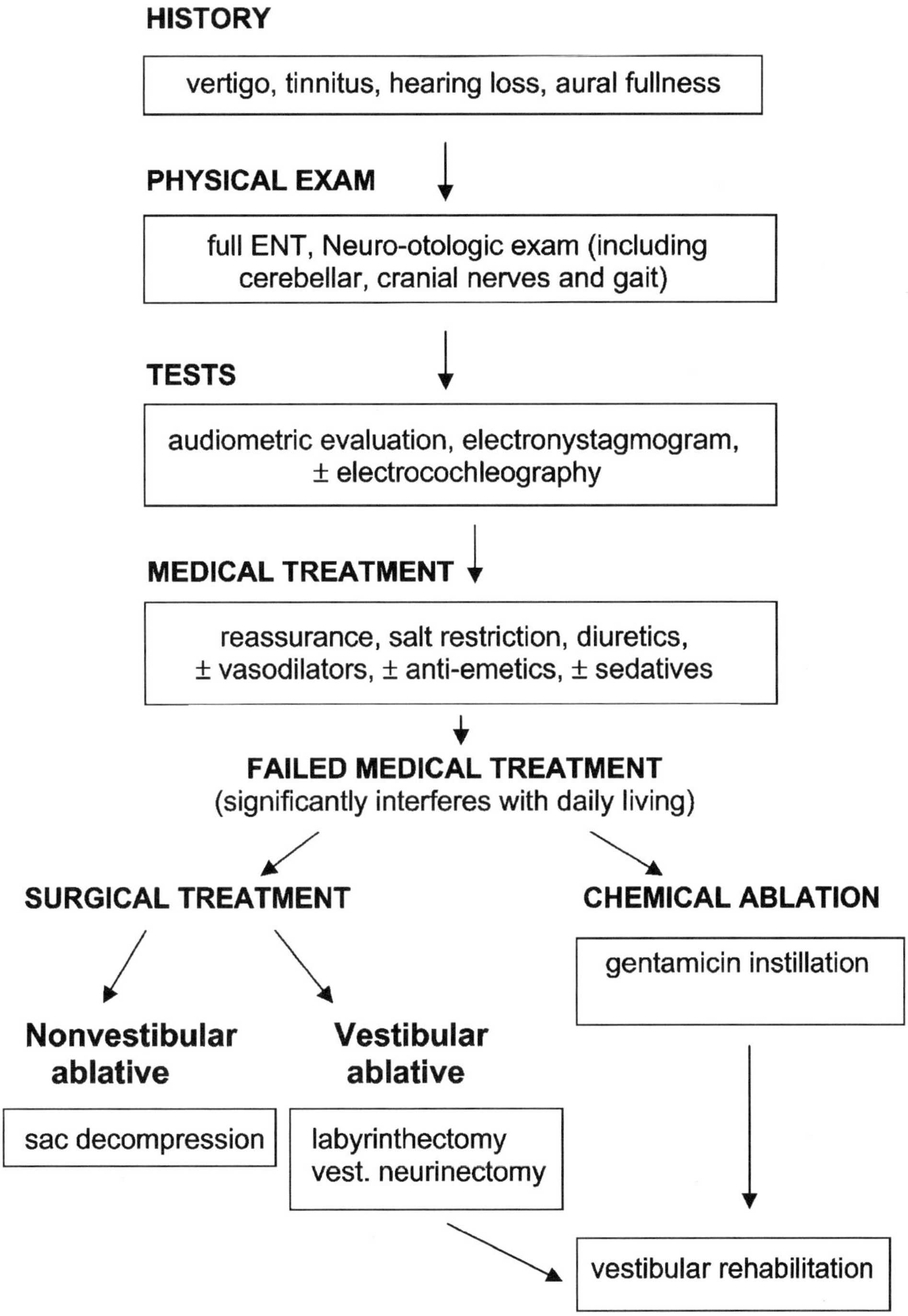

HISTORY

| vertigo, tinnitus, hearing loss, aural fullness |

PHYSICAL EXAM

| full ENT, Neuro-otologic exam (including cerebellar, cranial nerves and gait) |

TESTS

| audiometric evaluation, electronystagmogram, ± electrocochleography |

MEDICAL TREATMENT

| reassurance, salt restriction, diuretics, ± vasodilators, ± anti-emetics, ± sedatives |

FAILED MEDICAL TREATMENT
(significantly interferes with daily living)

SURGICAL TREATMENT

CHEMICAL ABLATION

| gentamicin instillation |

Nonvestibular ablative

Vestibular ablative

| sac decompression | | labyrinthectomy vest. neurinectomy |

| vestibular rehabilitation |

Scheme 1 The diagnosis and management flowchart.

The first line of medical treatment consists of salt restriction and diuretic therapy (48). At the dizziness clinic at Sunnybrook, hydrochlorothiazide is usually initially prescribed. A relatively large percentage of elderly patients are already under medical treatment for hypertension, which in some cases includes a diuretic.

Collaboration with the patient's family physician is sometimes required for possible modification of antihypertensive treatment to include a diuretic. It is important to monitor potassium levels. The rationale for this is to reduce endolymph volume. There are conflicting reports in the literature regarding the efficacy of this treatment (49,50).

Betahistine (serc) and other vasodilators have been used. They are given in the belief that Meniere's disease is a result of strial ischemia. The intent of their administration is to improve the blood flow to the labyrinth. Several studies show reduction of vertiginous attacks with these drugs, but again clear-cut efficacy has not been shown (51,52). These medications are very well tolerated by the elderly population with few side effects.

In many cases, symptomatic relief is sought by stronger anti-vertiginous medications, antiemetics, and sedatives. These drugs are not always tolerated well and in some cases cause depression in the elderly. Their use should be carefully monitored.

The emergence of chemical ablation in the last two decades has reduced the percentage of patients undergoing surgical procedures (53,54). Numerous protocols of gentamicin administration have been described. The protocol used at Sunnybrook involves insertion of a T-tube attached to a catheter in the clinic under local anesthesia. Three doses of gentamicin daily over four days are administered. Approximately 10% of the patients who underwent this treatment during the last 15 years were over 65 at the time of the treatment. Complete control of vertigo was achieved in 85% of individuals. Hearing was worse in 26%, unchanged in 48%, and improved in 26% (4). Control of vertigo in the elderly group was similar to younger individuals. However, the percentage of elderly individuals who realized a worsening of hearing was higher (37% vs. 26%).

In selected cases, notably patients experiencing drop attacks, labyrinthectomy may be the preferred treatment option. Other forms of surgical treatment include endolymphatic sac compression, cochleosacculotomy, and vestibular neurinectomy (55–57). Dayal and Proctor (58) specifically addressed labyrinthectomy for Meniere's in the elderly and concluded that while taking into account the chronologic as well as the physiologic age of the patient, labyrinthectomy is recommended for patients with incapacitating vertigo without serviceable hearing.

In all cases of deliberate ablation of peripheral vestibular function, it is imperative that patients undergo a course of intensive vestibular rehabilitation exercises.

SUMMARY

Although the incidence of Meniere's disease is thought to peak at middle age, its occurrence in patients over age 65 is not uncommon. The disease in the elderly may present initially over the age of 65 or may be a consequence of long-standing disease. Drop attacks in the elderly are a more frequent occurrence. They can be extremely debilitating and may result in trauma and fractures. Meniere's disease in the elderly is often confused with vertebrobasilar insufficiency. The hearing loss associated with the disease is frequently superimposed on presbycusis and leads to a more significant handicap. Caution should be practiced when using medications, which may be poorly tolerated by the elderly, i.e., sedatives. On the other hand, these patients frequently are a high surgical risk. Finally, although vertigo control is equal to that of younger individuals, hearing loss as a consequence of middle ear gentamicin instillation is higher in the elderly.

REFERENCES

1. Pfaltz CR, Thomsen J. Symptomatology and definition of Meniere's disease. In: Pfaltz CR, ed. Controversial Aspects of Meniere's Disease. New York: Georg Thieme, 1986.
2. Wladislavoski-Waserman P, Facer GW, Mokri B, Kurland LT. Meniere's disease: a 30-year epidemiologic and clinical study in Rochester, MN, 1951–1980. Laryngoscope 1984; 94:1098–1102.
3. Ballester M, Liard P, Vibert D, Hausler R. Meniere's disease in the elderly. Otol Neurotol 2002; 23:73–78.
4. Kaplan DM, Nedzelski JM, Chen JM, Shipp DB. Intratympanic gentamicin for the treatment of unilateral Meniere's disease. Laryngoscope 2000; 110:1298–1305.
5. Watanabe I. Meniere's disease in males and females. Acta Otolaryngol (Stockh) 1981; 91:511–514.
6. Parker W. Meniere's disease. Etiologic considerations. Arch Otolaryngol Head Neck Surg 1995; 121:377–382.
7. Oosterveld WJ. Meniere's disease, signs and symptoms. J Laryngol Otol 1980; 94: 885–894.
8. Paparella MM. The cause (multifactorial inheritance) and pathogenesis (endolymphatic malabsorbtion) of Meniere's disease and its symptoms (mechanical and chemical). Acta Otolaryngol (Stockh) 1985; 99:445–451.
9. Balkani T, Sizes b, Arenberg I. Bilateral aspects of Meniere's disease: an underestimated clinical entity. Otolaryngol Clin North Am 1980; 13:603–609.
10. Stahle J, Friedberg U, Svedberg A. Long term progression of Meniere's disease. Acta Otolaryngol (Stockh) Suppl 1991; 485:78–83.
11. Kitahara M, Matsubara H, Takeda T, Yazawa Y. Bilateral Meniere's disease. Adv Otorhinolaryngol 1979; 25:117–121.
12. Birgerson L, Gustavson KH, Stahle J. Familial Meniere's disease: a genetic investigation. Am J Otol 1987; 8:323–326.
13. Morrison AW. Meniere's disease. J R Soc Med 1981; 74:183–189.
14. Anatoli-Candela F. The histopathology of Meniere's disease. Acta Otolaryngol (Stockh) Suppl 1976; 340:1–42.
15. Schuknecht HF, Igarishi M. Pathophysiology of Meniere's disease. In: Pfaltz CR, ed. Controversial Aspects of Meniere's Disease. New York: Georg Thieme, 1986.
16. Paparella MM, Mancini F. Vestibular Meniere's disease. Otolaryngol Head Neck Surg 1985; 93:148–151.
17. Kimura RS, Schucknecht HF. Membranous hydrops in the inner ear of the guinea pig after obliteration of the endolymphatic sac. Pract Otorhinolaryngol 1965; 27:343–354.
18. Henriksson N, Igarishi M, Tonndorf J. Pathophysiology of Meniere's disease. In: Pfaltz CR, ed. Controversial Aspects of Meniere's Disease. New York: Georg Thieme, 1986.
19. Fukuda S, Keithley EM, Harris JP. The development of endolymphatic hydrops following CMV inoculation of the endolymphatic sac. Laryngoscope 1988; 98:439–443.
20. Derebery MJ, Rao VS, Siglock TJ, Linthicum FH, Nelson RA. Meniere's disease: an immune complex-mediated illness? Laryngoscope 1991; 105:225–229.
21. Gussen R. Vascular mechanisms in Meniere's disease. Otolaryngol Head Neck Surg 1983; 91:68–71.
22. Kimura RS. Fistulae in the membranous labyrinth. Ann Otol Rhinol Laryngol 1984; 93(suppl 112):36–43.
23. Schucknecht HF. Meniere's disease. Otolaryngol Clin North Am 1968; 1:331.
24. Jahnke K. Permeability barriers of the inner ear in respect to the Meniere's attack. In: Vosteen KH, ed. Meniere's Disease: Pathogenesis, Diagnosis, and Treatment. Stuttgart: Georg Thieme, 1981.
25. Zenner HP, Ruppersberg JP, Lowenheim H, Gummer AW. Pathophysiology: transduction and motor disturbances of hair cells by endolymphatic hydrops and transitory

endolymph leakage. In: Harris JP, ed. Meniere's Disease. The Hague: Kugler Publications, 1999.

26. Kimura RS, Schucknecht HF. Effect of fistulae on endolymphatic hydrops. Ann Otol 1975; 84:271–286.

27. Thomsen J, Bretlau P. General conclusions. In: Pfaltz CR, ed. Controversial Aspects of Meniere's Disease. Stuttgart: Georg Thieme, 1986.

28. Zanneti FR, Plester D, Klein R, Bursa-Zanneti Z, Berg PA. Immunological patterns of inner ear disease including Meniere's disease. In: Nadol JB Jr, ed. Meniere's Disease. Ansterdam/Berkely/Milano: Kugler and Ghedini Publ, 1989:133–137.

29. Hausler R, Arnold W, Schifferli J. C3 and C1q complement deposits in the membranous labyrinth of patients with Menierés disease. Adv Otorhinolaryngol 1988; 42:116–122.

30. Brookes GB. Circulating immune complexes in Meniere's disease. Arch Otol Laryngol Head Neck Surg 1986; 112:536–540.

31. Schucknecht HF, Nadol JB Jr. Temporal bone pathology in a case of Cogan's syndrome. Laryngoscope 1994; 104:1135–1142.

32. Jenkins HA, Pollak AM, Fisch U. Polyarteritis nodosa as a cause of sudden deafness: a human temporal bone study. Am J Otolaryngol 1981; 2:99–107.

33. Rauch SD, San Martin JE, Moscicki RA, Bloch KJ. Serum antibodies against heat shock protein 70 in Meniere's disease. Am J Otol 1995; 16:648–652.

34. Tomiyama S. Development of endolymphatic hydrops following immune response in the endolymphatic sac of the guinea pig. Acta Otolaryngol (Stockh) 1992; 112:470–478.

35. Kayan A, Hood JD. Neuro-otological manifestation of migraine. Brain 1984; 107: 1123–1142.

36. Gussen R. Vascular mechanisms in Meniere's disease. Theoretical considerations. Arch Otolaryngol 1982; 108:544–549.

37. Kimura RS, Trehey JA, Hutta J. Degeneration of vestibular sensori cells caused by ablation of the aqueduct in the gerbil ear. Ann Otol Rhinol Laryngol 1995; 104:155–160.

38. Barber HO. Meniere's disease: symptomatology. In: Oosterveld WJ, ed. Meniere's Disease: A Comprehensive Appraisal. New York: John Wiley, 1983.

39. Tumarkin A. The otolithic catastrophe: a new syndrome. Br Med J 1936; i:175.

40. Pillsbury HC III, Postma DS. Lermoyez' syndrome and the otolithic crisis of Tumarkin. Otolaryngol Clin North Am 1983; 16:197–203.

41. Odkvist LM, Bergenius J. Drop attacks in Meniere's disease. Acta Otolaryngol (Stockh) Suppl 1988; 455:82–85.

42. Morrison AW. Diagnostic and laboratory evaluation in Meniere's disease. In: Harris JP, ed. Meniere's Disease. The Hague: Kugler Publications, 1999.

43. Morrison AW, Moffat DA, O'Connor AF. Clinical usefulness of electrocochleography in Meniere's disease: an analysis of dehydrating agents. Otolaryngol Clin North Am 1980; 13:703–721.

44. Black O, Kitch R. A review of vestibular test results in Meniere's disease. Otolaryngol Clin North Am 1980; 13:631–642.

45. Stahle J, Klockhoff I. Diagnostic procedures, differential diagnosis and general conclusions. In: Pfaltz CR, ed. Controversial Aspects of Meniere's Disease. New York: Georg Thieme, 1986.

46. Baloh RW. Vertebrobasilar insufficiency and stroke. Otolryngol Head Neck Surg 1995; 112:114–117.

47. Epley J. New dimensions of benign positional vertigo. Otolaryngol Head Neck Surg 1980; 88:599–605.

48. Jackson CG, Glasscock ME III, Davis WE, Hughes GB, Sismanis A. Medical management of Meniere's disease. Ann Otol 1981; 90:142–147.

49. Klockhoff I, Lindblom U. Meniere's disease and hydrochlorothiazide—a critical analysis of symptoms and therapeutic effects. Acta Otolaryngol (Stockh) 1967; 63:347–365.

50. Klockhoff I, Lindblom U, Stahle J. Diuretic treatment of Meniere's disease. Arch Otolaryngol 1974; 100:262–265.

51. Wilmot TJ, Menon GN. Betahistine in Meniere's disease. J Laryngol Otol 1976; 90: 833–840.

52. Segers JM, Bedts D. Clinical trials of betahistine hydrochloride in the treatment of Meniere's disease. Acta Otorhinolaryngol Belg 1975; 29:814–821.

53. Nedzelski JM, Bryce GE, Pfeiderer AG. Treatment of Meniere's disease with topical gentamicine: a preliminary report. J Otolaryngol 1992; 21:94–101.

54. Nedzelski JM, Schessel DA, Bryce GE. Chemical labyrinthectomy: local application of gentamicin for the treatment of unilateral Meniere's disease. Am J Otol 1992; 13:18–22.

55. Glasscock ME III, Jackson CG, Poe DS, Johnson GD. What do I think of sac surgery in 1989. Am J Otol 1989; 10:230–233.

56. Schuknecht HF. Cochleosacculotomy for Meniere's disease: theory, technique and results. Laryngoscope 1982; 92:853–858.

57. Silverstein H, Norrell H, Rosenberg S. The resurrection of vestibular neurinectomy: a 10 year experience with 115 cases. J Neurosurg 1990; 72:533–539.

58. Dayal VS, Proctor T. Labyrinthectomy in the elderly. Am J Otol 1995; 16:110–114.

ANNOTATED BIBLIOGRAPHY

Ballester M, Liard P, Vibert D, Hausler R. Meniere's disease in the elderly. Otol Neurotol 2002; 23:73–78.

This is a particularly good reference. It is thorough and detailed and to our knowledge is the only paper specifically dealing with Meniere's disease in the geriatric population.

12

Dizziness in the Elderly

David E. Eibling
Department Otolaryngology—Head and Neck Surgery, University of Pittsburgh
School of Medicine, Pittsburgh, Pennsylvania, U.S.A.

INTRODUCTION

Dizziness is a common symptom that affects more than 30% of elderly individuals. In a study of 1622 elderly patients, dizziness accounted for *one-third* of all visits to primary care physicians for those older than 65, and was the most common complaint for those older than 75 (1). Seven percent of primary care visits by elderly patients were for symptoms of dizziness (2). Diagnosis of the underlying etiology and directed therapy is mandatory, since dizziness due to any number of causes can lead to falls with serious consequences in the geriatric population. Fear of falling results in disproportionate reductions in quality of life for the elderly, with nearly one-half of elderly dizzy patients reporting that they restrict their activities due to fear of falling versus 3% of age-matched controls (3).

The symptom of dizziness is often assumed by the patient, as well as the caregiver, to be due to a primary disorder of the vestibular end organ. However, many causes of dizziness arise from disorders of other organ systems, especially the cardiovascular and non-vestibular neurologic systems. Sloane points out that *most dizziness is non-vestibular*. Failure to correctly identify the cause will result in persistent symptoms and ineffective therapy. The challenge for the evaluating physician is to first rule out life-threatening causes of dizziness such as a cardiac arrhythmia or brainstem stroke, to then narrow the list of diagnoses to the most probable etiology(s), and then optimize treatment. An incomplete listing of some of the causes of non-vestibular dizziness that may be encountered in elderly dizzy patients are listed in Table 1.

Tinetti et al. (4) have proposed that dizziness in the elderly be considered a "geriatric syndrome" since dizziness is so prevalent in this population. In editorial remarks to Tinetti et al.'s paper, Drachman (5) expressed his concerns that the use of this term suggests that dizziness is an inevitable component of the aging process and reduces the incentive of the physician to seek a treatable cause. Indeed, Sloane et al. (1) point out that the cause(s) of dizziness in the elderly are often identifiable, and treatable.

Table 1 Some Non-vestibular Causes of Dizziness in the Elderly Listed in Order of Decreasing Severity

Life-threatening, possibly immediately
    Cardiac arrhythmia
    Cardiac failure
    Shock
    Hypoxia
    Impending seizure
    Incipient stroke
Serious, but not likely to be immediately life-threatening
    Anemia
    Vertebrobasilar insufficiency
      Subclavian Steal
    Cerebellar infarction
    Orthostatic hypotension
      Loss of volume (hypovolemia)
        Blood, fluid loss, diuretics
      Loss of vascular tone
        Autonomic dysfunction
        Prolonged bed rest
        Antihypertensive therapy
        Corticosteroid deficiency
          Iatrogenic or due to disease
      Loss of cardiac responsiveness
        Cardiac disease
          Chronotopic incompetence
        Medication
        Pacemaker
    Central lesion
      Encephalitis
      Degenerative disease
      Brain tumor
      Toxin exposure
Affecting mobility and quality of life
    Disequilibrium (may be vestibular)
      Disequilibrium of aging
      Multi-sensory deprivation
    Muscle weakness
      Sarcopenia
      CVA
      Spinal stenosis
    Central
      Parkinsons's disease
      Orthostatic tremor
      Degenerative disease
      Drugs
        Alcohol
        Sedatives
        CNS active medications
      Brain lesion
        Encephalitis
        Brain tumor
        Chronic degenerative disease

TAXONOMY OF DIZZINESS IN THE ELDERLY

More than 30 years ago (prior to the availability of noninvasive intracranial and vascular imaging), Drachman and Hart (6) suggested that the complaint of dizziness could be categorized based on symptom description. Current understanding of balance function and its disorders, as well as readily available diagnostic studies, permit more accurate identification of the underlying etiology and selection of more appropriate therapeutic modalities.

A careful history and focused physical examination will usually suggest one or more probable diagnoses, even in the elderly. Unfortunately, vague complaints of dizziness are quite common in this population and disorders of the vestibular end organ may be difficult to differentiate from unsteadiness related to other disease processes. Sloane points out that elderly patients are particularly difficult to categorize into a single category, since approximately one-half will have more than one cause for their symptom of dizziness. Even if a single likely etiology has been diagnosed and treated [for example, benign paroxysmal positional vertigo (BPPV)] the patient may remain symptomatic due to another etiology.

Orthostatic Hypotension

Orthostatic hypotension is a particularly common cause of non-vestibular dizziness in the elderly. The venous system in healthy adults contains a "reservoir" of 0.3–0.8 L of blood. When additional volume is required to maintain perfusion pressure, blood from this pool is added to the circulating volume by muscle contraction. Minimal changes in arterial pressure, primarily sensed by baroreceptors in the aorta and carotid arteries, increase sympathetic tone to maintain cerebral perfusion regardless of body position. The regulatory adjustments occur so rapidly in the young healthy individual that they cannot be measured without the use of invasive instantaneous monitoring.

A variety of factors can lead to significant slowing of this response in the elderly. The resultant temporary reduction in cerebral perfusion results in a number of symptoms such as light-headedness, true vertigo, blurring of vision or other visual changes, tremulousness, palpitations, cognitive dysfunction, or frank loss of consciousness. Symptoms are typically temporally related to movement to the upright position from a supine or sitting position. In the aggregate, these symptoms can also be described as "presyncopal," even in the absence of subsequent syncope. Underlying factors may be cardiac dysfunction, lack of vascular elasticity, reduced muscle tone, neurologic disorders, particularly involving the autonomic nervous system, and volume depletion. Although volume loss may be due to acute blood loss (such as from a gastrointestinal bleed), in the elderly patient it is more typically due to diuretic therapy.

In most instances, more than one factor is responsible for the fluctuation in perfusion pressure. For example, patients may be on a beta-blocker and a diuretic. The age-related changes of reduced muscle tone as well as possibly a mild peripheral neuropathy further aggravate the loss of vascular tone. Although each of these factors may be tolerated individually, in the aggregate they combine to create sufficient aberration in blood pressure homeostasis to result in reduced cerebral blood flow and symptoms of dizziness.

The most common underlying cause in the elderly is iatrogenic—due to medications, usually antihypertensives (5). Blood volume is reduced by diuretics, blood vessel reactivity is reduced by alpha-blockers, and cardiac responsiveness affected by beta-blockers and other medications. Sildenafil, nitrates, and other vasodilating medications can reduce blood pressure (BP) responsiveness and lead to orthostatic hypotension. Bradley and Davis (7) suggest that diagnosis is most easily verified by cautiously eliminating the suspected drug to determine whether it is the cause of the symptoms. On the other hand, the benefit of the drug may warrant its continuation, with care taken on the part of the patient to compensate for the anticipated light-headedness upon arising from a supine position.

Vertebrobasilar Insufficiency

Defective posterior fossa perfusion due to vascular disease of the basilar artery, one or both vertebral arteries, and inadequate collateral flow from the carotid system is termed vertebrobasilar insufficiency. Unfortunately, vertebrobasilar insufficiency can present with vertigo as the only symptom (4); therefore, the absence of other neurologic symptoms does not rule it out. Vertebrobasilar insufficiency is, in fact, a vestibular disorder, regardless of whether it is due to brainstem or peripheral end-organ ischemia. Evaluation requires vascular imaging, typically initially with a magnetic resonance angiogram (MRA). Current treatment algorithms are in flux due to the recent introduction of endovascular procedures designed to enhance cerebral blood flow, even in the posterior circulation.

A particular—and rare—form of vertebrobasilar insufficiency is subclavian steal syndrome, which occurs as a sequela of proximal subclavian artery stenosis. The distal subclavian artery is reconstituted by retrograde flow through the ipsilateral vertebral artery. This condition can be suspected by a history of dizziness brought on by arm exertion, with the diagnosis further supported by differential arm blood pressures. Trans-cervical Doppler study of the vertebral arteries may demonstrate retrograde flow, confirming the diagnosis.

ROLE OF THE OTOLARYNGOLOGIST IN NON-VESTIBULAR DIZZINESS

The most common setting in which an otolaryngologist is consulted to evaluate a patient with non-vestibular dizziness is due to the presumptive diagnosis of a vestibulopathy by the referring physician. The otolaryngologist may tend to assume that non-vestibular causes of dizziness have been already considered and ruled out, and that the patient therefore must be suffering from symptoms of a vestibular end-organ disorder. It is best that the consultant begin the evaluation by first assuming that no cause has been ruled out. The symptoms of dizziness and the patient's past medical history should be reviewed, especially any history of prior cardiovascular illnesses and current medications. Changes in medications, particularly antihypertensive medication, may provide specific clues to the diagnosis of orthostatic hypotension. Careful inquiry to the nature, duration, character, and timing of the episodes may provide important information. "Are you dizzy in bed before you get up, or after you stand up?" is a useful question that can effectively drive further questioning. An appropriate physical examination must be performed, with attention to other possible etiologies of the patient's symptoms as well as the common vestibulopathies. Finally, when evaluating patients with dizziness the otolaryngologist must assume the role of a general physician and assess other systems as well as the vestibular system. The emphasis in this setting should be on identifying possibly life-threatening processes, and rapidly referring the patient for appropriate management. If the patient is found to have a benign balance disorder, then management should be toward reducing the risk of falling, increasing activity levels, and improving the quality of life, usually via an exercise program including vestibular rehabilitation.

Management of the dizzy elderly patient is perhaps one of the most challenging problems faced by the primary care physician; hence, there is often a tendency to refer the elderly dizzy patient early in the diagnostic process. The knowledge and skills that are necessary for the diagnosis are not difficult, but in the busy primary care practice the assumption is often made that all dizziness is due to vestibular end-organ disease. The logical next step then is to abbreviate the evaluation and refer without having completed a careful search for a non-vestibular etiology. Empiric treatment with vestibular suppressants is often initiated before the patient is referred for otolaryngologic evaluation. All too often, the patient arrives for the consultation, already on vestibular suppressants, and still complaining of dizziness. The otolaryngologist should not only completely evaluate these patients, but should also use the referral as a teaching case for the primary care physician. Although formal teaching of the management of dizziness via lectures, books, web programs, etc. is useful, a discussion of the specific patient via a phone call may be the single most effective teaching modality for the primary care physician, and assist many more patients.

APPROACH TO THE PATIENT WITH NON-VESTIBULAR DIZZINESS

The patient with non-vestibular dizziness presents to the otolaryngologist with generic "dizziness and giddiness, not otherwise specified"; hence, the history will be exactly the same for dizziness whether of vestibular or non-vestibular causes. Orthostatic hypotension is a common source of dizziness in the elderly, and may be detected by questions regarding the timing of the onset: "Did it occur when you rolled over before arising, or shortly after standing up?" Occurrence of symptoms during specific head motion may suggest benign paroxysmal postural vertigo, but also may indicate vertebral-basilar insufficiency. Dizziness that accompanies upper extremity exercise may suggest subclavian steal. Associated neurologic symptoms such as syncope ("have you ever fainted or felt like you were going to faint?"), muscle weakness, tremor, or parathesias may provide an indication that the patients have some other cause of their complaint. A review of cardiac diseases, prior treatment, arrhythmias, medications, recent changes in medications, etc. may point to a cardiac cause. Questioning regarding the use of vestibular suppressants may assist in predicting the accuracy of a Dix-Hallpike or other vestibular testing. A wide variety of causes of dizziness may appear to respond to vestibular suppression, so a history of resolution following initiation of suppressant medication should not be perceived as prima facie evidence of vestibulopathy.

Geriatric patients, in particular, may present with dizziness of more than one cause; hence, it is probably safest to assume that any patient could have both a vestibular as well as a non-vestibular cause. The physical examination of any dizzy patient should therefore include a head and neck examination, and a basic cardiovascular examination to include an assessment of the cardiac rate and rhythm, and the status of the carotid arteries, as well as the BP. Pulse and BP should be obtained in both the supine as well as upright positions, especially in the elderly dizzy patient.

A drop in systolic blood pressure by 20 mm of mercury, or diastolic by 10, is sufficient for the diagnosis of orthostatic hypotension. The cardiac rate should increase to compensate; however, many elderly patients are on cardiac medications or a pacemaker that control cardiac rate, so a compensatory change in rate may not be observed.

A focused neurologic examination to include observation of gait, sensory and motor function, particularly of the lower extremities, and assessment of cerebellar function is required. Observation of gaze function, as well as testing for positional nystagmus should be performed. Recall that if the patient is already on vestibular suppression that the characteristic symptoms and physical findings of a Dix-Hallpike maneuver may be absent. Occasionally, patients with vertebrobasilar insufficiency may complain of symptoms reproduced by head position changes, making differentiation from BPPV challenging. The presence of other neurologic symptoms such as visual changes, perioral numbness, etc. suggests that the process is not BPPV and warrants careful neurologic examination and brain imaging.

If the history suggests BPPV, even in the absence of positional changes, some physicians routinely perform otolith repositioning in the hope that some benefit may ensue. Audiometry is considered standard in all cases of dizziness, and should be performed even if the initial impression is one of non-vestibular dizziness. Vestibular testing to include posturography is warranted in cases in which the history suggests a balance disorder but the diagnosis is unclear. Imaging is more likely to be required in the elderly dizzy patient than in younger patients, since the diagnosis is frequently less clear and may be confounded by a number of etiologies. In an elderly patient, the acute onset of severe vertigo should be considered to possibly represent a possible posterior fossa vascular event rather than vestibular neuronitis. Hence, urgent referral to an emergency department for evaluation and imaging is required in this population (8).

TREATMENT OF NON-VESTIBULAR DIZZINESS

Treatment of non-vestibular dizziness should first address the cause, if identified. In patients with orthostatic hypotension, this will mandate changes in medications, particularly antihypertensives and diuretics. The otolaryngologist will wish to refer the patient back to their primary care physician for adjustments in their medications. It is critical that patients be advised not to stop or reduce their antihypertensive medications without consulting their primary care physicians. The patient should be counseled that the risk of stroke or other disease due to discontinuation of their antihypertensive medications far outweigh any benefits in balance function they might appreciate.

Discontinuation of vestibular suppression should be an integral component of management in any elderly patient with non-vestibular (as well as vestibular) dizziness. Patients may be on several vestibular suppressants, including medication administered for management of dizziness as well as anxiolytic medications. Convincing the patient to reduce or discontinue these medications is often the most difficult component of treatment.

Treatment with a formal program of vestibular rehabilitation has been shown to be effective in a wide variety of balance disorders, whether or not they originate within the vestibular end organ. Hence, referral for vestibular rehabilitation should be part of any treatment plan for the dizzy elderly patient, regardless of etiology (with the possible exception of isolated BPPV). The details of this treatment modality are covered in the subsequent chapters in this text. Evidence suggests that an exercise program, whether or not it is specifically balance-oriented, will provide subjective and objective benefits for balance function as well (9). Patients should be encouraged to engage in a regular exercise program, preferably under the guidance of their primary care physician if they have been sedentary.

SUMMARY

Dizziness is common in the elderly, and more than one-half of affected patients suffer dizziness from non-vestibular causes. A taxonomy of possible etiologies assists in determining the most likely cause, but nearly one-half of the dizzy elderly patients will have more than one cause for their symptoms. Orthostatic hypotension due to loss of blood pressure responsiveness is one of the most common causes, and best managed by judicious adjustment of their antihypertensive regimen by the patient's primary physician. All patients should undergo a careful history, and physical examination with attention to the cardiovascular system, as well as a focused neurologic examination. BPPV should be considered, even in the presence of confusing symptoms, since the treatment of this condition with otolith repositioning may be gratifying. Further testing is required in most patients, with urgent imaging mandated in acute cases to rule out a posterior fossa vascular event. Treatment should focus on identified etiologic processes, discontinuation of vestibular suppressive medication, and formal vestibular rehabilitation. An age-appropriate exercise program will reduce the burden of the disorder in the majority of elderly patients, regardless of the underlying etiology. Finally, discussion of the diagnosis and management with the patient's referring physician may lead to prompt and appropriate evaluation and management of future elderly patients with dizziness.

REFERENCES

1. Sloane PD, Balzer D, George LK. Dizziness in a community elderly population. JAGS 1989; 37:101–108.
2. Sloane PD, Coeytaux RR, Beck RS, Dallara J. Dizziness: state of the science. Ann Intern Med 2001; 134:823–832.
3. Burker EJ, Wong H, Sloane PD, Mattingly D, Preisser J, Mitchell CM. Fear of falling in dizzy and nondizzy elderly. Psychol Aging 1995; 10:104–110.
4. Tinetti ME, Williams CS, Gill TM. Dizziness among older adults: a possible geriatric syndrome. Ann Intern Med 2000; 132:337–344.
5. Drachman DA. Occam's razor, geriatric syndromes, and the dizzy patient [editorial]. Ann Intern Med 2000; 132:403–404.
6. Drachman DA, Hart CW. An approach to the dizzy patient. Neurology 1972; 22:323–334.
7. Bradley JG, Davis KA. Am Fam Phys 2003; 68:2393–2398.
8. Furman JM, Cass SP. Vestibular Disorders: A Case-study Approach. New York: Oxford University Press, 2003.
9. Wolfson L, Whipple R, Derby CA, et al. A dynamic posturography study of balance in healthy elderly. Neurology 1992; 42:2069–2075.

13

Benign Paroxysmal Positional Vertigo

Joseph M. Furman
Division of Balance Disorders, Department of Otolaryngology, University of Pittsburgh,
Pittsburgh, Pennsylvania, U.S.A.

GENERAL DESCRIPTION OF THE CLINICAL PROBLEM

Benign paroxysmal positional vertigo (BPPV) is a common neurologic disorder that is particularly common in older individuals (1–3). The etiology of BPPV relates to free-floating otoconial debris in the vestibular labyrinth that causes the semicircular canals, especially the posterior semicircular canal, to become a gravity-sensitive organ (4). Normally, the semicircular canals sense rotational motion but are not sensitive to the orientation of the head with respect to gravity. Conversely, the otolith organs, namely the utricle and the saccule, are gravity sensitive. Patients with BPPV have an inappropriate sensitivity of one or more semicircular canals to the orientation of the head with respect to gravity. Patients with BPPV experience vertigo when they change their head position with respect to gravity. Typical provocative activities include turning in bed and looking up.

There are several different varieties of positional vertigo. The most common of these varieties of positional vertigo results from debris floating freely in the posterior semicircular canal. This form of positional vertigo has been called BPPV (5). Other types of positional vertigo can be caused by free-floating debris in the horizontal semicircular canal (6–9) and possibly in the anterior semicircular canal (10,11). Moreover, some forms of positional vertigo are thought to occur as a result of debris attaching itself to the cupula of one of the semicircular canals (12,13). In this circumstance, the debris is adherent rather than free-floating, and causes a variant of BPPV. The incidence of BPPV has been estimated to be between 10 and 100 cases per 100,000 individuals per year (3,14). A recent study has suggested that as many as 9% of geriatric patients have unrecognized BPPV (15). Common antecedents to BPPV include vestibular neuronitis and head trauma (1) but BPPV is often idiopathic especially in older persons. The recurrence rate of BPPV is approximately 1% per month, cumulatively suggesting that about 50% of patients will have a recurrence of BPPV at some time in the first four years following their initial episode (16,17). There are some data to suggest that recurrences of the BPPV are more likely in persons with post-traumatic BPPV.

BPPV affects adults of all ages but can be more troublesome in the elderly population for several reasons. Older individuals generally have impaired balance as compared to younger individuals, even in the absence of a specific balance disorder. Thus, BPPV probably increases the risk for falls and possibly injurious falls in the older population. Moreover, older individuals often have difficulty with other sensations that are important for balance, that is vision and somatosensation. Thus, BPPV may occur as part of a multisensory problem and thereby causes more of impairment with balance in an older individual than it would in a younger one. Also, recovery from BPPV in younger individuals often requires only a particle-repositioning maneuver (to be discussed below). However, older individuals may require vestibular rehabilitation therapy to more fully regain their balance function.

PATHOPHYSIOLOGY OF BPPV

It is now well established that BPPV is usually caused by displaced otoconial debris from the utricular macula that is floating freely in the posterior semicircular canal (Fig. 1). As a result, when patients with BPPV change their head position with respect to gravity, e.g., by looking up or rolling over in bed, the mobile otoconial debris moves inside the labyrinth. Movement of the debris presumably causes cupular motion and an associated stimulation of the labyrinth. Patients with BPPV experience spinning vertigo for a brief time after provocative head movements. If the head is kept in a new position, the debris reaches a new stable position and after a few seconds, the vertigo stops. Patients may, however, feel a sense of nausea and disequilibrium even after the vertigo stops. Also, patients with BPPV, especially older individuals, often experience imbalance, probably as a result of a malfunctioning labyrinth or central nervous system suppression of vestibular signals. Older

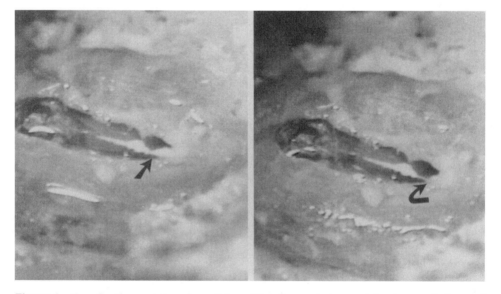

Figure 1 Free-floating endolymph particles within the posterior semicircular canal observed during surgery. The posterior semicircular canal had been opened in preparation for a canal plugging procedure. White debris was observed within the endolymph compartment of the posterior semicircular canal. These two photographs are sequential in time and show that the particles shifted during movement of the patient's head; compare shape and position of particles at straight arrow with the curved arrow. *Source*: From Ref. 18.

patients who have been placed on a vestibular suppressant medication for BPPV may have a worsening of their balance as a secondary effect of their medications, in addition to the underlying BPPV.

There are atypical forms of BPPV. In a small percentage of patients, free-floating debris apparently affects the horizontal semicircular canal rather than the posterior semicircular canal (6–9). Involvement of the anterior semicircular canal has been postulated but remains controversial (10,11). These atypical forms of BPPV also cause paroxysmal, that is, brief, episodes of positional vertigo. In some patients, debris apparently becomes adherent to the cupula of one of the semicircular canals and is thus fixed rather than free-floating (12,13). In these patients, vertiginous symptoms are typically not paroxysmal but rather persist for as long as the patient maintains the head tilted position.

CLINICAL PRESENTATION

Most patients with BPPV provide a clear history of vertiginous episodes during activities of looking up and turning in bed. In fact, without such a history, BPPV is unlikely. Many patients describe periods of time lasting from days to weeks during which they have positional symptoms but note having symptom-free intervals as well. Thus, many patients with a history characteristic for BPPV may not be suffering from the condition at the time of evaluation. Also, some patients relate experiencing an acute vestibular syndrome prior to the onset of symptoms typical for BPPV. Conditions such as vestibular neuritis, labyrinthine concussion (1), and possibly migraine-related vestibulopathy (19,20) may precede the onset of BPPV, but BPPV often occurs spontaneously. Vertiginous symptoms that occur without provocation, e.g., vertigo when someone is sitting still, argue against BPPV; in this case, other etiologies should be considered, e.g., Meniere's disease. Moreover, patients with auditory complaints or neurologic complaints other than dizziness or imbalance should be evaluated for conditions other than BPPV. The diagnosis of BPPV can be confirmed using the Dix-Hallpike maneuver (Fig. 2). This maneuver is most helpful for diagnosing typical BPPV, i.e., free-floating particles in the posterior semicircular canal. Performing the Dix-Hallpike maneuver can be more challenging in older individuals as a result of decreased range of motion of the neck. In such patients, a modified Dix-Hallpike maneuver may be required in which the patient's head is not extended over the edge of the examining table. Observing the patient's eye movements using Frenzel's glasses or infrared video-goggles rather than simply in a lighted room can increase the diagnostic accuracy of the Dix-Hallpike maneuver. Patients with BPPV will exhibit a nystagmus with a characteristic latency of onset, duration, and direction (Fig. 2; Table 1). The nystagmus of BPPV is typically accompanied by subjective vertigo. Any deviation from these characteristic findings should raise a concern that an alternative diagnosis may be present. Especially worrisome is downbeating nystagmus in the ear-down position as this may suggest a posterior fossa abnormality. In patients with negative Dix-Hallpike maneuver, an evaluation for lateral (horizontal) semicircular canal BPPV should be performed using the "roll test." The "roll test" actually uses yaw head movement and is performed by turning the patient from the supine to the head left or head right position and then to the opposite, i.e., head right or head left, position. Patients with lateral semicircular canal BPPV will experience vertigo after turning their head both to the left and to the right. Horizontal nystagmus beating toward the down ear will be observed while

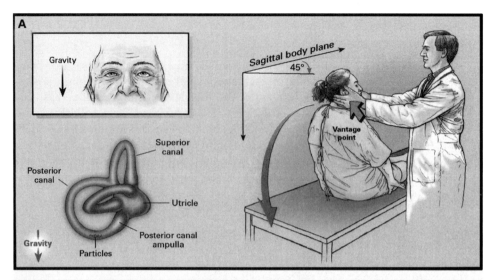

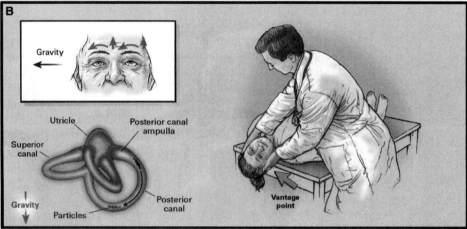

Figure 2 The Dix-Hallpike test of a patient with BPPV affecting the right ear. In panel (**A**), the examiner stands at the patient's right side and rotates the patient's head 45° to the right to align the right posterior semicircular canal with the sagittal plane of the body. In panel (**B**), the examiner moves the patient, whose eyes are open, from the seated to the supine right-ear-down position and then extends the patient's neck slightly so that the chin is pointed slightly upward. The latency, duration, and direction of nystagmus, if present, and the latency and duration of vertigo, if present, should be noted. The arrows in the inset depict the direction of nystagmus in patients with typical BPPV. The presumed location in the labyrinth of the free-floating debris thought to cause the disorder is also shown. *Abbreviation*: BPPV, benign paroxysmal positional vertigo. *Source*: From Ref. 16.

Table 1 Characteristics of Benign Paroxysmal Positional Vertigo

---

- Positionally induced vertigo and nystagmus using the Dix-Hallpike maneuver
- Latency of 1–40 sec (average 3–4 sec)
- Nystagmus is torsional—vertical
- Duration of signs and symptoms 10–60 sec
- Decreased signs and symptoms with repeated positioning
- Responds to particle repositioning

---

the patient is vertiginous. The vertigo and nystagmus is often severe, being worse when the patient is turned toward the involved ear. In the geriatric population, Dix-Hallpike maneuver may be confounded by the presence of other medical illnesses, especially orthostatic intolerance, which may lead to a sense of dizziness when the patient is moved from a recumbent to a sitting position. In these circumstances, patients typically do not report vertigo; rather, they report lightheadedness.

Patients with BPPV provide such a characteristic history and have such a characteristic physical examination in that no other disorder presents precisely in the same way. However, in some patients, the historical information is unclear and the Dix-Hallpike maneuver may be equivocal. Alternative diagnoses other than BPPV that should be considered as a cause of episodic vertigo include endolymphatic hydrops, i.e., Meniere's disease, vertebro-basilar insufficiency, migraine, and anxiety, particularly panic attacks. Usually, one or more aspects of the patient's presentation will allow differentiation between BPPV and one of these other disorders. However, there can be diagnostic uncertainty, especially in patients who are suffering from more than one condition.

Vestibular laboratory testing is not required for the diagnosis of BPPV. However, vestibular laboratory testing can provide information regarding whether the BPPV is an isolated problem or is an indication of more widespread vestibular disease. A unilateral caloric reduction suggests that the horizontal semicircular canal is involved in the patient's disorder. A directional preponderance on rotational testing or a spontaneous vestibular nystagmus suggests an ongoing vestibulo-ocular reflex asymmetry. Platform posturography testing may provide information regarding how a patient is using vestibular information for upright balance. Thus, although vestibular laboratory testing is not required for arriving at a diagnosis of BPPV, the tests are noninvasive and provide information that can overall be helpful in managing a patient's symptoms of dizziness and imbalance. Vestibular laboratory testing can be especially helpful for (i) deciding whether or not an individual should be referred for vestibular rehabilitation therapy, (ii) advising the patient regarding their activities, either at work or at home, and (iii) helping to prognosticate as to the length of time that will be required for recovery.

TREATMENT OF BPPV

The treatment of BPPV consists of repositioning the displaced otoconial debris from the posterior semicircular canal back to the region of the utricle where it no longer provokes symptoms. The particle-repositioning maneuver for patients with posterior canal BPPV, illustrated in Figure 3 (21), is highly successful, with a reported rate of success of approximately 90% (16,22,23). Performing this maneuver in elderly individuals is usually quite straightforward and can be performed without risk. An alternate particle-repositioning maneuver for patients with posterior canal BPPV, the so-called "liberatory maneuver", requires abrupt movements that are inappropriate for the elderly population (24). Since the liberatory maneuver has not been shown to be more successful than the particle-repositioning maneuver described in Figure 3, we do not advocate it. Following particle repositioning, many clinicians suggest that patients remain upright for 24 to 48 hours so that the otoconial debris is more likely to stay out of the posterior semicircular canal (16,21). However, remaining upright following particle repositioning is not recommended by all experts and has not been shown convincingly to alter treatment outcome (25,26). Thus, especially in older

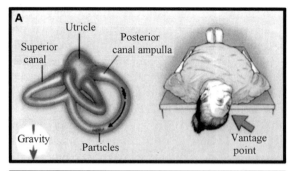

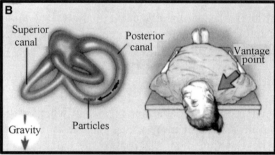

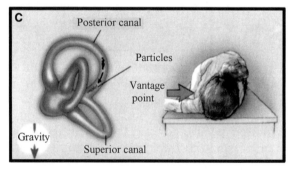

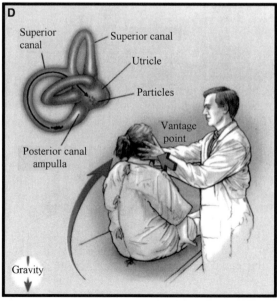

Figure 3 (*Caption on facing page*)

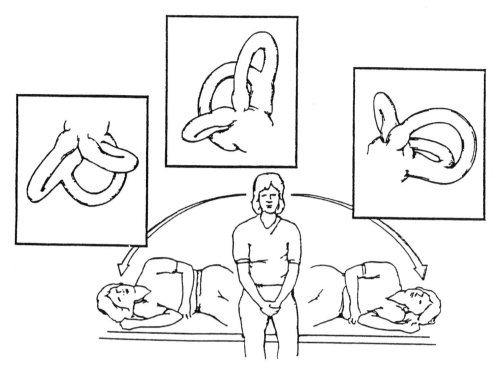

Figure 4 Brandt–Daroff exercises for benign paroxysmal positional vertigo. *Source*: From Ref. 31.

patients, recommending that the patient remain upright for 24 to 48 hours may not be appropriate. For lateral canal BPPV, there is a different kind of particle-repositioning maneuver that should be performed (27,28). A small percentage of patients with BPPV do not respond to particle repositioning initially and need to undergo a repeat particle-repositioning maneuver. Some patients cannot undergo particle repositioning either because of musculoskeletal problems, immobility, apprehension, or severe nausea at the time of assessment. For these individuals, Brandt–Daroff exercises (29,30), illustrated in Figure 4, should be prescribed. Rarely, patients with BPPV cannot be treated successfully with particle repositioning or Brandt–Daroff exercises or suffers from frequent recurrences. In these rare individuals, surgical

---

Figure 3 (*Facing page*) Bedside maneuver for the treatment of a patient with BPPV affecting the right ear. The presumed position of the debris within the labyrinth during the maneuver is shown in each panel. The maneuver is a three-step procedure. First, a Dix-Hallpike test is performed with the patient's head rotated 45° toward the right ear and the neck slightly extended with the chin pointed slightly upward. This position results in the patient's head hanging to the right (panel **A**). Once the vertigo and nystagmus provoked by the Dix-Hallpike test cease, the patient's head is rotated about the rostral–caudal body axis until the left ear is down (panel **B**). Then the head and body are further rotated until the head is face down (panel **C**). The vertex of the head is kept tilted downward throughout the rotation. The maneuver usually provokes brief vertigo. The patient should be kept in the final, face-down position for about 10 to 15 seconds. With the head kept turned toward the left shoulder, the patient is brought to the seated position (panel **D**). Once the patient is upright, the head is tilted so that the chin is pointed slightly downward. *Abbreviation*: BPPV, benign paroxysmal positional vertigo. *Source*: From Ref. 16.

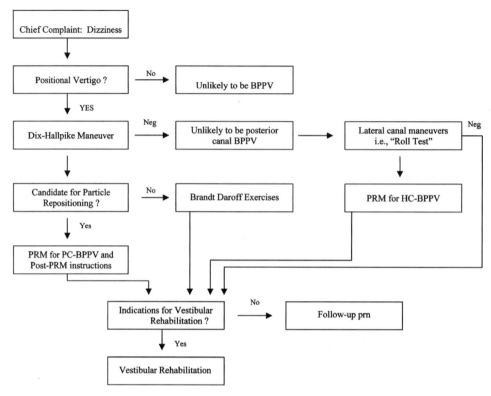

Figure 5 Algorithm for managing patients with benign paroxysmal positional vertigo.

intervention may be indicated. Posterior semicircular canal occlusion appears to be the surgical procedure of choice for such patients (32). However, advanced age is a relative contraindication for this elective surgery. Figure 5 provides an algorithm for managing patients presenting with positional vertigo. Note that many older patients with BPPV, even if treated successfully for their positional vertigo, will benefit from vestibular rehabilitation therapy.

REFERENCES

1. Baloh RW, Honrubia V, Jacobson K. Benign positional vertigo: clinical and oculographic features in 240 cases. Neurology 1987; 37(3):371–378.
2. Bourgeois PM, Dehaene I. Benign paroxysmal positional vertigo (Bppv). Clinical features in 34 cases and review of literature. Acta Neurol Belg 1988; 88(2):65–74.
3. Mizukoshi K, Watanabe Y, Shojaku H, Okubo J, Watanabe I. Epidemiological studies on benign paroxysmal positional vertigo in Japan. Acta Otolaryngol Suppl 1988; 447:67–72.
4. Hall SF, Ruby RR, McClure JA. The mechanics of benign paroxysmal vertigo. J Otolaryngol 1979; 8(2):151–158.
5. Lanska DJ, Remler B. Benign paroxysmal positioning vertigo: classic descriptions, origins of the provocative positioning technique, and conceptual developments. Neurology 1997; 48(5):1167–1177.
6. Baloh RW, Jacobson K, Honrubia V. Horizontal semicircular canal variant of benign positional vertigo. Neurology 1993; 43(12):2542–2549.

7. De la Meilleure G, Dehaene I, Depondt M, Damman W, Crevits L, Vanhooren G. Benign paroxysmal positional vertigo of the horizontal canal. J Neurol Neurosurg Psychiat 1996; 60(1):68–71.

8. Lempert T. Horizontal benign positional vertigo. Neurology 1994; 44(11):2213–2214.

9. Pagnini P, Nuti D, Vannucchi P. Benign paroxysmal vertigo of the horizontal canal. J Otorhinolaryngol Relat Spec 1989; 51(3):161–170.

10. Herdman SJ, Tusa RJ. Complications of the canalith repositioning procedure. Arch Otolaryngol Head Neck Surg 1996; 122(3):281–286.

11. Honrubia V, Baloh RW, Harris MR, Jacobson KM. Paroxysmal positional vertigo syndrome. Am J Otolaryngol 1999; 20(4):465–470.

12. Baloh RW, Yue Q, Jacobson KM, Honrubia V. Persistent direction-changing positional nystagmus: another variant of benign positional nystagmus? Neurology 1995; 45(7):1297–1301.

13. Schuknecht HF. Cupulolithiasis. Arch Otolaryngol 1969; 90(6):765–778.

14. Froehling DA, Silverstein MD, Mohr DN, Beatty CW, Offord KP, Ballard DJ. Benign positional vertigo: incidence and prognosis in a population-based study in Olmsted County, Minnesota. Mayo Clin Proc 1991; 66(6):596–601.

15. Oghalai JS, Manolidis S, Barth JL, Stewart MG, Jenkins HA. Unrecognized benign paroxysmal positional vertigo in elderly patients. Otolaryngol Head Neck Surg 2000; 122(5):630–634.

16. Furman JM, Cass SP. Benign paroxysmal positional vertigo. N Engl J Med 1999; 341(21):1590–1596.

17. Hain TC, Helminski JO, Reis IL, Uddin MK. Vibration does not improve results of the canalith repositioning procedure. Arch Otolaryngol Head Neck Surg 2000; 126(5):617–622.

18. Parnes LS, McClure JA. Free-floating endolymph particles: a new operative finding during posterior semicircular canal occlusion. Laryngoscope 1992; 102(9):988–992.

19. Ishiyama A, Jacobson KM, Baloh RW. Migraine and benign positional vertigo. Ann Otol Rhinol Laryngol 2000; 109(4):377–380.

20. Lempert T, Leopold M, von Brevern M, Neuhauser H. Migraine and benign positional vertigo. Ann Otol Rhinol Laryngol 2000; 109(12 Pt 1):1176.

21. Epley JM. The canalith repositioning procedure: for treatment of benign paroxysmal positional vertigo. Otolaryngol Head Neck Surg 1992; 107(3):399–404.

22. Lynn S, Pool A, Rose D, Brey R, Suman V. Randomized trial of the canalith repositioning procedure. Otolaryngol Head Neck Surg 1995; 113(6):712–720.

23. Steenerson RL, Cronin GW. Comparison of the canalith repositioning procedure and vestibular habituation training in forty patients with benign paroxysmal positional vertigo. Otolaryngol Head Neck Surg 1996; 114(1):61–64.

24. Semont A, Freyss G, Vitte E. Curing the Bppv with a liberatory maneuver. Adv Otorhinolaryngol 1988; 42:290–293.

25. Massoud EA, Ireland DJ. Post-treatment instructions in the nonsurgical management of benign paroxysmal positional vertigo. J Otolaryngol 1996; 25(2):121–125.

26. Nuti D, Nati C, Passali D. Treatment of benign paroxysmal positional vertigo: no need for postmaneuver restrictions. Otolaryngol Head Neck Surg 2000; 122(3):440–444.

27. Epley JM. Positional vertigo related to semicircular canalithiasis. Otolaryngol Head Neck Surg 1995; 112(1):154–161.

28. Nuti D, Agus G, Barbieri MT, Passali D. The management of horizontal-canal paroxysmal positional vertigo. Acta Otolaryngol 1998; 118(4):455–460.

29. Brandt T, Daroff RB. Physical therapy for benign paroxysmal positional vertigo. Arch Otolaryngol 1980; 106(8):484–485.

30. Brandt T, Steddin S, Daroff RB. Therapy for benign paroxysmal positioning vertigo, revisited. Neurology 1994; 44(5):796–800.

31. Herdman SJ. Assessment and management of benign paroxysmal positional vertigo. In: Herdman SJ, ed. Vestibular Rehabilitation. Philadelphia: FA Davis, 1999:20.

32. Parnes LS, McClure JA. Posterior semicircular canal occlusion in the normal hearing ear. Otolaryngol Head Neck Surg 1991; 104(1):52–57.

ANNOTATED BIBLIOGRAPHY

Furman JM, Cass SP. Benign paroxysmal positional vertigo. N Engl J Med 1999; 341(21):1590–1596.

An excellent review of benign paroxysmal positional vertigo.

Lanska DJ, Remler B. Benign paroxysmal positioning vertigo: classic descriptions, origins of the provocative positioning technique, and conceptual developments. Neurology 1997; 48(5):1167–1177.

A detailed account of the development of ideas concerning the pathogenesis, diagnosis, and treatment of benign paroxysmal positional vertigo. Issues regarding nomenclature are discussed.

Lynn S, Pool A, Rose D, Brey R, Suman V. Randomized trial of the canalith repositioning procedure. Otolaryngol Head Neck Surg 1995; 113(6):712–720.

A well-written account of particle repositioning for benign paroxysmal positional vertigo.

Parnes LS, Agrawal SK, Atlas J. Diagnosis and management of benign paroxysmal positional vertigo (BPPV). Can Med Assoc J 2003; 169(7):1–16.

Another excellent review of benign paroxysmal position vertigo.

14
Balance Rehabilitation

Horst R. Konrad
Division of Otolaryngology—Head and Neck Surgery, Southern Illinois University School of Medicine, Springfield, Illinois, U.S.A.

Meiho Nakayama
Department of Otolaryngology, Aichi Medical University, Aichigun Aichiken, Japan

Marian Girardi—In Memoriam

I had the privilege of working with Dr. Marian Girardi our former coauthor from November 1, 1993 to June 30, 2003. Dr. Girardi first joined our vestibular laboratory at a time when vestibular testing and balance rehabilitation was in its infancy. In the Southern Illinois University Vestibular Laboratory, she established normal values for elderly patients by testing many patients from the senior citizens groups in the Springfield area. These values are still used in most clinics in the evaluation and treatment of elderly patients with balance disorders. Dr. Girardi's academic life centered around the evaluation and management of patients with balance disorders, especially elderly patients. This subject also became her doctoral thesis. She taught extensively at SIU School of Medicine. She established and directed our first balance disorders and falls prevention clinic. She lectured extensively to medical students, residents, and faculty and developed a balance assessment and management team, which included otolaryngologists, audiologists, physical and occupational therapists, and fellows and residents from otolaryngology, neurology, and other services in the medical school. She also lectured extensively both nationally and internationally, and she was a pioneer in recognizing the usefulness of posturography and patient questionnaires to evaluate balance function and its impact on quality of life. She also published extensively in the medical literature on the subject of balance evaluation and treatment.

In addition to her academic achievements, she was very heavily involved in the 4-H Clubs of central and southern Illinois, where she taught horseback riding, dressage, cooking, baking, and many other 4-H activities.

She died on December 5, 2004, of complications of diabetes. She will be sorely missed by her colleagues, her students, and her many friends in our community.

Horst R. Konrad M.D.

INTRODUCTION

Balance rehabilitation relies on innate restorative mechanisms within the brain and the body to re-establish function lost through disease, injury, medication, surgical ablation, or disuse. Balance function requires: (i) sensory information from vision, vestibular, and proprioceptive systems, (ii) integration of this information by the central nervous system, and (iii) execution of motor activities by the musculoskeletal system. Many of these activities occur through reflexive action such as the spinal reflexes, the vestibulo-oculomotor reflexes, the visual oculomotor reflexes, and the vestibulospinal reflexes. Cerebral function controls and alters these reflexes while cerebellar activity "fine tunes" and adjusts the responses. Many of these systems are well known. The vestibulo-oculomotor reflex is one of the best examples.

Early work in rehabilitation is credited to Cooksey and Cawthorne in England in the 1940s. Cooksey, a physical therapist, and Cawthorne, an otolaryngologist, worked together to help patients with vestibular deficits improve their function through a physical therapy program. Later Brant Daroff exercises were popularized to help patients with balance impairment. Work by Makoto Igarashi et al. (1) at Baylor showed that the physiological basis of vestibular rehabilitation were dependent on head movement during vision. Experiments with cats and monkeys showed that animals with vestibular lesions did not compensate well when in the dark, compensated better when kept in the light and left to exercise at liberty, and improved even faster when forced to exercise in light. Igarashi et al. also showed that the neural elements for this improvement were the vestibular nuclei and the cerebellum where information from the visual system and the vestibular system could be utilized by cerebellar neurons to "reset" the sensitivity and gain of the vestibulo-ocular motor reflex. This improved understanding of the mechanisms involved in the resetting of the vestibulo-ocular motor reflex has been incorporated into exercise programs for patients who have uncompensated or inadequately compensated peripheral vestibular deficits.

Most patients with balance disorders benefit from a rehabilitation program. The magnitude of the benefit depends on many factors, including the characteristics of the disorder, age, and motivation. Evaluation of the patient's deficits as well as remaining function is critical in providing an efficient and effective rehabilitation program for the patients. Patients with stable, purely vestibular deficits have a high success rate with rehabilitation. Patients with a combination of peripheral sensory and central disorders or multisensory and central disorders are less likely to have full resolution of their problems, but are still likely to benefit from rehabilitation. These patients can particularly benefit by a reduction of falls and falls-related injuries. Rehabilitation includes the use and training with assistive devices such as canes and walkers, as well as an assessment and changes in the home. Often changes in lighting and floor surfaces, provision of handholds on steps and bathrooms, and an educational program for the patient's family and caregivers will lead to significant benefits.

Benign paroxysmal positional vertigo (BPPV) is a peripheral vestibular but paradoxical (unstable) disorder, which is very amenable to rehabilitation. It represents an excellent demonstration of the axiom that knowledge of the pathophysiology leads to treatment paradigms with very high success rates. It is probably the most common vestibular disorder affecting balance and is increasingly common in older populations.

BPPV was first described by Barany in 1921 (2) and further defined by Dix and Hallpike in 1952 (3). Dix and Hallpike described a provocative test maneuver that was diagnostic if it elicited torsional nystagmus directed to the undermost ear, with latency, limited duration, reversal upon reversing the maneuver, and response decline with repetition. In 1969, Schuknecht (4) documented the pathology of some cases of BPPV to be otolithic debris attached to the cupula of the posterior canal. This theory, cupulolithiasis, was believed as a mechanism of BPPV until other investigator documented cases of BPPV arose with a plug of material within the posterior canal itself, the so-called canalolithiasis, rather than material attached to the cupula (5,6). A paucity of temporal bone pathology cases with cupulolithiasis in this common disorder further suggests canalolithiasis as the probable cause of BPPV. It has since become apparent that the mechanism for BPPV is canalolithiasis, which are free-floating debris (or densities) collected within the posterior semicircular canal of the involved ear. This debris shifts in response to gravitational change, creating drag on the perilymph that is then imparted to the cupula. This triggers a nonphysiologic vestibulo-ocular reflex of the posterior semicircular canal, producing nystagmus in its plane. When the debris reach the limit of its descent, the cupula resumes its normal state and the nystagmus terminates. On reversal of the maneuver, the motion of the debris reverses, causing nystagmus with the same characteristics, but in the opposite direction. During the nystagmus period, patients complain of severe dizziness.

In 1992, Epley (7) described the canalith repositioning procedure of a five-position cycle of head movements. Epley postulated that the maneuver caused free canaliths to migrate by gravity out of the posterior semicircular canal to the vestibule, where they would no longer exert a rotational response. A high success rate was reported and the technique has become accepted by many as the first line of management of BPPV.

This describes most cases of BPPV. It is possible, although less common, for the debris to be in an anterior vertical, or the horizontal canal. In these cases, the positional nystagmus will be in the planes of these canals and can be treated by a maneuver in the planes of these canals. It is also possible for patients to have debris in more than one canal or for debris to be moved from one canal to another by the maneuver. For this reason, it is important to re-examine patients in two or more weeks after the performance of a maneuver. This is best done with the use of infrared goggles, which block the fixation reflex and allow the observer to see the eyes and their movements. In-depth discussion of BPPV can be found in the chapter in this text by Joseph Furman. Furthermore, it has been demonstrated that an exercise program following successful resolution of BPPV via the particle-repositioning maneuver reduces the recurrence of this condition (8).

GENERAL DESCRIPTION OF THE CLINICAL PROBLEM

Prevalence

Balance disorders are extremely common in all populations, accounting for 42% of physician visits. Approximately six million Americans annually seek medical help for dizziness or balance disorders. This is a particularly important issue in geriatrics since, as the populations age, balance disorders become increasingly common. For patients over age 65, this becomes the most common reason for visiting a physician, and even after that, balance problems continue to increase with advancing age. Balance disorders in the aging population not only lead to discomfort and limit the patient's activities, but also lead to falls and falls with injuries. In addition to this, the fear of falling associated with balance disorders severely affects the patient's quality of life. Fear of falling results in further limitation of movement, which, in turn, results in further weakness, stiffness, and a higher risk of falling with injury. In addition to changes in the patients' quality of life, balance disorders also affect other members of the family, since as these patients become progressively more incapacitated, children, spouses, or other family members and caregivers must assume roles in activities of daily living, including shopping, preparation of food, and even assisting in walking within the living area from bedroom to bathroom. Older populations, particularly women, are the most rapidly growing parts of the population in the United States and other developed countries. By 2010, more than 40 million Americans will be older than age 65. Both depression and anxiety states are common in patients with balance disorders and further result in limitation of activities.

Normal Aging Related to Balance

As we age, we lose sensitivity in the vestibular organs—both the rotational sensors, the semicircular canals, and the gravity receptors, the urtricle and saccule. This reduced sensitivity is due to a reduction in numbers of hair cells, particularly in the superior portion of the cupula of the semicircular canals (9). Aging also results in reduction of nerve fibers conducting vestibular information to the brain stem. Other normal changes that affect balance include slowing of central reflexes, particularly in the eye-movement control reflexes and in reflexes required to initiate body movements. Vision and hearing also decline in aging populations, and the function of proprioceptive sensory systems also declines. In addition to this, older patients tend to have less muscle mass and strength, and reduced flexibility and bone strength. Osteoporosis is particularly common in older women and further leads to more severe injuries when a fall occurs. In addition to these normal changes, there are also age-related disorders that significantly affect balance. Benign paroxysmal positional vertigo, described above, is much more common in aging populations. Vascular, carotid artery, vertebral basilar, and small vessel cerebrovascular disease can significantly affect circulation to important brain structures, which are required in eye, head, and limb movements. Transient ischemic attacks and cerebrovascular accidents can further damage brain structures important for balance. Coronary artery disease, cardiomyopathy, and cardiac arrhythmias can also result in decreased brain perfusion, which can add to problems in balance. Many neurological disorders including stroke, degenerative diseases, head injuries, and concussion are more common in the elderly and can lead to balance disorders. Parkinson's disease as well as degenerative cerebellar and brainstem ataxias also adversely affect balance. Diabetes mellitus reduces vision and proprioceptive function, and also increases arteriosclerosis in both small and large vessels. Hypertension leads to accelerated arteriosclerosis, and treatment leads to postural hypotension or labile blood pressure, which results in orthostatic changes, which can also increase risk of falling. Medications are more commonly used in the elderly populations, and many of the medications currently used can adversely affect balance. Benzodiazepines, such as Valium, and antihistamines such as Meclizine, can reduce vestibular sensitivity and adversely affect balance and recovery from vestibular injury. In younger populations, balance disorders are often characterized by episodes of dizziness or vertiginous episodes, while in the older population, the presenting symptom is generally a feeling of light-headedness, a feeling of disequilibrium or difficulty with walking. Positional vertigo is also a common symptom, and is often the first symptom in benign paroxysmal positional vertigo. The physical examination in patients complaining of balance disorders should focus on the sensory systems associated with balance, and also the functions of the cerebellum and cerebrum. Slowing of reflexes is a common cause of balance dysfunction in the elderly. Vision and eye movements need to be carefully assessed, and vision should be corrected when possible. Hearing and balance often go together, so clinical examination of both should be routine. Eye movements, including smooth pursuit, saccade, and observation for spontaneous nystagmus are part of the office examination. Positional tests can easily be done in the office and are very important in patients with symptoms of positional vertigo. Since balance disorders may be due to an intermittent disorder, every opportunity should be utilized to assess this problem at the time symptoms suggest its presence. Proprioception can be examined in the office and as part of the balance evaluation. In addition to this, general strength and flexibility and evaluation for the disorders, which affect balance, are part of the history and physical examination.

Electronystagmography, posturography, and audiometry are parts of the laboratory evaluation for these patients. Posturography is the best predictor of falls related to balance problems in the elderly, particularly the test conditions where vision and proprioception are impaired. Another valuable component of posturography testing is the limits of stability test, which determines how far patients can lean before becoming unstable. Electronystagmogram with particular attention to the saccadic latencies, the caloric sensitivity, and visual fixation suppression of caloric nystagmus is helpful in assessing the sensory systems related to inner ear and eye movement control and speed of central processing. Treatment is based on the specific patient's problem. The symptoms of many patients can be dramatically reduced by eliminating or changing medications that adversely affect balance, cause sedation, or impair reflexes. As a result, medications should be reviewed in all patients who complain of dizziness, particularly the elderly. This strategy is particularly valuable with patients who are on antihistamines, benzodiazepines, or other sedating medications.

Detailed description of rehabilitation exercises is beyond the scope of this chapter. Physicians would be advised to work with physical therapists, audiologists, or occupational therapists who are trained in the specific rehabilitation exercise programs. Not all therapists are trained in balance rehabilitation, but in most communities at least one or two therapists are knowledgeable and skilled in the techniques. Patients should be referred to these individuals, and encouraged to learn and practice regularly the techniques that they are taught.

Most patients with chronic disequilibrium can be significantly helped with balance rehabilitation. The basis of this benefit is adaptation, compensation, and restoration. In addition to improving strength and flexibility, vestibular balance rehabilitation training attempts to re-establish functions of the vestibular system by utilizing vision and balance exercises. Oculomotor skills can be improved through an exercise program aimed at eye movement control. Posture control can be improved through exercises, and strengthening and flexibility training. Patients are also taught better movement strategies so that the likelihood of falling is diminished. Some of the limitations of balance retraining include loss of vision, proprioception, and loss of vestibular sensitivity. However, balance retraining often can utilize one of these senses to overcome deficiencies in the others. The most difficult problems to manage are severe central nervous system (CNS) problems related to degenerative processes, strokes, or head injuries. Memory, cognitive abilities, and decision making are integral to balance retraining and are adversely affected by such disorders as Alzheimer's disease, small vessel atherosclerosis, and other degenerative

CNS disorders. Lack of motivation, anxiety disorder, and other psychological disorders can limit the efficacy of balance retraining and often need to be separately addressed during rehabilitation. Secondary gain and litigation can also be detrimental to good outcomes for balance retraining. It is important to assess not only the patient himself, but also family relationships, the potential for caregivers, and transportation options. Those who are likely to do well for the balance retraining exercises are those with stable vestibular dysfunction, in whom symptoms are persistent, but not progressing at a rapid rate. Poor individuals for vestibular rehabilitation are patients with rapidly progressing disease or with unstable lesions such as frequent attacks of Meniere's disease or those with demyelinating disorders and seizures. Patients with benign paroxysmal positional vertigo have an outstanding cure rate, in excess of 90%. Patients who have had vestibular neuronitis, labyrinthitis, or postsurgical vestibular damage; postvestibular ototoxicity patients; head trauma patients; and those who have suffered stroke or other forms of central toxicity but who are now stabilized are excellent candidates for rehabilitation. Patients with both central and peripheral disorders, such as head injury patients who received severe brain concussion and lost vestibular function from their head trauma, often suffer from persistent symptoms and may not benefit extensively.

Patients are best evaluated and treated through a falls risk assessment and treatment program. The treatment team often includes an otolaryngologist or a neurologist with a special interest in balance disorders. An audiologist, physical therapist, and occupational therapist are integral and equal members of the team. Each one of these individuals brings a special interest, knowledge, and training to benefit patients with balance disorders. Since many of these patients are elderly and have transportation problems, the team is best assembled at one time and placed to avoid separate appointments. Since family and other caregivers are very important for the success of this program, they should accompany the patients and participate in their evaluation and treatment. The use of a questionnaire mailed to the patient that outlines the history, list of medications, and previous treatments and evaluations is often very useful. Audiograms, electronystagmographic studies, imaging, and laboratory studies performed elsewhere are requested, as well as permission to obtain these studies prior to the first appointment.

At the first visit, an extensive history and physical examination is performed by the physician. The patient and caregiver or family are then evaluated by the physical therapist, occupational therapist, and audiologist. The treatment team reviews the findings and establishes a plan with specific recommendations for treatment. Additional tests may be necessary, and follow-up must be arranged. The final plan is discussed with the patient and caregivers and sent to the referring clinician. Therapy is instituted and the patient is usually re-evaluated in two to three months. For additional information on patients with multifactorial deficits causing balance dysfunction, see the chapter by Susan L. Whitney, Ph.D., "Multisensory impairment in older adults: evaluation and intervention."

SUMMARY

Balance rehabilitation is a critical part of the management of the dizzy elderly patient. Nearly all patients with dizziness from a variety of causes will benefit, as well as those with other balance disorders due to peripheral, central, or musculoskeletal etiologies. Balance rehabilitation therapy should be part of a falls-reduction program administered by a multidisciplinary team. Patients with balance disorders should be encouraged to be as active as physically possible in order to maintain and restore balance function. Elimination of sedative medication is often a critical adjunct to a program of balance rehabilitation. Communication and coordination with the patient's primary care physician is integral to any program of balance rehabilitation.

REFERENCES

1. Igarashi M, et al. Clinical pathological correlations in squirrel monkeys after suppression of semicircular canal function by streptomycin sulfate. Acta Otolaryngol 1966; 214:1–28.
2. Barany R. Diagnose von Krankheitserscheinungen im Bereiche des Otolithenapparates. Acta Otolaryngol 1921; 2:434–437.
3. Dix MR, Hallpike CS. The pathology, symptomatology and diagnosis of certain common disorders of the vestibular system. Ann Otol Rhinol Laryngol 1952; 61:987–1016.
4. Schuknecht HF. Cupulolithiasis. Arch Otolaryngol 1969; 90:765–778.
5. Hall SF. The mechanics of benign paroxysmal vertigo. J Otolaryngol 1979; 8:151–158.
6. Epley JM. New dimensions of benign paroxysmal positional vertigo. Otolaryngol Head Neck Surg 1980; 88:599–605.
7. Epley JM. The canalith repositioning procedure: for treatment of benign paroxysmal positional vertigo. Otolaryngol Head Neck Surg 1992; 107:399–404.
8. Amin M, Girardi M, Neill ME, et al. Effects of exercise on prevention of recurrence of BPPV symptoms. ARO Midwinter Meeting, in Feb. 14–18, 1999, St. Petersburg Beach, FL.
9. Nakayama M, Helfert RH, Konrad HR, Caspary DM. Scanning electron microscopic evaluation of age-related changes in the rat vestibular epithelium. Otolaryngol Head Neck Surg 1994; 111:799–806.

15
Olfaction and Aging

Karen J. Fong
Department of Otolaryngology—Head and Neck Surgery, Oregon Health and Science University, Portland, Oregon, U.S.A.

Mark A. Zacharek
Department of Otolaryngology—Head and Neck Surgery, Henry Ford Hospital, Detroit, Michigan, U.S.A.

INTRODUCTION

Olfaction is an important sensory function. Although it is known to decline with age, not all olfactory loss occurring in older adults can be attributed to aging (1–3). Sudden loss in olfaction should be cause for concern in all age groups. Olfactory loss has significant health implications and may increase an elderly individual's risk of injury or illness from inhalation of gaseous fumes, consumption of rotten food, and deficient caloric intake.

In the past decade, much interest has been focused on the changes that occur in the olfactory system during normal aging and the means by which these changes can be measured. This chapter will attempt to review the current understanding of the changes in the olfactory system during aging and the clinical approach to the elderly patient with an olfactory deficit.

Based on the National Health Interview Survey, approximately 2.7 million Americans suffer from chronic olfactory problems. The prevalence of this problem was found to be greatest in patients 75 years of age and older (46 per 1000). Adults aged 65–74 years reported the next highest rate at 26.5 per 1000. Taken together, these groups account for 40% of the 2.7 million adults in the United States reporting a chronic problem with their sense of smell (4). Traditionally, determining the prevalence of olfactory sensory changes has relied heavily on "self-reporting" by patients. This approach greatly underestimates the actual incidence of olfactory deficits in the elderly (5). A more recent study in which clinical olfactory testing was used revealed a much higher prevalence of olfactory impairment in older adults than previously identified by self-reporting: in the age groups of 60–69, 70–79, and 80–97, the prevalence rates of olfactory impairment were 17.3%, 29.2%, and 62.5%, respectively (6).

Table 1 Definition of Terms Relating to Olfactory Dysfunction

Anosmia	Complete olfactory loss
Hyposmia	Diminished sense of smell
Dysosmia	Distorted olfactory perception
Parosmia	In response to an olfactory stimulant
Phantosmia	In the absence of an olfactory stimulant
Hyperosmia	Enhanced olfactory perception

DEFINITIONS

Although multiple terms have been used to describe olfactory dysfunction, the use of standardized terminology is important (Table 1). *Anosmia* refers to a total absence of olfaction, whereas *hyposmia* refers to diminished smell sensitivity. *Dysosmia* refers to a distorted olfactory perception. This can occur in the presence of a sensory stimulus (*parosmia*) or in the absence of a sensory stimulus (*phantosmia*). *Hyperosmia* refers to increased odorant sensitivity.

ETIOLOGIES OF OLFACTORY LOSS

The etiologies of olfactory dysfunction are numerous (Table 2). The most common causes of olfactory loss are inflammatory in nature, occurring as a result of nasal and/or sinus disease, previous upper respiratory infection, and head trauma (7). Other potential causes of olfactory loss include toxic exposure, congenital conditions, systemic diseases, cigarette smoking, and aging itself. Despite a complete evaluation, the exact cause of olfactory loss often remains unknown (idiopathic). A number of conditions more prevalent in the elderly may contribute to chemosensory dysfunction; these include dementia, epilepsy, metabolic disorders (e.g., diabetes and hypothyroidism), and neurodegenerative disorders (e.g., Alzheimer's and Parkinson's) (8–11). The coexistence of multisystem disease, exposure to a broad range of toxins, and use of multiple medications also tend to be more common in the elderly. These factors taken in combination may affect chemosensory function and contribute to olfactory deficits (12).

PATHOPHYSIOLOGY OF OLFACTORY LOSS WITH AGING

A large body of literature indicates that the sense of smell declines with increasing age (1,3,6,13). Age-related changes to both the peripheral and central processes of olfaction are thought to be due to cumulative environmental insults with an associated reduction in regenerative capacity. Areas of the olfactory neuroepithelium, olfactory bulbs, and brain associated with olfactory processing show neuropathological changes with age. Some of these are more prominent in Alzheimer's disease and other neurodegenerative disorders. The relationship of olfactory loss and Alzheimer's disease is discussed in detail elsewhere in this text and will not be discussed here. Indeed, some have suggested that olfaction may be a good indicator of the integrity of the aging brain (14).

The olfactory neuroepithelium is unique in its ability to replace olfactory neurons throughout the lifetime of an organism. However, loss of olfaction suggests that the system is not perfect. Animal studies have shown an age-related decline in the number of olfactory receptor neurons and atrophy of the olfactory bulb (15). In part, this decline

Table 2 Etiology of Olfactory Dysfunction (Partial List)

Nasal and/or sinus inflammatory disease
   Allergic rhinitis
   Bacterial rhinosinusitis
   Viral rhinosinusitis
   Nasal polyposis
   Neoplasms (benign or malignant)
Post upper respiratory tract viral infection
Trauma
   Head injury
   Surgical
Toxic exposure
Age
Neurologic disease
   Alzheimer's disease
   Parkinson's disease
   Huntington's chorea
   Multiple sclerosis
   Dementia
   Schizophrenia
   Seizures
Metabolic
   Diabetes
   Hypothyroidism
   Liver disease
   Renal failure
Medications
Cigarette smoking
Radiation therapy to the head and neck
Malnutrition
Congenital (Kallman's syndrome)
Idiopathic

---

may be due to an increased rate of olfactory receptor neuron cell death (16). Histopathologic studies of human tissue have revealed that in aging, the olfactory neuroepithelium is gradually replaced with respiratory epithelium in a patchy distribution (17).

More centrally, human olfactory bulbs show atrophy with age (18). A decline in the number of mitral cells and glomeruli within the human olfactory bulb at an approximate rate of 10% per decade has also been noted during aging and may in part underlie the decline in olfactory abilities noted with age (19). Neuropathy in nondemented older adults has been described in the hippocampus, anterior olfactory nucleus, and entorhinal cortex (20). These regions are all involved in the central processing of olfactory information. Magnetic resonance imaging (MRI) has revealed age-related volume loss in areas of the brain associated with olfactory function (21,22). Functional MRI imaging studies in a cohort of elderly (mean age of 73) and young (mean age of 24) patients exposed to pulsed odorant stimuli revealed that younger subjects had a greater number of activated voxels in the regions of the frontal lobes, perisylvian, and cingulate gyri in comparison to elderly individuals (23).

The association of aging and dementia must be considered when determining olfactory change, as dementia is associated with impaired olfactory function (11,24). The incidence of dementia approaches nearly 50% beyond the age of 80.

While many earlier studies did not take this into account, more recent studies have attempted to focus on the differences in olfactory impairment between healthy aging subjects and those with dementia and other neurodegenerative disorders.

PATIENT EVALUATION

History

A presenting complaint of olfactory deficit in the geriatric population should be taken seriously, and not be dismissed as part of the normal aging process. A complete history should be elicited, including the degree of olfactory loss and/or the presence of a distorted perception, as well as a description of sudden versus gradual onset. Although many patients will present with a chief complaint of ageusia (loss of taste) rather than anosmia, it should be noted that the majority of *taste* complaints actually refer to a distortion of *flavor* perception, which in large part is dependent on olfaction. Patients who complain of loss of taste should be questioned specifically about the ability to distinguish between the four tastants: bitter, salty, sour, and sweet. If this perception remains intact, the problem is likely olfactory in nature. In a study of 750 patients presenting to the University of Pennsylvania Smell and Taste Center, 78.1% complained of a reduced ability to smell and 66.4% of a reduced ability to taste. After chemosensory testing was performed, however, less than 3% of patients had a taste loss, while 79.9% had an olfactory deficit (25).

The history should be directed at eliciting common causes of olfactory dysfunction. Patients should be questioned about nasal and sinus disease, including allergic rhinitis, chronic sinusitis, nasal polyps, and previous nasal or sinus surgery. A history of a preceding viral upper respiratory tract infection or head trauma should be elucidated. Concomitant medical conditions and current medications should be carefully reviewed. A history of toxic exposures or chronic exposures in the home or workplace is important. Smoking and previous radiation therapy to the head and neck may also be contributing factors.

Physical Examination

A complete head and neck examination should be performed. This includes both anterior rhinoscopy and nasal endoscopy to evaluate for the presence of allergic rhinitis, chronic rhinosinusitis, nasal polyps, masses, or other signs of inflammation. Signs of atrophic or vasomotor rhinitis should be noted.

If the history does not support a diagnosis of toxic exposure, or postviral or traumatic loss, and the physical examination does not support the presence of nasal or sinus disease, a full neurologic examination is important. As previously noted, olfactory deficits are found in a variety of neurological disorders, although they are seldom the primary complaint. Focal neurological findings may suggest the diagnosis of a central neoplastic process or stroke.

Chemosensory Testing

Olfactory function testing is an important step in evaluation of the geriatric patient with an olfactory complaint and usually consists of identification of specific odors, threshold detection, or both. As mentioned earlier, self-reporting alone significantly underestimates the prevalence of olfactory loss in older adults (6).

Several clinical olfactory identification tests have been developed, which can be administered in the office. The most widely used is the University of Pennsylvania Smell Identification Test (UPSIT, commercially available as the Smell Identification Test[TM], Sensonics, Inc., Haddon Heights, New Jersey, U.S.), a four-choice "scratch and sniff" odor identification test. Advantages of the UPSIT include the fact that it is self-administered, well validated, and based on a large body of normative data for males and females grouped according to age (26).

Olfactory function can also be assessed by threshold testing, which is used to measure the *detection* threshold (the lowest odorant concentration where a stimulus can be perceived). The two types of detection threshold testing currently used in clinical practice include the ascending method of limits and the single staircase; in both of these, odorants are presented to the patient in increasing concentrations. In the ascending method of limits procedure, stimuli are presented in increasing concentrations from undetectable levels to those concentrations where detection is reliably made. In the single staircase method, the stimulus concentration is increased following trials on which a subject fails to detect the stimulus and decreased following trials where correct detection occurs. Commonly used stimulants are phenyl ethyl alcohol and butanol, which have little trigeminal stimulation. Patients must choose between the solution with the stimulant, and one with water only. An advantage of this type of testing is that it allows for unilateral assessment. (For a more detailed description of the procedures, see Refs. 27,28).

Radiological Evaluation

Radiological evaluation is not always necessary in the evaluation of olfactory loss, but can be useful when the etiology is unclear. Computed tomographic scans of the paranasal sinuses are the most useful study when a conductive olfactory loss is suspected. Coronal computed tomographic scans of the paranasal sinuses provide the clearest detail of the bony and soft tissue anatomy and can demonstrate inflammatory disease or mass lesions of the nasal cavity and sinuses. MRI is the study of choice when an intracranial lesion is suspected. Olfactory groove meningioma, frontal lobe gliomas, and other lesions of the anterior cranial fossa can produce a gradually progressive olfactory loss, although it should be noted that such lesions rarely present with olfactory loss as their only symptom.

Other Diagnostic Tests

Routine laboratory tests are rarely helpful in the evaluation of the patient with olfactory loss. However, when clinical suspicion warrants, laboratory tests may help to confirm diagnoses such as hypothyroidism, diabetes, or renal or liver failure. It has been shown that some vitamin and mineral deficiencies such as B_{12}, zinc, and copper can be associated with olfactory or taste dysfunction, but these causes are so rare that evaluation for such deficiencies is rarely indicated unless patients demonstrate other clinical signs of severe malnutrition.

TREATMENT AND COUNSELING

In general, treatment of anosmia or hyposmia is extremely limited. Only olfactory loss due to nasal or sinus inflammatory disease is readily amenable to treatment, which is usually directed at controlling allergic rhinitis, or treating rhinosinusitis.

Nasal polyps are usually addressed initially with trials of topical and/or oral steroids. Surgery may be indicated in cases of anatomical obstruction, rhinosinusitis unresponsive to medical management, and severe nasal polyposis. A short trial of oral steroids can sometimes be helpful in determining the presence of reversible olfactory dysfunction secondary to inflammatory disease. In the rare instance that olfactory loss is thought to be due to an underlying medical condition, the latter should be corrected. Unfortunately, no effective treatment for postviral olfactory loss or olfactory loss due to head trauma is available. It is believed by many physicians that postviral olfactory loss that persists through the first year is permanent. However, in a long-term study following patients with postviral loss, 62–90% of patients showed some improvement in olfactory function at five years, depending on whether subjective or objective measures were assessed (29). Reduced regenerative ability of the aging olfactory epithelium to recover function after damage by a viral infection may explain the higher incidence of postviral olfactory deficits in the elderly population. The prognosis for patients with olfactory loss secondary to head trauma is poor and most post-traumatic deficits are permanent.

Regardless of etiology, appropriate counseling with patients and their family members is important in the management of olfactory deficits. This may be even more crucial in the elderly patient who may live alone and suffer from impairment of other sensory functions as well. Patients must be specifically counseled with regards to hazards such as smoke or leaking gas; installation and maintenance of working smoke detectors is therefore essential. Gas appliances should be equipped with natural gas detectors or changed in favor of electric ones whenever possible. These devices should be regularly checked and serviced by family members or facility personnel. Unfortunately, a disproportionate number of elderly dies from accidental gas poisoning (30). Patients are also at risk for food poisoning and must be counseled about spoiled items. They must adhere to a vigilant leftover policy and food should be regularly verified by a family member or friend.

Nutrition is another area of concern for older persons with olfactory loss. Since olfaction plays a large role in the perception of flavor, patients with diminished olfaction may have decreased enjoyment of food. Whether this influences overall food intake in the elderly population has yet to be fully determined, but in a population that may also be susceptible to changes in food intake regulatory mechanisms, the risk for nutritional deficits may be increased (31).

As in other chronic medical conditions, olfactory impairment may have a significant impact on quality of life. Results of a recent retrospective questionnaire sent to individuals with documented olfactory loss indicated a lower quality of life and higher level of disability in individuals with continued olfactory loss compared those with resolution of previous olfactory compromise (32).

It is estimated that approximately 14 million older adults in the United States have impairment of olfactory function. Although loss of olfactory function may occur as part of the normal aging process, it has been shown that older patients are largely unaware of their olfactory impairment. The impact of olfactory loss on the elderly patient may be especially great, when coexistent with diminished function in the other senses, or other systemic or physiologic changes. Perceived olfactory loss by an older individual should always be fully evaluated and treated when possible. Special attention should be devoted to appropriate counseling regarding the inability to detect hazards such as smoke, gas leaks, and spoiled foods. Reassurance and acknowledgement of the severity of impairment and impact on quality of life are also important components of management.

REFERENCES

1. Cain WS, Stevens JC. Uniformity of olfactory loss in aging. Ann N Y Acad Sci 1989; 561:29–38.
2. Cowart BJ. Relationships between taste and smell across the adult life span. Ann N Y Acad Sci 1989; 561:39–55.
3. Doty RL, Shaman P, Applebaum SL, et al. Smell identification ability: changes with age. Science 1984; 226:1441–1443.
4. Hoffman HJ, Ishii EK, MacTurk RH. Age-related changes in the prevalence of smell/ taste problems among the United States adult population. Results of the 1994 disability supplement to the National Health Interview Survey (NHIS). Ann N Y Acad Sci 1998; 855:716–722.
5. Nordin S, Monsch A, Murphy C. Unawareness of smell loss in normal aging and Alzheimer's disease: discrepancy between self-reported and diagnosed smell sensitivity. J Gerontol B Psychol Sci Soc Sci 1985; 50:187–192.
6. Murphy C, Schubert CR, Cruickshanks KJ, et al. Prevalence of olfactory impairment in older adults. JAMA 2002; 288:2307–2312.
7. Cowart BJ, Young IM, Feldman RS, et al. Clinical disorders of smell and taste. [review] [117 refs]. Occupational Med 1997; 12:465–483.
8. Royall DR, Chiodo LK, Polk MS, et al. Severe dysosmia is specifically associated with Alzheimer-like memory deficits in nondemented elderly retirees. Neuroepidemiology 2002; 21:68–73.
9. Hawkes CH, Shephard BC, Daniel SE. Is Parkinson's disease a primary olfactory disorder? [review] [60 refs]. Q J Med 1999; 92:473–480.
10. Hawkes C. Olfaction in neurodegenerative disorder [review] [68 refs]. Movement Disord 2003; 18:364–372.
11. Murphy C. Loss of olfactory function in dementing disease [review] [59 refs]. Physiol Behav 1999; 66:177–182.
12. Doty RL. Olfaction. Annu Rev Psychol 2001; 52:423–452.
13. Wysocki CJ, Gilbert AN. National Geographic Smell Survey. Effects of age are heterogeneous. Ann N Y Acad Sci 1989; 561:12–28.
14. Dulay MF. Olfactory acuity and cognitive function converge in older adulthood: support for the common cause hypothesis [article]. Psychol Aging 2002; 17:392–404.
15. Hinds JW, McNelly NA. Aging in the rat olfactory system: correlation of changes in the olfactory epithelium and olfactory bulb. J Comparative Neurol 1981; 203:441–453.
16. Conley DB, Robinson AM, Shinners MJ, et al. Age-related olfactory dysfunction: cellular and molecular characterization in the rat. Am J Rhinol 2003; 17:169–175.
17. Paik SI, Lehman MN, Seiden AM, et al. Human olfactory biopsy. The influence of age and receptor distribution. Arch Otolaryngol Head Neck Surg 1992; 118:731–738.
18. Smith CG. Incidence of atrophy of the olfactory nerves in man. Arch Otolaryngol Head Neck Surg 1941; 34:533–539.
19. Meisami E, Mikhail L, Baim D, et al. Human olfactory bulb: aging of glomeruli and mitral cells and a search for the accessory olfactory bulb. Ann N Y Acad Sci 1998; 855:708–715.
20. Price JL, Davis PB, Morris JC, et al. The distribution of tangles, plaques and related immunohistochemical markers in healthy aging and Alzheimer's disease. Neurobiol Aging 1991; 12:295–312.
21. Jernigan TL, Archibald SL, Fennema-Notestine C, et al. Effects of age on tissues and regions of the cerebrum and cerebellum. Neurobiol Aging 2001; 22:581–594.
22. Cerf-Ducastel B, Murphy C. FMRI brain activation in response to odors is reduced in primary olfactory areas of elderly subjects. Brain Res 2003; 986:39–53.
23. Yousem DM, Maldjian JA, Hummel T, et al. The effect of age on odor-stimulated functional MR imaging. Am J Neuroradiol 1999; 20:600–608.

24. Morgan CD, Nordin S, Murphy C. Odor identification as an early marker for Alzheimer's disease: impact of lexical functioning and detection sensitivity. J Clin Exp Neuropsychol 1995; 17:793–803.

25. Deems DA, Doty RL, Settle RG, et al. Smell and taste disorders, a study of 750 patients from the University of Pennsylvania Smell and Taste Center. Arch Otolaryngol Head Neck Surg 1991; 117:519–528.

26. Doty RL, Shaman P, Dann M. Development of the University of Pennsylvania smell Identification Test: a standardized microencapsulated test of olfactory function. Physiol Behav 1984; 32:489–502.

27. Doty RL. Practical approaches to clinical olfactory testing. In: Seiden AM, ed. Taste and Smell Disorders. New York: Thieme, 1997:38–51.

28. Seiden AM, Duncan HJ, Smith DV. Office management of taste and smell disorders. Otolaryngol Clin North Am 1992; 25:817–835.

29. Duncan HJ, Seiden AM. Long-term follow-up of olfactory loss secondary to head trauma and upper respiratory tract infection. Arch Otolaryngol Head Neck Surg 1995; 121:1183–1187.

30. Chalke H, Dewhurst J, Ward C. Loss of sense of smell in old people: a possible contributory factor in accidental poisoning from town gas. Publ Health 1958; 72:223–230.

31. Rolls BJ. Do chemosensory changes influence food intake in the elderly? [review] [35 refs]. Physiol Behav 1999; 66:193–197.

32. Miwa T, Furukawa M, Tsukatani T, et al. Impact of olfactory impairment on quality of life and disability. Arch Otolaryngol Head Neck Surg 2001; 127:497–503.

16

Olfactory Dysfunction in Neurodegenerative Diseases

Richard L. Doty
Smell and Taste Center, University of Pennsylvania Medical Center, Philadelphia, Pennsylvania, U.S.A.

INTRODUCTION

While it is widely known that the sense of smell declines with age (Fig. 1), it is less well known that this sense is altered in a number of neurodegenerative diseases whose phenotypes often become expressed in mid- to late-life, including Alzheimer's disease (AD), Huntington's disease (HD), idiopathic Parkinson's disease (PD), multiple sclerosis (MS), and the parkinsonism-dementia complex of Guam (PDC). Smell loss is also found in disorders associated with cerebellar degeneration (e.g., Friedreich's ataxia), and is a hallmark of schizophrenia (SZ), a disease commonly viewed as neurodevelopmental (for review, see Ref. 1). However, considerable variation in the prevalence and magnitude of olfactory dysfunction is present among such disorders. For example, AD, PD, and PDC are accompanied by marked alterations in the ability to smell, whereas HD, multi-infarct dementia, and SZ are accompanied by more moderate alterations. Progressive supranuclear palsy (PSP) and 1-methyl-4-phenyl-l,2,3,6-tetrahydropyridine–induced parkinsonism (MPTP-P) are associated with only minor, if any, changes in the ability to smell, in spite of the fact that they share major clinical features with PD.

It is not known to what degree the age-related decrements shown in Figure 1 reflect the earliest stages of an age-related neurodegenerative disease. Presumably a significant number of older persons experiencing smell dysfunction are, in fact, within the so-called preclinical stages of one or more of these diseases. Thus, when a nasal examination proves negative and smell loss is present in an older patient, it behooves the otorhinolarngologist to inquire about possible changes in motor function and cognition. If anomalies are noted by the patient or a close relative, or become apparent during the medical examination, referral to a neurologist or a memory disorders specialist may be in order. In the case of AD, there is both human and animal evidence that pharmacological interventions (e.g., with antioxidants, such as melatonin and vitamins C and E, as well as cholinergic agonists), if given early in the disease process, may mitigate to some degree the progression of elements of the disease process (e.g., Ref. 2).

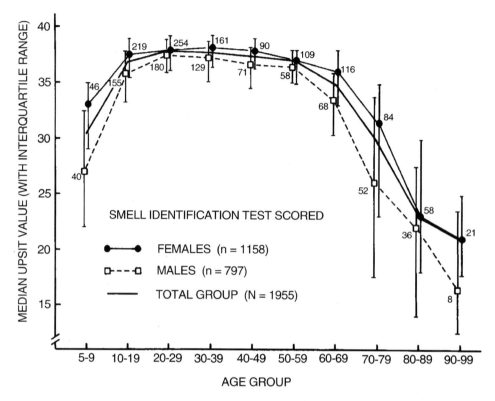

Figure 1 UPSIT scores as a function of age in a large heterogeneous group of subjects. Numbers by data points indicate sample sizes. *Abbreviation*: UPSIT, University of Pennsylvania Smell Identification Test. *Source*: From Ref. 3.

This chapter reviews the major neurodegenerative disorders for which olfactory dysfunction is present and provides details of the nature and magnitude of the dysfunction. The reader is referred elsewhere for a review of the possible neuropathological bases of the olfactory anomalies observed in such disorders (4).

NEURODEGENERATIVE DISEASES WITH MARKED OLFACTORY DYSFUNCTION

Alzheimer's Disease

AD is a pathological diagnosis made at autopsy. Nonetheless, the term "Alzheimer's disease" is commonly used synonymously with the term "probable Alzheimer's disease," which is diagnosed during life using a well-defined set of clinical inclusion and exclusion criteria (e.g., among others, an idiopathic slowly developing memory loss). Although olfactory dysfunction is perhaps the best predictor of conversion from mild cognitive decline to a diagnosis of probable AD, smell loss has not yet achieved orthodoxy in this regard.

Much is known about the olfactory phenotype of AD, although only recently have we begun to understand the physiological causes of the olfactory losses. Key features of the olfactory dysfunction are as follows: *First*, the loss, which is usually not total, typically presents bilaterally (i.e., in both nasal chambers). *Second*, it is present in 85–90% of early-stage patients. *Third*, its magnitude is generally greater in men than in women. *Fourth*, it is robust (Fig. 2) and detectable by a wide range of olfactory tests, including tests of odor identification, detection, discrimination, and memory. In a meta-analysis of 11 olfactory/AD studies, for example, effect sizes ranging from 0.98 to 12.15 (median = 2.17) were found for tests of odor identification, detection, and memory (5). *Fifth*, many AD patients are unaware of their olfactory deficit until formal testing. In one study, for example, only 6% (2/34) of early-stage AD patients responded affirmatively to the question, posed before olfactory testing, "Do you suffer from smell and/or taste problems?" despite the fact that over 90% exhibited lower scores on the 40-item University of Pennsylvania Smell Identification Test (UPSIT) than age-matched controls (6). *Sixth*, the olfactory loss of AD appears, on average, to be equivalent to that observed in PD and PDC, suggesting the possibility of a shared pathological substrate. *Seventh*, progression of dysfunction over time may occur in AD, conceivably reflecting the progression of pathology. *Eighth*, the smell loss observed in AD is often not present in disorders commonly misdiagnosed as AD, such as major affective disorder. Even a simple three-item odor

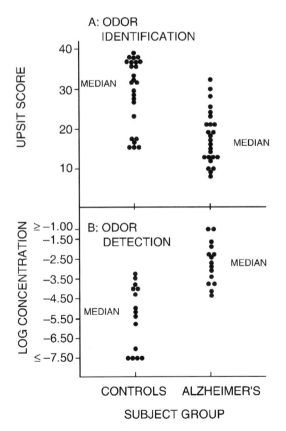

Figure 2 (**A**) UPSIT scores for patients with AD and for age-, gender-, and race-matched controls. (**B**) Detection threshold values for phenylethyl alcohol for AD patients and controls. Each dot signifies an individual subject's data point. Although some overlap appears between the AD and control subject data when plotted in this manner, very few of the AD subjects performed better than their matched controls. *Abbreviations*: UPSIT, University of Pennsylvania Smell Identification Test; AD, Alzheimer's disease. *Source*: From Ref. 6.

identification test more accurately makes the distinction between AD and depression than the widely used 30-item Mini-Mental State Examination (MMSE) (7). *Ninth*, genetic factors are involved in the smell loss of at least some cases of AD and smell loss seems to be one of the best predictors of future AD in at-risk populations. Thus, olfactory dysfunction (a) is present in some inherited forms of AD, (b) correlates with a family history of dementia, and (c) is more likely to occur in individuals with the apolipoprotein E (APOE) genotype. In a now classic study, Graves et al. (8) administered the 12-item Brief Smell Identification Test^{TM} (B-SIT) to 1604 nondemented community-dwelling senior citizens 65 years of age or older. Over a subsequent two-year time period, the B-SIT scores were found to be a better predictor of cognitive decline than scores on a global cognitive test. Persons who were anosmic and possessed at least one APOE-4 allele had 4.9 times the risk of having cognitive decline than normosmic persons not possessing this allele. This is in contrast to the 1.23 times greater risk for cognitive decline in normosmic individuals possessing at least one such APOE allele. When the data were stratified by sex, women who were anosmic and possessed at least one APOE-4 allele had an odds ratio of 9.71, compared to an odds ratio of 1.90 for women who were normosmic and possessed at least one allele. The corresponding odds ratios for men were 3.18 and 0.67, respectively.

Down Syndrome

Down syndrome (DS), a trisomy 21 disorder, accounts for ~17% of the mentally challenged population. A number of studies have demonstrated olfactory deficits in DS adults (for review, see Ref. 2). Given that the average smell loss observed in DS is similar to that observed in AD (i.e., UPSIT scores ~20), and DS patients who live into early adulthood inevitably develop the clinical and neuropathological features of AD, the question arises as to whether the smell loss is secondary to the AD-like neuropathology. One means of addressing this question is to determine at what age the olfactory loss expresses itself in DS. McKeown et al. (9) demonstrated olfactory dysfunction in 20 young DS subjects [mean age (SD) = 13.89 years (1.98)] equivalent to that observed in adult DS subjects. However, non-DS retarded children of the same IQ also exhibited such dysfunction. Thus, the olfactory loss appears to somehow be associated with retardation, rather than the development of AD-like amyloid pathology per se, since amyloid deposits do not emerge within the entorhinal cortex of DS subjects until ~19 years of age (10).

Parkinson's Disease

PD, since its first description by James Parkinson in 1817, has generally been considered to be a purely motor disease. It is now known, however, that some sensory changes accompany this disorder, including subtle alterations in vision and hearing and marked changes in olfaction. Like AD, much is known about the olfactory phenotype of PD. *First*, it occurs in ~90% of all cases, a frequency higher than that of tremor, one of the cardinal signs of the disorder (Fig. 3). In one study, the sensitivity and specificity of the UPSIT in differentiating between clinically diagnosed PD male patients and normal controls under the age of 61 was 0.91 and 0.88, respectively (11). *Second*, as in the case of AD, female PD patients generally have less dysfunction than male PD patients. *Third*, also as in AD, the loss is usually less than total and in some cases reflects difficulty in identifying, rather than detecting, the stimulus. Thus, in one report only 13% of 38 patients who received an odor detection threshold test

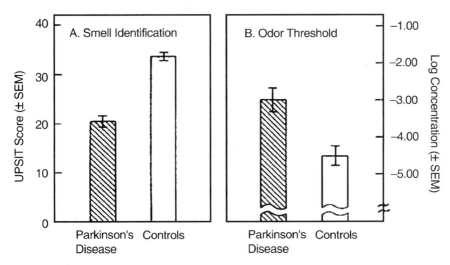

Figure 3 (**A**) UPSIT scores of PD patients and matched normal controls. (**B**) Phenyl ethyl alcohol odor detection threshold values of PD patients and matched normal controls. *Abbreviations*: UPSIT, University of Pennsylvania Smell Identification Test; PD, Parkinson's disease. *Source*: From Ref. 12.

were unable to detect the highest odorant concentration presented, and only 38.3% of 81 patients had UPSIT scores suggestive of anosmia (12). All but one of 41 PD patients asked if an odor was present on each of 40 UPSIT items answered affirmatively to 35 or more of the items, despite the fact that most were unable to identify the majority of the odors or felt that the perceived sensation did not correspond to the response alternatives. *Fourth*, the loss is generally bilateral, although there can be slight individual differences in the degree to which the left and right sides of the nose are involved. No association exists, however, between the side of relatively greater involvement and the side of hemiparkinsonism, as might be expected if asymmetrical damage to striatal dopamine systems were involved in the olfactory problem. *Fifth*, the smell loss is indistinguishable from that of AD and PDC, with UPSIT scores averaging around 20. *Sixth*, the smell loss is unrelated to the magnitude of the motor symptoms, although subtle variations among the so-called benign versus malignant forms may be present. *Seventh*, the smell loss is unrelated to performance on numerous neuropsychological measures, such as the Randt memory test, reaction time, a finger-tapping test, and selected verbal and performance subsets of the Wechsler Adult Intelligence Scale—revised (13). *Eighth*, the smell loss appears in both familial and sporadic forms of parkinsonism and may be a sign of the preclinical state of the disease. *Ninth*, unlike AD, there is no clear longitudinal progression in olfactory dysfunction as occurs in other elements of the disease process. *Tenth*, anti-PD medications (e.g., L-dopa, dopamine agonists, anticholinergic compounds) have no influence on the smell deficit, which occurs as severely in nonmedicated or never-medicated patients as in medicated ones. *Eleventh*, also like AD, many PD patients are unaware of their olfactory deficit until formal testing (12). *Twelfth*, olfactory testing is useful in the differential diagnosis of idiopathic PD from a number of other neurodegenerative diseases with motor symptoms, including disorders often misdiagnosed as PD (e.g., PSP, MPTP-induced PD, and essential tremor). *Finally*, as in the case with AD, some asymptomatic first-degree relatives of patients with either familial or sporadic forms of PD appear to exhibit olfactory dysfunction. Recently, Berendse (14) administered tests of odor detection, identification, and discrimination to 250 relatives of PD patients (~84% children, ~16% siblings, one parent). In 25 hyposmic and 23 normosmic individuals sampled from this group, nigrostriatal dopaminergic function was assessed using single photon emission computer tomography with $[^{125}I]\beta$-CIT as a dopamine transporter ligand. An abnormal reduction in striatal dopamine transporter binding was present in four of the 25 (16%) hyposmic relatives, two of whom subsequently developed clinical parkinsonism, and in none of the 23 normosmic relatives. These authors noted (p. 39), "The observation in the present study that significant reductions in dopamine transporter binding were found only in hyposmic relatives of PD patients suggests that olfactory dysfunction may precede clinical motor signs in PD." Such findings reiterate the point that olfactory testing, in conjunction with other measures, is likely useful in the early detection of PD.

Parkinsonism-Dementia Complex of Guam

Between 1957 and 1965, amyotrophic lateral sclerosis and parkinsonism-dementia accounted for at least 15% of adult deaths among the Chamorro populations of Guam and Rota (15). Although poorly understood, genetic susceptibility may be involved in producing this disorder. Even though no differences in APOE-4 frequencies have been found, persons with PDC have a lower frequency of APOE-2 than do controls (16).

Guamanian Chamorros with PDC have olfactory deficits similar to those observed in AD and PD. In one study, 24 PDC patients were administered the UPSIT (17). All were ambulatory and living with their families. At the time of testing, all evidenced some degree of rigidity and bradykinesia. Their scores did not differ significantly from those of 24 AD and 24 PD North American patients of similar age, gender, and smoking history. However, their scores were markedly lower than normals of the same age and gender. As in earlier studies, each subject was asked, prior to olfactory testing, whether or not he or she suffered from any smell or taste problems. Three of the PDC patients reported such problems (13%), as compared to two of the AD (8%) and three of the PD (13%) patients, indicating that the level of awareness of the problem is similar, if not identical, in these three disorders.

In a more recent study, an abbreviated version of the UPSIT was administered to nine Chamorros with symptoms of amyotrophic lateral sclerosis (ALS) alone, nine with symptoms of pure parkinsonism, 11 patients with pure dementia, and 31 patients with PDC, as well as to neurologically normal Chamorro Guamanians and 25 North American controls (18). The UPSIT scores were markedly depressed in the four disease groups relative to the controls, and did not differentiate among the four syndromes. Some of the control subjects had lower scores than North American counterparts, suggesting the possible presence of a subclinical neurogenerative disease process in nonsymptomatic individuals.

Huntington's Disease

HD, a progressive disorder of dysfunctional movement, cognitive deterioration, and altered behavior with autosomal dominant transmission, is often phenotypically expressed relatively late in life. As functional capacity worsens, chorea generally lessens and dystonia intensifies. Among its primary motor symptoms are hyperkinesias that take, initially, the form of chorea, being characterized by fleeting movements which, in some cases, appear semi-purposively within the context of overall heightened activity and motor restlessness. A number of studies have shown that HD patients exhibit deficits in odor identification, detection, discrimination, and memory, and that the problem is likely manifested by the time the classical phenotypic elements of the disorder appear. However, when the olfactory function occurs during the progression of the disease process is not presently known. In one study, UPSIT and phenyl ethyl alcohol (PEA) detection threshold scores were obtained from 25 probands with HD, 12 at-risk offspring, and 37 unrelated controls. Decreased olfaction was noted only in the HD group, with a mean UPSIT score of 24.8 (SD = 8.7) and a PEA threshold score of -4.4 log vol/vol (SD = 1.4) (19). More recently, these findings were extended by testing 20 HD patients who had the disease for a mean of eight years (range: 4–14 years), 20 normal subjects with the genetic mutation that causes HD, and 20 mutation-negative adults. Again, only the patients with clinical signs of HD exhibited depressed olfaction (mean UPSIT score = 27.4, SD = 6.5) (20).

NEURODEGENERATIVE DISEASES WITH LESS MARKED OR MINIMAL OLFACTORY DYSFUNCTION

1-Methyl-4-Phenyl-1,2,3,6-Tetrahydropyridine–Induced Parkinsonism

MPTP-P represents one syndrome with a PD-like phenotype that is not accompanied by significant alterations in olfactory function. Unlike most of the other disorders described in this chapter, the factor responsible for the neurological damage of patients with MPTP-P is well established. In this case, intravenous injection of MPTP, whose toxic metabolite 1-methyl-4-phenylpyridinium (MPP+) crosses the blood–brain barrier and damages brain regions critical for the coordination of motor movement, produces the parkinsonian symptoms (21). In the sole study addressing olfactory function in MPTP-P, UPSIT scores and detection threshold values for the odorant phenyl ethyl alcohol in six such patients did not differ significantly from those of 10 normal subjects of equivalent age (22). Thirteen rare young PD patients exhibited significantly lower test scores than both the MPTP-P and control subjects. Despite their major motor deficits, the MPTP-P patients evidenced no major decrements in cognitive function, could sniff adequately, and could respond verbally to the examiner's questions without difficulty. These data suggest that the functional integrity of the olfactory system of MPTP-P patients is greater than that of PD patients and demonstrate that olfactory dysfunction need not always be a concomitant element of parkinsonian syndromes.

Progressive Supranuclear Palsy

PSP (also termed the Steele, Richardson, and Olszewski syndrome) accounts for ~4% of patients with parkinsonian symptoms. Tremor is rarely present, although rigidity and bradykinesia frequently appear early in disease progression. The hallmark feature is vertical-gaze paresis (especially down-gaze paresis), which is of supranuclear origin and can be overcome by the oculocephalic maneuver. Commonly misdiagnosed as PD, PSP shares many motor features with PD. The parkinsonian features are, however, less responsive to anti-PD medications, and PSP typically has comparatively more frontal lobe dysfunction, more neuronal degeneration within the basal ganglia and upper brain stem, and less involvement of mesolimbic and mesocortical dopamine systems than PD (23).

Most patients with PSP have a relatively normal sense of smell, although slight to moderate losses are present in some individuals. In one study, the UPSIT and a phenyl ethyl alcohol odor detection threshold test were administered to 22 patients with PSP (24). The test scores of these individuals were compared to those from 22 PD patients and 22 neurologically normal age-, gender-, and race-matched controls. The performance was markedly superior to that of the PD patients [respective UPSIT means (SD): 31.59 (7.18) and 18.82 (6.94)], with approximately half scoring within the normal range. However, on average, the PSP patients did exhibit moderate deficits relative to the controls, whose mean (SD) UPSIT score was 35.60 (4.06).

Multiple System Atrophy

Wenning et al. (25) administered the UPSIT to 29 patients with multiple system atrophy (MSA), 15 PSP patients, 118 patients with idiopathic PD, seven patients with corticobasal degeneration (CBD), and 123 healthy controls. Relative to controls, the MSA patients had mild impairment. Normal test scores were noted for the PSP and CBD patients. The authors noted that "preserved or mildly impaired olfactory function in a parkinsonian patient is more likely to be related to atypical parkinsonism such as MSA, PSP, or CBD, whereas markedly reduced olfaction is more suggestive of idiopathic Parkinson's disease (IPD)." An UPSIT score of 25 was associated with a sensitivity of 77% and a specificity of 85% in differentiating PD from atypical parkinsonism.

Multiple Sclerosis

Until the mid-1980s, it was generally assumed that olfactory function was not altered at all in MS, since the primary olfactory neurons are unmyelinated. Indeed, the sole psychophysical study available at that time suggested no deficits were present (26). In 1984, we reported that 23% of 31 MS patients evaluated evidenced some degree of olfactory dysfunction on the UPSIT (27). A decade later, we presented case studies in which olfactory dysfunction was the presenting symptom of MS (28), and, more recently, demonstrated a strong inverse correlation ($r = -0.94$) between UPSIT scores and the number of MS-related plaques within the subfrontal and subtemporal lobes of patients (Fig. 4) (29,30). No such relationship was present between UPSIT scores and plaques in other brain regions. Subsequently, it has been shown that, in individual cases, UPSIT scores wax and wane in concert with the fluctuations in the number of plaques within olfaction-related brain regions (31).

ALS

As with the case of PD, ALS has been traditionally considered a motor neuron disease (MND). However, today we know that this is an oversimplification of this disorder. In 1991, Elian (32) reported that patients with MND exhibit decreased UPSIT scores bilaterally. Specifically, UPSIT scores from nine male and six female MND patients of varying severity were compared to those of age- and sex-matched controls, and proved to be significantly depressed. However, the magnitude of the deficit was more similar to that observed in schizophrenia than that observed in AD or PD, with the UPSIT scores falling around 30.

In a subsequent study, Sajjadian et al. (33) administered the UPSIT bilaterally to 17 female and 20 male ALS patients, and unilaterally to seven male and seven

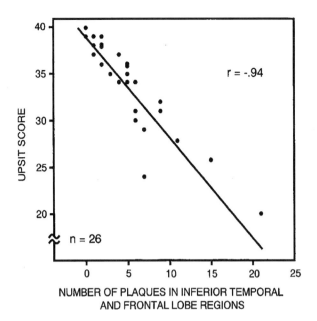

Figure 4 Relationship, in patients with MS, between number of plaques in subtemporal and subfrontal lobes and scores on the UPSIT. *Abbreviations*: UPSIT, University of Pennsylvania Smell Identification Test; MS, multiple sclerosis. *Source*: From Ref. 29.

female ALS patients. Age-, gender-, smoking-habit-, and race-matched controls were also evaluated. While the UPSIT scores of the ALS patients were significantly lower than those of the controls, the degree of dysfunction was similar to that seen by Elian. Thus, only 11% of the ALS patients had UPSIT scores indicative of total or near total anosmia. Despite the fact that nearly half of the ALS patients had UPSIT scores that fell within the normal range, 75.7% of the patients scored below their individually matched controls. Although no sex differences or laterality in the ALS-related test scores were observed, an age-related decrement was present and, interestingly, significant correlations were found between UPSIT scores and neurophysiological measures of peripheral nerve conductance. If the latter observation proves to be true, it is conceivable that a common pathophysiological process influences the motor neuron responses and segments of the afferent olfactory pathway.

More recently, Hawkes et al. (34) administered the UPSIT to 58 patients with MND and 135 controls. Additionally, olfactory event-related potentials (OERPs) in response to hydrogen sulfide (H_2S) were recorded in 15 patients, and the olfactory bulbs of eight MND cadavers were histologically examined. Although UPSIT scores were slightly worse in the MND patients, only the bulbar patients exhibited significant decrements. OERPs were normal in nine patients and delayed in one. OERPs from the remaining five subjects could not be recorded. Histological analysis of olfactory bulb tissue revealed excessive lipofuscin deposition in eight of eight cases examined.

Epilepsy

The earliest threshold studies of patients with epilepsy reported heightened, not lessened, overall bilateral sensitivity, particularly prior to an ictal event (e.g. Ref. 35).

This has not been observed in more recent studies, where detection thresholds for *n*-butanol and phenyl ethyl alcohol have been found normal (36). Suprathreshold deficits, however, have been reported, with several studies suggesting right-side foci are more disrupting. Thus, epileptic patients with right-side foci, but not left-side foci, have been found to exhibit decreased performance on an odor matching task, an odor memory test for nameable odors, and the UPSIT. Bilateral deficits have been reported for odor discrimination, short- and long-term odor memory, and odor naming (36). Prolonged odor event-related potential latencies have been reported in patients with both right- and left-side foci when the stimulation was made on the focal side (37).

CONCLUSIONS

It is apparent from the studies reviewed in this chapter that olfactory loss is a common element of many neurodegenerative diseases. Moreover, it is clear that the losses are (a) highly variable across diseases, (b) appear, in some cases, very early in the disease process, and (c) may or may not relate to disease stage, depending upon the disorder. As reviewed elsewhere (1), well over a hundred studies have now been published in the peer-reviewed literature demonstrating adverse influences of these diseases on the ability to smell.

Although the present study provides considerable information with respect to the olfactory dysfunction seen in a number of neurodegenerative diseases, it should be emphasized that this review is not comprehensive. At least some smell dysfunction has been demonstrated in a number of neurodegenerative disorders that are not discussed in detail, including Pick's disease, multi-infarct dementia, restless leg syndrome, and essential tremor (2). Although smell dysfunction is a hallmark of SZ, SZ is generally considered a neurodevelopmental, not a neurodegenerative, disease and for this reason was not reviewed in detail in this chapter. Nonetheless, UPSIT scores correlate inversely with the time since diagnosis, suggesting that there may be a progressive, possibly degenerative, element within brain regions associated with olfactory processing in this disease (38).

While it is quite possible that the lack of olfactory threshold deficits in some diseases is a real phenomenon, caution is warranted in interpreting a number of studies of olfactory threshold. Thus, thresholds based upon a single ascending series of stimuli or using non-forced-choice methodology can be extremely unreliable. Hence, such measures may not have the power to detect differences when small samples are employed. A case in point is a study that reported significant UPSIT, but not pyridine threshold, deficits in AD patients relative to controls (39). Based on this observation, the authors concluded that the olfactory deficit of AD is associated with a "central" rather than a "peripheral" anomaly. While, ultimately, their overall conclusion may be correct (i.e., that the cause of olfactory deficits in AD reflects damage in structures more central than the olfactory neuroepithelium), the basis upon which they arrive at this conclusion is suspect for three reasons. First, the vast majority of studies find threshold deficits in AD patients, and even their own data point to this conclusion. Thus, three of their subjects (30%) were either anosmic or hyposmic by their own criteria and, in fact, the average threshold value for the AD patients was higher (i.e., indicative of less sensitivity) than that of the controls, even though statistical significance at the 0.05 level was not achieved. Second, compared to other studies on this topic (see Ref. 1), their sample size was very small, compromising statistical power. In general, single ascending series detection threshold tests such as administered by them have test–retest reliability values on the order of 0.40, compared to those of the UPSIT, which are uniformly above 0.90. Third, the general assumption that threshold tests reflect peripheral damage and identification tests reflect central damage is questionable. Thus, central lesions have been associated with threshold deficits in some studies (e.g., Refs. 40,41) and peripheral (i.e., neuroepithelial) lesions are known to influence both detection threshold and odor identification tests (42).

ACKNOWLEDGMENTS

This work was supported, in part, by Grants RO1 DC 04278, RO1 DC 02974, RO1 AG 08148, and RO1 AG 27496 from the National Institutes of Health, Bethesda, Maryland, U.S.A. Disclosure: Dr. Doty is a major shareholder in Sensonics, Inc., the manufacturer and distributor of the UPSIT and other chemosensory test.

REFERENCES

1. Doty RL. Odor perception in neurodegenerative diseases. In: Doty RL, ed. Handbook of Olfaction and Gustation. New York: Marcel Dekker, 2003:479–502.
2. Sung S, Yao Y, Uryu K, et al. Early vitamin E supplementation in young but not aged mice reduces A beta levels and amyloid deposition in a transgenic model of Alzheimer's disease. FASEB J 2004; 18:323–325.
3. Doty RL, Shaman P, Applebaum SL, Giberson R, Siksorski L, Rosenberg, L. Smell identification ability: changes with age. Science 1984; 226:1441–1443.
4. Smutzer GS, Doty RL, Arnold SE, Trojanowski JQ. Olfactory system neuropathology in Alzheimer's disease, Parkinson's disease, and schizophrenia. In: Doty RL, ed. Handbook of Olfaction and Gustation. New York: Marcel Dekker, 2003:503–523.
5. Mesholam RI, Moberg PJ, Mahr RN, Doty RL. Olfaction in neurodegenerative disease: a meta-analysis of olfactory functioning in Alzheimer's and Parkinson's diseases. Arch Neurol 1998; 55:84–90.
6. Doty RL, Reyes PF, Gregor T. Presence of both odor identification and detection deficits in Alzheimer's disease. Brain Res Bull 1987; 18:597–600.
7. McCaffrey RJ, Duff K, Solomon GS. Olfactory dysfunction discriminates probable Alzheimer's dementia from major depression: a cross-validation and extension. J Neuropsychiatr Clin Neurosci 2000; 12:29–33.
8. Graves AB, Bowen JD, Rajaram L, et al. Impaired olfaction as a marker for cognitive decline: interaction with apolipoprotein E epsilon4 status. Neurology 1999; 53:1480–1487.
9. McKeown DA, Doty RL, Perl DP, Frye RE, Simms I, Mester. Olfactory function in young adolescents with Down's syndrome. J Neurol Neurosurg Psychiatry 1996; 61: 412–414.
10. Hof PR, Bouras C, Perl DP, Sparks L, Mehta N, Morrison JH. Age-related distribution of neuropathologic changes in the cerebral cortex of patients with Down's syndrome. Arch Neurol 1995; 52:379–391.
11. Doty RL, Bromley SM, Stern MB. Olfactory testing as an aid in the diagnosis of Parkinson's disease: development of optimal discrimination criteria. Neurodegeneration 1995; 4:93–97.
12. Doty RL, Deems DA, Stellar S. Olfactory dysfunction in parkinsonism: a general deficit unrelated to neurologic signs, disease stage, or disease duration. Neurology 1988; 38:1237–1244.

13. Doty RL, Riklan M, Deems DA, Reynolds C, Stellar S. The olfactory and cognitive deficits of Parkinson's disease: evidence for independence. Ann Neurol 1989; 25:166–171.
14. Berendse HWB. Subclinical dopaminergic dysfunction in asymptomatic Parkinson's disease patients' relatives with a decreased sense of smell. Ann Neurol 2001; 50:34–41.
15. Reed DM, Brody JA. Amyotrophic lateral sclerosis and parkinsonism-dementia on Guam 1945–1972. I. Descriptive Epidemiology. Am J Epidemiol 1975; 101:287–301.
16. Buee L, Perez-Tur J, Leveugle B, et al. Apolipoprotein E in Guamanian amyotrophic lateral sclerosis/parkinsonism-dementia complex: genotype analysis and relationships to neuropathological changes. Acta Neuropathol 1996; 91:247–253.
17. Doty RL, Perl DP, Steele JC, et al. Odor identification deficit of the parkinsonism-dementia complex of Guam: equivalence to that of Alzheimer's and idiopathic Parkinson's disease. Neurology 1991; 41:77–80.
18. Ahlskog JE, Waring SC, Petersen RC, et al. Olfactory dysfunction in Guamanian ALS, parkinsonism, and dementia. Neurology 1998; 51:1672–1677.
19. Moberg PJ, Doty RL. Olfactory function in Huntington's disease patients and at-risk offspring. Int J Neurosci 1997; 89:133–139.
20. Bylsma FW, Moberg PJ, Doty RL, Brandt J. Odor identification in Huntington's disease patients and asymptomatic gene carriers. J Neuropsychiatr Clin Neurosci 1997; 9:598–600.
21. Langston JW, Ballard PA, Tetrude JW, Irwin I. Chronic parkinsonism in humans due to a product of meperidine-analog synthesis. Science 1983; 219:979–980.
22. Doty RL, Singh A, Tetrude J, Langston JW. Lack of olfactory dysfunction in MPTP-induced parkinsonism. Ann Neurol 1992; 32:97–100.
23. Jankovic J. Parkinsonism-plus syndromes. Movement Dis 1989; 4:S95–S119.
24. Doty RL, Golbe LI, McKeown DA, Stern MB, Lehrach CM, Crawford D. Olfactory testing differentiates between progressive supranuclear palsy and idiopathic Parkinson's disease. Neurology 1993; 43:962–965.
25. Wenning GK, Shephard B, Hawkes C, Petruckevitch A, Lees A, Quinn N. Olfactory function in atypical parkinsonian syndromes. Acta Neurol Scand 1995; 91:247–250.
26. Ansari KA. Olfaction in multiple sclerosis. With a note on the discrepancy between optic and olfactory involvement. Eur Neurol 1976; 14:138–145.
27. Doty RL, Shaman P, Dann M. Development of the University of Pennsylvania Smell Identification Test: a standardized microencapsulated test of olfactory function. Physiol Behav 1984; 32:489–502.
28. Constantinescu CS, Raps EC, Cohen JA, West SE, Doty RL. Olfactory disturbances as the initial or most prominent symptom of multiple sclerosis. J Neurol Neurosurg Psychiatry 1994; 57:1011–1012.
29. Doty RL, Li C, Mannon LJ, Yousem DM. Olfactory dysfunction in multiple sclerosis. N Engl J Med 1997; 336:1918–1919.
30. Doty RL, Li C, Mannon LJ, Yousem DM. Olfactory dysfunction in multiple sclerosis: relation to plaque load in inferior frontal and temporal lobes. Ann N Y Acad Sci 1998; 855:781–786.
31. Doty RL, Li C, Mannon LJ, Yousem DM. Olfactory dysfunction in multiple sclerosis: relation to longitudinal changes in plaque numbers in central olfactory structures. Neurology 1999; 53:880–882.
32. Elian M. Olfactory impairment in motor neuron disease: a pilot study. J Neurol Neurosurg Psychiatry 1991; 54:927–928.
33. Sajjadian A, Doty RL, Gutnick DN, Chirurgi RJ, Sivak M, Perl D. Olfactory dysfunction in amyotrophic lateral sclerosis. Neurodegeneration 1994; 3:153–157.
34. Hawkes CH, Shephard BC, Geddes JF, Body GD, Martin JE. Olfactory disorder in motor neuron disease. Exp Neurol 1998; 150:248–253.
35. Santorelli G, Marotta A. La sogli olfattometrica dell'. La sogli olfattometrica dell'epilettico in condizioni di base e dopa crisi 1964; 32:185–190.

36. Martinez BA, Cain WS, de Wijk RA, Spencer DD, Novelly RA, Sass KJ. Olfactory functioning before and after temporal lobe resection for intractable seizures. Neuropsychology 1993; 7:351–363.

37. Hummel T, Pauli E, Schuler P, Kettenmann B, Stefan H, Kobal G. Chemosensory event-related potentials in patients with temporal lobe epilepsy. Epilepsia 1995; 36:79–85.

38. Moberg PJ, Doty RL, Turetsky BI, et al. Olfactory identification deficits in schizophrenia: correlation with duration of illness. Am J Psychiatry 1997; 154:1016–1018.

39. Koss E, Weiffenbach JM, Haxby JV, Friedland RP. Olfactory detection and recognition in Alzheimer's disease [letter]. Lancet 1987; 1:622.

40. Rousseaux M, Muller P, Gahide I, Mottin Y, Roman M. Disorders of smell, taste, and food intake in a patient with a dorsomedial thalamic infarct. Stroke 1996; 27:2328–2330.

41. Rausch R, Serafetinides EA. Specific alteration of olfactory function in humans with temporal lobe lesions. Nature 1975; 225:557–558.

42. Deems DA, Doty RL, Settle RG, et al. Smell and taste disorders, a study of 750 patients from the University of Pennsylvania Smell and Taste Center. Arch Otolaryngol Head Neck Surg 1991; 117:519–528.

17

Taste Changes in the Elderly

Natasha Mirza
*Department of Otolaryngology—Head and Neck Surgery, University of Pennsylvania
Health System and Philadelphia VA Medical Center, Philadelphia,
Pennsylvania, U.S.A.*

INTRODUCTION

The goal of the chemosensory system is the detection and discrimination of foods
and the initiation and sustenance of ingestion. This system is developed in both ver-
tebrates and invertebrates and is present even in the newborn infant. With aging,
there is a decline in chemosensory functions and while extensive research has conclu-
sively shown a decline in the olfactory system, the basis and extent of taste loss is
poorly understood. It is estimated that more than 2 million Americans have some
kind of chemosensory disorder (1).

Taste function in the elderly is rarely if ever lost completely because of the
redundancy in the mediation of taste, which occurs through several nerves.
Many confounding influences also come into play in older individuals like the effects
of medications, smoking, systemic illnesses, and decrease in cognitive functions.
What is proven so far has been that a loss or alteration of taste affects nutritional
intake in the elderly, in turn leading to multiple nutrition-related medical problems
(2). With a growing geriatric population in the country, it is important to identify
some of the effects of taste dysfunction and identify means of reducing them.

This chapter will briefly review the anatomy and physiology of taste including
taste transduction, and discuss some of the relevant research on aging and taste.
Methods to help decrease some of the harmful effects of taste loss on both nutrition
and quality of life will also be discussed.

DEVELOPMENT OF THE TASTE SYSTEM

Morphological evidence shows that there is a functional taste system present in
utero. Even premature infants respond pleasurably to sucrose and glucose. The
hedonic system of pleasantness is also well developed in infants (3). The acceptance
of sweet and rejection of bitter seem to be hard-wired while the effect associated with
odors depends much more on experience.

ANATOMY OF THE TASTE SYSTEM

In mammals, taste buds are located throughout the oral cavity, in the pharynx, the laryngeal epiglottis, and at the entrance of the esophagus. Taste buds on the dorsal lingual epithelium are the most numerous (approximately 4600 per tongue) and are contained within four major classes of papillae: the fungiform, foliate, circumvallate, and the non-gustatory filiform papillae (Fig. 1).

Fungiform papillae are located on the most anterior part of the tongue and generally contain one to several taste buds per papilla (4,5). They are innervated by the chorda tympani branch of the facial (VIIth cranial) nerve and appear as red spots on the tongue because they are richly supplied with blood vessels. The total number of fungiform papillae per human tongue is around 200. Foliate papillae are situated on the edge of the tongue slightly anterior of the circumvallate line. They are predominantly sensitive to sour tastes, and are innervated by the glossopharyngeal (IXth cranial) nerve and average five foliate papillae per side of the tongue with approximately 120 taste buds per foliate papilla.

Circumvallate papillae are sunken papillae, with a trough separating them from the surrounding wall. The taste buds are in tiers within the trough of the papillae. They are situated on the circumvallate line and confer a sour/bitter sensitivity to the posterior one-third of the tongue. They are innervated by the glossopharyngeal (IXth cranial) nerve. There are 3 to 13 circumvallate papillae per tongue with about 250 taste buds

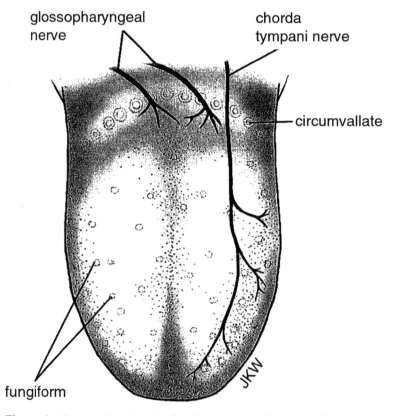

Figure 1 Tongue showing the distribution of the lingual papillae.

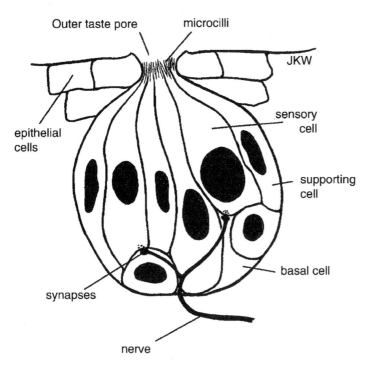

Figure 2 Anatomy of a taste bud.

per papilla. Filiform papillae are mechanical and non-gustatory. In addition, there are 2500 taste buds on the epiglottis, soft palate, laryngeal, and oral pharynx.

In mammals, taste buds are aggregations of 30 to 100 individual elongated "neuroepithelial" cells ($50 \mu m$ in height, $30–70 \mu m$ in width), which are embedded in the lingual papillae (6). At the apex of the taste bud, microvillar processes protrude through a small opening, the taste pore, ($4–10 \mu m$ in diameter) into the oral milieu. Just below the taste bud apex, taste cells are joined by tight junctional complexes. Taste cells are bipolar cells, which connect to the epithelial surface of the oral cavity via dendritic processes and to a nerve axon at the base, which invades the bud and ramifies extensively, with each fiber typically synapsing with multiple receptor cells within the taste bud (Fig. 2).

The lifespan of a mammalian taste cell is approximately 10 days. As a cell ages a nerve terminal detaches, finds a developing cell, and forms new synapses. The new cell has to be of the same taste specificity as the old dying cell; in other words, taste receptor cells act as surface markers to guide nerve fibers to the right cellular target.

Cells in each taste bud contain the sensory receptor cells, supporting cells, and basal cells, which differentiate into new receptor cells.

A single taste bud is all that is needed to provide sensation for all the four tastes so that even the decrease in number of lingual papillae does not necessarily lead to a significant loss of taste.

TASTE TRANSDUCTION

It is important to understand some of the basic science that is involved in taste transduction to understand the effects of aging on this mechanism (7). Taste receptors trigger transduction cascades, which then activate synapses and cause the excitation of nerve fibers. A signal is produced, which is then carried to the brain relaying information on the identity and intensity of the gustatory stimulus. Receptor proteins are located on the apical surface of cells and from there the stimulus enters the cell either via an ion channel, as it does for the salty and sour tastes or via second messenger systems like cyclic adenosine monophosphate (cAMP) for bitter and sweet. Once the stimulant enters the cell, there is a change in the internal electrical state of the cell, which leads to the secretion of a neurotransmitter and activation of a nerve fiber.

Each taste serves a specific purpose in the maintenance of health of an individual. Salt taste guides the intake of sodium chloride and thus the salt–water homeostasis. Sour helps with the recognition of complex foods. At low concentrations, it is pleasant but once it reaches high concentrations it becomes an unpleasant taste and leads to avoidance. It guides acid–base regulation and is sensitive to extracellular pH changes.

The sweet receptor is a classical proteinaceous molecule analogous to an olfactory receptor. It responds to soluble carbohydrates in the oral cavity and regulates caloric intake, nutrition, and energy balance. It uses a second messenger like cAMP to activate a cyclic nucleotide cascade. Sweet taste has a strong hedonic effect and is well developed in infants.

Bitter taste like sour is bearable and even to some extent pleasant in low concentrations but is repulsive when strong. Bitter receptors belong to the second messenger system of G proteins. They set off a G protein-coupled receptor-mediated signal, which leads to dual signaling of cAMP and cyclic guanosine monophosphate (cGMP) within the cell. Bitter taste serves as a warning system designed by nature to protect against the ingestion of harmful compounds. Again even newborn infants are seen to respond to bitter compounds like quinine with distaste.

Umami as a taste was discovered about 100 years ago and is somewhat similar to sweet taste. It is derived from L-glutamate and is the taste present in monosodium glutamate (MSG), chicken broth, meat extracts, and aging cheese. It guides the intake of peptides and proteins and the receptor contains GluR4.

INNERVATION OF THE TONGUE

Taste receptor cells do not have an axon. Information is relayed onto terminals of sensory fibers by transmitter. These fibers arise from the ganglion cells of three cranial nerves. Over the anterior tongue, the chorda tympani (a branch of the facial nerve) is sensory for taste and the lingual nerve, a branch of the trigeminal nerve, serves general sensation. Over the posterior tongue, taste is conveyed via the glossopharyngeal with some branches of the vagus providing additional taste sensation. In this region of the tongue, general sensation is also provided by the same two nerves. The trigeminal nerve is responsible for detecting the burning sensation caused by certain foods, e.g., peppers. Taste nerves normally inhibit one another across the midline. Therefore, when a nerve is damaged there is a decrease in inhibitory impulses from that side which in turn leads to an increase in responses from the opposite side. This disinhibition of the damaged nerve leads to an overall preservation of taste and total ageusia or loss of taste is very rare. On the other hand, the olfactory system depends on one nerve and is therefore more vulnerable to injury.

Central Pathways

Primary gustatory fibers synapse centrally in the medulla (in a thin line of cells called the nucleus of the solitary tract). From there the information is relayed to the somatosensory cortex for the conscious perception of taste and to the hypothalamus, amygdala, and insula, giving the so-called "affective" component of taste (1,2). This is responsible for the behavioral response, e.g., aversion, gastric secretion, and feeding behavior.

REVIEW OF LITERATURE

The influence of aging on taste has been investigated in a large number of studies. Verification of taste loss is an important aspect of testing when a patient comes to the doctor complaining of taste loss. It is often found that the sense of taste may be normal but the sense of smell is impaired leading to a loss of flavor. Flavor is a complete sensory experience arising from ingested stimulant molecules and involves taste, smell, texture, and temperature.

A review of more than 30 papers on this topic dating from 1959 on young and elderly subjects was conducted. Almost all the studies used similar stimulants, namely sodium chloride (NaCl) for salty, sucrose for sweet, acetic or citric acid for sour, and quinine sulfate for bitter. The type and extent of taste loss over the decades and which gender was most affected emerged as fairly inconsistent.

Taste studies looked at two primary aspects of taste: acuity and intensity.

Taste acuity measures two different parameters:

   a. taste detection or threshold testing, which is a measure of the concentration at which a distinction can be made between a taste substance (tastant) and water; and
   b. taste recognition, i.e., which is sweet, sour, salty, or bitter.

Taste intensity is a suprathreshold measure of taste qualities.

Whole mouth testing is used to assess the individual's ability to detect, identify, and evaluate the intensity of different concentrations of the four taste substances. Spatial taste testing is used to assess different areas of the tongue to identify if there is localized impairment of taste. At the Smell and Taste Center at the University of Pennsylvania, a drop of the tastant (sweet, sour, salt, and bitter) is placed on the tongue with a pipette and the subject is asked to identify the solution, to rate the confidence of their answer and also to rate the intensity of the solution on a nine-level scale of increasing shades of gray. In electrogustometry, a weak electrical current is delivered to the various taste regions in the oral cavity (8).

Most of the studies reviewed have discovered that with increasing age there is an increase in taste thresholds for all the four tastes (9). Cooper et al. (10) in 1959 used whole mouth testing and found that taste sensitivities remained stable till the age of 50 and after that there was an increase in all taste thresholds. In 1976, Murphy and Gilmore (11) found that taste thresholds were increased sevenfold in older individuals. In 1986, Bartoshuk et al. (12) used magnitude matching (comparing taste intensity to loudness intensity) and had similar results. In 1988, Lasilla et al. (13) found that the elderly had significantly higher identification and detection thresholds for all four tastants.

Several other studies found that the main effect of aging was on the salty taste (14,15). In 1979, Grzegorczyk et al. (16) found that there was a statistically significant increase in salt detection thresholds from the second to ninth decades of life. In 1982, Weiffenbach et al. (17) determined taste thresholds for all the four tastants using forced choice trials. They found a significant increase in detection thresholds for sodium chloride and a slight increase for quinine sulfate. Later in 1986, Weiffenbach et al. (18) used the direct scaling method (matched the linear extent of a tape to the perceived intensity of the stimulus) and found that there was a decrease in taste sensitivities for sodium chloride, quinine, and citric acid. Similar results were obtained by Spitzer (19) and Nordin et al. (20). In 2001, Mojet et al. (21), using the ascending staircase method of tastant identification, found that taste sensitivity was maximally affected in the elderly for NaCl and umami and least for sucrose. Osada et al. (22) and Bradley (23) in separate studies recorded the neuropsychological responses from the chorda tympani of young and old rats and found that responses to NaCl decreased significantly with aging.

Sweet taste in most of the studies reviewed seemed the most robust and survived the longest (24). Most studies have also found that males were much more vulnerable to the effects of aging compared with age-matched females both for taste thresholds and intensities.

Fungiform papillae are concentrated on the anterior tip of the tongue and anterior lateral margins in humans, and it has been demonstrated that NaCl threshold is inversely related to the number of fungiform papillae (more papillae = more sensitivity, lower threshold) (25).

Miller (26) in 1988 studied cadaveric tongues and looked at taste bud densities (the number of taste buds per surface area in cm^2). Miller looked at three age groups and found no differences in the mean taste bud densities across the age groups. There was a decrease in the thickness of the upper layer of the epithelium and a flattening of papillae with advancing age, and such changes did influence the number of fungiform papillae, but there was no proof of changes in taste receptor distribution or function. On the other hand, Arey et al. (27) found degenerative changes in taste receptors with a regression of gustatory papillae, a decrease in the number of papillae with age, and a decrease in the number of taste buds. Arey et al. found more than 250 taste buds in each circumvallate papilla in the young adult and less than 100 in persons over 70 years. Bradley found no significant change in the numbers of taste buds on the fungiform papillae of rats versus monkeys versus humans. However, the taste buds in the elderly were functionally impaired as indicated by electrophysiologic responses recorded form the chorda tympani. Bradley also suggested that there may be changes in the central nervous system (CNS) responses to these electrophysiologic stimuli in the aged.

Drawbacks in the studies reviewed were the lack of concordance in the various studies, procedural differences, and different psychophysical stimuli presented. Sample sizes were small and some studies were conducted either on cadaveric tongues or on animals and the results could not be directly related to human subjects.

REASONS FOR LOSS OF TASTE IN THE ELDERLY

Besides the loss of taste papillae and taste bud numbers and function discussed above, some of the other factors which lead to changes in taste perception in the aged population include the following:

    a. Decrease in the flow of saliva, which is also of increased salt concentration and increased viscosity. This in turn leads to decreased taste receptor stimulation.

    b. An increase in the incidence of gingivitis and periodontal disease in this population. This has been proven to increase taste thresholds. Also several studies have shown a lowering of taste thresholds with an improvement in oral hygiene. Trials of antifungal troches and antibiotics have also been tried in an effort to improve oral health.

    c. The use of dentures covers part of the soft palate where there are taste receptors, thereby decreasing taste.

    d. Systemic diseases like diabetes, gastric disease, hypothyroidism, liver disease, chronic renal failure, Alzheimer's, and Parkinson's disease. Gastric reflux is a common cause of dysgeusia and in the elderly can worsen problems with taste dysfunction.

    e. Use of medications, especially antihypertensive drugs and chemotherapeutic agents, affect taste. Medications are suspected of introducing tastable substances into the blood and thereby altering taste thresholds. Schiffman found that certain drugs could modify taste transduction or the turnover of cells and alter taste perception. The taking of more than one medication (the so-called polypharmacy) is common among older people and this compounds the problem with taste dysfunction.

    f. Smoking affects taste, especially the bitter sense. Hsu and Davis found that smoking decreased gustatory sensitivity.

    g. The elderly require longer stimulation to integrate the sensory information further impairing taste.

EFFECTS OF TASTE LOSS IN THE ELDERLY

What most elderly individuals complain of is a loss of flavor and enjoyment of foods, which is most often related to the well-known loss of olfaction combined with some taste loss (28). Added to this problem is a loss of memory and some cognitive changes and the effect is a loss of appetite in older individuals. This puts the elderly individual at higher risk for depression, anorexia, and weight loss.

When elderly individuals lose their sense of taste, they often blame the food and stop eating certain foods. Foods that are essential for nutritional balance often do not taste good enough and the elderly resort to eating unhealthy foods like candies and pastries instead of meats and vegetables. The decreased consumption of proteins and other nutrients leads to loss of bone mass, weakening of the immune system, and hypertension (29).

The increase in salty taste thresholds may be responsible for an increase in the intake of salt in the elderly. This is one of the causative factors contributing to the development of hypertension. Studies by Spitzer have shown that patients with hypertension demonstrate a greater preference for salt compared to younger individuals.

Institutionalized individuals also show an increase in taste thresholds, which may account for the poor intake and nutritional status of some of these people. Poor taste perception combined with olfactory loss puts the elderly individual at risk for food poisoning from the ingestion of spoiled foods.

THERAPY FOR TASTE LOSS

No specific therapy or pharmacological agents are available to reverse the loss of taste with aging and in general the prognosis is poor. Awareness of taste decrement in the aged is important to make sure that these individuals get a balanced diet and prevent health problems, which are secondary to a poor and unhealthy diet.

Flavor amplifiers have been developed to enhance the flavor by adding an extra ingredient to the food. Examples of these are seasoning salts, fruit juices, meat stocks, and gravy. MSG also helps as a flavor enhancer, especially for protein-based dishes because it adds a savory taste to these foods, e.g., meat loaf, casserole, etc. Other food enhancers include vinegars, sun-dried tomatoes, herbs, and spices. Color enhancers make the food more appealing and enjoyable to people who have a poor appetite.

Caregivers need to be educated in food preparation to prepare a nutritionally balanced diet with the appropriate addition of additives and flavor enhancers especially when helping to prepare meals for institutionalized individuals. Awareness of the fact that gastrointestinal irritation, if any of the additives is in too great a quantity, should also be created.

Anecdotal evidence also exists that lack of the trace elements can lead to decreases in metabolic functions. Chauhan et al. (30,31) have therefore suggested that zinc supplementation be tried to enhance taste along with vitamins A, B_{12}, and folic acid for the maintenance of taste bud integrity.

CONCLUSION

Current research is geared toward the development of drugs containing taste ligands, which activate or inhibit taste receptor proteins. These in turn can then increase or decrease specific tastes (e.g., artificial sweeteners like saccharin and aspartame). Awareness of the loss of taste with aging should be an important part of education both for caregivers of the elderly and for the geriatric population so that a conscious effort is made toward the preparation of a nutritionally balanced diet. When an individual notices a loss of taste a referral to a chemosensory center should be made, where a multidisciplinary team approach can help with the elimination of the reversible causes of taste loss. Protectants of taste should be researched for and avoidance of drugs and harmful habits like smoking should be encouraged, as they will help preserve the natural taste function longer. Keeping the sense of taste strong is essential for the enjoyment of life and for the survival of the human race as a whole.

ACKNOWLEDGMENT

The author would like to thank Ms. Juliette Watts of the Philadelphia Veteran's Administration Medical Media Department for her artistic help.

REFERENCES

1. Schiffman SS. Taste and smell in disease. N Engl J Med 1983; 308:1275–1279.
2. Bartoshuk LM. Taste. Robust across the age span. Ann NY Acad Sci 1989; 561:65–75.

3. Temple EC, Hutchison I, Laing DG, Jinks AL. Taste development: differential growth rates of tongue regions in humans. Dev Brain Res 2002; 135:65–70.

4. Satoh Y, Seluk LW. Taste threshold. Anatomical form of fungiform papillae and aging in humans. J Nihon Univ Sch Dent 1988; 30:22–29.

5. Sogovia C, Hutchison I, Laing DG, Jinks AL. A quantitative study of fungiform papillae and taste pore density in adults and children. Dev Brain Res 2002; 138:135–146.

6. Nelson GM. Biology of taste buds and the clinical problem of taste loss. Anat Rec (New Anat) 1988; 253(3):70–78.

7. Lindemann B. Receptors and transduction in taste. Nature 2001; 413:219–225.

8. Miller SL, Mirza N, Doty RL. Electrogustomertric thresholds: relationship to anterior tongue locus, area of stimulation, and number of fungiform papillae. Physiol Behav 2002; 75:753–757.

9. Schiffman SS, Hornack K, Reilly D. Increased taste thresholds of amino acids with age. Am J Clin Nutrition 1979; 32:1622–1627.

10. Cooper RM, Bilash I, Zubek JP. The effect of age of taste sensitivity. J Gerontol 1959; 14(1):56–58.

11. Murphy C, Gilmore MM. Quality specific effects of aging on the human taste system. Percept Psychophys 1989; 45:121–128.

12. Bartoshuk LM, Rifkin B, Marks LE, Bars P. Taste and aging. J Gerontol 1986; 41(1): 51–57.

13. Lasilla V, Sointu M, Raiha I, Lehtonen A. Taste thresholds in the elderly. Proc Finn Dent Soc 1988; 84(5–6):306–310.

14. Matsuda T, Doty RL. Regional taste sensitivity to NaCl: relationship to subject age, tongue locus and area of stimulation. Chem Senses 1995; 20:283–290.

15. Zallen EM, Hooks LB, O'Brien K. Salt taste preferences and perceptions of elderly and young adults. J Am Dietetic Assoc 1990; 90(7):947–951.

16. Grzegorczyk PB, Jones SW, Mistretta CM. Age related differences in salt taste acuity. J Gerontol 1979; 34(6):834–840.

17. Weiffenbach JM, Baum BJ, Burghauser R. Taste thresholds: quality specific variation with human aging. J Gerontol 1982; 37(3):372–377.

18. Weiffenbach JM, Cowart BJ, Baum BJ. Taste intensity perception in aging. J Gerontol 1986; 41(4):460–468.

19. Spitzer ME. Taste acuity in institutionalized and noninstitutionalized elderly men. J Gerontol Psychol Sci 1988; 43(3):71–74.

20. Nordin S, Razani JL, Markison S, Murphy C. Age associated increases in intensity discrimination for taste. Exp Aging Res 2003; 29:371–381.

21. Mojet J, Chris-Hazelhof E, Heidema J. Taste perception with age: generic or specific losses in threshold sensitivity to the five basic taste. Chem Senses 2001; 26:845–860.

22. Osada K, Komai M, Bryant BP, Suzuki H, Sunoda K, Furukawa Y. Age related decreases in neural sensitivity to NaCl in SHR-SP. J Vet Med Sci 2003; 65(3):313–317.

23. Bradley RM. Effects of aging on the anatomy and neurophysiology of taste. Gerondontics 1988; 4(5):244–248.

24. Schiffman SS, Lindley MG, Clark TB, Makino C. Molecular mechanism of sweet taste: relationship of hydrogen bonding to taste sensitivity for both young and elderly. Neurobiol Aging 1981; 2:173–185.

25. Doty RL, Bagla R, Morgenson M, Mirza N. NaCl thresholds: relationship to anterior tongue locus, area of stimulation, and number of fungiform papillae. Physiol Behav 2001; 72:373–378.

26. Miller IJ. Human taste bud density across adult age groups. J Gerontol 1988; 43(1): B26–30.

27. Arey LB, Tremaine MJ, Monzingo FL. Numerical and topographical relations of taste buds to circumvallate papillae throughout the life span. Anat Rec 1935; 64:9–24.

28. Deems DA, Doty RL, Settle RG, et al. Smell and taste disorders, a study of 750 patients from the University of Pennsylvania Smell and Taste Center. Arch Otolaryngol Head Neck Surg 1991; 117(5):519–528.

29. Mann NM. Management of smell and taste problems. Cleveland Clin J Med 2002; 69(4):329–336.

30. Chauhan J, Hawrysh ZJ, Gee M, Donald EA, Basu TK. Age related olfactory and taste changes and interrelationships between taste and nutrition. J Am Dietetic Assoc 1987; 87(11):1543–1550.

31. Chauhan J. Relationships between sour and salt taste perception and selected subject attributes. J Am Dietetic Assoc 1989; 89(5):652–657.

18

Sinusitis: Diagnosis, Treatment, and Complications

Berrylin J. Ferguson and Umamaheswar Duvvuri
*Division of Sino-Nasal Disorders and Allergy, Department of Otolaryngology,
University of Pittsburgh, Pittsburgh, Pennsylvania, U.S.A.*

INTRODUCTION

Sinusitis is a major public health concern, which affects approximately 20 million people. It is one of the main complaints that leads adults of any age to seek medical assistance (1). The diagnosis of sinusitis in the geriatric population is fraught with all the difficulties faced in the diagnosis in a younger population. These include lack of specificity of symptoms for rhinosinusitis (2) as well as the fact that different pathophysiologic conditions such as allergic rhinitis, vasomotor rhinitis, viral rhinosinusitis, bacterial rhinosinusitis, and even some headaches are collectively interpreted by many patients as "sinus trouble." Complicating the treatment of rhinosinusitis, regardless of cause, in the older population is the increased incidence of concurrent disease states, which increase the likelihood of adverse drug reactions or interactions with the patients' regular medications.

Sinus disease may present in either the acute or chronic forms. Acute sinusitis is defined as the persistence of symptoms for less than four weeks. Chronic sinusitis is defined as the persistence of symptoms for greater than 12 weeks. Subacute sinusitis falls between the two, lasting greater than four weeks but less than 12 weeks. Infectious causes of rhinosinusitis include viral, bacterial, and fungal etiologies and are a more common cause in acute sinusitis than chronic sinusitis. In general, chronic rhinosinusitis is less frequently due to an infectious etiology and more frequently caused by noninfectious inflammation, although there can be chronic bacterial or fungal rhinosinusitis. Chronic rhinosinusitis is frequently subdivided into chronic rhinosinusitis with polyps and chronic rhinosinusitis without polyps.

ACUTE SINUSITIS

Acute sinusitis has been better studied than chronic sinusitis. The majority of cases are caused by the common cold, a viral infection caused by a variety of different viruses, each with a multitude of serotypes. While upper respiratory tract infections are far more common in children than adults, the older adult can also have a cold. One risk factor for developing a cold is exposure to sick children, even though this may be somewhat reduced with hand washing. A viral infection cannot be reliably differentiated from a bacterial infection on the basis of symptoms, physical findings, or radiographs. In general, however, most cold symptoms will improve after three days although cough may persist for many weeks. The treatment of a cold is supportive. The use of decongestants may be problematic in the older population since decongestants may aggravate urinary retention from prostatic hypertrophy, exacerbate cardiac arrhythmias, or raise blood pressure. All of these comorbidities are more common in the older patient. Saline nasal sprays, mucolytics (such as increased hydration and high-dose guaifenesin), and chicken soup can be prescribed without fear of causing harm. Although analgesics such as nonsteroidal anti-inflammatory drugs can provide some symptomatic relief, caution should be utilized in patients taking anticoagulants or with a history of gastritis.

Diagnosis

Symptoms associated with acute sinusitis include facial pressure, pain of the maxillary teeth, postnasal drip, colored nasal discharge, and sometimes headaches. Facial pain or headache in the absence of other symptoms is rarely caused by sinusitis. Maxillary tooth pain is the most specific sign of bacterial sinusitis but is present in <15% of cases (3). Presence of unilateral purulent drainage is also more common in acute bacterial sinusitis; however, whether this is true for the geriatric population is unknown. Other more uncommon and nonspecific symptoms include halitosis, fever, nasal obstruction, cough, or otologic problems. In the elderly person who lacks dentition, a complaint of upper gum pain may be caused by maxillary sinusitis. Dental infection of the maxillary teeth can also lead to maxillary sinusitis. The pathogens of odontogenic sinusitis are more likely to consist of mixed microbial flora and include anaerobes.

The pertinent history should detail the severity of the complaints, precipitating and alleviating factors, associated symptoms, and a thorough past medical history. Obtaining a thorough past medical history and a list of medications, both prescription and over the counter, is particularly important in the geriatric patient. This allows the physician to evaluate for drug interactions and conditions that might mimic some feature(s) of sinusitis.

The physical examination by the otolaryngologist should consist of visualization of the nasal cavity. If the nose is so swollen that it cannot be adequately examined then it should be decongested with topical decongestants sprays or the placement of cotton pledgets impregnated with vasoconstrictors such as oxymetazoline or a few drops of 1:1000 epinephrine combined with 4% lidocaine. Local anesthetic of cocaine has fallen out of favor because of medical legal implications (i.e., patient drives home from the exam and has an accident in which the drug screen would be positive from the cocaine use in the exam). In addition, cocaine is associated with increased cardiac toxicity.

Frequently, a culture of purulent material from the middle meatus can be reliably obtained by a Calgi swab or aspirate. The correlation of endoscopically obtained bacteriologic findings is 70% to 90% with those obtained by maxillary puncture (4). Examination of the nasal cavity and acquisition of a culture is facilitated with the use of a rigid endoscope. The location of the purulent material in the nasal cavity correlates with the associated sinuses. Therefore, purulence in the middle meatus is associated with maxillary, anterior ethmoid, or frontal sinusitis. Pus streaming over the posterior superior aspect of the middle turbinate and above the eustachian tube orifice would indicate a posterior ethmoid sinusitis, while purulence coming from above the choana, 30° from the floor of the nose (the location of the sphenoid recess), would indicate a sphenoid sinusitis. A history of prior sinus surgery should be noted and may facilitate the aspiration of culture material. Cultures should be obtained using proper technique, which includes special care in avoiding contamination with the anterior nasal vestibule.

The presence of nasal polyps, vestibulitis, septal excoriation, turbinate hypertrophy, or evidence of prior surgery, scarring, and the character of the mucosa should all be noted during examination. The use of a 30° endoscope allows for improved visualization of the maxillary sinus ostia, and possibly the sinus contents, if the ostium is widely patent. If the patient has had prior sinus surgery, a flexible fiber-optic scope can be introduced into the maxillary sinus for visualization of the floor and lateral aspects of the sinus. Occasionally, purulent secretions will be seen in the floor of the maxillary sinus even when the nasal cavity examination is normal. Plain radiographs are usually obtained only if a maxillary puncture is required and there is a need to confirm presence of disease. An unenhanced coronal sinus computed tomography (CT) should be performed before surgical intervention. Another indication for sinus CT is the patient with persistent or puzzling symptoms despite appropriate treatment.

ANTIBIOTIC SELECTION

If the patient has symptoms that are worsening after three or four days or not improving after a week then clinically a bacterial sinusitis should be suspected. There is no information on whether the pathogens responsible for sinusitis in the older population differ in species or in antimicrobial resistance patterns from those found in younger adults. The 2004 sinus and allergy health partnership guideline recommendations for antimicrobial therapy in adults with mild symptoms include amoxicillin/clavulanate (1.75–4 g/250 mg/day), amoxicillin (1.5–4 g/day), cefpodoxime proxetil, cefuroxime axetil, or cefdinir. Trimethoprim/sulfamethoxazole (TMP/ SMX) (Bactrim or Septra), doxycycline, azithromycin, clarithromycin, erythromycin, or telithromycin may be considered in patients with β-lactam allergies, although bacteriologic failure rates of 20% to 25% may be encountered if treatment is not directed by culture and sensitivities. The recent guidelines are slightly different for adults with *mild* disease who have received antibiotics in the previous four to six weeks or for adults with moderate disease and include the following recommendations: respiratory fluoroquinolones (e.g., moxifloxacin, gatifloxacin, and levofloxacin, listed in order of potency) or high-dose amoxicillin/clavulanate (4 g/250 mg/day). The widespread use of respiratory fluoroquinolones for patients with milder disease may promote resistance to this broad-spectrum class of antibiotics and should be discouraged. The fluoroquinolones may, depending on the drug in the class, cause more disequilibrium in the geriatric age group compared to younger adults. Ceftriaxone (parenteral, 1–2 g/day × 5 days) or combination therapy with adequate gram-positive and -negative coverage is also an alternative. Examples of appropriate regimens of combination therapy include high-dose amoxicillin or clindamycin plus cefixime, or high-dose amoxicillin or clindamycin plus rifampin. Rifampin should not be used as monotherapy, or longer than 10–14 days as resistance to this agent quickly develops. Failure of a patient to respond to antimicrobial therapy after

72 hours of therapy should prompt either a switch to alternate antimicrobial therapy or re-evaluation of the patient (5).

If sinusitis is of odontogenic origin, then antibiotic coverage of anaerobes and oral flora is appropriate and includes penicillin and clindamycin. Antibiotics appropriate for sinusitis with their cautions/contraindications and drug interactions pertinent to the elderly are listed in Table 1. This table is not all-inclusive, particularly with regard to antibiotics undergoing hepatic metabolism.

IV antibiotics can be helpful in patients whose bacterial organism is resistant to oral antibiotics or in those with impaired host defenses and vascular insufficiency (e.g., diabetics) who may benefit from the higher antibiotic serum levels, which can be obtained intravenously. Laboratory monitoring of liver, renal, and hematological parameters depend on the antimicrobial agent selected.

In general, patients taking warfarin should have their international normalized ratio (INR) monitored while on any oral antibiotic, since risk of bleeding is increased

Table 1 Oral Antibiotics Appropriate for Acute Bacterial Sinusitis with Cautions/Contraindications and Drug Interactions Pertinent to the Elderly

	Possible drug interactions	Carry a caution for use in elderly patients
Fluoroquinolones (moxifloxacin, gatifloxacin, levofloxacin)	Possible with a number of antiarrhythmics and antihypertensives, list extensive	Yes Increased incidence of disequilibrium
Amoxicillin/clavulanate	Allopurinol, methotrexate	No but caution if impaired liver function or creatinine clearance <30
Amoxicillin	Allopurinol, methotrexate	No but caution if impaired renal function
Ceftriaxone		No but caution if renal dysfunction or hyperbilirubinemia
Oral cephalosporins	Antacids and proton pump inhibitors may decrease absorption	No
Macrolide	Numerous with other medications undergoing hepatic metabolism	No but caution if impaired liver function
Clindamycin	Neuromuscular blockers	No but caution if impaired liver or renal function or ulcerative colitis or history of antibiotic-associated colitis
Trimethoprim sulfamethoxazole	Digoxin, MAO 2 inhibitors, methotrexate, phenytoins, warfarin	Yes; also caution if bone marrow suppressed or if impaired liver function
Tetracycline	Numerous with other medications undergoing hepatic metabolism	No but caution if impaired renal or liver function
Rifampin	Numerous with other medications undergoing hepatic metabolism	No but caution if impaired liver function; hepatic enzyme inducer

secondary to altered vitamin K production by gut flora. Antibiotics increase risk for *Clostridia difficile* overgrowth in the gut. Many practitioners recommend that while the patient is taking oral antibiotics, yogurt, *Lactobacillus*, or probiotic administration be encouraged concurrent with the antibiotic (6). In addition, selection of an antibiotic with the narrowest spectrum targeted to the causative organism will reduce impact on the native microflora.

Fungal Sinusitis

Acute invasive fungal sinusitis should be suspected in the immunocompromised patient with objective evidence of sinus disease. Radiographs in invasive fungal sinusitis are indistinguishable from bacterial sinusitis and show no evidence of bony erosion until the disease is far advanced. An endoscopic culture or maxillary sinus puncture with lavage and culture should be obtained unless the latter is contraindicated because of coagulopathy. If the patient has poorly controlled diabetes, then mucormycosis should be suspected. The earliest symptom in mucormycosis is commonly anesthesia of the affected area followed by blackening of the mucosa (7). If invasive fungal sinusitis is suspected, a frozen section biopsy of the suspected tissue or immediate fungal stain of an aspirate along with culture should be obtained. If positive for invasive fungal sinusitis, then every effort should be made to reverse the patient's source of immunocompromise, and systemic antifungals should be selected appropriate to the fungus cultured or suspected histopathologically. Surgery should be conservative with debridement of necrotic areas. Acute invasive fungal rhinosinusitis may also be caused by a wide variety of fungi in addition to mucormycosis, with the most common being *Aspergillus fumigatus*, particularly in the nondiabetic immunocompromised patient.

CHRONIC SINUSITIS

Stankiewicz and Chow (2) looked prospectively at the relationship between the definition of chronic rhinosinusitis and the diagnosis of bacterial chronic rhinosinusitis in 78 patients ranging in age from 16 to 78. Patients who had a strong history of sinusitis by symptom score underwent same-day endoscopy and CT of the sinuses. Of those patients who had no polyps or purulence endoscopically, over half had normal CT scans. Moreover, there was no difference in symptom scores between CT(+) and CT(−) patients. Eighty percent of normal CT scans were associated with a normal nasal endoscopy (8). Thus, patients with symptoms suggestive of chronic sinusitis will have no objective evidence of sinusitis half of the time. Nasal endoscopy as the primary intervention, with only those patients with positive findings undergoing treatment, was calculated to be more cost effective than obtaining a CT scan on all patients and treating only those with disease or empirically treating all patients with broad-spectrum antibiotic and nasal steroid sprays for one month and only obtaining a CT scan on the failures (9).

Chronic sinus disease may be caused by bacteria and fungi or be independent of an identifiable infectious agent. The bacteria commonly implicated in chronic sinusitis are *Staphylococcus aureus* and gram-negatives (such as *Pseudomonas aeruginosa*) in patients who have had prior surgery or have impaired mucosal defenses. The role of anaerobes and coagulase negative staphylococcus in chronic sinusitis is controversial (1). Fungi can elicit an allergic reaction causing allergic fungal sinusitis. Allergic fungal sinusitis is far more common in younger people but has been reported to occur in patients in their 70s (10).

Diagnosis of chronic sinusitis requires objective evidence of sinus disease for at least three months. It is useful to divide patients into those with nasal polyps and those without. Patients with bilateral nasal polyposis are less likely to have a primary bacterial infection. If a bacterial pathogen is identified, then it should be treated with a culture-directed antibiotic. The course of therapy recommended is longer than that in acute bacterial sinusitis. A useful guideline is to continue the antibiotic for several days beyond symptom resolution or when symptom improvement plateaus. There are no controlled studies on the efficacy of antimicrobial therapy in chronic sinusitis.

Nasal steroid sprays are a cornerstone of medical therapy in patients with chronic sinusitis, particularly in the patient with nasal polyps, but are frequently used in any patient with symptoms of nasal congestion or postnasal drainage. The use of topical steroids reduces mucosal inflammation. Most topical steroid sprays have low systemic absorption and pose little risk of systemic steroid side effects. Although Beclomethasone nasal spray has been reported to cause increased intraocular pressure, this has not been reported in nasal sprays with less systemic bioavailability (11). There are no studies to date regarding the effect of nasal steroid sprays on ocular pressures in the elderly. Systemic steroid use is potentially more hazardous in the geriatric patient for the following reasons: glucose control may be compromised in diabetic patients, osteopenia/osteoporosis may be exacerbated, and steroids may affect blood pressure control and the progression of cataracts.

The majority of patients with sinus symptoms severe enough to require endoscopic sinus surgery are allergic. Whether this is true in the geriatric population is unknown. Allergies usually decrease with age but may be present even through the ninth decade. In general, first-generation sedating antihistamines are not suitable in elderly patients because of sedation and anticholinergic side effects.

CHRONIC FUNGAL RHINOSINUSITIS

Fungus Balls

Fungus balls of the paranasal sinuses comprise the most common chronic form of fungal sinusitis and are also a noninvasive form. Older individuals may be more susceptible although there are no definitive data to substantiate this (12–14). Ferreiro et al. (15) report a mean age of 64 years. There does appear to be a female predominance. Associated medical conditions such as allergic rhinitis and aspirin sensitive asthma are no higher than the general population. The clinical presentation of fungus balls is similar to that of chronic rhinosinusitis. Common symptoms include nasal obstruction, facial pain, and purulent discharge. Eighteen percent of patients were asymptomatic in the largest review and diagnosis was made incidentally on radiographs (14). The most commonly affected sinus is the maxillary followed by the sphenoid. Frontal sinus involvement is uncommon. Ethmoid sinus involvement is frequently contiguous with the maxillary.

The treatment of fungus balls of the sinus consists of surgical removal. With the advent of endoscopic instrumentation, most fungus balls can be approached endoscopically. Irrigation is also helpful in the debriding process. The management of the asymptomatic patients remains controversial and removal is often suggested to prove the diagnosis. Surgical resection may be advocated if the fungus ball is thought to precipitate asthma or if bony erosion is present on radiographs. If the asymptomatic patient becomes immunocompromised, the fungus ball may become invasive. Patients with a possible fungus ball, facing expected immunocompromise because of bone marrow transplant, for example, should have the fungus ball removed prior to becoming immunocompromised.

CHRONIC INVASIVE FUNGAL SINUSITIS

Chronic invasive fungal sinusitis is a rare entity that has been proposed by Stringer and Ryan (15) to describe nonfulminant invasive fungal disease in immunologically intact patients. In a case series of four patients, Stringer and Ryan reported a geriatric predominance, with three-fourths of patients being greater than 65 years of age. Symptoms directly related to the invasive disease may take several months to manifest and may only be apparent after the orbit or skull base is involved. Mucosal thickening is often noted, although signs of bony erosion or obliteration of fat planes around the maxillary sinus are also associated with invasive fungal disease. Chronic invasive fungal rhinosinusitis may mimic many other disorders including benign and/or malignant neoplasms, Wegener's granulomatosis, lymphoma, allergic fungal rhinosinusitis, and rhinoscleroma. Chronic invasive fungal rhinosinusitis has specifically been associated with *Mucor*, *Alternaria*, *Curvularia*, *Bipolaris*, *Candida*, *Drechslera*, *Sporothrix*, and *Pseudallescheria*.

Current treatment of chronic invasive fungal sinusitis consists of surgical debridement with adjuvant antifungal therapy. There is no consensus as to the extent of surgical debridement necessary to treat the disease, and recommendations have ranged from wide aeration of the diseased sinuses to a complete extirpation of the diseased tissue. It is also generally recommended that serial CT scans and nasal endoscopy be performed every three to four months after completion of therapy. Recurrent disease should be promptly addressed with further surgery and/or antifungal therapy.

Special Considerations in the Surgical Management of the Geriatric Patient

Geriatric patients with significant comorbidities require preoperative medical evaluation to minimize potential anesthetic and perioperative complications. In particular, perioperative and postoperative hypertension may increase the potential for epistasis and necessitate nasal packing. The geriatric male patient is more likely to have prostatic hypertrophy and suffer from postanesthetic urinary retention. Before discharge from the outpatient surgical suite all patients must be able to void on their own. Beyond this, sinus surgery is similar to that performed in the younger population.

Ramadan and VanMetre (16) compared endoscopic sinus surgeries (ESSs) in 46 geriatric patients (>65 years) to 522 younger patients (18–64 years). Approximately 33% of older patients required frontal sinusotomy as primary surgery compared to 21% of younger patients. Sphenoidotomy as either a primary or revision surgery was twice as common in the geriatric patient (68%) compared to the younger group. Revision ESS carried a higher risk of orbital injury (not blindness) (27% vs. 3%), and hemorrhage (18% vs. 3.4%) in geriatric patients compared to younger patients. There was no difference in complications between the two groups for primary surgery. None of the geriatric patients had a cerebrospinal fluid (CSF) leak compared to 2% in the younger group.

SUMMARY

Diagnosis of acute, subacute, or chronic sinusitis in the geriatric population must be based on a full history and physical examination, which includes rigid nasal endoscopy. Endoscopically guided cultures and appropriate use of CT scans may be helpful in guiding therapy. Special considerations regarding the use of antibiotics in the older adult include the presence of comorbidities, potential adverse effects, and interaction with other medications, as well as status of liver and renal function. Overall, sphenoid surgery is more common in the geriatric patient and there is a slight increase in minor complications with revision surgery.

REFERENCES

1. Benninger MS, Ferguson BJ, Hadley JA, et al. Adult chronic rhinosinusitis: definitions, diagnosis, epidemiology, and pathophysiology. Otolaryngol Head Neck Surg 2003; S129:S1–32.
2. Stankiewicz JA, Chow JM. A diagnostic dilemma for chronic rhinosinusitis: definition, accuracy and validity. Am J Rhinol 2002; 16:199–202.
3. Anon J, Jacobs MR, Poole MD, et al. Antimicrobial treatment guidelines for acute bacterial rhinosinusitis. Otolaryngol Head Neck Surg 2004; S130(1):S1–S45.
4. Williams JW Jr, Simel DL. Does this patient have sinusitis? Diagnosing acute sinusitis by history and physical examination. JAMA 1993; 270(10):1242–1246.
5. Talbot GH, Kennedy DW, Scheld WM, Granito K. Rigid nasal endoscopy versus sinus puncture and aspiration for microbiologic documentation of acute bacterial maxillary sinusitis. Clin Infect Dis 2001; 33:1668–1675.
6. Bergogne-Berezin E. Treatment and prevention of antibiotic associated diarrhea. Int J Antimicrob Agents 2000; 16(4):521–526.
7. Ferguson BJ. Mucomycosis of the nose and paranasal sinuses. Otolaryngol Clin North Am Fungal Rhinosinusitis Spectr Dis 2000; 33(2):349–365.
8. Stankiewicz JA, Chow JM. Nasal endoscopy and the definition/diagnosis of chronic rhinosinusitis. Otolaryngol Head Neck Surg 2002; 126:623–627.
9. Stankiewicz JA, Chow JM. Cost analysis in the diagnosis of chronic rhinosinusitis. Am J Rhinol 2003; 12:139–142.
10. Ferguson BJ. Eosinophilic mucin rhinosinusitis: a distinct clinicopathological entity. Laryngoscope 2000; 110(5 Pt 1):799–813.
11. Opatowsky I, Feldman RM, Gross R, Feldman ST. Intraocular pressure elevation associated with inhalation and nasal corticosteroids. Ophthalmology 1995; 102:177–179.
12. de Shazo RD, O'Brien M, Chapkin K, et al. Criteria for the diagnosis of sinus mycetoma. J Allergy Clin Immunol 1997; 99:475–485.
13. Ferreiro JA, Carlson BA, Cody DT. Paranasal sinus fungus balls. Head Neck 1997; 19: 481–486.
14. Klossek JM, Serrano E, Peloquin L, Percodani J, Fontanel JP, Pessey JJ. Functional endoscopic sinus surgery and 109 mycetomas of paranasal sinuses. Laryngoscope 1997; 107:112–117.
15. Stringer SP, Ryan MW. Chronic invasive fungal rhinosinusitis. Otolaryngol Clin North Am 2000; 33(2):375–387.
16. Ramadan HH, VanMetre R. Endoscopic sinus surgery in geriatric population. American Rhinologic Society meeting, Nashville, Tn., May 2003.

19

Allergic Rhinitis in the Elderly

Stephen J. Chadwick

*Department of Otolaryngology, Southern Illinois School of Medicine, Springfield, and
ENTA Allergy Head and Neck Institute, Decatur, Illinois, U.S.A.*

"Aging is a process that converts healthy adults into frail ones with diminished reserves in most physiologic systems and an exponentially increasing vulnerability to most diseases and to death" (1).

With improving American longevity and the maturing of the "Baby Boomers" (born in the 1940s and 1950s), health-related demands of the geriatric population continue to increase. Allergic rhinitis is common and increasing in this population. Some of this increase is related to pollutants and irritants as "... allergically predisposed parents are producing allergically predisposed progeny in an increasingly antigenic and irritant-laden environment" (2). This chapter summarizes the diagnosis and management of allergic rhinitis in the aged individual, and discusses these in the context of the patient with significant other medical problems. We assume the reader has a basic knowledge of the evaluation and management of allergic rhinitis, and the basic diseases, pathophysiologies, and constitutional milieu associated with the geriatric age group (3–8).

The proportion of people over age 65 in the United States is increasing faster than the general population (Table 1) (9). This is occurring despite continued socioeconomic incentives for smaller families! With the dramatic rise in the percentage of the population over 65, and over 85, there is a changing attitude toward health in the aged person (9–11).

Allergic rhinitis is a common disease, with nearly 50 million Americans afflicted (12). Of allergic asthmatics, 90% have concomitant allergic rhinitis. Between 35% and 70% of people presenting to a general otolaryngology practice have allergic factors in their symptom complex (13,14). Physicians of tomorrow will have a large expanding population of elderly patients with a continuum of physiologic cha and a complexity of medical problems impacting the management of co problems such as allergic rhinitis.

BACKGROUND

To better understand the approach to managing allergic rh
patient, we will look briefly at general changes that occur i

Table 1 Age Trends and Projections for the U.S. Population

Census year	U.S. population (million)	Percent over age 56
1900	76	4.1
1950	152.3	8.2
2000	276.1	12.6
2050 (projected)	403.7 (projected)	20.3 (projected)

Recently, interest and research in immunogerontology has accelerated as the role of the immunoneuroendocrine system in the aging process and its effect on survival became apparent. Immunosenescence involves a decline, deregulation, and remodeling of the immune system as it interacts with other systems. This complex field is challenged to determine whether abnormal findings are related to disease in aged unhealthy patients, "normal" changes in aging patients, or immune effects of exogenous factors such as medications or the state of physical conditioning (15).

Two approaches have helped sort out some of these conundrums: studying centenarians and the SENIEUR protocol. Anyone living to 100 years of age without major illness was assumed to be prototypic of a healthy, aged person (16). The immune systems of these centenarians appear to be more preserved, less deregulated, and at times, of different remodeling than aging people afflicted by cancer, infection, autoimmunity, and other diseases associated with old age (9). The SENIEUR protocol, on the other hand, uses rigid laboratory and clinical criteria to define a pool of healthy aged people for the purposes of study (16–18). Here are a few of the highlights of immunosenescence studies.

The thymus gland involutes with age, impacting both innate and adaptive immunity (19–22). Thymic involution accelerates after puberty, giving a 60-year-old less than 5% of the thymic mass of a newborn. Capacity to respond to new antigens depends on naïve T cells (quiescent lymphocytes) found in the thymus. These cells are activated as antigens are processed, as part of the body's attempt at antigen elimination. These cells become memory T cells, and are quiescent until re-exposure
_specific antigen. Young people have a high naïve-to-memory T-cell ratio,
_the ratio, as would be expected, with time and continued
_s involutes, the production of naïve
_igen response declines (16).
_ helper T-cell function to decline, but
_nclude modification in B-cell varietal
_action, and fluctuations in the ratio of
_(15,23–26). With aging, the circulating
_production of antigen-specific antibody
_reases. Susceptibility to infections such
_influenza (poor vaccination response),
_0). Other B-cell-related diseases such as
_mmopathy/myeloma, etc. become more

_oglobulin G (IgG) and IgA levels actually
_creasing except IgG$_4$ (15,32). Since IgG$_4$ is
_ with IgE in the allergic response, a decrease
_E production tends to decrease in the older
_llergy symptoms (33). Atopy may play an

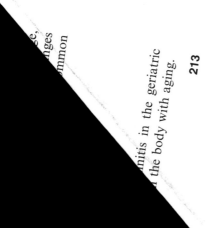

important role in complex respiratory complaints of geriatric patients. The paucity of knowledge in this area points to a need for research in geriatric allegroimmunology.

Changes in specific cellular immune response and T-cell response affect much of immunosenescence. In addition to thymic involution and decreasing naïve-to-memory T-cell ratio, T-cell receptor stimulation and response to receptor stimulation are decreased (31,34). Changes in CD4+ T cells and the subsequent alterations in interleukin (IL)-2 production favor a proliferation decline. Some studies suggest decreased IL-10 and increased IL-4 and IL-6 production. Changes in interferon (IFN)-γ have been variable. Cytotoxicity and delayed hypersensitivity do decline with age (27).

Innate immunity integrates with antigen-responsive T- and B-cell function (35). This includes phagocytosis, some cytotoxicity, production and release of cytoactive molecules such as adhesion molecules and cytokines, chemotaxis, and intercellular responses. Natural killer T cells usually increase with advancing age. Efficient natural killer activity is found in healthy geriatric individuals, while those with decreased activity often have increased morbidity and health problems.

The general decrease in cytokine production with advanced age impacts the T-helper-1 (Th1)/Th2 helper T-cell balance. IgE production and thus allergic symptoms depend on the Th2 lineage. The cell-related cytokine profiles shift with age. Th2-related immunity is prominent in infants, shifting to a Th1 profile in adulthood, and trending back to Th2 with advancing age. These immune changes parallel a common clinical presentation, of childhood allergy symptoms that were "outgrown," and then tend to recur with advancing age.

Age-related physiologic changes can worsen the impact of allergy symptoms. The geriatric population tends to be relatively dehydrated, causing more viscous mucus (36). Mucous-secreting glands decline and mucociliary transport is altered, so mucus is not transported efficiently. Atrophic changes are compounded by reduced nasal blood flow, and the nose becomes drier. The patient experiences more nasal congestion, stuffiness, and a perception of increased postnasal drainage, and becomes more susceptible to infection (37–46). Age-related structural nasal changes add to nasal obstruction and increased airway resistance. The nasal tip drops, and the columella retracts backward and upward (47). Thinning of upper and lower nasal cartilages paired with muscle atrophy promote nasal alar incompetence, and nasal obstruction.

PATIENT PRESENTATION AND HISTORY

Virtually every patient complaint relating to the nose or paranasal sinuses should prompt the taking of an allergic and environmental history (3,6). A well thought out patient questionnaire can be time efficient and promote thoroughness.

Medication: About 400 brand-name drugs have had rhinitis as a listed side effect (48,49). These drugs include some antihypertensives, aspirin and nonsteroidal anti-inflammatory agents, oral and parenteral contraceptives, conjugated estrogens, beta-blocking agents, some psychotropic drugs, cocaine, and legal topical vasoconstrictors commonly associated with rhinitis medicamentosa. Review of the patient's medication list will identify the possibilities. A suspect drug must be considered in consultation with the prescribing physician, weighing the importance of that medication in treating illness, and what options exist for alternate medications.

Head and Neck: Recurrent infections (rhinosinusitis, conjunctivitis, otitis, pharyngitis, laryngitis) can be exacerbated by inhalant allergies. IgE production increases in the allergic patient during viral infection, correlating with the clinical observation that the allergic patient often has a more prolonged illness and an increased risk of secondary bacterial infection (50). Dry eye syndrome can mimic or coexist with allergic conjunctivitis. A history of childhood allergic symptoms with an improvement in adulthood and a recrudescence at an older age is not uncommon.

Cardiovascular: Increased nasal congestion can occur with congestive heart failure. A history of hypertension, arrhythmia, valvular disease, cardiac surgery, peripheral vascular disease, etc. may affect the decision to use alpha-adrenergic drugs. Beta-blocker medications are a relative contraindication to allergy skin testing or immunotherapy, as they alter the effect of epinephrine if required to treat a systemic reaction or anaphylaxis. Angiotensin-converting enzyme (ACE) inhibitors can predispose to angioedema in allergy patients (51,52).

Respiratory: A patient with asthma (including cough-variant asthma) should be evaluated for allergies. A patient with allergic rhinitis has a 30% chance of developing asthma during a lifetime, and 90% of asthmatics have rhinitis. Asthma may have its onset in the geriatric age group (53,54). Recurrent bronchitis, bronchiectasis, chronic obstructive pulmonary disease (COPD) (including emphysema), and chronic cough may all have asthmatic/allergic components. Increased nasal airway resistance can contribute to obstructive sleep apnea and COPD (55).

Gastrointestinal: Laryngopharyngeal reflux and gastroesophageal reflux disease (GERD) occur frequently and can exacerbate asthma and voice or throat complaints. Food sensitivity is sometimes allergic in origin, so a history of colic in infancy, childhood gastrointestinal (GI) symptoms, or suspected food allergy should prompt further investigation. Some food allergens cross-react with other food or inhalant allergens, as seen in the "oral allergy syndrome." Nasal inflammation can occur with inflammatory bowel disease.

Genitourinary: Bladder outlet obstructive symptoms can influence the choice of medication used for allergy treatment. Childhood enuresis can suggest allergy (56).

Musculoskeletal: Rhinitis is increased with collagen vascular diseases such as rheumatoid arthritis and lupus erythematosus. It is similarly increased in granulomatous diseases such as sarcoidosis and Wegener's granulomatosis (57).

Integumentary: A history of eczema, hives, or angioedema (even if remote) suggests an allergic origin to a patient's rhinitis. Eczema or atopic dermatitis is associated with food allergy in children (30–80%) and inhalant allergies in adults. Atopic dermatitis is complex in character with other exacerbating factors including (but not exclusively) skin moisture/dryness, irritant exposure, and bacterial/fungal colonization (*Staphylococcus aureus, Malassezia* sp.) with possible super antigen effects (52,58).

Endocrine: Endocrine disorders associated with rhinitis include pregnancy, some birth control medications, diabetes, and thyroid dysfunction. Delivery or correction of the underlying problem may not lead to complete symptom resolution. Allergy evaluation and treatment can provide symptom improvement. Obesity can also contribute to nasal congestion.

Psychologic: Poor control of psychiatric problems such as anxiety and depression can magnify the effect of rhinitis symptoms on quality of life. Psychiatric medications may have nasal side effects (rhinitis, mucosal dryness). Tricyclic antidepressants and monoamine oxidase inhibitors are contraindications to allergy skin testing and immunotherapy.

Hematologic: While frequent rhinosinusitis may be suggestive of allergic factors, immunodeficiency and hematologic conditions need consideration.

Geriatric patients often have multiple medical problems, and take multiple medications. When undertaking evaluation and treatment of allergies, coordination of care with the patient's primary care physicians or other specialists will ensure the best possible treatment outcome.

DIAGNOSIS

It is often appropriate to begin an empiric trial of allergy pharmacotherapy based on the patient presentation. Suboptimal response of symptoms to initial pharmacotherapy is the most common reason for allergy testing. The information gained from allergy testing is used to design environmental changes to minimize allergen exposure, and as a basis for immunotherapy.

There are some age-related considerations in considering in vivo or in vitro allergy testing. Skin test reactivity declines with advancing age (39,59–64). This occurs despite a favored Th2 function, and is related to declining total IgE levels, tissue remodeling, and atrophic changes. Intradermal skin testing is more sensitive than epidermal (prick or scratch) testing, and may therefore be more appropriate in elderly patients. Systemic and intranasal antihistamine medication must be stopped three to five days prior to skin testing. In general, patients on beta-blocker medications, tricyclic antidepressants, or monoamine oxidase inhibitors are not skin tested.

Several classes of medication may interfere with the accuracy of allergy skin testing. These include antihistamines (both older and newer nonsedating types), some psychotropic drugs, especially the tricyclic antidepressants, nontopical corticosteroids in medium to higher doses, H2 blocking antihistamines, and some leukotriene modifying agents. Beta-blocking agents do not affect the accuracy of skin testing, but can impede epinephrine action if the patient requires treatment of a systemic or anaphylactic reaction due to skin testing. Topical beta-blockers such as ophthalmic preparations for glaucoma carry the same risk as oral beta-blockers (56). If these medications cannot be withdrawn for testing, in vitro testing, which is not affected by the patient's drug profile, is recommended.

In vitro antigen-specific IgE testing is sometimes a better choice for the geriatric patient. Many elders are on medications interfering with the accuracy or safety of allergy skin testing (as above, systemic dose steroids, antihistamines). Common comorbidities can impact the safety of allergy skin testing, such as the patient with rhinitis and asthma-factored COPD and little pulmonary reserve who could develop asthma during testing, or the brittle cardiac patient with suspected allergy and a relative contraindication to epinephrine use should an adverse reaction to testing develop. Other patient situations favoring in vitro testing include abnormal skin reactivity (dermatographism or urticaria), needle phobia, or a history of anaphylaxis.

MANAGEMENT

Elimination or avoidance of offending allergens is the cornerstone of allergy management. This can eliminate symptoms in a patient with limited sensitivities, and can reduce the allergic load in more complex patients. Environmental control may be difficult for some geriatric patients due to finances, an unfriendly domiciliary situation, or physical difficulties interfering with performing the required cleaning tasks. Living in a communal environment such as a nursing or retirement home may result in a limited say in controlling the surroundings.

For the dust mite-allergic patient, the key is making the bedroom and other frequently used areas as dust-free as possible. Strategies include allergen-proof mattress and pillow covers, weekly washing of bedclothes in hot water, meticulous dusting, and elimination of nonessential soft furnishings such as draperies and carpets. Laundry additives, carpet treatments, high-efficiency vacuum cleaners, and HEPA filters can also be helpful in minimizing dust exposure.

Mold-avoidance strategies include thorough frequent cleaning of all humid areas of the home (bathrooms, laundry rooms), routine emptying of drip pans (under refrigerators, air conditioners), elimination of houseplants, and dehumidification. Gardening and lawn mowing also expose the patient to heavy mold loads, and should be avoided.

Pet allergies can be controlled by giving away a pet or keeping the pet outdoors. When the pet in question is an important family member, however, such strategies will not work. Weekly washing and grooming of the pet and keeping the pet out of the bedroom will help with symptoms.

Pollen-allergic patients can avoid exposure by spending as little time outdoors as possible during pollination season. Broadly speaking, this is spring for tree pollens, summer for grass pollens, and fall for weed pollens. Local weather, plantings, and microclimates, however, provide much variation in pollination seasons. Wearing a mask covering the nose and mouth can minimize inhaled pollen. When coming in from outdoors, performing nasal irrigations, showering, shampooing, and completely changing clothes also reduce pollen exposure.

Pharmacotherapy for control of allergic symptoms has an annual "price tag" of several billion dollars in the United States (12,55,65–67). Successful drug choices for pharmacotherapy improve the symptoms, while not interfering with management of other medical problems, not causing serious side effects, and being affordable and easy to use. These choices become more complex in the context of the physical, psychological, and socioeconomic challenges of advancing age.

The general classes of medications used in management of allergic rhinitis include antihistamines (oral and topical), alpha-adrenergic decongestants (oral and topical), leukotriene modifying agents, topical anticholinergic agents, mast cell stabilizers, corticosteroids (oral, topical, and parenteral), and mucolytic agents.

Antihistamines improve symptoms of allergic mucosal inflammation and irritation. All antihistamines are equally efficacious. Side effects of first-generation antihistamines that may impact the elderly include mucosal dryness, increased mucus viscosity, altered mucociliary function, sedation and slowed reaction time, cardiotropic effects, hypertension, weight gain, hair loss, and bowel/bladder dysfunction. In the newer generation of antihistamines, these side effects are reduced or eliminated. Topical antihistamines also have some of these side effects, especially sedation and a local drying effect.

Oral decongestants help shrink edematous mucosa, improving nasal obstruction. Side effects include numerous cardiotropic effects, including hypertension, arrhythmias, and angina. Bladder, prostate, and bowel dysfunction are common, as are sleep disturbances. Topical preparations, including both the sympathomimetics and the imidazoline derivatives, cause some of the same systemic side effects, as well as carry the risk for rhinitis medicamentosa with prolonged use.

Corticosteroids have numerous side effects. Used as directed in recommended doses, intranasal steroids do not promote lasting hypothalamic–pituitary–adrenal axis changes, bone growth suppression, osteoporosis, or other worrisome effects (68,69). Airway dryness and epistaxis (especially in the anticoagulated or platelet-adhesive-treated patient) are not rare. Age-related physical and cognitive difficulties may render both use and compliance difficult, especially when using nasal sprays and eye drops. Some patients may be "steroid responders" from the standpoint of ophthalmic susceptibility to an increase in intraocular pressure, or cataracts, with the application of topical ophthalmic steroids, using on-label prescribed doses (70).

Lastly, a miscellany of thoughts on management medications is in order. While water is the best mucolytic agent for the dehydrated patient, guaifenesin is the most commonly used. If guaifenesin is not used with adequate hydration, it has a potential drying side effect. Data support the nasal decongestant effect of the leukotriene modifying agent, montelukast, which is attractive in the patient at risk for the cardiotropic effects associated with the alpha-adrenergic decongestants (71,72). Anticholinergic topicals, while safe and relatively free of side effects, are of limited use in allergic rhinitis and are most useful for vasomotor or idiopathic rhinitis factors. Saline topicals may not only be used for moisturizing, but may also have a symptomatic, therapeutic use. Zealous overuse of saline sprays may actually promote dryness due to an evaporative effect on the nasal mucosa. Saline gels may help reduce this consequence.

Drugs in development that may provide therapeutic alternatives for elderly patients include more potent intranasal steroids (indicated for younger and older patients), oral H1 plus H2 antihistamine combinations, oral antihistamines new to the U.S. market (tecastemizole, ebastine, mizolastine), more potent intranasal antihistamines, combination steroid plus antihistamine intranasal sprays, and leukotriene plus antihistamine combinations. Additional future options include pharmaceutical substances such as anti-IgE, which blend the lines between pharmacotherapy and immunotherapy.

IMMUNOTHERAPY

As with younger patients, immunotherapy is usually reserved for the patient with multiple sensitivities who is not responding well to pharmacotherapy and avoidance strategies. Since the geriatric patient's medical condition tends to be more complex, however, special attention is paid to risk and the patient's potential reserve for recovering from an adverse reaction to therapy, should one occur. Benefits of immunotherapy include better symptom control, and diminished need for medications. Sublingual immunotherapy has been used with success outside the United States, and is now coming under research scrutiny within the United States. Issues of cost (for example, eliminating charges for allergy injections), safety, drug interference issues, and compliance make this modality attractive to patients and payors. Tablet-based immunotherapy has been used with some success in Europe. Consideration for this single antigen, sublingual tablet will need appropriate U.S. research to complete development and obtain Food and Drug Administration (FDA) approval before launching in the United States. Anti-grass tablets will possibly be the first of potentially several formulations to be produced.

Anti-IgE therapy is now approved in the United States for the management of adult forms of moderate to severe IgE-mediated asthma (73). Omalizumab is the (rhu)mAb-E-25 antibody, which is a recombinant humanized monoclonal antibody to IgE-25 derived from the murine antibody MAE-1. Indications will be sought for the pediatric age group and then for allergic rhinitis (74). Studies for allergic rhinitis are making their way into the literature now (75–79).

Other mediator antagonists and immune modulators are in the earlier stages of research. Soluble IL-4 receptor antagonists, anti-IL-4 monoclonal antibodies, and mutated IL-4 receptor antagonists are being studied. Humanized anti-IL-5 antibodies for use in asthma, IL-5 synthesis inhibitors, and murine anti-IL-5 antibodies are works in progress. Other considerations include anti-IL-13 monoclonal antibodies, soluble IL-13 receptors-Fc fusion proteins, eosinophil receptor CCR-3 antagonists, adhesion molecule inhibitors, chemokine [RANTES, Eotaxin, monocyte chemotactic and activating factor (MCAF), monocyte chemotactic protein-1 (MCP)-1] modulation, action against mast cell secretory granule enzymes (tryptase, chymase), recombinant IL-12 (Th1 function suppresses Th2/allergic function) preparations, the nebulization of IFN-γ for topical asthma treatment, prostaglandin modifying agents, and more to come (80,81).

There is also a future in other forms of immunotherapy. Local nasal immunotherapy and peptide-based immunotherapy are nearing the horizon. Oligonucleotides are immune boosting molecules, which are attached to antigens and then the patient is injected. Enzyme-potentiated desensitization has been in use, but will need more research and regulatory alignment before becoming an easily available tool (82). While all of these modalities are provocative to thought, and may help reduce the need for conventional pharmacotherapy, consideration as to how these forms of allergy treatment will affect other aspects of the patient's medical make-up are critical, especially in the geriatric patient.

FOOD ALLERGY

Adverse reactions to foods are immunologically mediated (immediate IgE-mediated vs. delayed immune reactions). The most common immediate IgE-mediated reactions occur with peanuts and seafood. The diagnosis is usually made by history, and absolute avoidance is the only treatment. Patients with this condition should always carry self-injectable epinephrine (EpiPen®) for use in cases of inadvertent exposure.

The remainder of adverse reactions to food is best diagnosed by a careful history, a food diary, and withdrawal of the suspect food for five days, followed by reintroduction. Any foods that cause symptoms are eliminated from the diet completely for at least four to six months. After that time, patients can often tolerate occasional meals containing that food. If the food is eaten too frequently, however, symptoms will recur.

SUMMARY

Allergic rhinitis is a common and costly disease. A careful history will suggest an allergic etiology for the patient's symptom complex. Empiric pharmacotherapy often yields symptom resolution. When pharmacotherapy does not improve symptoms enough, allergy testing (skin or in vitro testing) can identify the specific allergen. Avoidance strategies can be planned, and, if needed, immunotherapy can be begun.

ACKNOWLEDGMENT

The author wishes to thank Ms. Karen Stoner, Chief Librarian of the Decatur Memorial Foundation Library for Ms. Stoner's tireless efforts, and the American Academy of

Otolaryngic Allergy Foundation library. Further thanks to Mr. George Smaistrla Jr., Clinic Administrator, and Ms. Julie Causey, transcriptionist, for their assistance. Lastly, the author's warm thanks goes to Melinda for donating time, and to Nicholson with whom the author divides the present with Vanderbilt University.

REFERENCES

1. Miller RA. The Biology of aging and longevity. In: Hazzard WR, et al. eds. Principles of Gerontology. Part I: Principles of Geriatric Medicine and Gerontology. New York: McGraw-Hill, 2003:3–15.
2. Chadwick SJ. Allergy in the contemporary laryngologist. Otolaryngol. Clin North Am 2003; 36:965.
3. Krouse JH, Chadwick SJ, Gordon BR, Derebery J. Allergy and Immunology–An Otolaryngic Approach. Philadelphia: Lippincott, Williams and Wilkins, 2002.
4. Kashima HK, Goldstein JC, Lucente FE. Clinical Geriatric Otorhinolaryngology. Philadelphia: B.C. Decker (Mosby-Yearbook), 1992.
5. Brocklehurst JC, Tallis RC, Fillit HM. Brocklehurst's Textbook of Geriatric Medicine Gerontology. 6th ed. New York: Churchill Livingston, 2003.
6. King HC, Mabry RL, Gordon BR, Marple BF, Mabry CS. Allergy in ENT Practice. The Basic Guide. 2nd ed. Thieme Medical Publishers, 2004.
7. Cassel CK, Cohen HJ, Larson EB, et al. Geriatric Medicine. 4th ed. Springer Verlag, 2003.
8. Adkinson NF, Yunginger J, Busse W, Boshner B, Holgate S, Middleton E. Middleton's Allergy: Principles and Practice Edition. 6th ed. C. B. Mosby, 2003.
9. Guralnik JM, Ferrucci L. Demography and Epidemiology. In: Hazzard WR, Blass JP, et al. eds. Part I: Principles of Geriatric Medicine and Gerontology. 5th ed. New York: McGraw-Hill, 2003:53–75.
10. Bunuel L. http://www.brainyquote.com/quotes/authors/l/luis_bunuel.html.
11. Butler RN. Economic and political implications of immunology and aging on tomorrow's society. Mech Aging Dev 1997; 93:7–13.
12. Fieneman SM. The burden of allergic rhinitis: beyond dollars and cents. Ann Aller Asthma Immunol 2002; 88:2–7.
13. Roecker EB, Kemnitz JW, ErshlerWB, Weindruch R. Reduced immune response on rhesus monkeys subjected to dietary restriction. J Gerontol A Biol Sci Med Sci 1996; 51:B276–B279.
14. Casale T, Amin B. Allergic rhinitis/asthma relationships. Clin Rev Allergy Immunol 2001; 21:27–49.
15. Ginaldi L, De Martins M, D'ostilio A, et al. The immune system in the elderly. Part I. Specific humoral immunity. Immunol Res 1999; 20(2):101–108.
16. Whitman DB. The Immunology of Aging. Cambridg Scientific Abstracts. http://www.casa.com/hottopics/immune-aging/oview.html. [Updated March 1999]. Accessed 11/28/03, 1999, all rights reserved, Cambridg Scientific Abstracts. NIAID Office of Communications, Bethsesda, MA, USA.
17. Ligthart GJ, Corberand JX, Fournier C, et al. Admission criteria for immunogerontological studies in man: the SENIEUR protocol. Mech Aging Dev 1984; 28:47–55.
18. Ligthart GJ, Corberand JX, Geertzen HG, Meinders AE, Knook DL, Hijmans W. Necessity of the assessment of health status in human gerontological studies: evaluation of the SENIEUR protocol. Mech Aging Dev 1990; 55:89–105.
19. Ligthart GH. The SENIEUR Protocol After 16 Years: the next step is to study the interaction of aging and disease. Mech Aging Dev 2001; 122(2):136–140.
20. Ershler WB. The value of the SENIEUR protocol: distinction between "ideal aging" and clinical reality. Mech Aging Dev 2001; 122(2):134–136.

21. Castle SC, Uyemura K, Makinodan T. The SENIEUR protocol after 16 years: a need for a paradigm shift? Mech Aging Dev 2001; 122(2):127–130.

22. Effros RB, Cai Z, Linton PJ. CD8 T-cells and aging. Crit Rev Immunol 2003; 23(1–2): 45–64.

23. Yang X, Stedra J, Cerny J. Repertoire diversity of antibody response to bacterial antigens in aged mice. IV. Study of VH and VL gene utilization in splenic antibody foci by in situ hybridization. J Immunol 1994; 152:2214–2221.

24. Stephan RP, Sanders VM, Witte PL. Stage specific alterations in murine B-lymphopoiesis with age. Int Immunol 1996; 8:509–518.

25. Yang X, Stedra J, Cerny J. Relative contribution of T and B cells to hypermutation and selection of antibody in general centers of aged mice. J Exp Med 1999; 183:959–970.

26. Klinman NR, Kline JH. The B-cell biology of aging. Immunol Rev 1997; 160:103–114.

27. Murasko DM, Gardner EM. Immunology of aging. In: Hazzard WR, Blass JP, Halter JB, Ouslander JG, Tinitti ME, eds. Part I: Principles of Geriatric Medicine Gerontology. 5th ed. New York: McGraw Hill 2003:35–52.

28. Callard RE, Basten A, Waters LK. Immune function in aged mice. II. B-cell function. Cell Immunol 1977; 31:26–36.

29. Miller RA. Aging and immune function. Int Rev Cytol 1991; 124:187–215.

30. Powers DC, Belsher B. Effective age on cytotoxic/lymphocyte memory as well as serum and local antibody response elicited by inactivated influenza virus vaccine. J Infect Dis 1993; 167:584–592.

31. Paganelli R, Scala E, Quinti I, Ansotequi IJ. Humoral immunity in aging. Aging Clin Exp Res 1994; 6:143–150.

32. Paganelli R, Quinti I, Fagiolo U, et al. Changes in circulating B-cells and immunoglobulin classes and subclasses in healthy age population. Clin Exp Immunol 1992; 90:351–354.

33. Stoy PJ, Roytman-Johnson B, Walsh G, et al. Aging and serum immunoglobulin E levels, immediate skin tests, RAST. J Allergy Clin Immunol 1981; 68:421.

34. Yang X, Stedra J, Cerny J. Relative contribution of T and B-cells to hypermutation and selection of the antibody repertoire in germinal centers of aged mice. J Exp Med 1996; 183:959–970.

35. Ginaldi L, De Martins M, D'ostilio A, Marini L, Coreto MF, Quaglino D. The immune system in the elderly: III. -Innate immunity. Immunol Res 1999; 20(2):117–126.

36. Boardley D, Fahlman M. Micronutrient supplementation does not attenuate seasonal decline of immune system indexes in well-nourished elderly women a placebo-controlled study. J Am Diet Ass 2000; 100(3):356–359.

37. Crameri R, Faith A, Hemmann S, Jayssi R, Ismail C, Merz G, Blaser K. Humoral and cell mediated autoimmunity in allergy to *Aspergillus fumigatus*. J Exp Med 1996; 184:265–270.

38. Bunikowski R, Mielke ME, Skarabis H, et al. Evidence for a disease-promoting effect of *Staphylococcus aureus*-derived exotoxins in atopic dermatitis. J Allergy Clin Immunol 2000; 105:814–819.

39. Tripathi A, Conley DB, Grammer LC, et al. Immunoglobulin E to staphylococcal and streptococcal toxins in patients with chronic sinusitis/nasal polyposis. Laryngoscope 2004; 114(10):1822–1826.

40. Conley DB, Tripathi A, Ditto AM, Reid K, Grammer LC, Kern RC. Chronic sinusitis with nasal polyps: staphylococcal exotoxin immunoglobulin E and cellular inflammation. Am J Rhinol 2004; 18(5):273–278.

41. Dennis DP. Chronic sinusitis: defective T-cells responding to superantigens, treated by reduction of fungi in the nose and air. Arch Environ Health 2003; 58(7):433–441.

42. Bernstein JM, Ballow M, Schlievert PM, Rich G, Allen C, Dryja D. A superantigen hypothesis for the pathogenesis of chronic hyperplastic sinusitis with massive nasal polyposis. Am J Rhinol 2003; 17(6):321–326.

43. Cryer J, Schipor I, Perloff JR, Palmer JN. Evidence of bacterial biofilms in human chronic sinusitis. J Otorinolaryngol Relat Spec 2004; 66(3):155–158.

44. Fakhri S, Christodoulopoulos P, Tulic M, et al. Role of microbial toxins in the induction of glucocorticoid receptor beta expression in an explant model of rhinosinusitis. J Otolaryngol 2003; 32(6)388–393.

45. Schubert MS. A superantigen hypothesis for the pathogenesis of chronic hypertrophic rhinosinusitis, allergic fungal sinusitis, and related disorders. Ann Allergy Asthma Immunol 2001; 87(3):181–188.

46. Roll A, Cozzio A, Fisher B, Schmid-Grendelmeier P. Microbial colonization and atopic dermatitis. Curr Opin Allergy Clin Immunol 2004; 4:373–378.

47. Slavin RG. Diagnosis and treatment of rhinitis and sinusitis in the elderly. Immunol Allergy Clin N Am 1997; 17(4):543–556.

48. Side effects report. Citings for sinusitis. PDR electronic library. Physicians' Desk Reference Publication. Thomas Medical Economics, 2003:1–5.

49. Side effects report. Citings for rhinitis. PDR electronic library. Physicians' Desk Reference Publication. Thomas Medical Economics, 2003:1–6.

50. International Rhinitis Management Working Group. International consensus report on the diagnosis and management of rhinitis. Allergy 1994; 49(suppl):1–34.

51. Gordon BR. Allergy and immunology- an otolaryngic approach. In: Krouse JH, Chadwick SJ, Gordon BR, Derebery MJ, eds. Anaphylaxis: Prevention and Treatment. Philadelphia: Lippincott, Williams and Wilkins, 2002:99–113.

52. Chadwick SJ. Allergy and immunology-an otolaryngic approach. In: Krouse JH, Chadwick SJ, Gordon BR, Derebery MJ, eds. The Pharynx and Larynx. Philadelphia: Lippincott, Williams and Wilkins, 2002:249–269.

53. Rogers L, Cassino C, Berger KI, et al. Asthma in the elderly-cockroach sensitization and severity of airway obstruction in elderly nonsmokers. Chest 2002; 122(5):1580–1586.

54. Mitsunobu F, Mifune T, Hosaki Y, et al. IgE-mediated and age-related bronchial hyperresponsiveness in patients with asthma. Relationship to family history of the disease. Age Ageing 2000; 29:215–220.

55. Schoenwetter WF, Dupclay L, Appajosyula MF, et al. Economic impact and quality-of-life burden of allergic rhinitis. Curr Med Res Opin 2004; 20(3):305–317.

56. Boyd EL. Patient history. In: Krouse JH, Chadwick SJ, Gordon BR, Derebery MJ, eds. Allergy and Immunology: An Otolaryngic Approach. Philadelphia: Lippincott, Williams and Wilkins, 2002:81–98.

57. Rinaldi RZ, Weisman MH. ENT manifestations of rheumatic diseases. In: Krouse JH, Chadwick SJ, Gordon BR, Derebery MJ, eds. Allergy and Immunology: An Otolaryngic Approach. Philadelphia: Lippincott, Williams and Wilkins, 2002:341–345.

58. Werfel T, Breuer K. Role of food allergy in atopic dermatitis. Curr Opin Allergy Clin Immunol 2004; 4:379–385.

59. Skassa-Brociek W, Manderscheid J, Michel FB, Bousquet J. Skin test reactivity dehistamine from infancy to old age. J Allergy Clin Immunol 1987; 90(5):711–716.

60. Poon AW, Goodman CS, Rubin RJ. In Vitro and skin testing for allergy: comparable clinical utility and cost. Am J Managed Care 1998; 4(7):969–985

61. Nielsen NH, Svendsen UG, Madsen F, Dirksen A. Allergen skin test reactivity in an unselected danish population. The Golstrup Allergy Study, Denmark. Allergy 1994; 49:86–91.

62. Salkie ML, Weimer N. The influence of season and of sex on the serum level of total IgE and on the distribution of allergen-specific IgE. Clin Biochem 1984; 17:362–366.

63. Nelson HS. Variables in allergy skin testing. Allergy Proc 1994; 15(6):265–268.

64. Friedhoff LR, Meyers VA, Marsh DG. A genetic-epidemiologic study of human immune responsiveness to allergens in an industrial population. J Allergy Clin Immunol 1984; 73(4):490–499.

65. Reed SB, Lee TA, McCorry DC. The economic burden of allergic rhinitis: a critical evaluation of literature. Pharm Econ 2004; 22(6):345–361.

66. Malone DC, Lawson KA, Smith DH, et al. Clinical aspects of allergic disease. J Allergy Clin Immunol 1997; 99(1):22–32.

67. Law AW, Reed SD, Sundy JS, et al. Direct costs of allergic rhinitis in the United States: estimates from the 1996 Medical Expenditures Panel Survey. J Allergy Clin Immunol 2003; 111(2):1–10.
68. Lipworth B, Jackson C. Safety of inhaled and intranasal corticosteroids. Lessons for the new millenium. Curr Opin Drug Safety 2000; 1(23):11–33.
69. Allen D. Systemic effects of intranasal steroids: an endocrinologist's perspective. J Allergy Clin Immunol 2000; 106(suppl 4):S179–S190.
70. Steroid induced glaucoma. http://www.eyemdlink.com/conditionasp?condition419.
71. Van Adelsberg J, Philip G, LaForce CF, et al. Randomized controlled trial evaluating the clinical benefit of Montelukast for treating spring season allergic rhinitis. Ann Allergy Asthma Immunol 2003; 90(2):214.
72. Philip G, Malstrom K, Hampel FC, et al. Montelukast for treating seasonal allergic rhinitis: a randomized, double-blind placebo-controlled trial performed in the spring. Clin Exp Allergy 2002; 32:1020–1028.
73. Busse W, Corren J, Lanier BQ, et al. Omalizumab-anti-IgE recombinant humanized monoclonal antibody, for the treatment of severe allergic asthma. J Allergy Clin Immunol 2001; 108(2): 184–189.
74. Soler M, Matz J, Townley R, et al. The anti-IgE antibody omalizumab reduces exacerbations and steroid requirement in allergic asthmatics. Eur Res J 2001; 18(2):254–261.
75. Corren J, Diaz-Sanchez D, Saxon A, et al. Effects of omalizumab, a humanized monoclonal anti-IgE antibody, on nasal reactivity to allergen in local IgE synthesis. Ann Allergy Asthma Immunol 2004; 93(3):243–248.
76. Lee DK. The role of omalizumab or rhuMAB-E 25 in the treatment of allergic rhinosinusitis. Eur Respir Aug 2004; 24(2):330.
77. Bez C, Schubert R, Kopp M, et al. Effect of anti-immunoglobulin E on nasal inflamation in patients with seasonal allergic rhinoconjunctivitis. Clin Exp Allergy 2004; 34(7): 1079–1085.
78. Hanf G, Noga O, O'Connor A, et al. Omalizumab inhibits allergian challenged-induced nasal response. Eur Resp J 2004; 23(3):1414–1418.
79. Lin H, Boesel KM, Griffith VP, et al. Omalizumab rapidly decreases nasal allergic response and Fcepsilon RI on Basophils. J Allergy Clin Immunol 2004; 113(2):297–302.
80. DeBuske LM. Mediator antagonist in the treatment of allergic disease. Allergy Asthma Proc 2001; 22(5):261–275.
81. Haydon R. New horizons in allergy management. In: American Academy of Otolaryngic Allergy Foundation Advanced Course. Washington, DC: American Academy of Otolaryngic Allergy Foundation, 2002:20036.
82. Mabry RL. Beyond Conventional Immunotherapy. Washington, DC: American Academy of Otolaryngic Allergy Foundation, 1990:20036.

20

Rhinitis in the Aging Patient

Margaret A. Chen and Terence M. Davidson
Division of Otolaryngology—Head and Neck Surgery, VA San Diego Healthcare System, and Department of Surgery, UCSD Medical Center, San Diego, California, U.S.A.

INTRODUCTION

Aging rhinitis, an atrophic rhinitis, is a common ailment in the elderly population and results from normal aging processes in the nose. Morbidity is significant, with patients complaining of throat tickle, thick postnasal drip, and chronic cough. Many do not seek medical treatment for this process, and those who do are frequently misdiagnosed or inappropriately managed. Fortunately, there is a simple and effective treatment. While medications and surgery have little utility in this disease, nasal irrigation with pulsatile, hypertonic nasal saline irrigation has been shown to be very effective in relieving symptoms and should be the standard of treatment. This chapter will discuss the pathophysiology, presentation, and treatment of aging rhinitis, including a comprehensive review of nasal irrigation.

OVERVIEW OF NORMAL NASAL PHYSIOLOGY

Nasal mucosa has two populations of cells responsible for secretory function. These are the nasal mucosal goblet cells, which produce a thick tenacious mucus, and submucosal serous glandular cells, which produce a thin watery mucus. The mucus itself is divided into two phases. The outer mucoid gel phase is viscous and traps particulate matter. The inner watery sol phase is thinner and less viscous. The mucus blanket floats on the watery sol layer. Ciliary beating in the sol layer propels the mucus blanket from the sinonasal cavity to the nasopharynx. Healthy nasal mucosa produces approximately 1 L of mucus each day, which is normally swallowed. Mucus properties are critical to nasal health. Changes in mucus viscosity disrupt the normal cycle of flow and cause troublesome nasal symptoms (1,2).

Turbinate vasculature is primarily responsible for warming and humidifying inspired air. This system is regulated by autonomic control and is highly sensitive to changes in temperature or circulating hormones. Changes in vascular health have severe consequences on normal mucosal function.

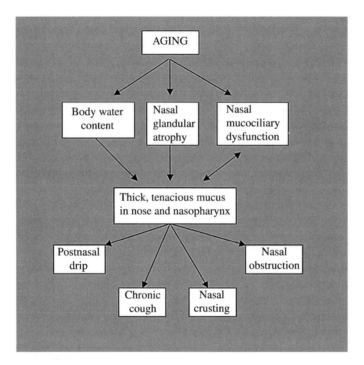

Figure 1   Pathophysiology of aging rhinitis.

PATHOPHYSIOLOGY OF AGING RHINITIS

Clinical Changes

Several factors contribute to the symptomatology of the aging nose (Fig. 1). The mucus becomes thick and tenacious secondary to generalized decreased body water content and local serous glandular atrophy (3). Change in the gel and sol layers impairs mucociliary function, resulting in mucosal stasis. The thick mucus is suspended in the nasopharynx and causes symptoms of throat tickle, snorting, postnasal drip, and cough (4,5).

An excellent clinical study by Edelstein involving 111 healthy subjects ages 21–94 showed that postnasal drip is 35% more prevalent with every 10 years of age (6). Other nasal complaints that occurred significantly more frequently with age were nasal drainage, sneezing, and coughing.

Autonomic dysfunction and atherosclerosis in aged individuals alter the vascular tone of the nasal turbinates. Decreased humidification of inspired air results in bothersome crusting. Thinner mucosa and fragility of vessels result in more frequent epistaxis. Ironically, turbinate atrophy can cause "empty nose-like syndrome," i.e., atrophic rhinitis, where nasal obstruction is falsely perceived secondary to disrupted perception of normal airflow.

Histopathologic Changes

In 1944, Hollender (7) published an extensive histopathologic comparison of nasal mucosa in 23 cadavers aged 50–90 years. Hollender was unable to find a correlation between epithelial morphology and age. However, older subjects demonstrated a relative decrease of lymphatic tissue in the subepithelial layer with abundant fibrosis. In 1992, a follow-up scanning electron microscopic study of aging human nasal epithelium demonstrated that the number of ciliated cells on the inferior turbinate did not decrease with age (8). Rather, the authors postulated that drying and crusting in the aging nose are likely due to changes in the viscoelastic properties of mucus.

Structural Changes

The structure of the nose significantly changes with aging. Degeneration of collagen and elastin in the skin with atrophy of subcutaneous tissues and facial musculature leads to drooping of the nose (9). Resorption of premaxillary fat and changes in dentition contribute significantly to this process. The result is a downward rotation of the lobule and retraction of the columella. The most important structural change occurs at the junction of the upper and lower lateral cartilages. Weakening of fibrous connective tissue at this location causes a significant loss of nasal tip support. Aging cartilage undergoes disorganization of its collagen fibril architecture and proteoglycan aggregates (10,11). Ultimately, degeneration of key support structures such as the septal, upper, and lower lateral cartilages and their fibrous connections results in collapse of the nasal valve. Consequent nasal obstruction is greatly exacerbated by any pre-existing septal deviation.

Mucociliary Changes

Mucociliary dysfunction in aging is more likely due to changes in mucus properties than to cellular derangement. Healthy elderly subjects were shown to have significantly impaired mucociliary transport relative to younger subjects, using the saccharin clearance test. Nevertheless, it should be noted that 70% of the elderly subjects had normal saccharin clearance times (12). While Edelstein's clinical study of 111 healthy subjects did not show a significant change in ciliary beat frequency with age, the standard deviation of the intrasubject beat frequency did vary significantly with age (6).

Immunologic Changes

Dysregulation of the immune system, or immune senescence, has been studied in rat nasal mucosa (13). Aging mucosa showed an alteration in the synthesis and release of cytokines with alterations at receptor sites, resulting in loss of control of inflammatory processes. These findings are interesting in light of the inflammatory mechanisms associated with many conditions of the aging nose.

Together, changes associated with aging result in disruption of mucus production and nasal airflow, causing symptoms of nasal obstruction and nasal dryness. Mouth breathing can result, which requires more physiological work than nasal breathing.

CLINICAL ASSESSMENT

Presentation

Commonly, patients who seek medical attention for aging rhinitis will complain of "allergies" or "sinus trouble." Direct questioning will reveal the major symptoms to be thick postnasal drainage with constant throat clearing, snorting, and cough. The patient will complain of nasal obstruction, especially when lying down, and may note nasal crusting which is particularly bothersome on first awakening.

Medical History

A thorough history should cover nasal and sinus surgery, nasal trauma, allergies, and concurrent medical illnesses. The patient will often have seen multiple medical professionals for this problem and all treatments, typically including nasal steroids and antihistamines, should be elicited. The patient's complete list of medications must be reviewed, particularly for medications that may exacerbate nasal dryness, such as antihistamines, antidepressives, diuretics, and antihypertensives (14).

Physical Examination

A thorough head and neck exam should be performed. On anterior rhinoscopy, it is common to see dry, irritated mucosa in a widely patent nasal passage, sometimes with crusting. Nasal airway obstruction should be evaluated. The nose should be examined endoscopically for infection, anatomic abnormalities, atrophic changes, and thick, viscous secretions. If a flexible endoscope is used, the postnasal secretions can often be seen stranding down the pharynx, often suspended over and into the larynx. If available, acoustic rhinometry will confirm that the nasal passages are widely patent.

Differential Diagnosis

Other chronic sinonasal disorders may manifest similarly, such as chronic sinusitis, allergic rhinitis, and other atrophic rhinitides. Chronic inflammatory diseases (sarcoid, lupus, Wegener's) and the irradiated nose may also demonstrate similar nasal physiology. These conditions should be considered during history and physical examination.

MANAGEMENT

General Principles

The primary goal of treatment for aging rhinitis is to wash out the thick nasal secretions. The most effective way to do this is with pulsatile, hypertonic, nasal saline irrigation. Other irrigation methods and adjunct treatments have also been widely used. While many controversies surround the issue of nasal irrigation, including saline tonicity, delivery of systems, and additives, the most important factor in symptom relief is frequent and regular irrigation. It must be emphasized to patients that control, not cure, is the goal of management for their disorder. The following section of the chapter will review literature evidence for the various aging rhinitis management strategies.

Aging rhinitis is commonly misdiagnosed as allergic rhinitis, and patients are commonly prescribed antihistamines. However, the basic problem in aging rhinitis is the drying and thickening of nasal secretions. Antihistamines, which decrease mucus secretion in the nose, are contraindicated and will exacerbate aging rhinitis.

Moreover, many antihistamines, particularly first-generation medications, have anticholinergic side effects that can cause significant morbidity in the elderly. Unless true allergic symptoms are present, antihistamines should be avoided in these patients. Nasal steroids are of no value in the treatment of aging rhinitis.

Guaifenesin at a moderate dose (under 2400 mg/day) has mucolytic and expectorant properties, and is commonly prescribed for upper respiratory disorders. However, a double-blind placebo-controlled crossover trial of guaifenesin in 10 subjects showed no measurable effect on mucociliary clearance (15). In our experience, we have not found this medication to be particularly useful; moreover, it is associated with a high rate of gastrointestinal side effects.

Nasal Saline Irrigation

The mainstay of treatment for aging rhinitis is nasal saline irrigation. Irrigation is used for many sinonasal disorders, and is thought to improve symptoms by several mechanisms. The primary mechanism is a mechanical clearance of inspissated secretions and crusts. Clearance of thick mucus improves mucociliary function, thereby improving mucosal health and function. Irrigation moisturizes the dry nasal cavity, while decreasing mucosal edema and clearing accumulated inflammatory mediators. There are no reported serious adverse effects to irrigation.

Abundant subjective and objective evidence exists that nasal saline irrigation is efficacious in the treatment of sinonasal disease. Papsin and McTavish (16) have written an excellent literature review summarizing that nasal irrigation is simple, effective, and safe. Moreover, prescribing saline irrigation can help conserve medical resources. Saline irrigation is associated with lower utilization of medications and office visits. Because patients are often prescribed antibiotics by primary care providers for sinonasal complaints, decreasing medication use in this population can help lower the prevalence of antibiotic resistance.

A clinical study of 93 chronic rhinitis patients showed significant improvement in patient symptoms with the use of metered-dose saline. Subjects also noted subjective improved efficacy of their pre-existing rhinitis medications, such as nasal steroids (17). A prospective, randomized, controlled, double-blinded trial of 40 sinusitis patients demonstrated that irrigation with saline solution resulted in significant improvement of subjective complaints, endoscopic appearance, and radiographic appearance (18).

In a randomized controlled trial evaluating the value of hypertonic saline irrigation in 76 sinusitis patients, subjects were randomized to irrigation with 2% hypertonic saline or no irrigation (19). Both groups continued their usual medical regimen for sinusitis. Subjects receiving irrigation had significant improvement of symptoms over the no-irrigation group by quality of life scores from two questionnaires. Of note, all patients who complied with a debriefing questionnaire indicated that they would recommend irrigation to friends and family, and 95% indicated that they would continue to use nasal irrigation.

A prospective controlled clinical study of 211 nasal dysfunction patients demonstrated that irrigation with pulsatile hypertonic saline significantly improved both severity and duration of patient-rated nasal symptoms (e.g., nasal congestion, postnasal drip, allergies, and nasal discharge) (20). Quality of well-being, assessed by the QWB questionnaire, also significantly improved. Moreover, compliance with irrigation was 92% after six weeks.

Irrigation Delivery

Methods of irrigant delivery may be as simple as a cupped hand or as elaborate as a top-of-the-line irrigating device. Other popular methods are bulb syringe, spray pump, nebulizer, and irrigation, or Neti, pot. Passive instillation differs from pressurized, or stream, delivery. Stream delivery may further be differentiated into laminar or pulsatile flow. The literature is rife with comparisons of efficacy among these methods.

A 99^{m}-technetium radio-labeled saline study demonstrated that a nebulizer is superior to a spray pump in distributing aerosol to the nasal cavity (21). A similar study using dye solution and endoscopy compared delivery among aerosolized spray, atomizer, nebulizer, and bulb syringe (22). While there was no demonstrable difference between aerosol and atomizer distribution, bulb syringe appeared to be statistically superior to other delivery methods in multiple sinonasal sites.

Other evidence further supports the efficacy of stream delivery. A randomized study of nasal irrigation in a post-rhinologic surgery population showed that stream delivery was significantly more effective than drops in improving both symptoms and endoscopic appearance (23). In a randomized controlled study, stream delivery by bulb syringe and by irrigation pot were equally effective in decreasing symptoms and medication usage among 150 chronic sinusitis patients (24).

Stream delivery of irrigant is most effective when delivered in a pulsatile as opposed to a laminar fashion. A study from the orthopedic literature demonstrated that pulsatile irrigation was 100 times more effective than bulb syringe in removing slime-producing *Staphylococcus* from implant surfaces, regardless of what irrigating solution was used (25). A radiologic study using contrast-labeled irrigation with computed tomography (CT) scan compared negative and positive pressure irrigation to nebulization (26). While both positive and negative pressure distributed contrast effectively, distribution was more even with positive pressure. Nebulization, however, distributed contrast poorly.

In 1974, Grossan (27) published a report of a new nasal irrigator tip to provide pulsatile irrigation from a Waterpik™ dental device. This new method made pulsatile nasal saline irrigation much more accessible to patients because it was inexpensive, readily available, and simple to use. To this day, it remains a very widely used and efficacious therapy.

The potential disadvantage of pulsatile irrigation involves trapping of fluid within the sinuses or the middle ear. Theoretically, this may result in serous otitis media or sinus pressure. If this occurs, the patient may need to change their method of irrigation to a laminar system, such as a Neti pot or syringe delivery system.

Irrigant Solutions

Saline Tonicity

A great deal of conflicting literature and opinion exists as to whether hypertonic saline is more efficacious in nasal irrigation than isotonic normal (0.9%) saline. Hypertonic saline has been studied in various concentrations and is believed to have several mechanisms of efficacy. First, salt has a topical antibacterial effect that is generally concentration-dependent. Second, the high ionic concentration disrupts ionic bonds in mucus, thus decreasing its viscosity. Third, diffusion of osmolar gradients may reduce mucosal edema. Fourth, hypertonic saline increases the mucinous response of nasal mucosa. Finally, high concentrations of salt stimulate release of intracellular calcium, possibly facilitating the use of adenosine triphosphate (ATP) at the ciliary axoneme. Increased ciliary beating improves mucociliary clearance.

The antimicrobial effect of hypertonic saline has been described in the surgical literature. One study described the use of different concentrations of saline to dress ulcers (28). Only ulcers dressed with hypertonic saline were culture-negative. Inoculation of *Staphylococcus* into different concentrations of saline showed that growth was not inhibited by normal saline, but was completely inhibited by 8.8% (3 Osm/L) saline. However, patients whose ulcers were dressed with 8.8% saline complained of itching at the site. The authors concluded that a moderate saline concentration of 4.4% (1.5 Osm/L) was the best compromise for antimicrobial effect and patient tolerance.

In a prospective crossover study comparing normal saline to hypertonic saline, 21 healthy subjects were randomized to a single irrigation with either normal or hypertonic (3%) saline (29). Subjects then underwent irrigation with the other solution the next day. Mucociliary transport, using the saccharin clearance test, was assessed at baseline and after each irrigation. There was a significant improvement in mucociliary transport only after irrigation with hypertonic saline. Although this study was conducted on healthy subjects, the authors predicted an even greater effect in symptomatic patients, where viscoelastic properties of mucus are likely altered.

A randomized, double-blind study of 30 children with chronic sinusitis compared normal and hypertonic (3.5%) saline nasal irrigation (30). Outcome was measured by three scores: cough score, nasal secretion/postnasal drip score, and radiologic Water's view score. Significant improvement in all three scores was seen with hypertonic saline, but only the nasal secretion/postnasal drip score was improved with normal saline.

The effect of hypertonic saline mucin secretion was studied in 16 healthy subjects (31). Subjects underwent hypertonic saline lavage, followed by histamine or methacholine challenge. Hypertonic saline alone was able to evoke global mucinous secretion, and also potentiated mucinous secretion after histamine or methacholine challenge.

One randomized, controlled, double-blind trial concluded that hypertonic nasal saline is not efficacious (32). One hundred forty-nine patients with colds or acute sinusitis were randomized to hypertonic or normal saline spray, or observation. Analysis of nasal symptom self-rating showed no difference in symptoms or duration of disease. Moreover, more than half of the patients indicated that they would not use hypertonic saline again because of burning discomfort on administration. These results are in contradiction to findings of patient tolerance in the majority of published studies. It is possible that these patients, suffering from self-limiting illnesses, were less likely to tolerate a new treatment for questionable gain. Our experience, as well as that evidenced in the bulk of the literature, indicates that patients with chronic disease overwhelmingly take to nasal irrigation when properly instructed, with excellent return on symptom resolution.

Base Solution

While most studies have examined the efficacy of hypertonic or normal saline in nasal irrigation, some studies suggest a re-examination of the base solution choice. An in vitro experimental study examined ciliary beat frequency in sinus mucosa in different solutions (33). Normal saline, hypertonic saline (7% and 14.4%), and Locke–Ringer's, an isotonic physiologic solution, were compared. While Locke–Ringer's solution had no inhibitory effect on ciliary beat frequency, normal and hypertonic saline had significant inhibitory effects proportional to salt concentration. In fact, 7% hypertonic saline caused a reversible ciliostasis, while 14.4% hypertonic saline caused irreversible ciliostasis and even cytotoxicity. It is important to note that these experiments were conducted in vitro and not in vivo. Nevertheless, the authors raise the question of whether nasal irrigation might be even more clinically effective if solutions without known ciliostatic effects, e.g., Locke–Ringer's, are used instead of saline.

An in vivo study of postoperative septoplasty patients compared mucociliary transport in patients irrigating with lactated Ringer's versus normal saline (34). Saccharin clearance was improved after irrigating with lactated Ringer's over normal saline. Because lactated Ringer's has the advantage of being more physiological in composition than normal saline, it may have less inhibitory effect on mucociliary function. Moreover, the solution, like saline, is inexpensive. However, given the composition of this solution [3.1 g sodium lactate, 6.0 g sodium chloride (NaCl), 0.3 g potassium chloride (KCl), and 0.2 g $CaCl_2 \cdot 2H_2O$], this solution would be difficult to make at home and would likely have to be purchased for long-term use.

Water Source

The use of tap water in homemade irrigation solution is important. Tap water commonly contains disinfectants such as chlorine, ozone, chlorine dioxide, and chloramines. Disinfection byproducts such as chloroform and trichloroacetic acid are also present. While some of these disinfectants and by-products are harmful in large doses, the amounts found in tap water are regulated closely by the Environmental Protection Agency to be at low levels such that the benefits of disinfection outweigh other risks (35).

Chlorine is a well-known broad-spectrum disinfectant that is a welcome addition to the nasal irrigation regimen. We recommend the use of tap water over bottled water for solution-making at home. Of note, the hardness of the water does not have a deleterious effect on its antibacterial action.

Additives and Antibiotics

Bicarbonate

The major indication for adding bicarbonate to irrigant solution is to ameliorate the burning sensation of hypertonic saline. If the patient finds irrigation uncomfortable for this reason, instructions should be given to add one-half teaspoon of baking soda to 500 cubic centimeters (cc) of solution. We believe that bacteria are more likely to thrive in an alkaline, rather than acidic, environment, and do not encourage the general use of bicarbonate in irrigant solutions. It should also be noted that chlorine is a more effective disinfectant at lower pH.

Nevertheless, patient compliance with the nasal irrigation regimen is of the utmost importance. Moreover, evidence is contradictory on this topic. Traditional teaching is that an alkaline environment causes mucus to be in a sol, rather than gel, state. However, a study of mucociliary clearance after nasal douching demonstrated no difference between unbuffered solution and solution buffered to pH 8 (36).

Antibiotics and Antifungals

Antimicrobial medications can be added to irrigant solutions for topical delivery to the nasal cavity and sinuses. Tobramycin irrigation (20 mg in 50 cc saline once daily) is a valuable adjunct in the treatment of cystic fibrosis-related sinusitis (37).

Table 1 Tonicity of Nasal Irrigant Solutions

	Normal saline (500 cc)	One teaspoon NaCl in 500 cc water	One heaping teaspoon NaCl in 500 cc water
% NaCl (g/100 mL)	0.9%	1.6%	2.3%
Weight Nacl (g)	4.5	8.0	11.5
Moles NaCl	0.077	0.137	0.197
Molarity (mol/L)	0.154	0.274	0.394

It is assumed that table salt is 100% NaCl (most table salt is reported to be > 99% NaCl and < 1% calcium silicate.
One teaspoon is 5 cc.
MW NaCl = 58.44 g/mol.
Abbreviation: MW, molecular weight.

Tobramycin has also been successfully used in the management of HIV sinusitis, difficult-to-manage chronic sinusitis, and atrophic rhinitis, including aging rhinitis (38,39). The use of topical gentamicin for purulent atrophic rhinitis has also been described (40).

The addition of antifungal agents for allergic fungal sinusitis is a relatively new advance. Nasal irrigation with amphotericin B suspension has been studied in 74 patients with nasal polyposis (41). After four weeks of twice-daily irrigation, nasal polyps disappeared in 39% of subjects. Efficacy was significantly higher in earlier-stage disease. Of note, there were no controls in this study, and the risk of systemic toxicity with use of topical amphotericin B was not addressed. The use of pulsatile and nebulized amphotericin B for the treatment of invasive fungal sinusitis has also been described (42).

Directions for Patients

A simple 1.6% hypertonic saline solution can be made by patients at home (Table 1). If burning is uncomfortable, one-half teaspoon of baking soda may be added. Patients should be instructed as follows:

1. Mix one level teaspoon of table salt in 500 cc (approximately two cups) of warm tap water (approximately body temperature).
2. Fill the nasal irrigator basin with the salt water.
3. Turn the unit on at the lowest setting.
4. Lean over the sink and place the irrigator up to the nose. Let the water run into the nose. It will run out the opposite side of the nose or the mouth.
5. Tilt and twist the irrigator side to side and up and down to direct the water flow into all portions of the nasal cavity until it feels clean on that side.
6. Repeat the procedure with the opposite side.
7. This can be repeated up to three times a day. The water pressure can be increased as the patient becomes accustomed to the sensation of nasal irrigation.

Multiple excellent irrigation devices are commercially available (Fig. 2). Patients unable to tolerate pulsatile irrigation may still benefit from a laminar system using Neti pot or syringe delivery.

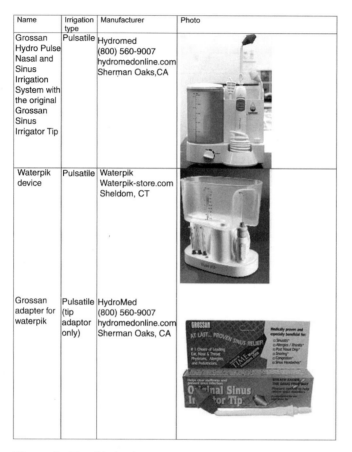

Name	Irrigation type	Manufacturer	Photo
Grossan Hydro Pulse Nasal and Sinus Irrigation System with the original Grossan Sinus Irrigator Tip	Pulsatile	Hydromed (800) 560-9007 hydromedonline.com Sherman Oaks,CA	
Waterpik device	Pulsatile	Waterpik Waterpik-store.com Sheldom, CT	
Grossan adapter for waterpik	Pulsatile (tip adaptor only)	HydroMed (800) 560-9007 hydromedonline.com Sherman Oaks, CA	

Figure 2 Nasal irrigation systems. (*Continued on next page*)

Other Treatments

Surgery

Surgery does not have a significant role in the management of aging rhinitis. In fact, overzealous mucosal resection and manipulation during surgery can contribute to tissue atrophy and accelerate the symptoms of aging rhinitis. The sole indication for surgical therapy is in the case of a severe septal deviation causing nasal obstruction and inability to irrigate the nose effectively. Septoplasty or septorhinoplasty may then be indicated; however, resection of tissue must be conservative.

Alternative Treatments

Several other therapies should be discussed for completeness. One alternative treatment is based on an ancient yogic treatment for rhinitis and involves the cleaning and rubbing of the nasal passages with a rubber catheter (43). This process likely works by eliciting a strong response of rhinorrhea, as well as the mechanical clearance of crusts and secretions. A study of reflexology massage on established sinus contact points on the fingertips and toes showed reflexology to be equally efficacious to nasal saline irrigation by bulb syringe or irrigation pot (24).

Ethicare adapter for Waterpik	Pulsatile (tip adaptor only)	Ethicare (800) 253-3599 www.ethicare.com Ft. Lauderdale, FL	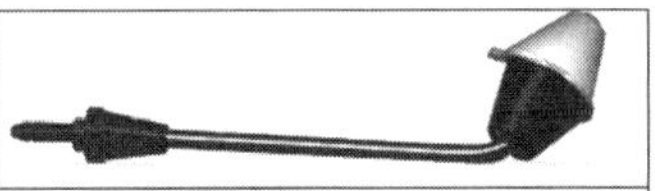
Kenwood adaptor for Waterpik	Pulsatile (tip adaptor only)	Kenwood Therapeutics, a division of Bradley Pharmaceuticals (800) 929-9300 www.brapharm.com Fairfield, NJ	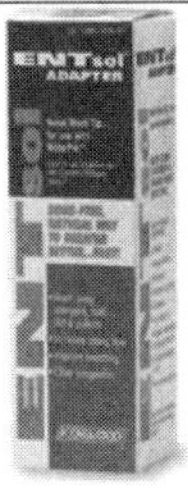
SinuCleanse	Laminar (neti pot, irrigatio pot)	Med-Systems, Inc. www.sinucleanse.com (888) 547-5492 Madison, WI	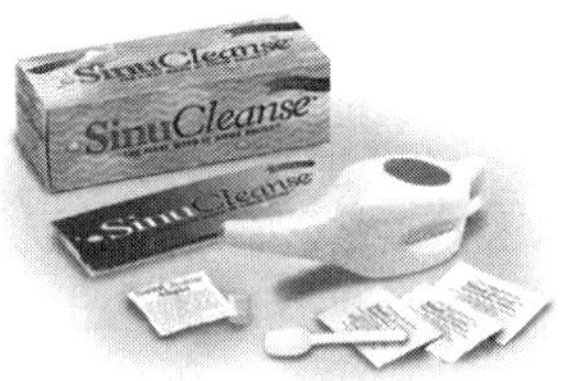
Nasaline	Laminar (syringe)	Camexco, Inc. www.camexco-inc.com (877) 226-3965 Bridgewater,NJ	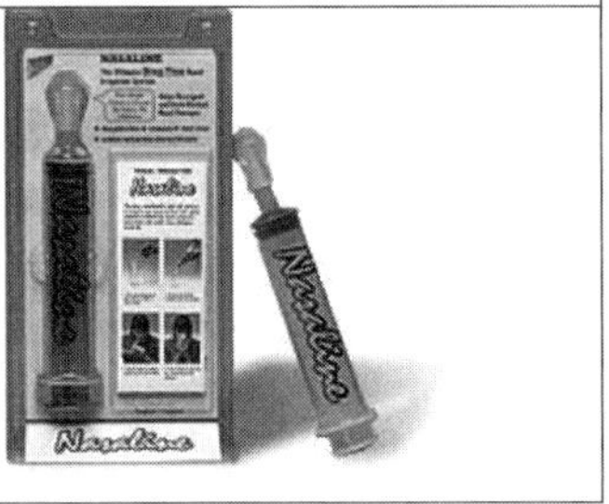

Figure 2 (*Continued*)

Lubricants

Little work has been done on the value of lubricating agents in the treatment of aging rhinitis. One randomized crossover study of sesame oil treatment in 79 subjects with nasal dryness demonstrated significant improvement in patient-rated nasal mucosa dryness, stuffiness, and crusting (44). Our experience is that, in general, lubricating agents are not terribly useful. While these may serve as a protective cover over the nasal mucosa, they do nothing to rid the nose of the tenacious mucus secretions responsible for the majority of patient symptoms. At best, they are a useful adjunct to nasal saline irrigation. Our favorite nasal lubricant, developed at the Massachusetts Eye and Ear Infirmary and brought to California by Dr. Jeffrey Harris, is a suspension of menthol, eucalyptus, and camphor in a mineral oil base.

CONCLUSION

Aging rhinitis is a common disorder in the elderly and results from natural aging processes in the nose. The pathophysiology is based on the thickening and drying of nasal secretions, leading to a perceived increase in mucus and symptoms in the nose and pharynx. It is important not to misdiagnose this ailment as allergic rhinitis, since antihistamine medications commonly contribute to nasal dryness. The disease is chronic, and treatment is based on control rather than cure. The mainstay of treatment is nasal irrigation with pulsatile, hypertonic, saline tap water. While many irrigation methods have been described and debated in the literature, patient compliance with regular irrigation is the key to successful management of symptoms.

REFERENCES

1. Bassichis BA, Marple BF. Dry mouth and nose in the older patient: what every PCP should know. Geriatrics 2002; 57(10):22–35.
2. Jordan JA, Mabry RL. Geriatric rhinitis: what it is, and how to treat it. Geriatrics 1998; 53(6):76–81.
3. Janzen VD. Rhinological disorders in the elderly. J Otolaryngol 1986; 15(4):228–230.
4. Davidson TM. Handbook of nasal disease. (Internet. http://www.surgery.ucsd.edu/ent/DAVIDSON/NASHAND/nasal.htm.)
5. Davidson TM. Otolaryngic gerontology (issues of aging). (Internet. http://www.surgery.ucsd.edu/ent/DAVIDSON/AGING/Aging.htm.)
6. Edelstein DR. Aging of the normal nose in adults. Laryngoscope 1996; 106(9 Pt 2):1–25.
7. Hollender AR. Histopathology of the nasal mucosa of older persons. Arch Otolaryngol 1944; 40:92–100.
8. Kushnick SD, Pelton-Henrion K, McCormick SA, Kimmelman CP. A scanning electron microscopic study of smoking and age-related changes in human nasal epithelium. Am J Rhinol 1992; 6:185–190.
9. Patterson CN. The aging nose: characteristics and correlation. Otolaryngol Clin N Am 1980; 13:275–288.
10. Hwang WS, Li B, Jin LH, Ngo K, Schachar NS, Hughes GN. Collagen fibril structure of normal aging and osteoarthritic cartilage. J Pathol 1992; 167:425–433.
11. Roughley PJ, Nguyen Q, Mort JS. Mechanisms of proteoglycan degradation in human articular cartilage. J Rheumatol 1991; 18(suppl 27):52–54.
12. Sakakura Y, Ukai K, Majima Y, Murai S, Harada T, Miyoshi Y. Nasal mucociliary clearance under various conditions. Acta Otolaryngol 1983; 96(1–2):167–173.
13. Himi T, Yoshioka I, Kataura A. Influence of age on the production of interleukin-8-like chemokine (GRO/CINC-1) in rat nasal mucosa. Eur Arch Otorhinolaryngol 1997; 254(2):101–104.
14. Mabry RL. Nasal stuffiness due to systemic medications. Otolaryngol Head Neck Surg 1983; 91(1):93–94.
15. Sisson JH, Yonkers AJ, Waldman RH. Effects of guaifenesin on nasal mucociliary clearance and ciliary beat frequency in healthy volunteers. Chest 1995; 107(3):747–751.
16. Papsin B, McTavish A. Saline nasal irrigation: its role as an adjunct treatment. Can Fam Phys 2003; 49:168–173.
17. Nuutinen J, Holopainen E, Haahtela T, Ruoppi P, Silvasti M. Balanced physiological saline in the treatment of chronic rhinitis. Rhinology 1986; 24(4):265–269.
18. Bachmann G, Hommel G, Michel O. Effect of irrigation of the nose with isotonic salt solution on adult patients with chronic paranasal sinus disease. Eur Arch Otorhinolaryngol 2000; 257(10):537–541.
19. Rabago D, Zgierska A, Mundt M, Barrett B, Bobula J, Maberry R. Efficacy of daily hypertonic saline nasal irrigation among patients with sinusitis: a randomized controlled trial. J Fam Pract 2002; 51(12):1049–1055.
20. Tomooka LT, Murphy C, Davidson TM. Clinical study and literature review of nasal irrigation. Laryngoscope 2000; 110(7):1189–1193.

21. Suman JD, Laube BL, Dalby R. Nasal nebulizers versus aqueous nasal spray pumps: a comparison of deposition patterns in human volunteers. Resp Drug Deliv 1998; 6:211–218.

22. Miller TR, Muntz HR, Gilbert ME, Orlandi RR. Comparison of topical medication delivery systems after sinus surgery. Annual meeting of the Western Section of the Triologic Society, Indian Wells, Ca., Jan 31–Feb 2, 2003.

23. Seppey M, Schweri T, Hausler R. Comparative randomized clinical study of tolerability and efficacy of Rhinomer Force 3 versus a reference product in postoperative care of the nasal fossae after endonasal surgery. ORL J Otorhinolaryngol Relat Spec 1996; 58(2): 87–92.

24. Heatley DG, McConnell KE, Kille TL, Leverson GE. Nasal irrigation for the alleviation of sinonasal symptoms. Otolaryngol Head Neck Surg 2001; 125(1):44–48.

25. Anglen JO, Apostoles S, Christensen G, Gainor B. The efficacy of various irrigation solutions in removing slime-producing *Staphylococcus*. J Orthop Trauma 1994; 8:390–396.

26. Olson DE, Rasgon BM, Hilsinger RL Jr. Radiographic comparison of three methods for nasal saline irrigation. Laryngoscope 2002; 112(8 Pt 1):1394–1398.

27. Grossan M. A device for nasal irrigation. Trans Am Acad Ophthalmol Otolaryngol 1974; 78(4):ORL279–280.

28. Mangete EDO, West D, Blankson CD. Hypertonic saline solution for wound dressing. Lancet 1992; 340:1351.

29. Talbot AR, Herr TM, Parsons DS. Mucociliary clearance and buffered hypertonic saline solution. Laryngoscope 1997; 107(4):500–503.

30. Shoseyov D, Bibi H, Shai P, Shoseyov N, Shazberg G, Hurvitz H. Treatment with hypertonic saline versus normal saline nasal wash of pediatric chronic sinusitis. J Allergy Clin Immunol 1998; 101(5):602–605.

31. Greiff L, Andersson M, Wollmer P, Persson CG. Hypertonic saline increases secretory and exudative responsiveness of human nasal airway in vivo. Eur Respir J 2003; 21(2): 308–312.

32. Adam P, Stiffman M, Blake RL Jr. A clinical trial of hypertonic saline nasal spray in subjects with the common cold or rhinosinusitis. Arch Fam Med 1998; 7(1):39–43.

33. Boek WM, Keles N, Graamans K, Huizing EH. Physiologic and hypertonic saline solutions impair ciliary activity in vitro. Laryngoscope 1999; 109(3):396–399.

34. Ünal M, Gorur K, Ozcan C. Ringer-lactate solution versus isotonic saline solution on mucociliary function after nasal septal surgery. J Laryngol Otol 2001; 115(10):796–797.

35. Simmons JE, Richarson SD, Speth TF, et al. Development of a research strategy for integrated technology-based toxicological and chemical evaluation of complex mixtures of drinking water disinfection byproducts. Environ Health Perspect 2002; 110(suppl 6): 1013–1024.

36. Homer JJ, England RJ, Wilde AD, Harwood GRJ, Stafford ND. The effect of pH of douching solutions on mucociliary clearance. Clin Otolaryngol 1999; 24:312–315.

37. Davidson TM, Murphy C, Mitchell M, Smith C, Light M. Management of chronic sinusitis in cystic fibrosis. Laryngoscope 1995; 105(4 Pt 1):354–358.

38. Murphy C, Davidson TM, Jellison W, et al. Sinonasal disease and olfactory impairment in HIV disease: endoscopic sinus surgery and outcome measures. Laryngoscope 2000; 110(10 Pt 1):1707–1710.

39. Desrosiers MY, Salas-Prato M. Treatment of chronic rhinosinusitis refractory to other treatments with topical antibiotic therapy delivered by means of a large-particle nebulizer: results of a controlled trial. Otolaryngol Head Neck Surg 2001; 125(3):265–269.

40. Dudley JP. Atrophic rhinitis: antibiotic treatment. Am J Otolaryngol 1987; 8(6):387–390.

41. Ricchetti A, Landis BN, Maffioli A, Giger R, Zeng C, Lacroix J. Effect of anti-fungal nasal lavage with amphotericin B on nasal polyposis. J Laryngol Otol 2002; 116:251–263.

42. Rubenfeld GD, Clark BD, Candage R, Kass ES. A novel approach to invasive fungal sinusitis-use of adjuvant topical and nebulized amphotericin B. Annual meeting of the Triological Society, Naples, Fl., Jan 9–11, 2003.

43. Sim MK. Treatment of disease without the use of drugs. VI. Treatment of rhinitis by a yogic process of cleaning and rubbing the nasal passage with a rubber catheter. Singapore Med J 1981; 22(3):121–123.

44. Johnsen J, Bratt B, Michel-Barron O, Glennow C, Petruson B. Pure sesame oil vs. isotonic sodium chloride solution as treatment for dry nasal mucosa. Arch Otolaryngol Head Neck Surg 2001; 127:1353–1356.

21

Epistaxis in the Geriatric Population

Dana S. Smith and Mark K. Wax
Department of Otolaryngology/Head and Neck Surgery, Oregon Health and Science University, Portland, Oregon, U.S.A.

INTRODUCTION

Epistaxis is a problem that the otolaryngologist commonly encounters in the office. Although epistaxis occurs in all age groups, its incidence increases sharply in the elderly (1). The common usage of medications in the elderly, which impair coagulation, such as aspirin and warfarin, may contribute both to the high incidence and severity of the problem. Several local factors, such as dry nasal mucosa, stiff vessels from arteriosclerosis, and nasal trauma from frequent falls also contribute to the higher incidence in older individuals. While management in younger individuals is usually straightforward and in an office setting, the geriatric population typically presents to the emergency room and requires more complex treatment and/or procedures. This chapter will start with a description of the anatomy of the nasal cavity followed by a discussion of the otolaryngological management of epistaxis in the elderly.

ANATOMY

The blood supply of the nasal cavity is derived from the internal and external carotid arteries. The internal carotid artery gives rise to the ophthalmic artery, which divides into a number of branches within the orbit, including the posterior and anterior ethmoid arteries. The posterior ethmoid artery exits the orbit through the posterior ethmoid foramen to cross medially along the roof of the ethmoid cavity to the anterior cranial fossa. It then passes through the cribriform plate and divides into septal and lateral nasal wall branches. These supply the posterior superior part of the septum in the back of the nose. The anterior ethmoid artery takes a similar route, traveling through the anterior ethmoid foramen, then crossing medially along the roof of the ethmoid cavity to the anterior cranial fossa. It passes through the cribriform plate before dividing into septal and lateral nasal wall branches. These branches supply the superior anterior part of the nose. This blood supply is important to understand, since the area of concern is usually high up in the nose and not accessible to conservative treatment. The intracranial course and relationship to the optic nerve are important in the surgical management. Management of bleeding from these sources is usually via an external approach.

The external carotid artery gives rise to a number of branches including the facial artery and the internal maxillary artery. The facial artery branches include the superior labial artery, which in turn supplies the caudal septum via a septal branch. The internal maxillary artery divides into multiple terminal branches within the pterygopalatine fossa, including the sphenopalatine and descending palatine arteries. The sphenopalatine artery branches near the sphenopalatine foramen. One branch supplies the turbinates and lateral nasal wall, while the other crosses the face of the sphenoid sinus and supplies the nasal septum. The descending palatine artery travels through the greater palatine foramen, becoming the greater palatine artery. This continues anteriorly along the hard palate, then through the incisive foramen to supply the anterior septum.

Kisselbach's plexus (also known as Little's area) is situated at the anterior nasal septum and consists of the anastamosis of the terminal branches from the several arteries supplying the nasal cavity. It includes the anterior and posterior ethmoids, the sphenopalatine, greater palatine, and superior labial septal branch. This area is especially significant since it is the most common site of epistaxis.

ETIOLOGY

As in the overall population, epistaxis in older patients has multiple causes. These may be divided into local, medical, and pharmaceutical causes. It is important to note that multiple factors often contribute simultaneously to an episode of epistaxis, such that management is often more difficult in the elderly. For instance, epistaxis secondary to trauma in a younger patient may be easily managed, while the same problem in an elderly patient with hypertension and dry mucosa secondary to medication use is much more challenging.

Local Causes

Mechanical causes are often responsible for mucosal injury leading to epistaxis. The elderly have a high rate of falls, many of which lead to nasal trauma. Even in the absence of a nasal fracture, mucosal lacerations may occur and result in profuse bleeding. In addition, many medical procedures such as the introduction of a nasogastric tube or feeding tube through the nasal cavity may disrupt the delicate mucosa of the septum or turbinates. Any surgical procedure involving the nose, such as functional endoscopic sinus surgery, may lead to epistaxis.

The elderly often have dry mucous membranes, frequently as a result of generalized dehydration. Many medications may contribute to this. Dryness is also common in patients with general functional impairment such as residents of assisted living facilities. In addition, the common use of oxygen by nasal cannulas, often without the addition of humidification, may desiccate the nasal mucosa. Dry nasal mucosa can be fragile and prone to significant bleeding, even from seemingly minor mucosal trauma. Digital trauma (nose picking) is a frequently overlooked cause of epistaxis, which, by its repetitive nature, fuels the epistaxis/trauma cycle. Occasionally, despite a diligent search, epistaxis may start without any evident immediate cause.

Medical Causes

Many medical conditions, such as hypertension and various deficiencies in coagulation that include liver disease, are encountered in older patients and may contribute to epistaxis.

Although hypertension has not been shown by itself to lead to a greater incidence of nosebleeds, it is far more prevalent in older patients, and may contribute to the severity and persistence of epistaxis; medical attention is required because the higher pressure bleeding vessels are less likely to spontaneously coagulate (2–4). Active epistaxis at presentation to the emergency department has been associated with hypertension (5). Exacerbating this is the effect of the "invasive treatment" on the blood pressure. Use of vasoconstrictors, tension, and stress all contribute to an increase in blood pressure and more bleeding. It is especially important to control blood pressure in order to control epistaxis in the acutely bleeding hypertensive patient.

Coagulation deficiencies are common in the geriatric population as a result of the frequency of systemic diseases, which affect coagulation. Liver diseases such as hepatitis B, hepatitis C, and alcoholic cirrhosis may cause a decrease in production of coagulation factors. In the seriously ill patient, disseminated intravascular coagulation leads to a consumption of circulating coagulation factors, and may manifest as epistaxis. In addition, platelet disorders from systemic disease, such as thrombocytopenia from osteogenic malignancy or myelodysplasia, may cause epistaxis.

Hereditary hemorrhagic telangectasia (also known as Osler–Weber–Rendu Syndrome) is another potential cause of epistaxis, which may be encountered in all age groups.

Pharmaceutical causes of epistaxis are especially important to consider in the older population due to the multitude of medications taken by older patients that impair coagulation; these include aspirin, nonsteroidal anti-inflammatory drugs (NSAIDs), and warfarin, as well as platelet aggregation inhibitors. Increasingly, more patients are taking over-the-counter herbal medications, which may impair coagulation, such as gingko biloba. In the seriously ill hospitalized patient, heparin-induced thrombocytopenia, in which an autoimmune reaction consumes platelets, may cause epistaxis.

EVALUATION OF EPISTAXIS

In order to effectively treat epistaxis, the location and the underlying etiology must be considered. A directed history should be taken. Although this does not need to be lengthy, especially if the patient requires rapid treatment for brisk bleeding, certain points should be elicited. The past medical history, including previous nosebleeds, bleeding disorders, liver disease, renal disease, and hypertension should be elucidated. The past surgical history, especially recent nasal operations such as endoscopic sinus surgery, should be obtained. The patient's medications should be reviewed for the potential to impair coagulation. A family history of important disorders such as hemophilia and hereditary hemorrhagic telangectasia may be significant.

Physical examination should include a directed head and neck examination for which the patient should be thoroughly prepared. A frank discussion and possible sedation is mandatory. All equipment needed for visualization and coagulation (cautery—either chemical or electrical) should be readily available. Cotton pledgets for nasal packing should be accessible and prepared in large numbers ahead of time. Anterior rhinoscopy should be performed with a nasal speculum, headlight, and Frazier tip suction. Often, this reveals the source of bleeding since most nosebleeds are located on the anterior septum. If the source of bleeding is still unclear, it is helpful to suction the nose and spray topical anesthetic (containing lidocaine and a vasoconstrictor) in order to perform rigid nasal endoscopy. The authors' preference is a 1:1 mixture of 4% lidocaine and oxymetazoline. Endoscopy is then performed with a 2.7 mm 30° rigid nasal endoscope and Frazier tip suction. Transoral inspection of the posterior oropharynx is also performed to assess the extent of postnasal passage of blood from the nasal cavity.

Laboratory examination includes a complete blood count, prothrombin time, and partial thromboplastin time in order to determine if excessive bleeding or coagulation deficiencies are present.

TREATMENT OF EPISTAXIS

Conservative Measures

Most episodes of epistaxis experienced by the elderly can be resolved with relatively simple measures. Often, a vasoconstrictor nasal spray such as oxymetazoline is sufficient to stop epistaxis (6). However, this should be used cautiously as many geriatric patients may become hypertensive, which may actually exacerbate bleeding. Silver nitrate cautery can also be used, and is most useful when the source of bleeding is on the anterior septum and the site is not briskly bleeding (6). Good preoperative vasoconstriction and anesthesia allow for placement of the silver nitrate stick. The bleeding site as well as the vessels leading to it should be cauterized. Silver nitrate should not be applied to the same site of both sides of the nasal septum due to the risk of septal perforation from devascularization of the cartilage and subsequent chondronecrosis. Absorbable cellulose sponges placed over the site may help with hemostasis and will protect the area while it heals from the cauterization. Unipolar electrocautery may also be used if the site is easily accessible via anterior rhinoscopy. Heat cautery may also be effective in this situation (7). This requires injection with topical anesthetic with epinephrine, which often slows the bleeding temporarily due to its vasoconstrictive effect.

If the above measures fail, nasal packing is the next step (8,9). Packs provide hemostasis by their compressive effect. Packs come in a variety of materials, including preformed cellulose sponges, inflatable balloons, and strip gauze. Solid packs, such as balloon packs, will work best for anterior bleeding along the septum or medial aspect of the turbinates where the packs can directly compress the bleeding vessel. More posterior bleeding, often arising from the sphenopalatine arterial branches, may require anterior–posterior packing in order to provide adequate tamponade of the vessel (10). The posterior pack is positioned in the nasopharynx in order to give support to the anterior pack and to prevent it from falling into the nasopharynx. A gauze roll or Foley catheter may be used for the posterior pack. For the anterior pack, petroleum strip gauze layered from the nasal floor to the roof can be used. Often, bleeding in coagulopathic patients or hypertensive patients is difficult to control initially, so nasal packing may serve to slow or stop bleeding, while blood pressure is lowered and/or the coagulopathy corrected. Antibiotics with good *Staphylococcus* coverage are given to prevent bacterial overgrowth and possible toxic shock syndrome, and packs are generally removed after three days (11). Hypoxia and hypercarbia may also occur with packing in place, and monitoring with pulse oximetry may be warranted (12). In patients with several comorbidities, admission to the intensive care unit for observation may be necessary. Mucosal necrosis from pack pressure is another potential complication (13). Having anterior packs in place is relatively uncomfortable to the patient. If they are hypertensive, the placement of the packs and their continued presence will exacerbate the bleeding. Most patients will tolerate a unilateral pack once. If bilateral or repeated packing is required, then ancillary measures should be considered (14).

Greater palatine artery injection, warm water irrigation of the nasal cavities, and fibrin glue application may also be effective in controlling epistaxis (9,15–17). Finally, it must be stressed that the hypertension and the high systolic pressure that is inevitably present must be controlled.

Considerations in Anticoagulated Geriatric Patients

Deciding whether or not to correct the coagulopathy depends on the difficulty in controlling bleeding versus the risk of correcting the coagulopathy. For instance, a patient with atrial fibrillation and brisk bleeding may be corrected, as there is not a significantly elevated stroke risk for a short period of time; however, the risk of reversing coagulation in a patient with an artificial valve is significantly higher and may not be warranted unless the patient is having life-threatening epistaxis, which cannot be controlled by other measures. One small study demonstrated no advantage in reversing warfarin anticoagulation for control of epistaxis if the international normalized ratio (INR) was in therapeutic range (18). In these instances, use of an absorbable pack such as Gelfoam or Surgicel, which does not require removal, may be the best option.

Surgical Management of Recalcitrant Epistaxis

The majority of epistaxis is controlled either by the patient in their home setting, in the physician's office, or in the emergency room setting by local measures. Occasionally, patients will present with severe epistaxis that is not controllable with any of the simple measures mentioned above. It is difficult to get a grasp on the incidence of this intractable epistaxis, since the majority of centers that report on surgical or other invasive methodology for treatment of epistaxis are seeing a highly biased patient population. For instance, our institution has developed interest and expertise in angiographic embolization (19). All patients that present to our institution are so treated, yet we realize that this patient population is a small subset of the patients seen in the greater community.

When medical management fails, patients are usually referred to the otolaryngologist for secondary procedures. Elderly patients who are hospitalized and fail more conservative management such as repeated nasal packing, blood transfusions, and control of comorbid medical conditions may require invasive procedures (10).

The most common invasive procedures currently performed in the United States include internal maxillary artery ligation, angiographic embolization, anterior/posterior sphenoid artery ligation, and external carotid artery ligation (19–22). Success rates for these options are similar, with the choice depending on the available expertise and/or experience in a particular institution.

Angiographic Embolization

The major cause of bleeding in the geriatric population is from branches of the internal maxillary artery. In the early 1970s, as angiographic techniques improved, various centers began to explore and utilize angiography in diagnosing, and ultimately treating epistaxis with embolization. This paradigm has continued with a number of centers obtaining expertise in the management of patients with this problem. A recent report from our institution describes 70 patients who were admitted with intractable epistaxis. All of the patients had been previously treated with nasal packing. A small minority underwent surgery or cauterization. A significant number (34%) had required blood transfusions prior to being admitted. Patients were admitted and brought to the angiography suite, where embolization of the internal maxillary arteries was performed. Epistaxis was controlled in >90% of patients, allowing for discharge within 24 hours. The embolization is carried out in the angiography suite under local anesthesia, and there is very little medical or local morbidity from the procedure itself (19). Complications, when they do occur, include pain, persistent bleeding, and neurologic events such as cerebrovascular accidents. In 10% of patients, epistaxis was not controlled with embolization, and operative intervention was required.

Internal Maxillary Artery Ligation

All that can be said for arteriographic embolization can be reiterated for surgical approaches (20). These require a general anesthetic for identification of branches of the internal maxillary artery in the pterygopalatine fossa, which are ligated with small hemoclips. While under anesthesia, an incision is made in the buccal mucosa overlying the maxillary sinus. The anterior and posterior walls of the maxillary sinus are removed. The pterygopalatine fossa is identified and the terminal branches of the internal maxillary arteries are identified and clipped. An endoscopic nasal approach may also be used to identify and clip branches of the internal maxillary artery. Reports of success, as well as morbidity, for this technique are identical to that for embolization with success rates between 85% and 95%. Patients are often discharged within 24 hours. In skilled surgical hands, this technique carries little local morbidity and has excellent short- and long-term control rates. Patients who fail this procedure do so because the bleeding is from the anterior or posterior ethmoid arteries or small unidentified branches. Continued bleeding from these small branches can be handled with angiographic embolization. The incidence of local complications due to maxillary sinus violation, as well as numbness secondary to the infraorbital nerve traction, runs upward to 25%.

Anterior/Posterior Ethmoid Artery Ligation

Occasionally, one encounters a patient whose epistaxis originates high in the nasal vault. These areas are supplied by the anterior or posterior ethmoid arteries. Bleeding in this area is difficult to visualize endoscopically. Obtaining sufficient pressure with a nasal pack is problematic in an awake patient. Since the origin of these vessels is from the internal carotid, embolization of the internal maxillary artery will not control the bleeding. Embolization through the internal carotid system is not undertaken due to the risk of intracranial complications and blindness. Unfortunately, the diagnosis of bleeding from these vessels is often that of exclusion. Most patients who require intervention due to bleeding from these arteries have either failed angio-graphic embolization or some other surgical approach. It is difficult to anatomically pinpoint these vessels during a physical or endoscopic examination.

The technical approach is through a small incision in the medial canthus of the eye, along the lamina papyracea. The anterior and posterior ethmoid arteries are anatomically in a very predictable location, and technically the procedure is easy to perform. Particular care must be exercised in approaching the posterior ethmoid artery because of its proximity to the orbital nerve. The morbidity of the surgical procedure, other than the general anesthetic, is low, and control rates for epistaxis have been reported in >90% of cases (21).

External Carotid Artery Ligation

The external carotid artery is the feeding vessel for the internal maxillary artery, as well as the facial artery. Thus, ligation of the external carotid artery should devas-cularize the ipsilateral nasal cavity. Flow from collaterals, as well as connections from the contralateral side, will prevent tissue necrosis. Success rates with external carotid artery ligation are reported in up to 50% of patients (22). The same factors that prevent soft tissue necrosis on the ipsilateral side also contribute to failure of this procedure. Collateral flow from the contralateral side, as well as from intra-cranially, will lead to failure in controlling the epistaxis.

This method is rarely undertaken today because of low success rates and the availability of superior surgical, angiographic, and endoscopic techniques.

Endoscopic Sphenopalatine Artery Ligation

Recently, a small number of centers have begun to explore the use of endoscopic sinus surgical techniques for control of epistaxis (23). The majority of posterior epi-staxis is felt to be due from branches of the sphenopalatine artery that are branches of the internal maxillary artery. Endoscopic sinus surgery, which is a technical approach to sinus diseases, has seen an explosion in popularity due to improvements in both technique and instrumentation. With this has come an ability to approach the foramen of the sphenopalatine artery in the posterior aspect of the nose. The nose is approached as for an endoscopic nasal procedure. Landmarks consist of the middle turbinate and basal lamella. In this area, a small mucosal flap is elevated and posterior dissection is undertaken to identify the foramen and the sphenopala-tine artery. Once it has been visualized it is clipped. Rarely is it necessary to pack the nose. Postoperative care is as for any patient who has undergone endoscopic sinus surgery. A small number of centers have reported expertise with patients who have had recalcitrant epistaxis and had the sphenopalatine artery ligated through a trans-nasal endoscopic approach. As with most other surgical techniques, success rates in the authors' hands have been in the 90% range. As more and more centers, as well as otolaryngologists, are trained in this method, the low morbidity and ease of the procedure may see the emergence of this new technique as the preferred treatment for recalcitrant epistaxis.

SUMMARY

While medical management of epistaxis is satisfactory in the majority of cases, in patients where simple medical means do not control the bleeding, surgical intervention should be considered. Several surgical approaches are available for the treatment of recalcitrant epistaxis, and the choice depends on the experience and preference of the attending surgeon. Success rates are high for all methods in well-trained hands.

REFERENCES

1. Tomkinson A, Roblin DG, Flanagan P, Wunie SM, Backhouse S. Patterns of hospital attendance with epistaxis. Rhinology 1997; 35(3):129–131.
2. Fasce E, Flores M, Fasce F. Prevalence of symptoms associated with blood pressure in normal and hypertensive population. Revista Medica de Chile 2002; 130(2):160–166.
3. Lubianca-Neto JF, Bredemeier M, Carvalhal EF, et al. A study of the association between epistaxis and the severity of hypertension. Am J Rhinol 1998; 12(4):269–272.
4. Mendelson G, Ness J, Aronow WS. Drug treatment of hypertension in older persons in an academic hospital-based geriatrics practice. J Am Geriatr Soc 1999; 47(5):597–599.
5. Herkner H, Havel C, Mullner M, et al. Active epistaxis at ED presentation is associated with arterial hypertension. Am J Emergency Med 2002; 20(2):92–95.
6. Krempl GA, Noorily AD. Use of oxymetazoline in the management of epistaxis. Ann Otol Rhinol Laryngol 1995; 104(9 Pt 1):704–706.
7. Quine SM, Gray RF, Rudd M, von Blumenthal H. Microscope and hot wire cautery management of 100 consecutive patients with acute epistaxis—a superior method to traditional packing. J Laryngol Otol 1994; 108(10):845–848.
8. Pringle MB, Beasley P, Brightwell AP. The use of Merocel nasal packs in the treatment of epistaxis. J Laryngol Otol 1996; 110(6):543–546.
9. Stangerup SE, Dommerby H, Lau T. Hot-water irrigation as a treatment of posterior epistaxis. Rhinology 1996; 34(1):18–20.
10. Shaw CB, Wax MK, Wetmore SJ. Epistaxis: a comparison of treatment. Otolaryngol Head Neck Surg 1993; 109:60–65.
11. Aeumjaturapat S, Supanakorn S, Cutchavaree A. Toxic shock syndrome after anterior-posterior nasal packing. J Med Assoc Thailand 2001; 84(3):453–458.
12. Hady MR, Kodeira KZ, Nasef AH. The effect of nasal packing on arterial blood gases and acid–base balance and its clinical importance. J Laryngol Otol 1983; 97(7):599–604.
13. Uslu SS, Ileri F, Koybasioglu A, Celik H, Sargon M, Ozbilen S. Scanning electron microscopy of hydroxylated polyvinyl acetal and conventional gauze strip nasal packing materials. Am J Rhinol 2001; 15(2):91–94.
14. Monte ED, Belmont MJ, Wax MK. Management paradigms for posterior epistaxis: a comparison of costs and complications. Otolaryngol Head Neck Surg 1999; 121:103–106.
15. Bharadwaj VK, Novotny GM. Greater palatine canal injection: an alternative to the posterior nasal packing and arterial ligation in epistaxis. J Otolaryngol 1986; 15(2):94–100.
16. Vaiman M, Segal S, Eviatar E. Fibrin glue treatment for epistaxis. Rhinology 2002; 40(2):88–91.
17. Walshe P, Harkin C, Murphy S, Shah C, Curran A, McShane D. The use of fibrin glue in refractory coagulopathic epistaxis. Clin Otolaryngol Allied Sci 2001; 26(4):284–285.
18. Srinivasan V, Patel H, John DG, Worsley A. Warfarin and epistaxis: should warfarin always be discontinued? Clin Otolaryngol Allied Sci 1997; 22(6):542–544.
19. Christensen NP, Smith DS, Barnwell SL, Wax MK. Arterial embolization in the management of posterior epistaxis. Presented at the Western Section of Triologic Society, January 31, 2004, Otolaryngol Head Neck Surg. Submitted March 2004.
20. Strong EB, Bell DA, Johnson LP, Jacobs JM. Intractable epistaxis: transantral ligation vs. embolization: efficacy review and cost analysis. Otolaryngol Head Neck Surg 1995; 113(6):674–678.
21. Douglas SA, Gupta D. Endoscopic assisted external approach anterior ethmoidal artery ligation for the management of epistaxis. J Laryngol Otol 2003; 117(2):132–133.

22. Spafford P, Durham JS. Epistaxis: efficacy of arterial ligation and long-term outcome. J Otolaryngol 1992; 21(4):252–256.
23. Kumar S, Shetty A, Rockey J, Nilssen E. Contemporary surgical treatment of epistaxis. What is the evidence for sphenopalatine artery ligation? Clin Otolaryngol 2003; 28(4):360–363.

22

Oral Mucosal Pathology in the Geriatric Population

Bobby M. Collins
Oral Medicine and Pathology, University of Pittsburgh School of Dental Medicine, Pittsburgh, Pennsylvania, U.S.A.

Mucosal diseases are relatively common in the geriatric population. Systemic diseases that compromise liver or renal function can contribute to mucositis, and any number of medications taken for chronic disease can affect the integrity of the oral mucosa. Xerostomia, epithelial atrophy, ulceration, and vesiculation are some of the more common oral findings associated with medication usage. Radiation therapy, chemotherapy, drug "allergy," and paraneoplastic syndromes are reported to cause clinical mimics (such as desquamation) to a number of mucocutaneous diseases discussed in this chapter.

Vesiculobullous diseases, though rare, are problematic for both patient and practitioner. Patients suffer through bouts of oral pain that worsen with the consumption of hot, spicy foods and acidic beverages. Speech and oral hygiene are compromised when desquamation or ulceration occur. Effective treatment relies upon an accurate diagnosis. Some of the more common oral diseases associated with ulceration are: herpetic stomatitis, erythema multiforme, lichen planus, pemphigoid, pemphigus, and aphthous ulcers. Aphthous ulcers do not pass through a vesicular stage. They simply arise as ulcers and do not represent vesiculobullous disease. Their discussion here is due to common occurrence and frequent confusion with vesiculobullous disease.

While the clinical presentation will be similar in a number of the vesiculobullous diseases, duration and distribution often differ, as well as the presence of associated mucosal and cutaneous changes in other anatomic areas. Desquamative gingivitis (Fig. 1) is a clinical description of the gingival sloughing seen in erosive lichen planus, pemphigoid, pemphigus, and as a reaction to certain ingredients in toothpastes (pyrophosphates, peroxides, surfactants, and preservatives).

The virally induced vesiculobullous lesions are often so characteristic as to make biopsy unnecessary. A clinical diagnosis is made. However, the majority of the vesicular lesions require a representative biopsy. The excised tissue is divided and submitted in 10% neutral buffered formalin for hematoxylin and eosin staining (H and E), and the remaining tissue is placed in phosphate-buffered saline (Michel's solution) or Zeus® tissue fixative for immunofluorescence studies. In the submitted

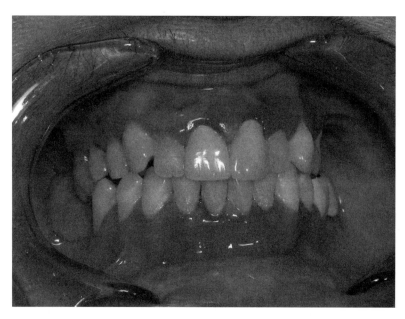

Figure 1 Clinical photo of maxillary and mandibular gingival erosions or "desquamative gingivitis" in a patient with mucous membrane pemphigoid.

tissues, the epithelium must be attached to the underlying connective tissue. As the tissue is fragile, this requires careful tissue manipulation on the part of the surgeon performing the biopsy.

HERPES SIMPLEX

The most common of the vesiculobullous diseases are virally related. Herpes simplex virus (HSV) antibodies are estimated to be as high as 80–85% in the general population. While the initial infection is largely asymptomatic, about 30% of those infected may present with primary herpetic gingivostomatitis. The clinical features of malaise, cervical lymphadenopathy, fever, and oral pain are coincident with clustered vesicular eruptions perinasally, periorally, and along the lips and mucosa. Fiery red gingiva are seen on intraoral examination. Oral discomfort will limit eating, speaking, and adequate oral hygiene. Resolution occurs in 7 to 14 days, with the virus traveling in a retrograde fashion to the sensory ganglion, where it lies dormant until reactivation (viral latency). Each vesicle has about a three-day life cycle, with new vesicle eruptions occurring synchronously, until immunosurveillance eventually controls the infection in about two weeks. Two viral forms exist, with HSV I affecting the oral region and HSV II affecting the genital region. However, the forms may exist at either site. Both forms may coexist, as HSV I provides minimal immunologic protection for infection with HSV II. HSV II infection outbreaks tend to persist for longer than 14 days.

The age of presentation varies from 5 to 10 years, but any previously unexposed person can present with the primary infection. Recurrences commonly are noted periorally and are heralded by a tingling, itching, or burning sensation as the virus travels from the sensory ganglion down the sensory nerve. The resulting viremia causes infection or reinfection of keratinized mucosal epithelium. Intraorally, the herpetic lesions are seen as clustered, punctate shallow ulcerations on the attached gingiva and palate. Fragile vesicles coalesce, burst, and ulcerate in an area coinciding with the initial infection. The vesicle fluid is highly contagious, and scratching may subsequently autoinnoculate other anatomic sites such as the eyes or genitalia. The ulcers are shallow with a punctate round appearance commonly, but trauma and coalescence can produce large ulcers with ragged, irregular borders. Vesicles that burst are responsible for the amber brown crusts that are a common sight in recurrent herpes labialis.

Histologically, ballooning degeneration and keratinolysis are observed. The lytic cells merge and fuse to produce giant cells. The nuclei of adjacent cells merge and show nuclear molding. These nuclei are large and have a "smudged" or "ground glass" appearance. Viral inclusions are seen within the nuclei and are called Lipshütz bodies or Cowdry type A inclusions.

L-lysine consumption, topical vitamin A application, and ice serve as anecdotal preventives and possibly palliatives, but antiviral medications are more effective in treatment of the disease. Abreva® (doconasol cream 10%) is available over the counter and is reported to accelerate healing time. Denavir® (pencyclovir), available by prescription, is slightly more effective than Zovirax® (acyclovir). Valtrex® (vala-cyclovir), which is prescribed for genital herpes, has also been used for oral herpes simplex and herpes zoster infections.

Other viral infections are more rare than herpes simplex. Coxsackie viral outbreaks are seasonal and commonly occur in clusters of school-aged children. In herpangina (caused by Coxsackie group A), vesicles and shallow ulcers are noted on the soft palate and tonsillar complex. The soft palate, tonsillar area, buccal mucosa, and palmar and plantar skin are affected in hand, foot, and mouth disease (Coxsackie A 12). Varicella zoster virus gives rise to "chicken pox" in children as the initial or primary infection, and to herpes zoster or "shingles" in older adults as the latent disease.

ERYTHEMA MULTIFORME

Erythema mutiforme (EM) is an acute vesiculoulcerative disease characterized by bloody crusting of mucosal surfaces. The disease is most common in young adults, and males are affected more often than females. Erythema multiforme is self-limiting and is thought to be a type of hypersensitivity reaction to certain drugs and infections. Drugs like sulfonamides and barbiturates, as well as preceding infections by herpes simplex virus and Mycoplasma pneumonia, are considered precipitating factors. There is a spectrum of disease that may be as mild as shallow oral ulceration and bloody crusting of the lips, or as severe as the bloody crusting of the oral mucosa, lips, eyes, and genitalia of Stevens–Johnson syndrome. The most severe form is life threatening. It shows sloughing of large segments of skin and mucosal surfaces, and is called toxic epidermal necrolysis or Lyell's disease. This form is commonly associated with medication ingestion (antibiotics, analgesics, antihypertensives, and antianginals).

The oral ulcerations of erythema multiforme are sudden in onset and sufficiently painful to limit eating and drinking. Topical anesthetics and supportive care are necessary to ensure adequate hydration and nutrition. When EM follows recurrent herpetic eruptions, consideration must be given to treating the preceding herpes infection to prevent the EM outbreak. The skin lesions of EM show central erythema and a pale ring at the periphery resembling a "bullseye" or "iris."

Histologically, necrotic keratinocytes and epithelial edema are noted. Edematous separation may be intraepithelial or subepithelial, and a nonspecific inflammatory infiltrate is present. The clinical presentation is distinctive enough to render a diagnosis. Corticosteroids are used in the management of EM, but care must be taken if there was a preceding herpetic infection. The use of corticosteroids for the treatment of Stevens–Johnson syndrome or toxic epidermal necrolysis is controversial, as some cases are linked to a previous or coincident infection. The possibility of secondary or superinfection is considered a great risk. However, treatment success with controlled trials of corticosteroid therapy has been reported.

PEMPHIGOID

Pemphigoid is an autoimmune disease that occurs in older adults, with female occurrence about 2:1 over males. The mean age of presentation is 60 years. There are two forms of the disease: (i) bullous pemphigoid, which is largely a cutaneous disease causing tense bullae that rarely affects the oral mucosa, and (ii) mucous membrane or cicatricial pemphigoid that commonly has oral lesions as the initial presentation.

In mucous membrane pemphigoid, any mucosal surface can be affected, including soft palate, buccal mucosa, and gingiva. The bullae may present with straw-colored fluid, or they may be hemorrhagic. The bullae are fragile and rupture easily, giving rise to irregular erosions with a gray-white coating in areas representing sloughed, necrotic surface epithelium. These erosions may be chronic and are accompanied by slow healing and often scarring. The areas of desquamation are indistinguishable from those of pemphigus. Eye lesions in mucous membrane pemphigoid often scar down, leaving a fibrous attachment between the globe and eyelid. This is called symblepheron (or ankyloblepheron, if complete) and is the reason patients diagnosed with mucous membrane pemphigoid should see an ophthalmologist.

Immunologic attack occurs on antigenic proteins in the basement membrane zone leading to a subepithelial separation. Histologically, the epithelium separates cleanly from the lamina propria and maintains its rete peg architecture (Fig. 2A and B). Immunofluorescent stains [immunoglobulin G (IgG), C3, and to a lesser extent, IgA] decorate the attachment interface between the epithelium and the lamina propria/connective tissue, thus highlighting the area of immunologic attack.

Pemphigoid is treated with steroids and steroid-sparing agents (dapsone, cyclophosphamide), tetracycline, and niacinamide, and more recently tacrolimus and intravenous immunoglobulin. Pemphigoid has a good prognosis with occasional long periods of remission. Dapsone usage requires frequent assessment of liver function and hematologic reactions to evaluate hemolysis and methemoglobulinemia.

PEMPHIGUS

Pemphigus is an uncommon autoimmune acantholytic disease in which oral lesions are often the presenting feature. The average age of onset is 49 years. Many clinical forms exist, but pemphigus vulgaris is the most severe form and will be discussed here. The disease occurs most often in middle-aged women and those of Eastern European Jewish ancestry. Extensive bullous eruptions involve the skin and mucosal surfaces and rupture to yield ragged ulcers. The remnants of surface epithelium are gray-white and necrotic and, unlike pemphigoid, do not tend to heal without treatment. Pemphigus is a serious disease, and prior to the advent of steroid therapy, survival averaged about two years.

(A)

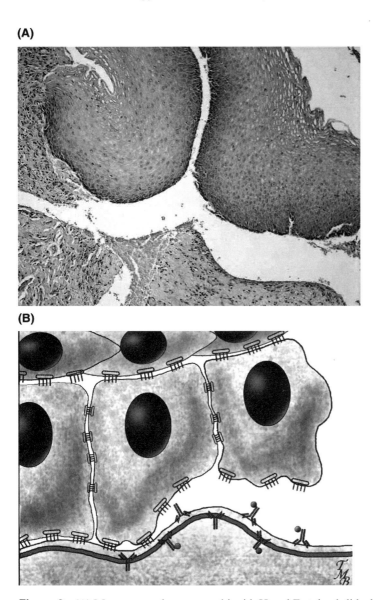

(B)

Figure 2   (**A**) Mucous membrane pemphigoid: H and E stained slide demonstrates sub-basilar separation of the epithelium in pemphigoid. Direct immunofluorescence will demonstrate auto-immune attack along the basement membrane zone. (**B**) Diagram of sub-basilar discohesion resulting from immunologic attack on the hemidesmosomes in the basement membrane zone.

Histologically, pemphigus characteristically shows acantholysis or epithelial separation within the spinous layer (Fig. 3A and B). The immunologic attack occurs on desmogleins that serve as intercellular attachment proteins. Acantholytic cells float free of contact inhibition and spread out to resemble "fried eggs," and are called Tzanck cells. The basal cell layer remains adherent to the connective tissue and resembles "tombstones." Tzanck cells are noted between the adherent basal cells and the superficial epithelium. Immunofluorescence decorates antigenic desmosomal proteins between the epithelial cells. The basal cells remain adherent, because they lack the particular desmoglein that serves as the autoantigen.

(A)

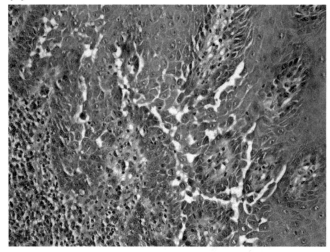

(B)

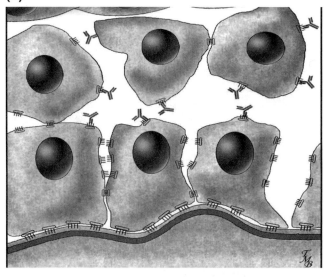

Figure 3 (**A**) Pemphigus vulgaris: An H and E stained slide demonstrates suprabasilar acantholysis due to dissolution of intercellular bridges in pemphigus. Direct immunofluorescence will highlight the intraepithelial immunologic attack. (**B**) Diagram of epithelial discohesion or suprabasilar acantholysis resulting from immunologic attack on desmosomal desmogleins.

The treatment for pemphigus is long-term steroid therapy, or therapy with steroid-sparing agents (azathioprine). This has vastly improved the formerly dismal prognosis. Promising new drugs for the treatment of pemphigus include intravenous immunoglobulin and mycophenolate.

LICHEN PLANUS

Lichen planus (LP) is a common mucocutaneous disease. Although the cause is unknown, its chronic nature and prevalence in females is suggestive of an autoimmune process. Adults over the age of 35 are most often affected, and the disease is largely asymptomatic. Those affected are commonly unaware of the condition until it is brought to their attention by a dentist, hygienist, or other health care provider during an oral exam. Symptoms exist in the erosive form of disease or when there is a super-imposed fungal infection. Lichen planus and lichenoid reactions are exacerbated by contact with amalgam restorations and are noticed frequently in the buccal mucosa that is in contact with the restoration.

The classic appearance of oral lichen planus is radiating white lines that intersect in a "lacy" pattern most noticeable in the buccal mucosa (Fig. 4). These Wickham's striae are also seen on the ventral tongue. The dorsal tongue shows white plaque-like lesions when affected by lichen planus. The gingiva show desquamation and shallow ulceration, commonly along the tips of the papillae. Lichen planus is the most com-mon cause of desquamative gingivitis because LP is more prevalent than pemphigoid. Bullous lesions and ulceration are known to occur with LP. These clinical features may represent the erosive form of the disease. Although it is controversial, erosive lichen planus is felt to have the greatest potential for malignant transformation at 1.2% to 1.4%.

Histologically, hyperkeratosis is responsible for the appearance of Wickham's striae. Vacuolar or hydropic degeneration of the epithelial basal cell layer is noted over a band-like, T-lymphocytic infiltrate and angular "sawtoothing" of the rete pegs can be seen. The sawtooth rete peg appearance is more common in cutaneous biopsies. The degeneration of the basal cell layer results in spinous cells approximat-ing the basement membrane zone. This is referred to as squamatization. The T-cell lymphocytic infiltrate "hugs" the basement membrane zone. This is the characteristic histologic picture of interface mucositis. Gingival biopsies will contain abundant plasma cells.

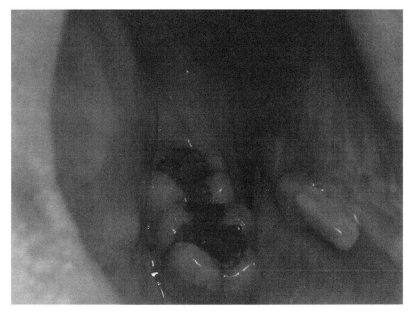

Figure 4   Clinical photo: Buccal mucosal ulcer and radiating, white linear "Wickham's striae" in a patient with lichen planus with ulceration.

The treatment for symptomatic lichen planus includes topical "swish and spit" steroids, steroid gels, and systemic steroids depending on the severity. Topical tacrolimus and tetracycline with niacinamide also provide relief in erosive lichen planus. When lichen planus is symptomatic due to candidiasis, fluconazole is an effective therapy.

LICHENOID DRUG REACTION

The clinical and histologic appearance of lichenoid drug reactions are identical to lichen planus. This striking similarity has caused some authorities to propose that lichen planus is a patterned response to various antigens rather than a specific disease. Numerous medications have been identified as causing the lichenoid eruption, and include nonsteroidal anti-inflammatory drugs, antimalarials, antibiotics, and antiarthritics. Allopurinol can precipitate erosive or ulcerative lichenoid lesions. These lesions can be extensive, and discontinuing the allopurinol provides relief in about two weeks. Amalgam restorations also exacerbate lichenoid lesions in mucosa in contact with the material. Removal of the dental amalgam can cause the lesions to resolve, but replacement dental materials may also precipitate the lichenoid reaction.

The association of lichen planus and hepatitis C is more likely a lichenoid reaction to the interferon or ribavirin therapy for the hepatitis. A perusal of the patient's medical and medication history can be quite beneficial in diagnosing lichenoid drug eruptions. Consultation with the patient's primary care physician and a search of a drug information reference is both necessary and informative. Treatment of lichenoid drug reactions is simple when the suspected medication can be changed or suspended. However, in some cases, this is not possible without adverse systemic health effects. In this instance, topical steroid therapy is attempted. As in lichen planus, if erosions are not present, remember that a candidal infection can cause symptoms.

APHTHOUS ULCERS

Aphthous ulcers are a common cause of oral discomfort found in 10–20% of the general population, but with a reported incidence as high as 40% in some populations (college students at exam time). The etiology is unknown, but is likely an immunologic irregularity. Aphthae exist in three forms: minor, major, and herpetiform or clusterform. Minor ulcers are the most common and account for 80% of the lesions. They have a regular round or oval border, surrounded by a fiery red halo, and are surfaced by a tan-gray pseudomembrane (fibrin clot). The ulcers are 4–6 mm in diameter, occur on loose, nonkeratinized mucosa, and are exquisitely painful for their size. One to 10 minor ulcers may be present, and there is a tendency for recurrence, therefore the clinical diagnosis of recurrent aphthous stomatitis. Each ulcer lasts from 7 to 10 days.

The major ulcers are larger than 1 cm, typically single, and can extend onto keratinized tissue. These persist for four to six weeks and heal with scarring.

Clusterform aphthae resemble the punctate ulcers of recurrent herpetic stomatitis. They are 2–3 mm in diameter and number from 10 to 100. They extend onto keratinized mucosa and into the oropharynx and esophagus. AIDS and other immunocompromised patients are frequently affected with clusterform lesions. Each ulcer lasts 7 to 10 days, but the multiple ulcers account for disease persistence for a month or more.

Histologically, aphthae are nonspecific ulcers with a surface fibrin clot. The clot overlies granulation tissue containing a mixed inflammatory infiltrate that is rich with lymphocytes and histiocytes. The peripheral epithelium is edematous.

Aphthous ulcers or aphthous-like ulcers are also seen in systemic diseases, such as Crohn's disease (a chronic granulomatous disease with "skip" lesions from mouth to anus) and Behçet's disease (oral and genital ulcers and occular inflammation).

Aphthous ulcers are treated with palliation or topical corticosteroids. Laser coagulation is said to immediately halt the discomfort with aphthae, but may cause scarring. Chemical cautery may cause scarring, and often the materials are toxic.

BIOPSY

A representative biopsy can be a difficult task in vesiculobullous disease. First, a nonulcerated site must be located, and care must be taken on biopsy to ensure that the epithelium remains attached to the connective tissue. The clinician should obtain a positive Nikolsky sign, then biopsy the area adjacent to it. Using either the bow or straight surface of a dental explorer, rub lightly for about a minute. A positive Nikolsky sign is obtained when the epithelium slides over the underlying tissue. This separation and slide is due to the loss of epithelial attachment and edema created by immunologic attack on the cellular "cementing" proteins within the desmosomes in pemphigus and hemidesmosomes in pemphigoid. Look at the tissue color and surface texture to be sure that epithelial integrity exists (pink and stippled, as opposed to red, shiny, and easily bleeding). Anesthetize the area with block anesthesia, if possible, to avoid the edematous tissue distension that is obtained with infiltration. Place a black silk traction suture centrally within the tissue to be excised to assist in tissue adherence and ease of manipulation. Tissue forceps tend to crush and separate the tissues. With sharp scalpel dissection, remove an ellipse that is at least 5–6 mm in length, 4–5 mm in width, and 3 mm in depth. Scalpel biopsy is the least traumatic for this fragile tissue. Laser and electrosurgery generate heat and edema that hasten epithelial separation and mask or destroy significant microscopic architecture. The traction suture facilitates the excision laterally and deep.

When the tissue is removed it is carefully divided to provide tissue for hematoxylin and eosin staining (H and E) and direct immunofluorescence staining. The tissue for H and E submission is placed in 10% neutral buffered formalin. The formalin fixation destroys tissue antigenicity, but prevents cellular degradation, preserving the cellular and tissue detail that existed at excision. The tissue for immunoflurescence is placed in a special solution that preserves tissue antigenicity, either Michel's solution (a phosphate-buffered saline) or Zeus® tissue fixative (N-ethylmaleimide ammonium sulfate and citrate buffer). These solutions are shelf-life sensitive and should be requested from your lab shortly before the surgical biopsy. If a white precipitate is present at the specimen jar lid, then the solution is not optimal for tissue transport.

Direct immunofluorescence provides a method of determining the site of immunologic attack and assists in the diagnosis of pemphigus, pemphigoid, and erosive lichen planus, as well as many other immune-mediated vesiculobullous processes. The tissues are processed, sectioned, and reacted with a panel of antibodies to human immunoglobulins, fibrinogen, and C3. These antibodies are labeled or "tagged" with a dye (fluorescein). This dye will fluoresce under ultraviolet (UV) light reflected through the tissue on the microscopic slide, highlighting the site of attack. The common panel of antibodies is IgG, IgA, IgM, fibrinogen, and C3 (a component of complement). When the tissues are examined with a special microscope equipped with a UV light source, the location and pattern of fluorescence determine the diagnosis. Pemphigus vulgaris shows deposition between the epithelial cells, as the attack is on the epithelial desmosomal cementing substances (desmogleins). IgG, C3, and IgA highlight or decorate more intensely between epithelial cells or interepithelially. In pemphigus, the basal cells adhere to the basement membrane and resemble "tombstones." The interepithelial separation gives rise to acantholytic Tzanck cells that float in the edema fluid above the firmly attached basal cell layer. The split or separation is up and can be remembered by the presence of the letter "u" in pemphigus.

Pemphigoid shows a linear pattern of fluorescence at the basement membrane zone. IgG and C3 stain more intensely in the area of epithelial attachment to the basement membrane zone. Epithelial rete pegs with an intact basal layer are preserved, and the lamina propria extensions are cleanly separated from the overlying epithelium. The split or separation is down and is remembered by the presence of the letter "d" in pemphigoid. Lichen planus shows a sub-basilar deposition of fibrinogen. The other antibodies are unreactive. Lichen planus is characterized by vacuolar degeneration of the basal cell layer, "sawtoothing" of the rete pegs, and a band-like T-lymphocytic infiltrate in the superficial lamina propria.

SELECTED SUGGESTED MEDICATIONS[a]

1. *1-2-3 Mouthwash* [30 mL of 2% viscous lidocaine, 60 mL of benadryl elixir (12.5 mg benadryl per 5 mL) and 90 mL Maalox]. Mix thoroughly. Dispense 180 cm^3.
   Rinse with one teaspoonful for 30 seconds as needed for pain.
   Comment: Sterile water can be substituted for lidocaine if the patient does not desire profound numbness. To better remember the formulation, all ingredients can be mixed in equal amounts. This mouthrinse works well for traumatic ulcers, aphthous ulcers, and occasionally for sore and burning mouth as palliation until a definitive diagnosis is rendered.

Aphthous Ulcers, Lichen Planus, Pemphigoid

1. *Decadron elixir* (dexamethasone elixir) 0.5 mg/5 mL.
   Dispense one pint bottle.
   Rinse with one teaspoonful for full two minutes, then expectorate; four times daily. Do not swallow. Do not eat or drink for 20 minutes after usage.
2. *Prelone syrup* (prednisolone) 15 mg/5 mL.
   Dispense one pint bottle.
   Rinse with one-third teaspoonful for full two minutes, then expectorate; four times daily.
   Comment: Works well for generalized ulcerations like aphthae. Can be used for symptomatic lichen planus. Use of a steroid preparation will make your patient prone to develop a fungal infection. Follow your patients regularly

---

[a] Changes in disease treatment and drug therapy require vigilant monitoring of product information. One should always consult a drug reference for accuracy in dosing, administration, interactions, and contraindications.

when they are using a steroid. A history of diabetes, peptic ulcer disease, osteoporosis, or tuberculosis will obviate systemic steroid use, but topical "swish and spit" preparations are tolerated.

3. *Lidex gel* (fluocinonide) 0.05%.
   Dispense one 15 g tube.
   Apply thin coat to oral ulcers up to QID.
   Comment: Works well for one or few ulcers. Warn patients about the potential bitter taste. Do not use on facial skin. Steroids will predispose to fungal infections.

Recurrent Herpetic Lesions

1. *Denavir* cream 1%.
   Dispense one 2 g tube.
   Apply thin coat to herpetic lesions every two hours for four days.
   Comment: Used to shorten the course of recurrent herpes simplex virus lesions of lips, commissure. Works best when application begins at first sign of tingling prodrome.
2. *Valtrex* (valacyclovir) 500 mg.
   Dispense eight tablets.
   Take four tablets when "tingling or itching" occurs, then four tablets 12 hours later.
   Do not take this medication for herpes labialis/oralis any longer than one day.

Oral Candidiasis

1. *Diflucan* 100 mg tablets.
   Dispense 11 tablets.
   Take two tablets to start, then one tablet each morning until gone.
   Comment: Use of thiazide diuretics potentiates the effect of fluconazole. Severe oropharyngeal and esophageal candidiasis will require a two-week course. If there are frequent, recurrent candidal infections, immunosuppression or systemic disease should be suspected.

BIBLIOGRAPHY

Anhalt G. Pemphigoid: bullous and cicatricial. Dermatol Clin 1990; 8:701.

Aslanzadeh J, Heim K, Espy M, et al. Detection of HSV-specific DNA in biopsy tissue of patients with erythema multiforme by polymerase chain reaction. Br J Dermatol 1992; 126:19.

Farthing PM, Maragou P, Coates M, et al. Characteristics of the oral lesions in patients with cutaneous recurrent erythema multiforme. J Oral Pathol Med 1995; 24:9.

MacPhail L, Greenspan D. Herpetic gingivostomatitis in a 70-year old man. Oral Surg Oral Med Oral Pathol Oral Radiol Endod 1995; 79:50.

Mydlarski PR, Mittman N, Shear NH. Intravenous immunoglobulin: use in dermatology. SkinTher Lett 2004; 9:1.

Robinson JC, Lozada-Nur F, Frieden I. Oral pemphigus vulgaris: a review of the literature and a report on the management of 12 cases. Oral Surg Oral Med Oral Pathol Oral Radiol Endod 1997; 84:349.

Scully C. Orofacial herpes simplex virus infections: current concepts in the epidemiology, pathogenesis and treatment, and disorders in which the virus may be implicated. Oral Surg Oral Med Oral Pathol 1989; 68:701.

Vincent SD, Lilly GE, Baker KA. Clinical, historic, and therapeutic features of cicatricial pemphigoid: a literature review and open therapeutic trial with corticosteroids. Oral Surg Oral Med Oral Pathol 1993; 76:453.

23

Halitosis in the Elderly

David E. Eibling

Department of Otolaryngology—Head and Neck Surgery, University of Pittsburgh School of Medicine, Pittsburgh, Pennsylvania, U.S.A.

INTRODUCTION

One of the more embarrassing problems faced by any individual is an unacceptable odor that accompanies their person. Halitosis is the most ubiquitous of these odors, is common in individuals of all ages, and usually originates from within the oral cavity. Essentially every individual has some degree of "morning breath" upon arising prior to oral cleansing. Ingesting food and drink and/or formal oral care rapidly reduce the odor in most individuals. Oral odor may persist throughout the day and may be noted by the patient themselves or their families. Occasionally, detection of halitosis will prompt an evaluation by an otolaryngologist in a search for the cause as well as recommendations for therapy.

Problems with objectionable odor are more often encountered in the elderly since many suffer from varying degrees of hyposmia or even anosmia. As a result, many are unaware of the odors that emulate from their bodies or clothing. Moreover, their spouses and caregivers may also suffer from reduced ability to sense foul odors, leading to persistent difficulties. As more elderly individuals actively wish to engage in community activities, the impact of the social disability increases. Odors due to poor personal hygiene or urinary or fecal incontinence are well recognized, and even more problematic from a social standpoint than halitosis.

Halitosis accompanies a number of disorders of the head and neck in individuals of all ages. Not all oral odor originates within the oral cavity. Some of these are the odors associated with nasal foreign bodies, ulcerated, necrotic cancers of the oral cavity or pharynx, foods such as garlic, or exhaled odor from systemic disease such as ammonia or ketones. Some medications can result in breath odor (1). The identification and management of these entities is not different in the elderly from that in the younger population. It must be remembered that the differential diagnosis of halitosis extends beyond the tonsillar pillars.

The oral odor of halitosis most frequently arises from anaerobic and microaerophillic gram-negative organisms that release volatile sulfur compounds (VSC), chiefly methyl mercaptan and hydrogen sulfide. These organisms include *Treponema denticola, Porphyromonas gingivalis, Prevotella intermedia, Bacteroides forsythus,* and *Fusobacteria* (2). These organisms reside deep in periodontal crevices, in the debris trapped by the papillae on the dorsum of the tongue, and in tonsillar crypts. A study of healthy subjects suggests that a quarter of healthy individuals are colonized with organisms that release volatile sulfur compounds. Occasionally patients will present with severe periodontal disease such as necrotizing ulcerative gingivitis (Vincent's disease), but more commonly there is no specific oral lesion identified (3). Tongue coating varies among individuals as well as varies from time to time within the same individual. The thickness of the coating correlates with the degree of colonization of VSC-releasing organisms. Any lesion in the oral cavity that results in bleeding will lead to halitosis, including tumors, gingivitis, or dental care such as extractions or periodontal surgery.

A study of institutionalized elderly in Japan demonstrated that there were higher levels of malodor as well as increased numbers of patients with oral colonization of *Candida* sp. and *Staphylococci* when compared with age-matched community dwellers (4). The authors correlate these changes with the poor oral care often provided to institutionalized elderly patients as well as the likelihood that many of the institutionalized are unable to perform their own oral care. They also note that *Candida* sp. are particularly adept at adhering to denture material; hence, *Candida* overgrowth on dentures often occurs in an institutional environment without adequate denture management policies. These investigators also measured sulfur compounds in saliva and noted that the levels were twice as high in institutionalized than community-dwelling elderly (4). Although both *Candida* overgrowth and VSC-related oral malodor were found in higher numbers in the institutionalized, it was not clear whether any cause and effect relationship existed.

APPROACH TO THE PATIENT WITH HALITOSIS

As with any complaint, the investigation of halitosis begins with a history and physical examination. Duration, timing, and character of the halitosis should be determined. The history of dental care and dental diseases should be obtained, particularly any recent dental work. A history of oral bleeding, as well as any symptoms that suggest the presence of specific oral or pharyngeal lesions should be elicited. The patient should be questioned regarding xerostomia as well as medications, particularly those that may result in xerostomia.

The physical examination will include not only inspection of the oral cavity, but nasal endoscopy and examination of the hypopharynx as well. A search for adherent oral debris or other evidence of poor swallowing function should be done. The condition of the remaining teeth and presence of deep periodontal pockets or root caries should be noted. If the patient wears dentures they should be removed and examined for adherent debris. Throughout the exam, the physician should be alert to tell-tale odors that may indicate other diseases, such as necrotic tumor or ammonia due to liver failure.

Laboratory testing is generally not required. Cultures are of little use, except perhaps in immunocompromised patients or others with unusual circumstances.

TREATMENT OF HALITOSIS

Halitosis is best managed by mechanical means. In nearly all patients, this means standard oral care to include brushing, flossing, and mouth rinses. Elderly patients who are being fed by tube represent a particular problem as the lack of oral feeding results in reduced mechanical cleansing of the oral cavity by mastication and rinsing. Moreover, in many instances, these individuals suffer from other disabilities that make it unlikely that they would be able to administer their own oral care.

Systemic antibiotics are not indicated for the management of halitosis. It is important to recognize that the oral cavity cannot be sterilized, and that systemic antibiotic therapy will only result in a temporary alteration of the flora. Topical antibacterial agents are, however, effective, and are used widely for a variety of oral indications. The most commonly used by dentists is chlorhexidine (Periodex[®]) which is highly effective, reducing VSC levels by more than 50% when combined with brushing (5). Unfortunately, over half of patients using chlorhexidine report a change in the taste of food and a quarter report burning, and it has been reported to cause staining. Hence, this product is better reserved for short-term use following dental work than for chronic use. Most individuals with halitosis chose to use an over-the-counter (OTC) mouth rinse, of which dozens exist. Most of these do reduce levels of VSC temporarily, although the duration varies. A blinded comparison of four commercially available OTC products with 0.2% chlorhexidine in normal subjects revealed that all resulted in lower levels of VSCs than did a water–alcohol control group; however, none were as low as the chlorhexidine group (6). There was minimal variability among the commercially available products. Based on the side effects of chlorhexidine, the authors recommend that patients use of any of the OTC commercial products instead.

Mechanical cleaning of teeth and interdental crevices with brushing and flossing is the most effective treatment strategy. If there are marked levels of calculus and plaque, dental referral for cleaning and scaling is necessary. Mechanical cleansing of the tongue has been demonstrated to be effective in reducing oral malodor (5). Tongue scrapers (Fig. 1) are commercially available and should be recommended to patients with extensive tongue coating. The scraper should be placed as far

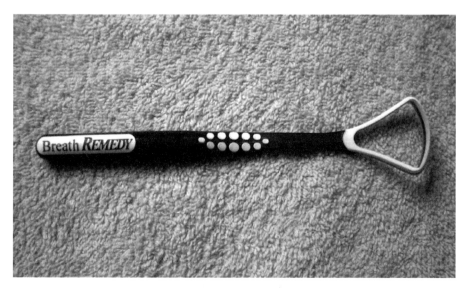

Figure 1 Photograph of a commercially available tongue scraper. The device is placed as far posteriorly as tolerated and drawn forward to scrape the debris off the papillae of the dorsum of the tongue.

posteriorly as feasible, and then lightly drawn forward. The process is repeated until no further debris is brought out. Their use is uncomfortable for some due to gagging, but with practice most patients can find a location which is tolerable.

CONCLUSION

Halitosis is a common problem affecting all individuals at some time. Elderly individuals are at greater risk due to xerostomia, dental disease, and reduced ability to perform oral care. The resultant social disability can be severe and impair functioning within society; hence, evaluation and management are warranted. The odor of halitosis is due to volatile sulfur compounds that are fermentation products produced by a number of anaerobic and microaerophillic gram-negative organisms. These organisms reside in dental crevices, tonsillar crypts, and in the coating on the dorsum of the tongue. Evaluation of affected individuals should include a complete head and neck examination to rule out other causes of the malodor. Mechanical cleansing of oral cavity surfaces is the mainstay of treatment, and is temporarily aided by limited use of OTC mouthwashes. Dental evaluation is required for some patients, particularly those with necrotizing ulcerative gingivitis. Daily oral care by caregivers is necessary for patients with inability to perform these activities of daily living on their own.

REFERENCES

1. Murata T, Fujiama Y, Yamaga T, Miyazaki H. Breath malodor in an asthmatic patient caused by side-effects of medication: a case report and review of the literature. Oral Dis 2003; 9:273–276.
2. Scully C, El-Maaytah M, Porter SR, Greenman J. Breath odor: etiopathogenesis, assessment and management. Eur J Oral Sci 1997; 105:287–293.
3. Coventry J, Griffiths G, Scully C, Tonetti M. ABC of oral health: periodontal disease. BMJ 2000; 321:36–39.
4. Honda E. Oral microbial flora and oral malodour of the institutionalized elderly in Japan. Gerodontology 2001; 18(2):65–72.
5. Quorynen M, Zhao H, van Steenberghe D. Review of the treatment strategies for oral malodour. Clin Oral Invest 2002; 6:1–10.
6. Garvalho MD, Tabchoury CM, Cury JA, Toledo S, Nogueira-Filho GR. Impact of mouth rinses on morning bad breath in health subjects. J Clin Periodontol 2004; 31:85–90.

24

Oral Health Care of the Elderly Patient

Azfar A. Siddiqui
School of Dental Medicine, Department of Maxillofacial Prosthetics, University of Pittsburgh, Pittsburgh, Pennsylvania, U.S.A.

INTRODUCTION

The quality of life for the geriatric adult is often impaired by poor oral health. Oral diseases and disorders affect health and well-being throughout life; however, they have a disproportionate effect in vulnerable populations such as the aged. The elderly geriatric population in the United States is the most rapidly growing population segment in the country. Currently, over 12% (32 million) of the U.S. population is aged 65+ years and this population will increase to 23% by the year 2040 (68 million). Nearly two million of those over the age of 65 are dependent for at least part of their care and reside in nursing homes. Many of these elderly will have remaining teeth, and the rest will have dentures. Dental conditions will affect their quality of life, nutritional status, and the management of chronic illnesses.

DENTAL LOSS IN THE ELDERLY

In developed countries, elderly patients no longer accept the removal of natural teeth and provision of dentures as a component of normal aging. Over the past century, there has been a steadily increasing number of elderly people with retention of heavily restored natural teeth, even into old age due to improved dental care. A recent report from the Division of Oral Health at the Centers for Disease Control (CDC) notes that more than one-half of elderly adults have retained most of their teeth (missing five or less), with a range of 27% in West Virginia to 64% in Utah (1). Elderly patients today are much better informed of the various treatment options available to retain natural teeth and have the time, resources, and willingness to devote to their maintenance.

CHANGES IN ORAL DENTAL HEALTH WITH AGING

Common pathologic conditions of the oral cavity occur with aging due to a combination of systemic, local, and lifestyle factors. Apart from the aging process itself, these factors include diseases of the teeth, bony supporting structures, gingival tissue, and salivary glands, all of which lead to dental loss. Caries in remaining teeth may result from poor nutrition, poor manual dexterity and inability of keep teeth clean, and failure of routine dental treatment. Xerostomia contributes to caries, and may be due to systemic disease or prior radiotherapy for head and neck cancer. Disease of the musculoskeletal structures, such as periodontal disease or apical cysts and abscesses, may promote alveolar bone resorption. Systemic conditions such as diabetes, stroke, HIV/ AIDS, and Alzheimer's can predispose patients to develop oral disease. Social factors that contribute to dental disease and tooth loss include history of smoking, alcohol, and drug abuse. Poor oral health, often related to hygiene, leads to caries and periodontal disease. Infective organisms colonizing the oral disease can gain entrance to the bloodstream, seeding distant vulnerable sites such as damaged heart valves. Oral secretions with high concentrations of pathogenic bacteria may be aspirated into the lungs and result in life-threatening lung abscesses or pneumonia. Recent data suggest that some chronic degenerative diseases, such as endovascular disease, may be causatively related to a chronic inflammatory response to ongoing periodontal disease. Regardless of causation, oral disease is often correlated with a wide variety of systemic illnesses, lifestyles, and substances.

Treatment needs of dentate patients are considerably greater than those who are edentulous, where maintenance can be relatively straightforward. The medical team caring for the patient must be able to evaluate, diagnose, and refer the patient for management of their dental needs if necessary. In the care-dependent population of elderly, caregivers must be instructed in oral care. Providing this care becomes both more critical as well as more difficult as aging progresses, due to increased xerostomia, increased retention of oral food particles following meals, and increased fragility of oral tissues. Otolaryngologists who are asked to evaluate the geriatric patient for other conditions should also routinely evaluate the status of oral care, and recommend intervention if necessary.

DENTURES IN THE ELDERLY

Any oral examination must include removal of the dentures as well as an examination of the prosthesis that the patient may be wearing. These can range from fixed partial dentures or bridges to removable dentures. With poor oral hygiene or inability to keep the oral environment clean, this prosthesis can become a focus of bacterial and fungal colonization and can thus lead to undesirable oral conditions. Fixed partial dentures that have been placed for many years may predispose to recurrent caries, which if left unchecked can result in the loss of the prosthesis. Similarly, removable partial dentures and obturators need to be evaluated for proper fit so as not to cause chronic tissue trauma. Clips that attach to remaining teeth may result in erosion, leading to tooth loss, loss of fixation of the denture, and secondary tissue trauma secondary to chronic movement. Appropriate refitting may be necessary. If new fixation points cannot be identified, often full-mouth extraction and denture fitting may be the only viable option.

TREATMENT OF DENTURE PROBLEMS IN THE ELDERLY

Mandibular height decreases as aging progresses in the edentulous patient due to loss of alveolar bone. This loss results in reduction of sulci adjacent to the mandible.

Dentures that fit well following healing after extractions will need to be refit (relined) on multiple occasions during the life of the patient. Wear of dentures that do not fit results in excessive motion and pressure-induced ulceration from the denture flange. There is often significant adjacent reactive hyperplastic mucosa resembling neoplastic disease. These typically occur adjacent to the mandible in the depths of the buccal-gingival and labial-gingival sulci. Pain is often a prominent complaint, and may impair eating to such a degree that weight loss ensues. Examination may initially suggest malignancy; however, if the patient leaves the dentures out for several weeks these lesions will resolve. Failure to resolve mandates biopsy. Comparison of the concave fitting surface of the denture with the shape of the remaining mandible will usually demonstrate the source of the pathology. Most edentulous patients require relining of their dentures every three to five years. Attempts to extend this interval lead to the development of secondary complications due to poor fit.

Bone grafting to restore alveolar height is usually performed only on younger (fifth and sixth decade) edentulous patients due to donor-site morbidity. However, healthy elderly patients with severe bone loss and secondary denture dysfunction may occasionally be considered for grafting. Each patient should be considered individually, taking quality of life issues, comorbidities, and desires of the patient into account.

DENTAL CARIES

Caries can develop at any age, but may be more problematic in the elderly. Loss of enamel is a result of etching caused by toxins secreted by gram-positive bacteria and is the first step in the process of decay. Caries can develop on either the occlusal surface or the sides of the teeth, as well as on roots exposed by loss of gingival and alveolar bone (gingival recession). If left untreated it will expose the dental pulp, resulting in dental nerve exposure with resultant pain, which can be severe. The open pulp cavity provides access for pathogenic organisms with the development of periapical abscess, spread of infection in the facial planes, and even cellulitis such as Ludwig's angina.

Root surface caries are more common than occlusal caries in the elderly population and occur due to exposure of the tooth roots, which are not protected by enamel. The elderly have many predisposing factors such as poor filling margins placed close to the gums, loss of alveolar bone, poor oral hygiene, and poor manual dexterity that contribute to rapid progression of root caries. One of the most important factors that can lead to the rapid development of caries and tooth decay is xerostomia. This can be a result of poor salivary function due to systemic conditions such as Sjogren's disease or Alzheimer's disease, or salivary dysfunction due to radiation therapy required for treatment of head and neck cancer. More than 400 drugs have been reported to decrease salivary flow, some of which may not be intuitive to the treating physician. In addition to diuretics, drugs such as tricyclic antidepressants, sedatives, tranquilizers, and antihistamines may contribute. A large number of elderly patients are on a variety of combinations of these and other medications that contribute to xerostomia; hence, they are more susceptible to rapidly developing tooth caries.

Prevention of tooth loss becomes most important in patients who have received head and neck radiation. This is due to the fact that any extraction in the immediate post-radiation period can potentially result in osteoradionecrosis (ORN). Thus, a thorough and complete evaluation of the patient's oral health prior to radiation therapy cannot be overemphasized. Management of the teeth in patients with cancer is discussed in a later section of this chapter.

TREATMENT

Treatment of caries includes removal of decayed tooth structures, and replacement with restorative filling materials. Fluoride releasing filling materials are often employed when restoring root surface caries. Preventive measures should include regular follow-up evaluation and patient education, as well as educating caregivers or family members providing care to the elderly person. Fluoride mouth rinses, as well as custom fabricated fluoride delivery trays, are most useful for patients at high risk, such as those who have received radiation therapy to the head and neck region or have xerostomia of other causes. A thin bead sodium fluoride gel is placed in the tray, which is worn over the teeth for a minimum of five minutes daily before bedtime. The patient should avoid eating and rinsing for 30 minutes following treatment.

PERIODONTAL DISEASE

Periodontal disease is a disease of the supporting structures of the teeth, namely the gingival tissues, alveolar bone, cementum, and the periodontal ligament. Periodontal disease can broadly be classified as either gingivitis or periodontitis. Gingivitis involves only the gingiva, whereas periodontitis involves the alveolar bone, periodontal ligament, and cementum. The major causative organisms are anaerobic gram-positive and -negative bacteria found in dental plaque. The quantity of organisms in this plaque is quite high, approaching the number that would be found in a pure culture of bacteria. Once entry to the soft tissues is obtained, local tissue sepsis ensues.

Although age in itself is not a factor, multiple comorbidities common in the elderly can contribute to periodontal disease. These include systemic disease, medications, and patient's ability to maintain good oral hygiene. Patients with diabetes demonstrate a higher prevalence of periodontal disease due to their propensity for slower healing. The prevalence of periodontal disease in the elderly population is possibly since more elderly patients are retaining their original dentition and are on more medications. Several medications frequently prescribed to the elderly may cause gingival enlargement including calcium channel blockers and the well-known phenytoin.

Periodontal disease may affect both the oral and systemic well-being of the patient. Consequences of untreated periodontal disease include loosening of teeth with eventual tooth loss, pain, local sepsis, and systemic disease due to sepsis or reduced nutrition. Patients may be entrapped in the vicious cycle of periodontal disease leading to pain, reduced oral intake, nutritional deficiencies, immunosuppression, and poor healing, resulting secondarily in increased periodontal disease.

TREATMENT OF PERIODONTAL DISEASE

Treatment of active periodontal disease includes topical and systemic antimicrobial therapy, mechanical removal of plaque by scaling/root planning, and surgical elimination of periodontal pockets if possible. However, patients who are immunocompromised, are frail and elderly, or have systemic diseases may be poor candidates for such procedures. In these patients, treatment should be limited to conservative therapy of superficial prophylaxis/root planning, and antimicrobial therapy. Extraction may often be the most conservative therapeutic option. Antimicrobial therapy for severe periodontal disease includes twice-daily mouth rinses with chlorhexidine gluconate 0.12% (Periodex™) and systemic therapy with an antibiotic with coverage of oral anaerobes such as metronidazole or clindamycin.

ORAL HEALTH OF CANCER PATIENTS

A particularly vulnerable population is those elderly patients who have been diagnosed with head and neck cancer and are scheduled for either surgical or nonoperative therapy. These patients require a thorough oral evaluation prior to starting any treatment to ensure that needed prophylactic oral treatment is provided in order to minimize post-treatment complications.

Patients with cancer of other sites who require systemic chemotherapy frequently develop severe oral sequellae, particularly mucositis. The intense mucositis and painful ulcerations of chemotherapy are usually relatively short-term and resolve over several weeks as the antiproliferative and immunosuppressive effects of the chemotherapy abate. However, over the short term the pain of the mucositis will impair the ability of the patient to maintain proper oral hygiene measures, resulting in worsening of any underlying periodontal disease. Oral care of these patients is difficult, but vital to their recovery.

Immunosuppression and loss of the mucosal barrier predispose the patient to oral fungal infections, recurrent herpetic lesions, oral infections, gingival bleeding, or inflammation. Gingival conditions encountered in normal healthy individuals may require surgical intervention; however, such treatment may not be possible in an immunocompromised patient. Timing of needed dental treatment must be coordinated with other therapy, and is usually limited to that which is most necessary. Treatment-related complications can often be avoided or their severity reduced with a thorough dental evaluation and treatment prior to the initiation of either local radiation and/or systemic chemotherapy.

The dentist evaluating a patient prior to therapy should be informed of the diagnosis as well as the planned treatment. Nonrestorable teeth and those with periodontal disease should be extracted. Dento-alveolar infections and oral mucosal conditions that may be asymptomatic at this stage should be addressed and effective treatment rendered prior to starting any cancer treatment. Failure to do so can result in complication arising during or in the immediate post-treatment period, when the patient is immunocompromised, and can be life-threatening. In most instances, the patient should be closely followed during and following therapy by a dentist familiar with the oral manifestations of cancer treatment.

Patients scheduled to receive radiation therapy to the head and neck should be evaluated by a dentist prior to the initiation of treatment. The usual dose of head and neck radiation exceeds 6000 cGy, sufficient to result in long-term complications such as poor healing, osteoradionecrosis, and xerostomia. Any teeth with even minimal probability of causing problems within the next two years should be restored or extracted prior to radiation therapy. Extractions performed following radiotherapy have a potential to precipitate osteoradionecrosis and result in severe morbidity. Teeth with large carious lesions, periapical disease, and periodontal infections should be extracted.

A decision regarding preservation of some teeth should be made based on the patient's motivation and life expectancy, as well as the potential need for a future prosthesis for postoperative rehabilitation. If it is felt that the patient is highly motivated to keep his teeth clean, then required restorative treatment should be completed. Custom fluoride trays should be provided to the patient to reduce the incidence of radiation-induced caries. It is recommended that the fluoride trays should be worn after normal brushing for a period no less than five minutes every day, using sodium fluoride gel applied to the fitting surface of the trays.

Extractions in the immediate post-radiation period should be avoided due to the possibility of developing ORN. The risk of ORN is greater in the mandible than in the maxilla and depends on the total dose of radiation, fraction size, and energy levels, as well as the direction of the beam and shielding used. Newer techniques (such as intensity-modulated radiotherapy) may reduce the dose to the bone and reduce the risk. If extractions or preprosthetic dento-alveolar surgery is performed prior to radiation therapy, a minimum delay of two to three weeks should be allowed prior to starting radiation therapy.

Extractions that become necessary following completion of therapy present a significant problem. If possible, these should be performed within several months following completion of therapy during the hyperemic phase. Following this phase, however, radiation-induced microangiopathy results in reduced vascularity, relative tissue hypoxia, and reduced capacity for healing, particularly bone. Treatment with hyperbaric oxygen therapy has been demonstrated to be useful by increasing tissue oxygenation, promoting bone healing, and reducing complications in patients who require late extractions. Standardized protocols typically require 20 dives prior to surgery and 10 dives post surgery. Cost is often a significant issue for these patients. Perioperative antibiotics have been demonstrated to reduce the risk of ORN and are strongly recommended.

Treatment of chemotherapy-induced mucositis is symptomatic and consists of analgesics, local irrigations, and mouth rinses. One common "magic swizzle" rinse is an emulsion made up of equal parts of Benadryl™ solution, Kaopectate™, and viscous lidocaine. Patients are instructed to keep the emulsion in the mouth for one minute, expectorate, and not to rinse.

Treatment of oral fungal infections in immunocompromised patients should first aim at improving oral hygiene. If the patient is wearing removable dentures or obturators, these should be removed and worn only for meals. Often improvement in oral hygiene can result in resolution of the problem. If fungal infections still persist, the patient can be treated with a variety of medications including topical Nystatin™ or Clotrimazole™, in suspension or troches, or systemic antifungal agents such as fluconazole.

DENTURE CARE

Wearing a removable prosthesis is often uncomfortable for the patient during radiation/chemotherapy as well as in the postoperative period following surgery. However, in order to maintain swallowing and nutrition, their minimal use may be necessary. During this period, the patient may complain of loose or ill-fitting dentures. To help solve this problem while the patient is recovering, the dentures can be relined with a temporary soft liner. This is usually sufficient to improve function. Dentures may need to be relined several times to help the patient adjust to their prosthesis. If anatomic relationships have been altered by treatment, a new prosthesis may need to be fabricated after the patient has recovered. Denture wear is problematic for post-radiation patients due to lack of the lubricating effect of saliva. Denture wear can also lead to traumatic abrasions and ulcerations. Artificial salivary substitutes as well as constant sipping of water can improve the condition to some extent.

Specialized prostheses such as obturators and mandibular repositioning appliances require care similar to that of conventional dentures. It should be noted that all dentures, no matter how well they are fabricated, accumulate plaque and provide an area for bacterial and fungal growth. Maintenance of oral hygiene becomes of paramount importance. Dentures and obturators should not be worn at night and should be cleaned and allowed to soak in either water or antiseptic mouthwash. This allows the tissues to recover as well as assists in mechanically removing bacteria from the denture surface. However, patients recovering from treatment are often unable to comply with oral hygiene measures. Under these circumstances, patients can develop fungal colonization of the oral appliances. Application of a few drops of nystatin oral suspension or a thin film of nystatin oral ointment to the fitting surface of the dentures after each meal often helps to reduce this colonization.

SUMMARY

Oral health significantly impacts the quality of life as well as general well-being of geriatric patients. Elderly patients are particularly vulnerable to the development of oral and dental diseases, and may be adversely affected in a variety of ways.

More elderly patients now retain their teeth into old age, and avoidance of dental and periodontal disease requires on-going maintenance, either by the patient, or, as they age, their caregivers. Those without teeth and dentures require periodic relining of their dentures to accommodate the changes in oral anatomy that accompany aging. Finally, those elderly patients who require treatment for cancer have even greater needs for oral care and prophylaxis to prevent serious complications.

REFERENCE

1. Gooch BF, Eke PI, Malvitz DM. Public health and aging: retention of natural teeth among older adults—United States, 2002. MMWR 2003; 52:1226–1229.

25

Burning Mouth

David E. Eibling
Department of Otolaryngology—Head and Neck Surgery, University of Pittsburgh School of Medicine, Pittsburgh, Pennsylvania, U.S.A.

INTRODUCTION

Burning mouth syndrome (BMS) is a chronic pain condition of unknown etiology involving the mouth, usually the tongue, with no obvious source. In classic BMS, no cause for the symptom can be identified by history, physical examination, or laboratory testing. A neuropathic pain process involving the distribution of the fifth and ninth cranial nerves is the most likely etiology.

REPRESENTATIVE CASE

A 72-year-old lady presents with complaints of a "burning mouth." This pain has been present for more than a year, and has not changed appreciably since it was first noted. The lady has seen the primary care physician as well as the dentist and no known cause has been identified. Over-the-counter medications including topical anesthetics were unsuccessful in relieving the pain, and in fact seemed at times to make the pain worse. The patient cannot remember exactly when the pain began, although does believe that a viral upper respiratory infection might have occurred at the time of onset. The pain is more or less constant but seems to be worse at the time of awakening at night. The patient has no symptoms of sore throat, dysphagia, reflux, swelling, ulcerations, or bleeding, and relates no past history of herpes infections nor apthous ulcers.

The past medical history of the patient is unremarkable and no medications other than Fosamax were used by the patient. Specifically there is no history of arthritis, hypertension, cancer, diabetes, or cardiac disease. The patient does not associate the onset of pain to the medication, which has been taken for a number of years. The patient is a lifetime nonsmoker and nondrinker. The lady is widowed, her husband having died approximately five years ago. All children of the patient live out of state, but the patient keeps in contact with them with weekly telephone calls. The patient is active in church activities and is also a member of several volunteer organizations in the community. The patient is not believed to be depressed and describes the pain as more of a "giant frustration" that adversely affects her quality of life but is not debilitating.

EPIDEMIOLOGY OF BMS

BMS is a frustrating (and often debilitating) condition to both the patient and physician. By the time the average patient arrives at the otolaryngologist office, they have usually tried a number of over-the-counter medications, been treated by their primary physician with a variety of treatments, and may have seen their dentist. In typical cases, the physical examination is completely normal and no underlying cause can be identified. Specifically, there is no past history of herpetic ulcerations, prior oral cavity lesions, surgery, or radiation therapy. Salivary flow is normal, with moist mucosal surfaces, although the patients may complain about a subjective sensation of a dry mouth and occasionally mild dysguesia. Physical examination reveals no evidence of mucosal abnormality, angioneurotic edema, submucosal fibrosis, or swelling. In many instances, patients may have tried discontinuing medications on their own in order to determine whether the BMS might be secondary to a drug reaction.

The condition most commonly affects postmenopausal women; however, it also occurs in premenopausal women as well as men. The prevalence increases with increasing age. In a sample of over 1400 randomly selected individuals, Bergdahl and Bergdahl identified BMS in 3.6% of the oldest group of men, whereas in the oldest age group of women the prevalence was 12% with only 0.6% of women under age 40 experiencing the symptom. The mean age was 59 for men, and 57 for women (1). Other authors report different age averages, based on the age of their sampled population.

The term burning mouth syndrome implies that the oral cavity examination is normal. The symptom of burning mouth can be associated with a wide variety of disease processes, including xerostomia, Stevens–Johnson syndrome, atrophic glossitis, iron deficiency or pernicious anemia, or post-herpetic neuralgia. However, in these instances, the symptom is due to the underlying cause, and the term BMS should not be used.

ETIOLOGY

The etiology of BMS is not known. It has been proposed that the underlying process can be subdivided into four major categories, including local mucosal disease, systemic disease, psychiatric disorder, or idiopathic causes. Local diseases include conditions associated with xerostomia, atrophic glossitis, and lichenoid reactions. Since there is a mucosal abnormality, however, these do not really represent BMS. Approximately two-thirds of patients with BMS complain of subjective dry mouth symptoms, usually without objective evidence of xerostomia. In these cases with xerostomia, the symptoms of dry mouth and BMS are secondary to a systemic disorder, or caused by administration of specific medication.

Pajukoski et al. (2) screened for symptoms of both *burning* mouth and *dry* mouth in more than 400 hospitalized and outpatient elderly patients. They noted an association between the use of psychiatric medications and both dry mouth and BMS. These authors also determined salivary quantity and pH, and correlated it with both symptoms. Hospitalized patients had significantly lower salivary flow as well as lower salivary pH, likely due to medication administration. Although there was an association between the symptoms of dry mouth and BMS among their outpatient group, there was no association with salivary volume, saliva character, or yeast count.

An association between burning mouth syndrome and dental materials has been suggested. Purello et al. (3) reported a patient who developed BMS thought to be secondary to cadmium in her denture. They confirmed the sensitivity with cutaneous patch testing, and the symptoms of the patient resolved after discontinuation of denture use. It is a general consensus that dental restorations are not responsible for BMS; however, some dentists have recommended removal and replacement in patients with BMS. This treatment is controversial and not recommended by most dental authorities.

Systemic causes of BMS include a number of chronic illnesses, often associated with xerostomia as well. In these situations, differentiation of BM from symptomatic xerostomia may be impossible. Thyroid disease, atrophic glossitis due to anemia, and a number of vitamin deficiencies may be associated with BMS.

Some have attempted to associate BMS with specific infections. An investigation of the possible role of *Helicobacter* colonization of the tongue in patients with BMS utilizing polymerase chain reaction was reported by Gall-Troselj et al. (4). One in five of the population with BMS (in the absence of oral mucosal changes) demonstrated the presence of *Helicobacter* colonization using polymerase chain reaction, but the authors questioned whether the finding related to the BMS symptoms (4).

Known psychiatric illness is found in a significant number of patients with BMS (1,2,5). It is likely that at least some of these have developed BMS due to medication. Treatment with mild anxiolytics as well as cognitive therapy has been reported as beneficial (1). Carlson et al. (6) studied the association in more detail, however, and could not demonstrate an association with depression, anxiety, or somatization scores in 80% of the BMS patient group. They hypothesized that the association, when present, may represent a reaction to chronic pain (effect, not cause).

Over the past several years, a consensus has developed that attributes burning mouth syndrome to chronic neuropathic pain. The response of BMS to clonazepam, a gamma-aminobutyric acid agonist, supports this hypothesis, as does the fact that the use of topical anesthetics may *increase* the pain whereas topically applied capsaicin has been reported to *reduce* the pain. White et al. (7) reported successful use of gabapentin in the management of BMS. They hypothesized that BMS represents a phantom pain syndrome due to disinhibition of pain fibers in cranial nerves V and IX, and that increases in nerve excitation by gamma-aminobutyric acid result in pain relief. Although this report gives us additional information about the likely etiology of BMS, the authors point out that gabapentin should not be used as first-line therapy.

EVALUATION AND MANAGEMENT OF PATIENTS WITH BMS

A standard focused history and head and neck examination are prerequisites in the diagnosis of BMS. The history should address prior oral mucosal disease, systemic illnesses, and current medications. Any changes in symptoms associated with institution or discontinuation of medication should be noted as well as associated symptoms of dry mouth. A brief mental status examination is also warranted, although attribution of BMS to psychiatric causes should be withheld as a diagnosis of exclusion. Laboratory studies may be warranted, particularly thyroid function studies and evaluation for possible iron deficiency or pernicious anemia. Other laboratory studies may be warranted based on additional history. Imaging is typically not required, unless the history suggests a localized neuropathy, in which case appropriate imaging may be required in order to evaluate the course of the involved cranial nerve.

Treatment is largely supportive and aimed at symptom resolution. Initial trials of topical anesthetics are warranted, although may paradoxically *increase* the pain. Discontinuation of medications that cause xerostomia as well as selective serotonin reuptake inhibitors may be considered, after consultation with the patient's primary care physician. Systemic disorders amenable to management such as anemia or thyroid disease can be treated. Treatment of xerostomia with salivary substitutes or pilocarpine may relieve associated burning. Low doses of clonazepam can be initiated, with care to avoid over-sedation, particularly in the elderly. As of this writing, gabapentin should probably be reserved for severe cases. Psychiatric evaluation and management may be warranted in selected patients.

SUMMARY

Burning mouth syndrome is enigmatic to the patient, primary care physician, and otolaryngologist. The etiology is unknown, but it probably represents a neuropathic pain syndrome. The diagnosis is one of exclusion, so that evaluation should consist of ruling out identifiable and treatable causes. Treatment is via appropriate adjustment of medications, salivary substitutes, and judicious use of anxiolytics and possibly gabapentin. Selected patients may benefit from referral for psychiatric evaluation and therapy.

REFERENCES

1. Bergdahl M, Bergdahl J. Burning mouth syndrome: prevalence and associated factors. J Oral Pathol Med 1999; 28(8):350–354.
2. Pajukoski H, Meurman JH, Halonen P, Sulkova R. Prevalence of subjective dry mouth and burning mouth in hospitalized elderly patients and outpatients in relation to saliva, medication, and systemic diseases. Oral Surg Oral Med Oral Pathol Oral Radiol Endod 2001; 92(6):641–649.
3. Purello-D'Ambrosio F, Gangemi S, Minciullo P, Ricciardi L. Burning mouth syndrome due to cadmium in a denture wearer. J Invest Allergol Clin Immunol 2000; 10(2):105–106.
4. Gall-Troselj K, Mravak-Stipetic M, Jurak I, Ragland WL, Pavelic J. *Helicobacter pylori* colonization of tongue mucosa–increased incidence in atrophic glossitis and burning mouth syndrome (BMS). J Oral Pathol Med 2001; 30(9):560–563.
5. Drage LA, Rogers RS III. Burning mouth syndrome. Dermatol Clin 2003; 21(1):135–145.
6. Carlson CR, Miller CS, Reid KI. Psychosocial profiles of patients with burning mouth syndrome. J Orofac Pain 2000; 14(1):59–64.
7. White TL, Kent PF, Kurtz DB, Emko P. Effectiveness of gabapentin for treatment of burning mouth syndrome. Arch Otolaryngol Head Neck Surg 2004; 130(6):786–788.

26
Effects of Aging on Swallowing

JoAnne Robbins
Sections of Geriatrics and Gastroenterology, Departments of Medicine and Radiology, University of Wisconsin–Madison, and Geriatric Research Education and Clinical Center, William S. Middleton Veterans Hospital, Madison, Wisconsin, U.S.A.

Nadine Connor
Division of Otolaryngology, Department of Surgery, University of Wisconsin–Madison, Madison, Wisconsin, U.S.A.

Steven Barczi
Section of Geriatrics, Department of Medicine, University of Wisconsin–Madison, and Geriatric Research Education and Clinical Center, William S. Middleton Veterans Hospital, Madison, Wisconsin, U.S.A.

INTRODUCTION

Swallowing requires the coordination of a complex series of psychological, sensory, and motor behaviors that are both voluntary and involuntary. *Dysphagia* refers to any difficulty in these processes and may encompass both oropharyngeal or esophageal problems. Such problems may involve a number of physiological events at any point in the process of preparing a bolus in the oral cavity, transporting that bolus from the mouth to the esophagus, and then further transporting the bolus from the esophagus to the stomach.

Although the anatomical, physiological, psychological, and functional changes that occur in the dynamic process we refer to as "aging" place older adults at risk for dysphagia, a healthy older adult's swallow is not inherently impaired. However, older adults appear to be more vulnerable to dysphagia than younger adults. Older adults readily can cross over from a healthy older swallower to a person with dysphagia in association with certain perturbations, such as acute illness, surgery, chemoradiation, and other factors.

The term *presbyphagia* refers to characteristic changes in the mechanism of swallowing in otherwise healthy older adults (1). We review normal swallowing briefly in this chapter to set the stage for changes that may be observed with presbyphagia. In addition, we discuss promising strategies for rehabilitation of dysphagia that are based upon the recognition that swallowing disruption may be a manifestation of "sarcopenia," the age-related loss of skeletal muscle mass, organization, and strength (2).

THE IMPACT OF DYSPHAGIA

The care of elderly persons with dysphagia represents a significant clinical problem (2,3). It is estimated that 6 million to 15 million elderly Americans have dysphagia (2,4–6). More than 40% of those within institutional settings such as assisted living or nursing homes are dysphagic (7). In institutional settings, eating dependency has been shown to be associated with multiple impairments and early mortality (7,8).

The consequences of dysphagia vary from social isolation due to the embarrassment of choking or coughing at mealtime, to physical discomfort (e.g., food sticking in the chest), to potentially life-threatening conditions. The more ominous sequelae include dehydration, malnutrition, and aspiration.

We define aspiration as the entry of material into the airway *below* the level of the true vocal folds. When this type of event does not trigger overt signs of aspiration, such as coughing or throat clearing, the term *silent aspiration* applies. Both overt and silent aspiration may be risk factors for serious illnesses, such as pneumonitis, pneumonia, exacerbation of chronic lung diseases, or even asphyxiation and death (9,10).

Dysphagia can have a profoundly negative effect on quality of life. Patients with swallowing difficulties, especially those with compromised oral eating, manifest significant changes in psychosocial status, functional status, and emotional well-being. Eating and drinking are social events that relate to friendships, acceptance, entertainment, and communication. As such, major adjustments in the process of feeding and eating can lead to distressing responses such as shame, anxiety, depression, and isolation. Recent recognition of the effect of swallowing disruption on a patient's perception of their health and functioning have led to the inclusion of swallowing-related items on general health quality of life instruments, such as those for head and neck cancer (11,12). Dysphagia-specific quality of life instruments are also available (13–15). Use of these questionnaire instruments allows health care providers to monitor functional outcomes in their patients before and after surgery or other treatments provided in their clinical practice to more objectively assess and adjust their treatments for dysphagia care.

NORMAL SWALLOWING

A basic understanding of the relationship of the anatomic components and functional interaction of the normal swallowing mechanism is essential to the understanding of the effects of age and age-related diseases.

Swallowing is an integrated neuromuscular process that combines volitional and relatively automatic movements. The process of deglutition can be described as occurring in two, three, or four phases or stages, or horizontal versus vertical subsystems related to the direction of bolus flow (Fig. 1) (17).

The horizontal subsystem is largely volitional and is comprised anatomically by structures within the oral cavity. Within this subsystem, food is accepted, contained, and manipulated. Labial, buccal, and lingual actions, in combination with enzyme-rich intraoral fluids, allow manipulation of the texture of food to mechanically formulate a bolus. The cohesive bolus is moved posteriorly (and, horizontally when the subject is in a normal upright seated posture) to the inlet of the superior aspect of the pharynx (Fig. 2). To accomplish this, the intrinsic and extrinsic tongue muscles change the shape and the position of the tongue,

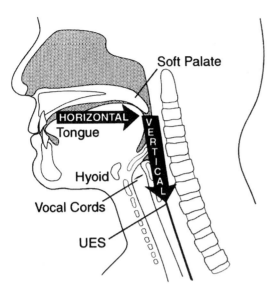

Figure 1 The oropharyngeal swallowing mechanism may be divided into two basic structural subsystems, horizontal and vertical, that mirror direction of bolus flow. *Source*: From Ref. 16.

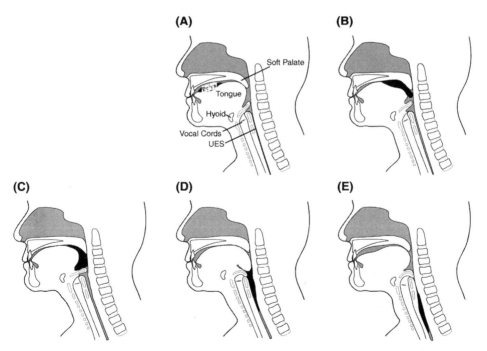

Figure 2 Lateral view of bolus propulsion during swallowing. (**A**) Voluntary initiation of the swallow by tongue "loading." (**B**) Bolus propulsion by tongue dorsum and UES opening anticipating bolus arrival. (**C**) Bolus entry into pharynx associated with epiglottal downward tilt, hyolaryngeal excursion, and UES opening. (**D**) Linguapharyngeal contact facilitating bolus passage through the pharynx and (**E**) UES and completion of oropharyngeal swallowing, then the entire bolus is on the esophagus. *Abbreviation*: UES, upper esophageal sphincter. *Source*: From Ref. 16.

and stimulate oropharyngeal receptors that trigger ensuing portions of the swallow sequence (16–18).

The pharyngeal and laryngeal components, in conjunction with the tongue dorsum, comprise the superior aspect of the vertical subsystem where gravity begins to assist in the transport of the bolus. The anatomical juxtaposition of the entrance to the airway (laryngeal vestibule) and the pharyngeal aspect of the upper digestive tract demand biomechanical precision to ensure simultaneous airway protection and bolus transfer or propulsion through the pharynx. As lingual–palatal contact sequentially moves the bolus against the posterior pharyngeal wall, the contact contributes to the positive pressures imparted to the bolus propelling it downward (19,20). Simultaneously, the pharyngeal constrictors begin contracting in a descending sequence, first elevating and widening the entire pharynx to engulf the bolus (Fig. 2D, E) (19,21). A descending peristaltic wave then cleanses the pharynx of residue. The tongue is the primary propulsive mechanism responsible for plunging the bolus into the vertical subsystem, but other mechanisms such as velopharyngeal closure also contribute to pressure gradients facilitating the bolus transfer.

Airway protection is ensured during the swallow by three levels of sphincteric closure: (i) aryepiglottic folds, (ii) the false vocal folds, and (iii) the true vocal folds. The hyolaryngeal complex is also lifted upward and forward by the combined contraction of the suprahyoid and thyrohyoid muscles, and pharyngeal elevators. This hyolaryngeal elevation and anterior movement, coupled with tongue base retraction, covers the laryngeal vestibule, diverts the bolus laterally around the airway, and also provides the traction pull on the cricoid cartilage moving it anteriorly, an important aspect of upper esophageal sphincter (UES) opening (20,22).

Timely relaxation and opening of the UES permits continuous vertical passage of the bolus into the esophagus, and the pharyngeal transport stage of the swallow terminates when the UES returns to its hypertonic, closed "resting state."

NEUROPHYSIOLOGY OF OROPHARYNGEAL SWALLOW

Sensorimotor control of swallowing requires the coordinated activity distributed across both cranial and spinal nerve systems, including peripheral nerves, their central nuclei, and neural centers. More specifically, the neural control of swallowing involves five major components: (i) afferent sensory fibers contained in cranial nerves, (ii) cerebral and midbrain fibers that synapse with the brainstem swallowing centers, (iii) paired swallowing centers in the brainstem, (iv) efferent motor fibers contained in cranial nerves and the ansa cervicalis, and (v) muscles. This distributed neural network spans all levels of the neuraxis from the cerebrum superiorly to the brainstem and spinal nerves inferiorly and muscles at the periphery to integrate and sequence both volitional and automatic activities of swallowing.

Healthy persons depend on a highly automated neuromuscular sensorimotor process that intricately coordinates the activities of chewing, swallowing, and airway protection. To accomplish a normal swallow in two seconds or less, the muscles of chewing (masseters, temporalis, pterygoids—innervated by cranial nerve V), the lip and buccal musculature, obicularis oris and buccinator (innervated by cranial nerve VII), and the intrinsic and extrinsic lingual muscles (cranial nerve XII) interact with 26 pairs of striated pharyngeal and laryngeal muscles. In healthy young individuals, the outcome of optimal structural integrity and precise neural mediation is continuous and rapid bolus flow from the mouth to the esophagus that accommodates variation in bolus size, texture, temperature, and the individual's intent to swallow, chew, or just hold the bolus in the mouth (Fig. 3A–C).

SENESCENT SWALLOWING

Changes in swallowing function can occur with healthy aging. A progression of change appears to put members of the older population at increased risk for dysphagia, particularly when they are faced with stressors such as medications that affect the nervous system, mechanical perturbations (e.g., nasogastric tubes or tracheostomy), or chronic medical conditions (e.g., frailty) that might not elicit dysphagia in a less vulnerable system.

Older healthy swallowing occurs more slowly. Longer swallowing duration occurs in older individuals largely before the more automatic vertical subsystem of the swallow is initiated. Delays in the onset of components that comprise the vertical phase are also apparent. In those over age 65, the initiation of laryngeal and pharyngeal events, including laryngeal vestibule closure, maximal hyolaryngeal excursion, and UES opening are significantly delayed relative to durations recorded in adults younger than 45 years old (23–26). In older healthy adults, it is not uncommon for the bolus to be adjacent to an open airway by pooling or pocketing in the pharyngeal recesses, for more time than in younger adults (Fig. 4A–C). This situation may be associated with greater risk for airway penetration or aspiration.

Aspiration and airway penetration are believed to be the most significant adverse clinical outcomes of misdirected bolus flow. In older adults, penetration of the bolus into the airway occurs more often and to a deeper and more severe level than in younger adults (23,27). When the swallowing mechanism is functionally altered or perturbed in older people, such as with the placement of a nasogastric tube, airway penetration can be even more pronounced. A study examining this issue found that liquid penetrated the airway significantly more frequently when a nasogastric tube was in place in men and women older than 70 years (23). Thus, it appeared that under stressful conditions or system perturbations, older individuals were less able to compensate and were more at risk to experience airway penetration or aspiration.

Age-related changes in lingual pressure generation also define presbyphagia. Healthy older individuals demonstrate significantly reduced isometric tongue pressures compared with younger counterparts. In contrast, maximal lingual pressure generated during swallowing (which is a submaximal pressure requirement task) remained normal in magnitude. Because peak lingual pressures used in swallowing are lower than those generated isometrically, healthy old individuals managed to achieve pressures necessary to effect a successful swallow, but achieved these peak swallowing pressures more slowly than young swallowers (28,29). We have suggested previously that as people get older, slower swallowing may permit increased time to recruit the necessary number of motor units for pressures critical for adequate bolus propulsion through the oropharynx (16,29). However, it must be again considered that perturbations or functional alterations in the swallowing mechanism, or perhaps general age-related or disease-related frailty, may not allow safe swallows in older adults. That is, the compensation of slower swallowing may not be enough for these individuals in whom *presbyphagia* crosses over into *dysphagia* at which point there will be a need for compensatory or rehabilitatory interventions to promote safe swallowing.

(A)

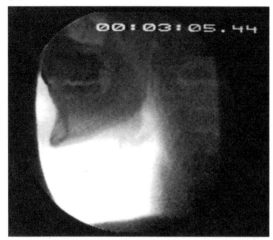

(B)

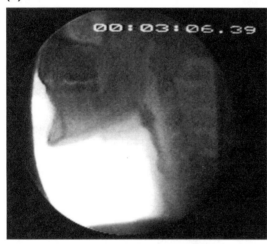

(C)

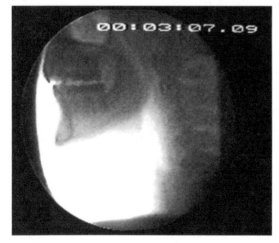

Figure 3   (*Caption on facing page*)

Neurophysiologic Correlates of Senescent Swallowing

Slowing of performance in fine and gross motor tasks is well documented in elderly persons. The reaction time to sensory stimuli declines with increasing age (30,31).

Magnetic resonance imaging (MRI) is highly sensitive in detecting periventricular white-matter hyperintensities (PVHs) in the cerebral white-matter tracts. Neuroimaging studies using cranial MRI in normal adults show a relationship between slower swallowing and increased number and severity of PVHs in the brain, supporting the concept that voluntary control of swallowing is mediated by corticobulbar pathways that travel within the periventricular white matter (32). The occurrence and degree of these PVHs increase with age and may explain, at least in part, the relatively asymptomatic decline in oropharyngeal motor performance observed in older people. Cerebral atrophy, blood flow changes, and other age-related conditions also must be factored into the process underlying presbyphagia.

Changes in the peripheral nervous system as well as central changes are documented with age and may be related to sarcopenia in muscles of the head and neck. Structurally, sarcopenia is associated with reductions in muscle mass and cross-sectional area, a reduction in the number or size of muscle fibers, and a transformation or selective loss of specific muscle fiber types (33–36). Reductions in tongue muscle fiber diameter are reported for the superior longitudinal muscle from 50 human tongues. Reductions in fiber diameters began at age 40 in males and age 30 in females (37). In addition, an increase in fatty and connective tissue and increased amyloid deposits in the blood vessels of the tongue have also been reported (38). In the larynx, changes in human laryngeal muscle specimens (thyroarytenoid) from autopsy or laryngectomy show a tendency for decreasing Type II (fast) muscle fibers and increasing Type I (slow) fiber composition with increasing age (39). Accordingly, there are reports in our literature of sarcopenia-like changes in muscles of the upper aerodigestive tract. However, most of the work performed in the area of sarcopenia has been performed in the limb musculature and further work is certainly indicated in cranial muscles.

Muscle disuse, which may be better termed as "reduction" or "alteration" in use, has been proposed as the cause of muscular atrophy observed in the aged (40). This hypothesis has intuitive appeal, due to the assumption that elderly people are less active. However, the fact that muscles of speech, swallowing, and respiration undergo changes associated with aging argues against this hypothesis since aged individuals speak, swallow, and breathe frequently within any given day (41). Further, "disuse" has not been proven as a simple causative factor in animal studies (33,40,42). Again, it is clear that mechanisms underlying sarcopenia in muscles of the head and neck must be defined to allow the design and implementation of appropriate treatments.

The morphological changes observed in aged muscle and at nerve–muscle connections may have physiological or functional consequences such as a diminished ability to sustain synaptic transmission, reduced force generation per unit of muscle fiber cross-sectional area, and altered or disorganized patterns of muscular contraction during complex movements (42–47). Reduced muscle forces and altered

---

Figure 3 (*Facing page*) Healthy young swallowing documented with videofluoroscopy. (**A**) Bolus in mouth initiating swallow. (**B**) Bolus appears as "column" of material swiftly moving through pharynx. (**C**) Oropharynx cleared of material when swallow completed. *Source*: From Ref. 16.

(A)

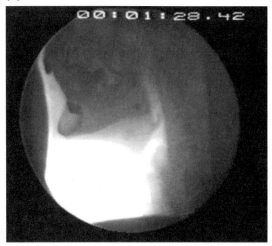

(B)

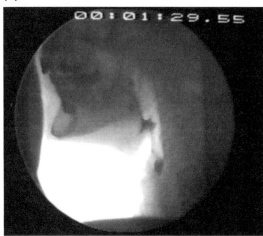

(C)

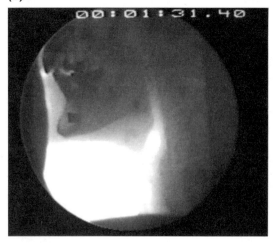

Figure 4 (*Caption on facing page*)

temporal properties have been reported in human and animal studies and indicate that aged laryngeal muscle contractions are generally of reduced force, require more time to reach peak contraction, and also more time for recovery prior to initiation of the next contraction (48,49). These factors could contribute to reductions in motor performance required for swallowing actions.

In summary, the differences in swallowing function for elderly and young individuals appear dependent on age-associated changes of both central and peripheral mechanisms. It can be hypothesized that slowed swallowing that remains coordinated and effective, as found in most healthy old people, may not reflect central nervous system (CNS) deterioration as much as it represents a compensatory strategy for achieving pressure-generation values that may be critical to successful bolus propulsion.

DIFFERENTIAL CONSIDERATIONS FOR DYSPHAGIA AND ASPIRATION

Etiologies

Older adults are at increased risk for developing dysphagia due to a number of age-associated phenomena (50). Comorbid processes increase the chances for older adults to suffer the adverse consequences of dysphagia such as dehydration, malnutrition, or aspiration pneumonia. By targeting high-risk groups and intervening with acceptable compensatory and rehabilitative approaches, it is hoped that the ultimate burden of dysphagia on the geriatric population will decline.

Age-Related Conditions

Age-related difficulties and comorbidities can develop throughout the upper aerodigestive tract and have the potential of influencing the integrity of the swallow. In the horizontal subsystem, the food bolus may be inadequately prepared due to poor or absent dentition, periodontal disease, ill-fitting dentures, or inappropriate salivation from xerostomia (51,52). Musculoskeletal factors such as weakness of the muscles of mastication, arthritis of the temporomandibular joint or larynx, osteoporosis of the jaw, changes in tongue strength, and discoordination of oropharyngeal events can deter efficient swallowing. Sensory input for taste, temperature, and tactile sensation changes in many older adults (53–55) and may impair sensorimotor interaction required for proper bolus formation and timely response of the swallowing sequence. All of these factors may detract from the pleasure of eating.

Age-Related Disease

Neurological and neuromuscular disorders are principal risks for dysphagia (Table 1). Neurological diseases rise in prevalence in older cohorts of the population. Conditions of stroke, head injury, Alzheimer's and other dementia syndromes, and Parkinson's disease all place older adults at increased risk for dysphagia with its

---

Figure 4 (*Facing page*) Healthy old swallowing documented with videofluoroscopy. (**A**) Bolus in mouth initiating swallow. (**B**) Bolus pooled in vallecula and pyriform sinus during delayed onset of pharyngeal response. (**C**) Bolus cleared of material when swallow completed. *Source*: From Ref. 16.

Table 1 Neurologic Disorders Causing Dysphagia

Stroke
Head trauma
Parkinson's disease and other movement and neurodegenerative disorders
Progressive supranuclear palsy
    Olivopontocerebellar atrophy
    Huntington's disease
    Wilson's disease
Torticollis
    Tardive dyskinesia
Alzheimer's disease and other dementias
Motor neuron disease (amyotrophic lateral sclerosis)
Guillain–Barre syndrome and other polyneuropathies
Neoplasms and other structural disorders
    Primary brain tumors
    Intrinsic and extrinsic brainstem tumors
    Base of skull tumors
    Syringobulbia
    Arnold–Chiari malformation
    Neoplastic meningitis
Multiple sclerosis
Postpolio syndrome
Infectious disorders
    Chronic infectious meningitis
    Syphilis and Lyme disease
    Diphtheria
    Botulism
    Viral encephalitis, including rabies
Myasthenia gravis
Myopathy
    Polymyositis, dermatomyositis, inclusion body myositis, and sarcoidosis
    Myotonic and oculopharyngeal muscular dystrophy
    Hyper- and hypothyroidism
    Cushing's syndrome
Iatrogenic conditions
    Medication side effects
    Postsurgical neurogenic dysphagia
    Neck surgery
    Posterior fossa surgery
    Irradiation of the head and neck

incipient consequences. For example, cerebrovascular conditions such as stroke increase steadily with advancing age with incidence ranging from 9 to 12 per 1000 individuals by age 75. Between 50% and 75% of acute stroke patients develop eating and swallowing problems with ensuing complications of aspiration in 50%, malnutrition in 45%, and pneumonia in 35% of these individuals. Six clinical features are associated with increased risk for aspiration post-stroke (56). These include (i) abnormal volitional cough, (ii) abnormal gag reflex, (iii) dysarthria, (iv) dysphonia, (v) cough after trial swallow, and (vi) voice change after trial swallow. The presence of any two of these findings had a sensitivity of 92% and specificity of 67% that there would be penetration and aspiration of material as evidenced with videofluoroscopy.

A host of common problems within the head and neck can directly damage effector muscles of swallowing and increase the risk for dysphagia. Head and neck injury, carcinoma, complex infections and thyroid conditions, and diabetes are associated with age-related dysphagia. Head and neck cancer surgeries, some spinal cord surgeries, thyroid surgeries and any intervention that may jeopardize the recurrent laryngeal nerve may incite dysphagia. A number of chemotherapy and radiotherapy regimes can lead to swallowing impairment, but tend to improve with time post treatment (57). The prospective outcome of dysphagia should be incorporated into the risk-benefit discussions of these procedures.

DYSPHAGIA INTERVENTION–PREVENTION PARADIGMS

Treatment for dysphagia usually is either rehabilitative or compensatory in nature. Rehabilitative interventions have the capacity to directly improve the dysphagia at the biologic level. That is, aspects of anatomical structures or neural circuitry are the targets of rehabilitative therapy that may have direct influence on physiology, biomechanics, and bolus flow. On the other hand, compensatory interventions avoid or reduce the effects of the impaired structures or neuropathology and resultant disordered physiology and biomechanics on bolus flow, for instance, by modification of the environment, the patient's position during mealtime, or the texture of the food.

Traditionally, interventions for dysphagia in the elderly are most often compensatory in nature and are directed at modifying bolus flow, by targeting biomechanical features of the swallow or by adapting the environment; the latter of which is something that the care provider can accomplish for patients who are unable to do so for themselves. Examples of compensatory strategies for dysphagia treatment are postural adjustment, slowing the rate of eating, limiting bolus size, adaptive equipment, and the most commonly used environment adaptation, diet modification.

Rehabilitative exercises are, by nature, more active and rigorous. During the past 20 years, a body of literature has emerged that suggests that loss of muscle strength with age is, to a great extent, reversible through incorporating exercise and strength training into rehabilitative programs.

The research in the area of exercise for elderly people has typically been applied to reducing falls in elderly persons, rather than swallowing impairment (58). However, both clinical and animal studies examining this issue are currently underway and results will be forthcoming. In studies of progressive resistance exercise in the limbs, results demonstrated that elderly men and women can increased muscle size and strength with training, even subjects who were 90 years old or older (59–62). According to Evans (63), "There is no pharmacologic intervention that holds a greater promise of improving health and promoting independence in the elderly than does exercise."

There are compelling preliminary data to suggest that increased muscle activation and/or strength and effort training may play an important role in swallowing rehabilitation (64–69). For example, reports in the clinical literature are suggestive of improvements in swallowing function following performance of tongue exercises in combination with other factors (70). In a randomized trial, young, healthy adults significantly increased maximum tongue strength with either standard strength exercises using a tongue depressor or the Iowa oral performance instrument, compared to a group that received no treatment (67). In one study of asymptomatic, healthy, elderly subjects, significant increases were found in magnitude of laryngeal excursion, and cross-sectional area of UES opening after performance of a head-raising exercise (68). Two other recent reports, one using a small number of elderly subjects and the other a head and neck cancer patient, were indicative of improved force and temporal characteristics of the swallow after eight weeks of progressive lingual resistance training (66,69). These changes generalized to improvements in the subjects' nutritional intake and quality of life. Perhaps even more hopeful for the future is a study demonstrating that even healthy elders, after eight weeks of progressive resistance training, not only increased lingual strength but also had direct carry over of the strength training to functional increased pressures during swallowing (71). Thus, while there is substantial literature in limb systems to date, some preliminary data in head and neck systems are pointing to the potential benefits of strength training as a possible intervention for swallowing disorders. Exercise targeting sarcopenia with or without additional impairment deserves further clinical study, because such an approach holds the promise of prevention of age-related dysphagia for individuals who employ exercise regimes focusing on head and neck musculature.

SUMMARY

As our population ages, strategies for treating elderly persons with dysphagia will be of crucial importance. Research into the underlying pathophysiology of age-related swallowing disorders is of primary importance to allow development of interventions with sound scientific bases to encourage prevention, slowing, or reversal of these conditions. Certainly, the state of the evidence calls for more research with a need for randomized clinical trials in this area.

Contributions by all team members involved in the care of these patients are valuable in the challenging decision-making process, with the patient's family or care provider's point of view perhaps the most critical contribution.

ACKNOWLEDGMENT

Grant E20641R from the Department of Veterans Affairs supported a portion of this work. This is manuscript number 2004–0002 from the Geriatric Research Education and Clinical Center (GRECC) of the William S. Middleton VA Hospital. Thanks to Alisa Bergman, Abby Duane, B.S., and Stephanie Kays, M.S., Certificate of Clinical Competence in Speech Language Pathology (CCC-SLP) for assisting with manuscript preparation.

REFERENCES

1. Robbins JA. Old swallowing and dysphagia: thoughts on intervention and prevention. Nutr Clin Pract 1999; 14:S21.
2. Rosenberg RH. Sarcopenia: origins and clinical relevance. J Nutr 1997; 127:990S–991S.
3. Barczi SR, Sullivan PA, Robbins JA. How should dysphagia care of older adults differ? Establishing optimal practice patterns. Semin Speech Lang 2000; 21(4):347–361.
4. Feinberg MJ, Knebl J, Tully J, et al. Aspiration and the elderly. Dysphagia 1990; 5:61–71.

5. ECRI report: diagnosis and treatment of swallowing disorders (dysphagia) in acute-stroke patients. Evidence Report/Technology Assessment No. 8 (Prepared by ECRI Evidence-Based Practice Center under Contract No. 290–97–0020). AHCPR Publication No. 99-E024. Rockville, Md.: Agency for Health Care Policy and Research, 1999.

6. Lindgren S, Janzon L. Prevalence of swallowing complaints and clinical findings among 50–79 year old men and women in an urban population. Dysphagia 1991; 6:187–192.

7. Trupe EH, Siebens H, Siebens A. Prevalence of feeding and swallowing disorders in a nursing home. Arch Phys Med Rehabil 1984; 65:651–652.

8. Williams MJ, Walker GT. Managing swallowing problems in the home. Caring Mag 1992; 11:59–63.

9. Siebens H, Trupe E, Siebens A, et al. Correlates and consequences of eating dependency in institutionalized elderly. J Am Geriatr Soc 1986; 34:192–198.

10. Langmore SE, Terpenning MS, Schork A, et al. Predictors of aspiration pneumonia: how important is dysphagia? Dysphagia 1998; 13:69–81.

11. Lundy DS, Smith C, Colangelo L, et al. Aspiration: cause and implications. Otolaryngol Head Neck Surg 1999; 120:474–478.

12. Bjordal K, Hammerlid E, Ahlner-Elmqvist M, et al. Quality of life in head and neck cancer patients: validation of the European Organization for Research and Treatment of Cancer Quality of Life Questionnaire-H & N35. J Clin Oncol 1999; 17:1008–1019.

13. Chen AY, Frankowski R, Bishop-Leone J, et al. The development and validation of a dysphagia-specific quality-of-life questionnaire for patients with head and neck cancer. Int J Radiat Oncol Biol Phys 2001; 53:23–28.

14. McHorney CA, Bricker DE, Kramer AE, et al. The SWAL-QOL outcomes tool for oropharyngeal dysphagia in adults: I. conceptual foundation and item development. Dysphagia 2000; 15:115–121.

15. McHorney CA, Bricker DE, Robbins J, et al. The SWAL-QOL outcomes tool for oropharyngeal dysphagia in adults: II. Item reduction and preliminary scaling. Dysphagia 2000; 15:122–133.

16. Robbins JA. Normal swallowing and aging. Semin Neurol 1996; 16(4):308–317.

17. Kennedy J, Kent RD. Anatomy and physiology of deglutition and related functions. In: Logemann J, ed. Seminars in Speech and Language: The Relationship Between Speech and Swallowing. Vol. 6. New York: Thieme-Stratton, 1985:1–12.

18. Kier WM, Smith KK. Tongues, tentacles and trunks: the biomechanics of movement in muscular-hydrostats. Zool J Linn Soc 1985; 83:307–324.

19. Dodds WJ. The physiology of swallowing. Dysphagia 1989; 95:171–178.

20. McConnel FMS. Analysis of pressure generation and bolus transit during pharyngeal swallowing. Laryngoscope 1988; 87:71–78.

21. Doty RW, Bosma JF. An electromyographic analysis of reflex deglutition. J Neurophysiol 1956; 19:44–60.

22. Logemann J, Kahrilas PJ, Cheng J, et al. Closure mechanisms of the laryngeal vestibule during swallow. Am J Physiol 1992; 262:G338–G344.

23. Robbins JA, Hamilton JW, Lof GL, et al. Oropharyngeal swallowing in normal adults of different ages. Gastroenterology 1992; 103:823–829.

24. Tracy JF, Logemann JA, Kahrilas PJ. Preliminary observations on the effects of age on oropharyngeal deglutition. Dysphagia 1989; 1:3–6.

25. Shaw DW, Cook IJ, Dent J. Age influences on oropharyngeal and upper esophageal sphincter function during swallowing. Gastroenterology 1990; 98:A390.

26. Shaw DW, Cook IJ, Gabb M, et al. Influence of normal aging on oral-pharyngeal and upper esophageal sphincter function during swallow. Am J Physiol 1995; 268:G389–G396.

27. Robbins JA, Coyle J, Roecker E, Rosenbek J, Wood J. Differentiation of normal and abnormal airway protection during swallowing using the penetration-aspiration scale. Dysphagia 1999; 14(4):228–232.

28. Robbins JA, Levine RL, Wood J, et al. Age effects on lingual pressure generation as a risk factor for dysphagia. J Gerontol Med Sci 1995; 50A(5):M257–M262.

29. Nicosia MA, Hind JA, Roecker EB, et al. Age effects on temporal evolution of isometric and swallowing pressures. J Gerontol Med Sci 2000; 55A:M340–M640.

30. Welford AT. Reaction time, speed of performance, and age. Ann NY Acad Sci 1988; 515:1–17.

31. Birren IE, Woods AM, Williams MV. Speed of behavior as an indicator of age changes and the integrity of the nervous system. In: Hoffmeister F, Mueller C, eds. Brain Function in old age. Berlin: Springer-Verlag, 1979:10–44.

32. Levine R, Robbins JA, Maser A. Periventricular white matter changes and oropharyngeal swallowing in normal individuals. Dysphagia 1992; 7:142–147.

33. Brown M, Hasser EM. Differential effects of reduced muscle use (hindlimb unweighting) on skeletal muscle with aging. Aging (Milano) 1996; 8:99–105.

34. Carlson BM. Factors influencing the repair and adaptation of muscles in aged individuals: satellite cells and innervaton. J Gerontol 1995; 50:96–100.

35. Lexell J. Human aging, muscle mass, and fiber type composition. J Gerontol 1995; 50: 11–16.

36. Lexell J, Taylor CC, Sjostrom M. What is the cause of ageing atrophy? Total number, size and proportion of different fiber types studied in whole vastus lateralis muscle from 15 to 83-year-old men. J Neurol Sci 1988; 84:275–294.

37. Nakayama M. Histological study on aging changes in the human tongue. J Otolaryngol Japan 1991; 94:541–555.

38. Yamaguchi A, Nasu M, Esaki Y, et al. Amyolid deposits in the aged tongue: a post mortem study of 107 individuals over 67 years of age. J Oral Pathol 1982; 11:237–244.

39. Rodeno MT, Sanchez-Fernandez JM, Rivera-Pomar JM. Histochemical and morphometrical ageing changes in human vocal cord muscles. Acta Otolaryngol (Stockh) 1993; 113:445–449.

40. Cartee GD. What insights into age-related changes in skeletal muscle are provided by animal models? J Gerontol 1995; 50A:137–141.

41. Prakash YS, Sieck GC. Age-related remodeling of neuromuscular junctions on type-identified diaphragm fibers. Muscle Nerve 1998; 21:887–895.

42. Faulkner JA, Brooks SV, Zerba E. Muscle atrophy and weakness with aging: Contraction-induced injury as an underlying mechanism. J Gerontol 1995; 50A:124–129.

43. Rosenheimer JL. Ultraterminal sprouting in innervated and partially denervated adult and aged rat muscle. Neuroscience 1990; 38:763–770.

44. Balice-Gordon RJ. Age-related changes in neuromuscular innervation. Muscle Nerve 1997; 5:S83–S87.

45. Smith DO. Actylcholine storage, release and leakage at the neuromuscular junction of mature and aged rats. J Physiol (Lond) 1984; 347:161–176.

46. Light KE, Spirduso WW. Effects of adult aging on the movement complexity factor of response programming. J Gerontol 1990; 45:P107–P109.

47. Yan JH, Thomas JR, Stelmach GE. Aging and rapid aiming arm movement control. Exp Aging Res 1998; 24:155–168.

48. Baker KK, Ramig LO, Luschei ES, et al. Thyroarytenoid muscle activity associated with hypophonia in Parkinson disease and aging. Neurology 1998; 51:1592–1598.

49. Mardini IA, McCarter RJ, Neal GD, et al. Contractile properties of laryngeal muscles in young and old baboons. Am J Otolaryngol 1987; 8:85–90.

50. Sonies BC, Stone M, Shwker T. Speech and swallowing in the elderly. Gerontology 1984; 3:115–123.

51. Carlsson GE. Masticatory efficiency: the effect of age, the loss of teeth, and prosthetic rehabilitation. Int Dent J 1984; 34:93–97.

52. Ship JA, Duffy V, Jones JA, Langmore S. Geriatric oral heatlh and its impact on eating. J Am Geriatr Soc 1996; 44:456.

53. Schiffman SS. Perception of taste and smell in elderly persons. Crit Rev Food Sci Nutr 1993; 33:17–26.

54. Weiffenbach JM, Bartoshuk LM. Taste and smell. Clin Geriatr Med 1992; 8:543–555.

55. Kenshalo DR. Somesthetic sensitivity in young and elderly humans. J Gerontol 1996; 41:732–742.

56. Daniels SK, Brailey K, Priestly D, et al. Aspiration in patients with acute stroke. Arch Phys Med Rehabil 1998; 79:14–19.

57. Eisbruch A, Lyden T, Bradford CR, et al. Objective assessment of swallowing dysfunction and aspiration after radiation concurrent with chemotherapy for head-and-neck cancer. Int J Radiat Oncol Biol Phys 2002; 53:23–28.

58. Fiatarone MA, Evans WJ. The etiology and reversibility of muscle dysfunction in the aged. J Gerontol 1993; 48:77–83.

59. Fiatarone MA, Marks EC, Ryan ND, et al. High intensity strength training in non-agenarians. Effects on skeletal muscle. JAMA 1990; 263:3029–3034.

60. Frontera WR, Meredith CN, O'Reilly KP. Strength conditioning in older men: skeletal muscle hypertrophy and improved function. J Appl Physiol 1988; 64:1038–1044.

61. Grimby G, Aniansson A, Hedberg M, et al. Training can improve muscle strength and endurance in 78–84 year old men. J Appl Physiol 1992; 73:2517–2523.

62. Tracy BL, Ivey FM, Hurlbut D, et al. Muscle quality. II. Effects of strength training in 65- to 75-year-old men and women. J Appl Physiol 1999; 86:195–201.

63. Evans WJ. Exercise, nutrition, and aging. Clin Geriatr Med 1995; 11:725–734.

64. Burnett TA, Mann EA, Cornell SA, et al. Laryngeal elevation achieved by neuromuscular stimulation at rest. J Appl Physiol 2003; 94:128–134.

65. El Sharkai A, Ramig L, Logemann JA, et al. Swallowing and voice effects of Lee Silverman voice treatment (LSVT[R]): a pilot study. J Neurol Neurosurg Psychiatry 2002; 72:31–36.

66. Hind JA. The effects of lingual exercises on swallowing. Peer-reviewed paper presented at the annual convention of the American Speech Language and Hearing Association, Washington, D.C., 2000.

67. Lazarus C, Logemann JA, Huang CF, et al. Effects of two types of tongue strengthening exercises in young normals. Folia Phoniatr Logop 2003; 55:199–205.

68. Shaker R, Kern M, Bardan E, et al. Augmentation of deglutitive upper esophageal sphincter opening in the elderly by exercise. Am J Physiol 1997; 272:G1518–G1522.

69. Sullivan P, Hind J, Robbins JA. Lingual exercise protocol for head and neck cancer. Poster presented at the annual meeting of the Dysphagia Research Society, Savannah, Ga., 2000.

70. Neumann S, Bartolome G, Buchholz D, et al. Swallowing therapy of neurologic patients: correlation of outcome with pretreatment variables and therapeutic methods. Dysphagia 1995; 10:1–5.

71. Robbins J, Hind J, Theis S, Kays S. Effects of lingual exercise on swallowing in older adults, 2004 (submitted).

27

Dysphagia Evaluation

Jonathan E. Aviv and Thomas Murry
*Voice and Swallowing Center, Department of Otolaryngology—Head and Neck
Surgery, College of Physicians and Surgeons, Columbia University, Columbia University
Medical Center, New York–Presbyterian Hospital, New York, New York, U.S.A.*

INTRODUCTION

Dysphagia, or difficulty swallowing, is one of the most common problems affecting
the geriatric population in this country and is one of the most likely reasons an
elderly individual will consult with an otolaryngologist. Swallowing can be thought
of as an interaction between two related physiologic entities: airway protection and
bolus transport (1). Airway protection is determined by assessment of the sensory
component of swallowing and bolus transport is determined by assessment of the
motor component of swallowing. This chapter will discuss the magnitude of swallowing problems in the elderly: the likely reasons elderly individuals have swallowing difficulties, and the diagnostic and therapeutic techniques available to address
geriatric dysphagia.

EPIDEMIOLOGY

Why is the study and treatment of dysphagia in the elderly important? One reason is
that it is an extraordinarily common problem affecting millions of the geriatric
population every year. The best example of the ubiquitous nature of swallowing
problems in the elderly is demonstrated by the frequency with which they occur after
stroke. Dysphagia is very common in the 400,000 people each year who develop
a stroke, primarily affecting those over 70 years of age with an incidence ranging
from 35% to 47% (2,3). The primary reason for death following stroke is related to
pulmonary complications, specifically aspiration pneumonia. Approximately 50,000
people die each year as a result of aspiration pneumonia after stroke (4,5). While
the development of aspiration pneumonia is a multifactorial process, several studies
have demonstrated a significant association between dysphagia and aspiration pneumonia. Dysphagia often results in difficulty handling food and secretions, which in
turn leads to soiling of the lungs with foreign material (6–10).

Aspiration pneumonia is also a significant cause of chronic illness in the elderly
residing in U.S. nursing homes and is the most common reason for residents of

293

nursing homes to be transferred to a hospital (11,12). In American nursing homes, the prevalence of aspiration pneumonia has been reported as high as 8% (13–16). The cost of treating a single episode of pneumonia in a hospital, including intravenous antibiotics and a stay in an intensive care unit, with or without respiratory support, averaged $19,000 in 1991 (17). This treatment cost has escalated in proportion to other medical costs since that time. Extrapolating to the current population of approximately two million elderly in nursing homes, the annual health care costs related to aspiration pneumonia from the nursing home population is over three billion dollars per year. The mortality from aspiration pneumonia approaches 40%, and is usually associated with recurrent pneumonias over several years in patients over 70 (4,5). The goals of therapy for the geriatric patient with dysphagia are to improve swallowing safety and to improve the quality of life while at the same time keeping the instances of aspiration pneumonia to a minimum. Therefore, the emphasis of the diagnostic and treatment plan for the elderly with dysphagia is not so much an obsession with whether or not the patient is aspirating, but rather to determine whether the patient can sustain him/herself nutritionally with oral intake alone.

ETIOLOGY

As one ages, dysphagia and aspiration during swallowing are more likely to occur (18,19). The primary explanations for these observations have been oral and pharyngeal motor dysfunctions, which include abnormal lingual activity, poor lingual-palatal seal, and pharyngeal pooling (18,20). While oropharyngeal motor dysfunction contributes to swallowing difficulties in the elderly, it has also been shown that oral cavity sensory discriminatory ability diminishes with advancing age (21,22). Over the past decade, laryngopharyngeal sensory capacity has been studied in the elderly and it has been demonstrated that airway protective capacity also diminishes as people get older. Specifically, as healthy individuals age there is a progressive increase in the stimuli required to elicit fundamental airway protective reflexes, with patients 61 years and older requiring significantly greater stimuli than those 60 and younger (23). Basic scientific data support the clinical observations that airway protective reflexes mediated by the superior laryngeal nerve (SLN) diminish in the elderly. The SLN provides afferent fibers to the hypopharyngeal tissues from the laryngeal surface of the epiglottis to the level of the true vocal folds. The changes in sensory nerve composition that take place with increasing age in the human SLN were examined in fresh cadavers. It was found that there is an extensive and statistically significant decrease in the number of sensory nerve fibers in subjects over 60 years of age (24).

While the healthy elderly develop a progressive diminution in both airway protective capacity and motor capabilities as they age, the unhealthy elderly, such as those that suffer from a stroke or progressive neuromuscular diseases, have even more of an assault to their airway protective capacity and muscular coordination (25–27). Studies evaluating sensory capacity of the laryngopharynx in supratentorial or brainstem stroke patients who presented with dysphagia showed that stroke patients had either unilateral or bilateral laryngopharyngeal sensory deficits (25). These sensory deficits were significantly greater than age-matched controls and contribute evidence that impairment of airway protective capacity contributes to dysphagia after stroke. The point of these studies is that in the elderly with swallowing problems, attention must be paid not only to how food moves from the lips to the esophagus, but how one senses the food in the upper aerodigestive tract.

DIAGNOSTIC TECHNIQUES

Swallowing difficulties in the elderly can be evaluated with two basic techniques: non-instrument-based methods and instrument-based methods. The non-instrument-based method is an office or bedside physical examination generally performed as an initial screening exam to determine symptoms and signs of a swallowing problem in the elderly individual. Because of the limited nature of reliable information obtainable without some type of instrumentation, a bedside evaluation is generally eschewed for an instrument-based exam (28–30).

The two primary means of assessing swallowing problems in the elderly with an instrument-based approach are video fluoroscopy, or X-ray-based tests, such as modified barium swallow (MBS) and barium swallow and video endoscopy-based tests such as fiber-optic endoscopic examination of swallowing (FEES), flexible endoscopic evaluation of swallowing with sensory testing (FEESST), and transnasal esophagoscopy (31–39). MBS, FEES, and FEESST give detailed information regarding the oropharyngeal and hypopharyngeal structures and physiology during the swallow. The barium swallow, or esophagram, and transnasal esophagoscopy are primarily focused on the esophagus and esophageal disease and really study a separate series of anatomic issues and concerns than MBS and FEESST.

Unlike the MBS, FEES and FEESST do not involve X-ray exposure, barium administration, or the presence of a radiologist or a radiology technician. Instead, FEES and FEESST involve endoscopy, and give direct evidence regarding the handling of secretions (40). Moreover, FEESST provides an objective assessment of hypopharyngeal sensitivity, which, in turn, gives the clinician information regarding a patient's ability to protect their airway during the ingestion of food. Like MBS, FEES and FEESST require the participation of a speech language pathologist, and are extremely useful in guiding the dietary and behavioral management of patients with difficulty swallowing.

The importance of sensation as it relates to swallowing and airway protection in healthy individuals has been recently and elegantly studied (41,42). The idea that sensation might be critical in the assessment of swallowing problems in stroke patients was first studied by Kidd et al. (43), who demonstrated that impaired pharyngeal sensation is related to the development of pneumonia after stroke. Kidd assessed pharyngeal sensation in a somewhat crude way with the tip of a stick applied to the oropharynx. A method and technique of measuring sensory discrimination was then developed, which circumvented the mouth by transnasal passage of a flexible endoscope to the laryngopharynx. Through a port in the endoscope, discrete air pulse stimuli were delivered to the mucosa innervated by the SLN in order to elicit the laryngeal adductor reflex, a brainstem-mediated, fundamental sensory-motor airway protective reflex (36,41,44). FEESST combines the elicitation of the laryngeal adductor reflex with food administration trials so that both the sensory and motor components of the swallow can be analyzed.

In the office, at the bedside, or even at the home setting, endoscopic swallowing evaluations are convenient, efficient ways to assess swallowing problems in the elderly (45). With the recent introduction of single-use, disposable endosheaths that can be applied to existing flexible laryngoscopes, thereby obviating the need to carry around potentially toxic scope cleaning agents (46,47), the portability of endoscopic swallowing evaluations makes it an ideal method to reach elderly individuals with impaired ability to ambulate. Furthermore, a prospective, randomized outcome study investigating whether FEESST or MBS was superior as the diagnostic test for evaluating and guiding the behavioral and dietary management of outpatients with dysphagia has shown that overall pneumonia incidence and pneumonia-free interval are essentially the same (48). The only difference in outcomes was seen in a small cohort of patients with stroke whose pneumonia incidence was less in those whose management was guided by FEESST.

There are two possible reasons for better outcomes in patients whose dietary and behavioral management was guided by FEESST versus MBS. One relates to the greater amount of time allowed for a FEESST relative to an MBS, so that patient fatigue and its sequelae are more readily identified and managed. Fatigue as a meal progresses is not unusual in the geriatric patient in general, and can be severely exacerbated after stroke. Patients with stroke have been shown to experience fatigue of the pharyngeal phase of swallowing as they progress through a meal (26,27). The other reason for the marked difference in stroke patient outcomes may be related to the fact that information regarding the sensory or afferent component of the swallow is rigorously assayed with FEESST while only indirectly addressed with MBS. As a result, the clinician using FEESST has a heightened awareness of potential aspiration and pneumonia risks that might otherwise have been overlooked.

TREATMENT

Nonsurgical

Current treatment of swallowing disorders in the elderly requires an understanding of both the sensory and motor systems of the swallowing mechanism. What the sensory test provides for the elderly patient with dysphagia is a guide to manage the patient's oral intake. For instance, if a patient is aspirating a small amount of material during the food administration trials of a FEESST examination but has an intact laryngeal adductor reflex, then the general goal should be to push oral intake, knowing that the patient's airway protective reflexes are functioning (Fig. 1). In contradistinction, if a patient is penetrating food particles into the endolarynx, not aspirating during the FEESST examination yet has an absent laryngeal adductor reflex (i.e., no response to continuous air pulse stimulation) then that patient is likely at risk for aspiration. Extreme caution should be used for such patients. Supervised feeding, temperature monitoring, and the use of a swallow–cough–swallow sequence may be necessary to keep the patient on an oral diet. Once a sensory assessment is completed, the assessment of motor control during the swallow can be made with accuracy and with a plan to improve swallow safety and oral intake.

The treatment of swallowing disorders in the elderly may include dietary modification or restriction, behavioral techniques to improve oral intake consisting of swallow postures and maneuvers, and medications or surgical intervention. For example, if a unilateral sensory deficit is found during sensory testing, a head turn to the sensory impaired side of the hypopharynx results in the less sensate portion of the hypopharynx being closed off to the incoming food bolus. The type of treatment depends on the cognitive status of the patient, their level of treatment involvement, the sensory and motor deficits identified in the swallow assessment, and the availability of rehabilitation support.

A general approach to dietary modification and restriction in the elderly is summarized in Table 1. The goals for the elderly are to facilitate oral transport, sense and slow down the oropharyngeal swallow and move the bolus through the esophageal phase of swallowing. Therapeutic intervention for swallowing disorders in the

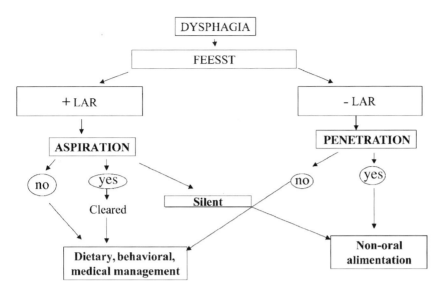

Figure 1 Algorithm for endoscopy-based diagnosis and management of dysphagia in the elderly. *Abbreviations*: FEESST, flexible endoscopic evaluation of swallowing with sensory testing; LAR, laryngeal adductor reflex.

elderly may also include various postural adjustments and maneuvers, which have been reported by Logeman et al. (49–52). Murry (53) has summarized therapeutic swallowing exercises in the elderly for lip strength and awareness, tongue strength and movement, and vocal fold closure and laryngeal elevation. Specific maneuvers to increase swallow safety and bolus propagation have also been developed and reviewed by Logeman (54).

Swallow rehabilitation in the elderly must always account for issues related to the patient's cognitive abilities; level of sensory awareness; medications; comorbid, anatomic, and neurologic conditions; and diseases and level of motivation (55). Diseases such as diabetes, hypertension, and renal or liver disease may require certain diets or nutritional loads that are not easily managed by the patient with a swallowing disorder. For example, patients with diabetes and a swallowing disorder who require high fluid intake may be at higher risk for aspiration than those diabetics with normal swallow function.

Additional concerns in the elderly exist when a patient is transferred to a nursing care facility. Increased risks of nutritional deficiencies, aspiration, and nosocomial infections have been reported in the elderly who reside in nursing care facilities (55,56). For these reasons, dietary management and nutrition must be monitored carefully. Conservative management and awareness of the level of supervision should be considered when devising a swallowing/nutrition plan for a patient who will be discharged to a long-term care facility.

Surgical Management

The surgical management of the elderly patient with dysphagia is limited and dependent upon the reason the patient has dysphagia. One of the most common surgically treatable etiologies of dysphagia in the elderly is a Zenker's diverticulum. While a diverticulectomy and cricopharyngeal myotomy via an open neck approach is

Table 1 Bolus, Size, Consistency, and Other Modifications Based on the Underlying Swallowing Problem

Problem	Proposed modifications	Avoid
Decreased sensation	Oral intake with extreme caution. Try cold or sour consistencies in small amounts. Use cough	Large boluses. Unsupervised meals or drinking thin liquids
Decreased tongue mobility	Thicken liquids. Place food on posterior tongue; clean oral cavity after meals	Thick, sticky, or dry foods
Decreased tongue coordination	Thicken liquids; clean oral cavity after meals	Thick, sticky, crumbly, or dry foods
Pharyngeal delay	Thicken liquids. Thick foods with single consistency; small bolus size	Thin liquids
Lack of laryngeal elevation	Thicken liquids. Combine diet modification with chin tuck; multiple swallows	Bolus with high viscosity
Cricopharyngeal dysfunction	Liquids; small boluses. Evaluate for myotomy or Botulinum toxin injection	Bolus with high viscosity
Reduced base of tongue movement	Thin liquids	Bolus with high viscosity
Vocal fold closure	Puree consistency. Use vocal fold adduction exercises	Thin liquids. Drinking any consistency with a straw or from bottle
Cognitive impairment	Remove distractions. Select single best bolus consistency and size	Unsupervised eating

readily performed in healthy patients, in the frail, debilitated elderly individual, diverticulopexy, combined with cricopharyngeal myotomy, may be preferable (57). With the diverticulopexy, the hernia sac is isolated and tacked with permanent suture to the prevertebral fascia, such that the mouth of the sac is in a dependent position (57). Diverticulopexy avoids a pharyngotomy, reducing the risk of a pharyngocutaneous fistula or injury to the recurrent laryngeal nerves.

Another surgical option for treatment of a Zenker's diverticulum in the elderly is endoscopic division of the party wall between the sac and the esophagus, performed via the mouth using specialized diverticuloscopes (58,59). Recent techniques employing an endoscopically applied enteric stapler have gained increasing acceptance, especially for elderly and ill patients in whom an open procedure might pose great risks (58).

Motility disorders of the esophagus are often seen in elderly patients, either in those with multiple systems atrophy after surgery or after stroke. Cricopharyngeal dilation and cricopharyngeal myotomy have been successful for treating disorders of the cricopharyngeus. Recently, Murry, Carrau, and Castillo reported on the success of injecting botulinum toxin into the cricopharyngeus muscle in the office. Their report of the procedure and long-term follow-up suggests that this procedure is an acceptable alternative to intraoperative myotomy or dilation (60).

In general, cricopharyngeal myotomy is primarily useful for true cricopharyngeal achalasia such as after vagus nerve injury at the base of the skull where pharyngeal motor function remains otherwise intact (61,62). Cricopharyngeal myotomy is contraindicated in conditions when there is impaired pharyngeal peristalsis such as advanced amyotrophic lateral sclerosis and scleroderma (63). In many disease entities such as myopathy and brainstem stroke, where cricopharyngeal myotomy was thought to be useful in improving dysphagia, the procedure is of no benefit (61).

In clinical situations where elderly individuals are continually contaminating their upper airways with food and saliva, there are surgical measures to divert debris from the airway. In patients with vocal fold weakness as the etiology of their repeated aspiration, injection laryngoplasty can be performed under local anesthesia as a means of enhancing mechanical closure of the vocal folds (64). Other procedures include tracheotomy, laryngeal stents, reversible laryngeal closure procedures, laryngotracheal separation, and total laryngectomy (65–68). Clearly, the decision to have an elderly individual undergo a surgical procedure to prevent aspiration must take into account a myriad of social and medical factors that require intense discussion with the patient, family, and caregivers.

In those elderly individuals who are becoming malnourished as a result of swallowing problems, the issue of gastrostomy tubes must be discussed. Endoscopically placed gastrostomy or jejunostomy tubes are safe ways to immediately provide nutritional support for patients who are unable to sustain themselves with oral intake alone. While the technical details of gastrostomy are straightforward, the social and medical issues involved in this type of decision making are complex at best and often need to be addressed on a case by case basis.

SUMMARY

Early intervention and appropriate management of the elderly patient with a swallowing disorder, especially those patients in nursing homes, provides nutritional, rehabilitative, and social benefits to patients, their families, and their friends. In all cases of elderly with swallowing disorders, the first concern is swallow safety, which begins with the functional assessment of the sensory and motor components of swallowing. The otolaryngologist who treats elderly patients must always follow a protocol of treatment ranging from conservative nutritional, behavioral, and swallowing rehabilitative techniques to properly selecting nonoral nutritional management. This may be with a feeding tube or with surgical management to reduce or eliminate the risk of aspiration.

REFERENCES

1. Zamir Z, Ren J, Hogan W, Shaker R. Coordination of deglutitive vocal cord closure and oral-pharyngeal swallowing events in the elderly. Eur J Gastro Hepatol 1996; 8:425–429.
2. Veis S, Logemann J. Swallowing disorders in persons with cerebral vascular accident. Arch Phys Med Rehabil 1985; 66:372–375.
3. Horner J, Massey EW, Riski JE, Lathrop DL, Chase KN. Aspiration following stroke: clinical correlates and outcome. Neurology 1988; 38:1359–1362.
4. Brown M, Glassenberg M. Mortality factors in patients with acute stroke. JAMA 1983; 224:1493–1495.

5. Scmidt EV, Smirnov VE, Ryabova VS. Results of the seven year prospective study of stroke patients. Stroke 1988; 19:1942–1949.

6. Schmidt J, Holas M, Halvorson K, Reding M. Video-fluoroscopic evidence of aspiration predicts pneumonia but not dehydration following stroke. Dysphagia 1994; 9:7–11.

7. Martin BJW, Corlew MM, Wood H, et al. The association of swallowing dysfunction and aspiration pneumonia. Dysphagia 1994; 9:1–6.

8. Johnson ER, McKenzie SW, Sievers A. Aspiration pneumonia in stroke. Arch Phys Med Rehab 1993; 74:973–976.

9. Holas MA, DePippo KL, Reding MJ. Aspiration and relative risk of medical complications following stroke. Arch Neurol 1994; 51:1051–1053.

10. Smithard DG, O'Neill PA, Park C, et al. Complications and outcome after acute stroke. Does dysphagia matter? Stroke 1996; 27:1200–1204.

11. Marrie TJ, Durant H, Kwan C. Nursing home-acquired pneumonia. J Am Geriatr Soc 1986; 34:697–702.

12. Norman DC, Castle SC, Cantrell M. Infections in the nursing home. J Am Geriatr Soc 1987; 35:796–805.

13. Alvarez S, Shell CG, Woolley TW, Berk SL, Smith JK. Nosocomial infections in long-term facilities. J Gerontol 1988; 43:M9–M17.

14. Back-Sague C, Villarino E, Giuliano D, et al. Infectious diseases and death among nursing home residents: results of surveillance in 13 nursing homes. Infect Control Hosp Epidemiol 1994; 15:494–496.

15. Scheckler WE, Peterson PJ. Infections and infection control among residents of eight rural Wisconsin nursing homes. Arch Int Med 1986; 146:1981–1984.

16. Hoffman N, Jenkins R, Putney K. Nosocomial infection rates during a one-year period in a nursing home care unit of a Veterans Administration hospital. Am J Infect Control 1990; 18:55–63.

17. Boyce JM, Potter-Boyne G, Dziobek L, Solomon SL. Nosocomial pneumonia in medicare patients: hospital costs and reimbursement under the prospective payment system. Arch Int Med 1991; 151:1109–1114.

18. Feinberg MJ, Ekberg O. Videofluoroscopy in elderly patients with aspiration: importance of evaluating both oral and pharyngeal stages of deglutition. AJR 1991; 156: 293–296.

19. Zavala DC. The threat of aspiration pneumonia in the aged. Geriatrics 1977; 32:46–51.

20. Feinberg MJ, Knebl J, Tully J. Prandial aspiration and pneumonia in an elderly population followed over 3 years. Dysphagia 1996; 11:104–109.

21. Aviv JE, Hecht C, Weinberg H, Dalton JF, Urken ML. Surface sensibility of the floor of mouth and tongue in healthy controls and radiated patients. Otolaryngol Head Neck Surg 1992; 107:418–423.

22. Calhoun KH, Gibson B, Hartley L, Minton J, Hokanson JA. Age-related changes in oral sensation. Laryngoscope 1992; 102:109–116.

23. Aviv JE, Martin JH, Jones ME, et al. Age related changes in pharyngeal and supraglottic sensation. Ann Otol Rhinol Laryngol 1994; 103:749–752.

24. Mortelliti AJ, Malmgren LT, Gacek RR. Ultrastructural changes with age in the human superior laryngeal nerve. Arch Otolaryngol Head Neck Surg 1990; 116:1062–1068.

25. Aviv JE, Martin JH, Sacco RL, et al. Supraglottic and pharyngeal sensory abnormalities in stroke patients with dysphagia. Ann Otol Rhinol Laryngol 1996; 105:92–97.

26. Hamdy S, Aziz Q, Rothwell JC, et al. Explaining oropharyngeal dysphagia after unilateral hemispheric stroke. Lancet 1997; 350:686–692.

27. Hamdy S, Aziz Q, Rothwell JC, et al. The cortical topography of human swallowing musculature in health and disease. Nat Med 1996; 11:1217–1224.

28. Leder SB, Espinosa JF. Aspiration risk after acute stroke: comparison of clinical examination and fiberoptic endoscopic evaluation of swallowing. Dysphagia 2002; 17(3): 214–218.

29. Aviv JE. The bedside swallowing evaluation when endoscopy is an option: what would you choose? Dysphagia 2002; 17:219.

30. Splaingard M, Hutchins B, Sulton L, Chaudhuri G. Aspiration in rehabilitation patients: videofluoroscopy vs. bedside clinical assessment. Arch Phys Med Rehabil 1988; 69: 637–640.

31. McConnel FMS, Cerenko D, Hersh T, Weil LJ. Evaluation of pharyngeal dysphagia with manofluorography. Dysphagia 1988; 2:187–195.

32. Logemann JE. Evaluation and Treatment of Swallowing Disorders. San Diego: College Hill Press, 1983:214–227.

33. Langmore SE, Schatz K, Olsen N. Fiberoptic endoscopic examination of swallowing safety: a new procedure. Dysphagia 1988; 2:216–219.

34. Bastian RW. Videoendoscopic evaluation of patients with dysphagia: an adjunct to modified barium swallow. Otolaryngol Head Neck Surg 1991; 104:339–350.

35. Hiss SG, Postma GN. Fiberoptic endoscopic evaluation of swallowing. Laryngoscope 2003; 113(8):1386–1393.

36. Setzen M, Cohen MA, Mattucci KF, Perlman PW, Ditkoff MK. Laryngopharyngeal sensory deficits as a predictor of aspiration. Otolaryngol Head Neck Surg 2001; 124:622–624.

37. Aviv JE, Johnson LF. Flexible endoscopic evaluation of swallowing with sensory testing (FEESST) to diagnose and manage patients with pharyngeal dysphagia. Practical Gastro 2000; 24:52–59.

38. Belafsky PC, Postma GN, Daniel E, Koufman JA. Transnasal esophagoscopy. Otolaryngol Head Neck Surg 2001; 125:588–589.

39. Aviv JE, Takoudes T, Ma G, Close LG. Office-based esophagoscopy—a preliminary report. Otolaryngol Head Neck Surg 2001; 125:170–175.

40. Murray J, Langmore SE, Ginsberg S, Dostie A. The significance of accumulated oropharyngeal secretions and swallowing frequency in predicting aspiration. Dysphagia 1996; 11:99–103.

41. Jafari S, Prince RA, Kim DK, Paydarfar D. Sensory regulation of swallowing and airway protection: a role for the internal superior laryngeal nerve in humans. J Physiol 2003; 550:287–304.

42. Sulica L, Hembree A, Blitzer A. Sensation and swallowing: endoscopic evaluation of deglutition in the anesthetized larynx. Ann Otol Rhinol Laryngol 2002; 111:291–294.

43. Kidd D, Lawson J, Macmahon J. Aspiration in acute stroke: a clinical study with videofluoroscopy. Q J Med 1993; 86:825–829.

44. Aviv JE, Martin JH, Kim T, et al. Laryngopharyngeal sensory discrimination testing and the laryngeal adductor reflex. Ann Otol Rhinol Laryngol 1999; 108:725–730.

45. Spiegel JR, Selber JC, Creed J. A functional diagnosis of dysphagia using videoendoscopy. ENT J 1998; 77:8–11.

46. Silberman HD. Non-inflatable sheath for introduction of the flexible nasopharyngolaryngoscope. Ann Otol Rhinol Laryngol 2201; 110:385–387.

47. Srinivasan A, Wolfenden LL, Song X, et al. An outbreak of *Pseudomonas aeruginosa* infections associated with flexible bronchoscopes. NEJM 2003; 348:221–227.

48. Aviv JE. Prospective, randomized outcome study of endoscopy versus modified barium swallow in patients with dysphagia. Laryngoscope 2000; 110:563–574.

49. Logemann JA. Speech and swallowing rehabilitation for head and neck tumor patients. In: Myers EN, Suen J, eds. Cancer of the Head and Neck. 2nd ed. New York: Churchill Livingston, 1997:1021–1043.

50. Logeman JA, Kahrilas PJ, Kobara M, Vakil N. The benefit of head rotation on pharyngoesophageal dysphagia. Arch Phys Med Rehab 1989; 70:767–771.

51. Welch M, Logeman JA, Rademaker AW, Kaharilas P. Change in pharyngeal dimensions effected by chin tuck. Arch Phys Med Rehab 1993; 74:178–181.

52. Mendelsohn MS. New concepts in dysphagia management. J Otolaryngol 1993; 22 (suppl 1):9.

53. Murry T. Therapeutic intervention for swallowing disorders. In: Carrau RL, Murry T, eds. Comprehensive Management of Swallowing Disorders. San Diego: Singular Publishing Group, 1999:243–248.

54. Logeman JA. Therapy for oropharyngeal swallowing disorders. In: Pearlman AL, Schultz-Delrieu K, eds. Deglutition and Its Disorders. San Diego: Singular Publishing Group, 1997:449–462.

55. Sullivan DH, Walls RC. Impact on nutritional status on morbidity in a population of geriatric rehabilitation patients. J Am Gerontol Soc 1994; 42:471–477.

56. Pick, McDonald A, Bennett N, et al. Pulmonary aspiration in a long term care setting; clinical and laboratory observations and an analysis of risk factors. J Am Gerontol Soc 1996; 44:763–768.

57. Laccourreye O, Menard M, Cauchois R, Huart J, Brasnk D, Laccourreye H. Esophageal diverticulum: diverticulopexy versus diverticulectomy. Laryngoscope 1994; 104:889–892.

58. Scher RL, Richtsmeier WJ. Endoscopic staple-assisted esophagodiverticulostomy for Zenker's diverticulum. Laryngoscope 1996; 106:951–956.

59. Van Overbeek JJM. Meditation on the pathogenesis of hypopharyngeal (Zenker's) diverticulum and a report of endoscopic treatment in 545 patients. Ann Otol Rhinol Laryngol 1994; 103:178–185.

60. Murry T, Wasserman TL, Carrau RL, Castillo B. Injection of Botulinum A for the treatment of dysfunction of the upper esophageal sphincter. Laryngoscope 2004, in press.

61. Wisdom G, Blitzer A. Surgical therapy for swallowing disorders. Otol Clin North Am 1998; 31:537–560.

62. Pou AM. Surgical treatment of swallowing disorders: cricopharyngeal myotomy. In: Carrau RL, Murry T, eds. Comprehensive Management of Swallowing Disorders. San Diego, CA.: Singular Publishing Group, Inc., 1999.

63. Lebo CP, Sang K, Norris FH. Cricopharyngeal myotomy in amyotrophic lateral sclerosis. Laryngoscope 1976; 86:862–868.

64. Chu PY, Chang SY. Transoral teflon injection under flexible laryngovideostroboscopy for unilateral vocal fold paralysis. Ann Otol Rhinol Laryngol 1997; 106(9):783–786.

65. Eliachar I, Nguyen D. Laryngotracheal stent for internal support and control of aspiration without loss of phonation. Otolaryngol Head Neck Surg 1990; 103:837–840.

66. Castellanos PF. Method and clinical results of a new transthyrotomy closure of the supraglottic larynx for the treatment of intractable aspiration. Ann Otol Rhinol Laryngol 1997; 106:451–460.

67. Lindeman RC, Yarington CT, Sutter D. Clinical experience with the tracheoesophageal anastomosis for intractable aspiration. Ann Otol Rhinol Laryngol 1976; 85:609–613.

68. Cannon CR, McClean WC. Laryngectomy for chronic aspiration. Am J Otolaryngol 1982; 3:145–149.

28

Xerostomia in the Elderly

Karen M. Kost
*Department of Otolaryngology, McGill University, Montreal General Hospital,
Montreal, Quebec, Canada*

INTRODUCTION

Xerostomia, or dry mouth, is the abnormal reduction of saliva. Normal salivary
function plays an important role in the maintenance and preservation of several
bodily functions. It is well known that salivary fluids facilitate food breakdown
and bolus formation, and enhance taste by diffusing food particles to tongue papillae. Saliva also acts as a buffer to acids from both external and internal environments. Finally, salivary fluids participate in the preservation, protection, and
repair of oral mucosal tissues, remineralization of teeth, and the modulation of viral,
fungal, and bacterial populations (1). Individuals with reduced salivary output from
whatever reason are much more prone to dental caries, oral mucositis (e.g., candidiasis),
dysphagia, oral infections, and altered taste (2).

PHYSIOLOGY

The average individual produces at least 500 mL of saliva over a 24-hour period.
Salivary flow rates vary substantially during a 24-hour period as a function of
demand and/or patient status. The resting (unstimulated) flow rate is 0.3 mL/min,
decreasing to 0.1 mL/min during sleep, and increasing to 4.0–5.0 mL/min while
eating or chewing (3). Saliva is hypotonic to plasma, with sodium and chloride concentrations lower than those of plasma. As the secretory flow rate increases, so does the
tonicity of saliva. Salivary gland secretion is principally under autonomic control,
although a number of influences, including hormones, may modulate function either
through a cyclic adenosine monophosphate or calcium-dependent pathway (3).

Saliva consists of two components secreted by independent mechanisms. The
first component is fluid in nature, and includes ions produced by parasympathetic
stimulation. The second component is a protein arising from secretory vesicles in
acini and released in response to sympathetic stimulation. Although excitation of
both sympathetic and parasympathetic nerves stimulates salivary flow, the effects
of the parasympathetic nerves are more pronounced and longer-lasting. In general,
parasympathetic stimulation produces copious saliva of low protein concentration,

whereas sympathetic stimulation produces little saliva with a high protein concentration, which on occasion may give a sensation of dryness (3).

Histomorphometric examinations of "normal" salivary gland tissue have revealed age-associated decreases in the number of acinar cells and as such a gradual loss in reserve capacity (4). Although it was originally thought that salivary function declined with age, results of cross-sectional and longitudinal studies have shown that parotid salivary function in healthy individuals is generally age-independent (5–12). This indicates a large "reserve capacity" allowing for normal salivary function in the presence of nonpathologic, "normal" aging changes (13). Physiologically stressful circumstances strain this reserve capacity, thereby hindering its ability to compensate for increased metabolic demand, resulting in compromised function (14). In the presence of acute and/or chronic stress, functional decline occurs more quickly and recovery takes longer in the older population (15). A study was done by Ghezzi and Ship in 2003 (15) comparing responses of the major salivary glands in young (age 20–38) and older (age 60–77) healthy subjects to anticholinergics. The results indicated that salivary gland output was significantly more adversely affected in healthy older subjects. Dry mouth is a common complaint in the elderly. In a Swedish study involving 1148 subjects over the age of 70, 16% of men and 25% of women reported symptoms of a dry mouth. In a study by Pajukoski et al. (16), the incidence of subjective xerostomia was high for both outpatients (57%) and hospitalized patients (63%). In the latter group, the complaint is significantly associated with the use of medications. Interestingly, these symptoms often occur in the presence of normal measured salivary flow rates (17,18). Subjective complaints of dry mouth have also been noted in a high proportion of diabetics and postmenopausal women in the presence of normal objectively measured salivary flow rates (19–21). While the reasons for this discrepancy between symptoms and objective findings are unclear, it has been proposed that qualitative changes in salivary composition and/or changes in mucosal sensory receptors may play a role. Dentate status is not associated with a complaint of xerostomia (16).

ETIOLOGY

Several medical conditions, medications (e.g., chemotherapy, diuretics), and other treatments such as radiotherapy to the head and neck may contribute to salivary gland dysfunction in elderly subjects (2,22–25). The causes of long-standing xerostomia are summarized in Table 1. Of these, the most common cause of xerostomia is related to medication use; a partial list of these drugs is found in Table 2.

Iatrogenic

Drugs

Over 500 different medications are associated with xerostomia. Many of these may potentiate each other's drying effect in a synergistic fashion, which is particularly problematic in the elderly, who tend to be on multiple medications, and are at risk for xerostomia (26). There is normally a recognizable temporal relationship between the development of xerostomia and initiation of medication and/or increasing the dose. The principal mechanism of drug-induced xerostomia is an anticholinergic or sympathomimetic action. Examples include tricyclic antidepressants,

Table 1 Etiology of Xerostomia

Iatrogenic
    Medications
    Radiotherapy to the head and neck
    Chemotherapy
Conditions of the salivary glands
    Sjogren's syndrome
    Sarcoidosis
    HIV salivary gland disease
    Hepatitis C
    Primary biliary cirrhosis
    Diabetes mellitus
Other
    Amyloidosis
    Hemochromatosis
    Wegener's syndrome

antipsychotics, benzodiazepines, atropinics, beta-blockers, and antihistamines. More recent drugs such as omeprazole, anti-human immunodeficiency virus (HIV) protease inhibitors, the nucleoside analog HIV reverse transcriptase inhibitor didanosine, trospium chloride, elliptinium, tramadol, and new-generation antihistamines may all be responsible for drug-induced xerostomia (3).

Some medications such as hydralazine, busulfan, quinidine sulphate, and thiabendazole can induce a Sjogren-like illness, which is transient in nature and is not associated with the typical immunologic markers.

Radiation

Although all salivary tissues are at risk for radiation damage, the parotid glands are particularly vulnerable. The degree of xerostomia depends on the extent of salivary

Table 2 Medications Causing Xerostomia

Medications with anticholinergic effects
    Antimuscarinics (e.g., atropine)
    Tricyclic antidepressants
    Serotonin reuptake inhibitors
    Antihistamines
    Antiemetics
    Antipsychotics
Medications with sympathomimetic effects
    Decongestants
    Bronchodilators
    Appetite suppressants
    Amphetamines
Other
    Lithium
    Omeprazole
    Oxybutinin
    Disopyramide
    Diuretics
    Protease inhibitors

gland exposure. A single dose as low as 20 Gy can cause permanent damage; doses above 52 Gy are associated with severe salivary dysfunction. Radiation therapy is commonly used in the treatment of head and neck carcinomas, with total doses of 60–70 Gy. The result is complete cessation of salivary flow by five weeks, with, at best, partial recovery, which is maximal by one year post-treatment.

Unilateral fields of radiation are associated with an approximate reduction in salivary flow of 50%, while bilateral fields are linked to an 80% reduction in flow. More recent cone radiation techniques narrow the radiation field to one side, thereby preserving contralateral function.

Chemotherapy

Xerostomia is a common and distressing symptom in patients treated with either chemotherapy alone or in combination with radiotherapy (27). The severity is associated with the total number of drugs used, and correlates with the severity of oral discomfort, dysgeusia, dysphagia, and dysphonia. Examples of chemotherapeutic agents used in the treatment of head and neck cancer include paclitaxel, carboplatin, and 5-fluorouracil.

Disorders of the Salivary Glands

Sjogren's Syndrome

Sjogren's syndrome (SS) is a chronic multisystem immune-mediated disorder characterized by inflammation of exocrine glands resulting in frequently severe clinical symptoms of dryness, particularly to the eyes and mouth (Table 3). It is the second most common autoimmune connective tissue disorder. The eye and mouth symptoms are caused by profound lymphocytic infiltration of the salivary and lacrimal glands.

Primary SS is characterized by signs and symptoms affecting only the eyes and mouth. It is frequently associated with B-cell hyper-reactivity manifested by hypergammaglobulinemia and anti-Ro or anti-La autoantibodies. Secondary SS is characterized by xerostomia, xerophthalmia, and an associated connective tissue disorder, most often rheumatoid arthritis or systemic lupus erythematosis.

Table 3 Clinical Manifestations of Sjogren's Syndrome

Fatigue; normocytic anemia
Sicca complex; xerophthalmia and xerostomia
Rheumatoid arthritis and other connective tissue diseases
Salivary gland enlargement
Polymyopathy
Neuropathy
Central nervous system disease
Chronic liver disease
Chronic pulmonary disease
Lymphoma
Purpura; hyperglobulinemia; vasculitis
Cryoglobulinemia; macroglobulinemia

Source: From Ref. 3.

Criteria required to make the diagnosis include the subjective symptoms of dry eyes and dry mouth, as well as the following objective findings: (i) positive Schirmer's test or elevated rose Bengal dye score, (ii) focal lymphocytic sialadenitis, (iii) salivary gland involvement by salivary scintigraphy, and (iv) presence of Ro/Sjogren's syndrome antigen (SSA) and/or La/Sjogren's syndrome B antibody (SSB) autoantibodies.

Sarcoidosis

Xerostomia and salivary gland enlargement may affect up to 9% of patients with sarcoidosis, usually in the context of Heerfordt's syndrome, which is characterized by uveitis, parotid swelling, and facial neeve paralysis (28). Sarcoidosis may be distinguished from SS based on clinical, laboratory, and histopathologic findings. Patients with sarcoidosis usually have pulmonary and skin involvement, elevated levels of angiotensin-converting enzyme, and on minor salivary gland biopsy demonstrate non-caseating granulomas. Patients with SS demonstrate elevated autoantibodies and focal lymphocitic sialadenitis on minor salivary gland biopsy.

HIV Disease

HIV salivary gland disease (HIV-SGD) most frequently affects the parotid glands and is characterized by recurrent or persistent salivary gland enlargement and xerostomia. HIV-SGD may present a clinical picture similar to SS, but may be distinguished from the latter by the lack anti-Ro and anti-La autoantibodies, and the presence of CD8 T-cell infiltrates on minor salivary gland biopsies.

Hepatitis C Virus Infection

In contradistinction to hepatitis A and B infections, hepatitis C may be associated with salivary gland disease and xerostomia in up to 10% to 33% of patients (29). Minor salivary gland biopsy demonstrates a lymphocytic infiltrate with a predominance of CD20-positive cells.

Other Causes

Other unusual causes of xerostomia include primary biliary cirrhosis, diabetes mellitus, salivary gland agenesis, amyloidosis, and hemochromatosis.

CLINICAL CONSEQUENCES OF XEROSTOMIA

It is clear from Table 4 that the effects of prolonged xerostomia are multiple and significant. Results of quality-of-life assessments in patients with xerostomia have indicated a reduced quality of life compared with healthy individuals, underscoring the impact and importance of this symptom. In the elderly, who frequently suffer from additional comorbidities, the effect is even more pronounced, and may compound swallowing and nutrition problems.

THE WORK UP OF XEROSTOMIA

Arriving at the correct diagnosis begins with a thorough history followed by a complete physical examination. This allows the investigations to be directed toward

Table 4 Effects of Xerostomia

Increased tendency to dental caries
Increased risk of gingivitis
Dysarthria
Dysphagia
Dysgeusia
Laryngopharyngeal reflux
Candidal infections; stomatitis, angular cheilitis
Oral mucosal sensitivity
Dry, tender, cracked lips

a focused differential diagnosis. In the elderly, it is particularly important to inquire about the past medical history, and use of prescription and over-the-counter medications, as well as the use of tobacco and alcohol. A history of radiation to the head and neck indicates that the xerostomia is permanent, while the presence of autoimmune disease such as rheumatoid arthritis or systemic lupus erythematosis may suggest the presence of Sjogren's syndrome. Tobacco is an irritant and has a desiccating effect on oral mucosa, and should be discouraged. A host of medications, including diuretics (for hypertension or congestive heart failure) and antihistamines are commonly used medications in the elderly, and frequently contribute to xerostomia. A gradual onset indicates a slowly evolving process, while an acute onset may be temporally related to a new medication.

A complete examination focused on the head and neck may reveal clues as to the underlying etiology. The salivary glands should be carefully examined, looking for signs of enlargement, obstruction, previous surgery, or infection. Objective evidence of xerostomia and xerophthalmia should be sought.

Investigations required may include blood work (hematology, biochemistry, immunology), imaging, and histopathology. A complete blood count indicating anemia and an elevated erythrocyte sedimentation rate may be nonspecific findings associated with chronic disease. Angiotensin-converting-enzyme levels may be elevated in sarcoidosis. Patients with SS may have positive/elevated levels of rheumatoid factor, antinuclear antibodies, anti-Ro and anti-La antibodies, antiphospholipid antibodies, and abnormal thyroid function tests.

Sialography demonstrates ductal structure and sialectasis, while salivary scintigraphy shows function; both may be useful for the diagnosis of SS. Ultrasound, computed tomography, and magnetic resonance imaging may all illustrate structural details indicative of SS. Gallium scans may be useful in the diagnosis of sarcoidosis. Histopathology may be extremely helpful in distinguishing SS (lymphocytic infiltrate) from sarcoidosis (non-caseating granulomas), lymphomas (lymphoplasmacytic infiltrate), HIV (CD8+ T lymphocytes), and amyloidosis (amyloid protein deposit). Ophthalmology tests such as Schirmer's and rose Bengal staining are specifically useful in the diagnosis of SS.

MANAGEMENT OF XEROSTOMIA

The paucity of randomized, controlled trials, and the use of different, unvalidated measures of disease assessment and outcome is such that evaluation of success of available treatments of xerostomia is difficult at best.

Management of xerostomia in the elderly consists of addressing causative factors (underlying illness, medications) when possible, and preventing complications related to the disorder. Patients must be carefully instructed as to proper and meticulous oral hygiene, which includes dental flossing and brushing as well as regular visits to the oral hygienist. Daily use of chlorhexidine or fluoride mouthwashes may help minimize the risk of caries. Xerostomia frequently results in dysphonia from lack of lubrication of the vocal folds and exposure to acid reflux. Aggressive vocal hygiene consisting of adequate hydration, smoking cessation, avoiding vocal abuse, and an antireflux diet with or without medication may eliminate these sequelae of xerostomia. Preventative measures and treatment options are summarized in Table 5.

ORAL CARE—TOPICAL AGENTS

Salivary substitutes may provide short-term symptom relief by improving lubrication of the oral cavity. However, they lack the protective effect of saliva. Lubricating agents in the form of gels, mouthwashes, and lozenges have been used with varying results. In the elderly, compliance increases as a function of taste, duration of action, the delivery system, severity of symptoms, and cost (30). Salivary substitutes administered through a "slow-release" intraoral device may provide longer benefits. In one study, a mucin spray was found to be particularly helpful in elderly patients with prior radiation to the head and neck (31). Sugar-free gum, candies, and/or lozenges are inexpensive, easy to use, and may stimulate salivary output. The above therapies may also be used in combination and tailored to patients' needs and preferences.

ORAL CARE—SYSTEMIC AGENTS

Cholinergic Agonists

Pilocarpine is a parasympathetic agonist of acetylcholine muscarinic M3 receptors. It stimulates secretion by exocrine glands such as the salivary, sweat, lacrimal, and

Table 5 Treatment of Xerostomia

Oral hygiene
    Regular dental visits, plaque control, brushing, and flossing
    Chlorhexidine or fluoride mouthwash
Antifungals
    Nystatin or amphotericin lozenges, miconazole gel
Topical saliva substitutes
    Sugar-free gum and candies
    Lubricating gels, mouthwashes, lozenges, and toothpaste
    Salivary stimulant pastilles
    Mucin spray
    Humidifiers
    Saliva substitute in intraoral device
Systemic therapies
    Pilocarpine
Cevimeline
Others

respiratory mucus glands. In addition, it promotes contraction of smooth muscle and enhances motility of the gastrointestinal and urinary tracts (32). Systemic pilocarpine is indicated in the management of xerostomia resulting from SS or head and neck radiation. Unfortunately, it is probably not effective in drug-induced xerostomia. Adverse effects associated with pilocarpine reflect its other cholinergic effects. These include sweating, headache, nausea, mild abdominal pain, gastrointestinal upset, urinary frequency, chills, rhinitis, flushing, excessive lacrimation, and palpitations. Despite this impressive list, it is generally safe and well tolerated, with no serious drug interactions. It should be avoided in patients suffering from respiratory conditions such asthma, chronic bronchitis, and chronic obstructive pulmonary disease.

The optimal dose of pilocarpine is 5 mg orally four times daily or 10 mg given three times daily. Clinical response can vary significantly among patients, and there is no way of predicting who will respond best. Pilocarpine increases salivary flow from the major salivary glands, and also enhances minor salivary gland function.

Cevimeline

Cevimeline is an acetylcholine analog with a high affinity for M3 muscarinic receptors of both lacrimal and salivary glands (33). It is less well known than pilocarpine and has been less well studied. At a dosage of 30 mg orally three times daily, cevimeline has been shown to increase salivary flow and improve both the subjective and objective symptoms of xerostomia. Adverse effects associated with cevimeline are similar to those described for pilocarpine.

OTHER TREATMENTS

A number of other drugs including carbacholine, anethole trithone, pyridostigmine, bromhexene, and hydroxychloroquine have been proposed as possible treatments for xerostomia, but all remain unproven.

Preliminary studies have shown that alpha interferon, administered as an oral lozenge, may increase salivary flow without the adverse effects associated with systemic therapy (34). Further study in this area is needed to define the possible benefits of this drug.

Electrostimulation, acupuncture, and dietary supplements have all been suggested in the treatment of xerostomia, but further study is required to establish what, if any, role these modalities play.

SUMMARY

Xerostomia is a frequent problem in the elderly. In otherwise healthy individuals, it is associated with substantial morbidity, giving rise to dental caries, dysphagia, and dysphonia. In the elderly with comorbidities, xerostomia may compound these problems and exacerbate poor nutrition, swallowing difficulties, and hoarseness. Diagnosis begins with a good history and physical exam, followed by appropriately directed testing. Treatment is directed at correcting the underlying problem when possible, and identifying and changing drugs, which may be responsible for the problem. Medical therapy consists primarily of local measures such as adequate hydration, sialogogues, sugar-free gum, salivary substitutes, and lubricants. When these steps are insufficient, a trial of cholinergic agonist medications may be warranted.

REFERENCES

1. Mandel JD. The role of saliva in maintaining oral homeostasis. J Am Dent Assoc 1989; 119:298–304.
2. Atkinson JC, Wu A. Salivary gland dysfunction: causes, symptoms, treatment. J Am Dent Assoc 1994; 125:409–416.
3. Porter SR, Scully C, Hegarty AM. An update of the etiology and management of xerostomia. Oral Surg Oral Med Oral Pathol Oral Radiol Endod 2004; 97:28–46.
4. Scott J, Flower EA, Burns J. A quantitative study of histological changes in the human parotid gland occurring with adult age. J Oral Pathol 1987; 16:505–510.
5. Baum BJ. Evaluation of stimulated parotid saliva flow rate in different age groups. J Dent Res 1981; 60:1292–1296.
6. Heft MW, Baum BJ. Unstimulated and stimulated parotid salivary flow rate in individuals of different ages. J Dent Res 1984; 63:1182–1185.
7. Aguirre A, Levine MJ, Cohen RE, et al. Immunochemical quantitation of alpha-amylase and secretory IgA in parotid saliva from people of various ages. Arch Oral Biol 1987; 32:297–301.
8. Percival RS, Challacombe SJ, Marsh PD. Flow rates of resting whole and stimulated parotid saliva in relation to age and gender. J Dent Res 1994; 73:1416–1420.
9. Challacombe SJ, Percival RS, Marsh PD. Age-related changes in immunoglobulin isotypes in whole and parotid saliva and serum in healthy individuals. Oral Microbiol Immunol 1995; 10:202–207.
10. Ship JA, Baum BJ. Is reduced salivary flow normal in old people? Lancet 1990; 336:1507.
11. Wu AJ, Atkinson JC, Fox PC, et al. Cross-sectional and longitudinal analyses of stimulated parotid salivary constituents in healthy, different aged subjects. J Gerontol Med Sci 1993; 48:M219–M224.
12. Ship JA, Nolan N, Puckett S. Longitudinal analysis of parotid and submandibular salivary flow rates in healthy, different aged adults. Gerontol Med Sci 1995; 50A: M285–M289.
13. Introduction. In: DiGiovanna AG, ed. Human Aging: Biological Perspectives. New York: McGraw-Hill, Inc., 1994:9.
14. Evers BM, Townsend CM, Thompson JC. Organ physiology of aging. Surg Clin North Am 1994; 74:23–39.
15. Ghezzi EM, Ship JA. Aging and secretory reserve capacity of major salivary glands. J Dent Res 2003; 82:844–848.
16. Pajukoski H, Meurman JH, Halonen P, et al. Prevalence of subjective dry mouth and burning mouth in hospitalized elderly patients and outpatients in relation to saliva, medication, and systemic diseases. Oral Surg Oral Med Oral Pathol Oral Radiol Endod 2001; 92:641–649.
17. Thompson WM, Chalmers JM, Spencer AJ, et al. The occurrence of xerostomia and salivary gland hypofunction in a population-based sample of older South Australians. Spec Care Dentist 1999; 19:20–23.
18. Närhi TO, Meurman JH, Ainamo A. Xerostomia and hyposalivation: causes, consequences, and treatment in the elderly. Drugs Aging 1999; 15:103–116.
19. Ben-Aryeh H, Serouya R, Kanter Y, et al. Oral health and salivary gland composition in diabetic patients. J Diabetic Comp 1993; 7:57–62.
20. Ben-Aryeh H, Miron D, Berdicevsky I, et al. Xerostomia in the elderly: diagnosis, complications and treatment. Gerodontology 1985; 4:77–82.

21. Ben-Aryeh H, Gottlieb I, Ish-Shalom S, et al. Oral complaints related to menopause. Maturitas 1996; 24:185–189.
22. Mandel JD. Sialochemistry in diseases and clinical situations affecting salivary glands. Crit Rev Clin Lab Sci 1980; 12:321–366.
23. Atkinson JC, Fox PC. Salivary gland dysfunction. Clin Geriatr Med 1992; 8:499–511.
24. Wu AJ, Ship JA. A characterization of major salivary gland flow rates in the presence of medications and systemic diseases. Oral Surg Oral Med Oral Pathol 1993; 76:301–306.
25. Sreebny LM, Schwartz SS. A reference guide to drugs and dry mouth. 2nd ed. Gerodontology. 1997:14:33–47.
26. Porter SR, Scully C. Adverse drug reactions in the mouth. Clin Dermatol 2000; 18: 525–532.
27. Pow EH, McMilan AS, Leung WK, et al. Salivary gland function and xerostomia in Southern Chinese following radiotherapy for nasopharyngeal carcinoma. Clin Oral Investig 2003; 7:230–234.
28. Ohtsuka S, Yanadori A, Tabata H, et al. Sarcoidosis with parotomegaly. Cutis 2001; 68:199–200.
29. Mariette X, Loiseau P, Morinet F. Hepatitis C virus in saliva. Ann Intern Med 1995; 122:556.
30. Epstein JB, Stevenson-Moore P. A clinical comparative trial of saliva substitutes and radiation-induced salivary gland hypofunction. Spec Care Dentist 1992; 12:21–23.
31. Momm F, Guttenberger R. Treatment of xerostomia following radiotherapy: does age matter? Support Care Cancer 2002; 10:505–508.
32. Ferguson MM. Pilocarpine and other cholinergic drugs in the management of salivary gland dysfunction. Oral Surg Oral Med Oral Pathol 1993; 75:186–191.
33. Iwabuchi Y, Masuhara T. Sialogogic activities of SN1-2011 compared with those of pilocarpine and McN-A-343 in rat salivary glands: identification of a potential therapeutic agent for treatment of Sjörgren's syndrome. Gen Pharmacol 1994; 25:123–129.
34. Ship JA, Fox PC, Michalek JE, et al. Treatment of primary Sjörgren's syndrome with low-dose natural human interferon-alpha administered by the oral mucosal route: a phase II clinical trial. IFN Protocol Study Group. J Interferon Cytokine Res 1999; 19:943–951.

29
Zenker's Diverticulum

Daniel H. Coelho, Douglas A. Ross, and Clarence T. Sasaki
Section of Otolaryngology, Yale University School of Medicine, New Haven, Connecticut, U.S.A.

GENERAL DESCRIPTION OF THE CLINICAL PROBLEM

Zenker's diveriticulum (ZD), the protrusion of esophageal mucosa through a defect in the hypopharyngeal wall, is among the most common causes of dysphagia in the elderly. The constellation of symptoms is nearly pathognomonic and radiographic findings are unmistakable. Treatment, although surgical, is trending toward less invasive techniques, making the cure available to both the elderly and infirm.

WHY IS ZENKER'S DIVERTICULUM PARTICULARLY IMPORTANT IN THE GERIATRIC POPULATION?

Age is undoubtedly a factor of importance in the pathogenesis of ZD. Rarely found in patients below 40 years old, it is generally assumed that the loss of tissue elasticity and decrease in muscle tone that occur during aging directly contribute to the formation of ZD.

Until recently, pharyngeal pouch surgery had long been associated with significant morbidity—due to the surgery itself and also to the high incidence of comorbidities in this typically geriatric patient population. However, recent advances in surgical techniques have made ZD a condition easily treated with low morbidity, low recurrence, and tremendous patient satisfaction.

BASIC SCIENCE

Historical Perspective

Ludlow first described the pharyngeal pouch in 1769. The author reported a posterior pharyngeal wall diverticulum in the postmortem examination of a patient who had complained of dysphagia. Yet, the eponym itself derives from an 1878 reclassification by Friedrich Albert Zenker, who along with Von Ziemssen described the clinical features so well that Zenker's name has since adhered to this disorder. Zenker and von Ziemssen (1) described a protrusion of pharyngeal mucosa on the dorsal wall, immediately proximal to the transition from hypopharynx into the esophagus. In 1908, Killian further characterized the site of herniation occurring between the thyropharyngeal and cricopharyngeal fibers of the inferior constrictor, which has since eponymously come to be known as Killian's triangle.

Pathology

Pharyngeal diverticuli may be posterior, posterolateral, or lateral. By far, the most commonly encountered type is the posterior pulsion diverticulum. This usually is through a single opening through a dehiscence of Killian's triangle, although the presence of a double pharyngeal pouch has been reported (2). The diverticuli can range in size from less than a centimeter to over 20 cm, with varying severity of symptomatology.

Although fairly rare, diverticular carcinoma has been described. A Mayo Clinic retrospective analysis of 1249 patients treated for ZD from 1932 to 1982 revealed six squamous cell carcinomas in the sac (3). van Overbeek (10) had a total of two patients with carcinoma in the sac in the series of 646 patients. Chronic irritation and inflammation of the diverticular wall as a result of food retention are factors believed to predispose to carcinoma in a diverticulum. Once carcinoma is formed in the sac, regurgitated food can often be blood-tinged. Filling defects on barium esophagram, such as loss of smooth contour of the interior of the pouch, usually due to retained food, can also point to the presence of carcinoma in the sac. Constant presence of a filling defect on radiographs taken at intervals would more strongly suggest the presence of a diverticular malignancy. When present, carcinoma usually forms at the lower end of the sac. Therefore, special care must be taken to clean and carefully examine the complete diverticulum prior to endoscopic repair.

Pathogenesis

No general consensus exists with regard to the exact pathogenesis of ZD. Patients usually experience coexistent gastroesophageal reflux disease, historically supported by convincing statistical association (4). However, a cause and effect relationship between these two remains unclear. There is now convincing evidence that patients with ZD demonstrate increased resting tone of the cricopharyngeus muscle (CPM) and that abnormally high CPM resting tone may be the primary factor contributing to ZD (5). It is also recognized, however, that there are many patients with increased CPM resting tone who never develop ZD. Is there the possibility that an important cofactor may provide increased risk for the development of ZD?

Studies have suggested that intraluminal acid perfusion in an opossum induces short-term esophageal long axis shortening, while others note that recurrent acid-induced injury produces permanent shortening of the esophagus (6–8). For those interested in hiatus hernia, this observation provides an attractive hypothesis implicating long axis shortening as the causative factor in the development of hiatus hernia as the stomach is pulled intrathoracically with shortening of the esophagus.

One could raise the possibility that a similar unifying hypothesis may be suggested for the development of ZD. The key to this hypothesis is the understanding that the CPM is a muscle unit that is continuous dorsally without a median raphe. On the other hand, pharyngeal constrictors immediately cephalad to it not only possess a median raphe, but are vertically anchored by it to the prevertebral fascia. The absence of an anchoring raphe in the CPM allows it to be displaced inferiorly away from the constrictors above it, as the esophagus undergoes long axis shortening (9). A developing gap between these structures readily allows herniation to occur in a high-pressured hypopharynx caudal to the constrictors but cephalad to the CPM, resulting in a typical ZD deformity that enlarges over time.

HISTORY

ZDs are most commonly seen in the sixth through ninth decades of life, with a mean age of 71.3 (10). It rarely occurs in patients under 40 years old. Males tend to outnumber females at approximately 1.5:1 (2). The estimated annual incidence of ZD is two per 100,000, although true incidence of the condition may be markedly higher, as many older patients with ZD may have minimal symptoms and/or thus do not seek medical advice (11,12). It is equally likely that referrals to surgeons may have previously been tempered by the higher rates of surgical complications using open rather than newer endoscopic techniques.

The constellation of symptoms seen in patients with ZD is so characteristic as to be virtually pathognomonic. ZD should be suspected in any patient who presents with some or all of the following symptoms: regurgitation of undigested food, dysphagia for solid food, borborygmi arising from the throat, choking spells, postprandial or nocturnal coughing attacks, globus sensation, halitosis, malnutrition, dehydration, and aspiration pneumonia. As the diveriticulum grows, it can compress the normal esophageal lumen immediately distal to it, increasing dysphagia by producing symptoms of obstruction. The duration of symptoms may range from a few weeks to many years.

Of interest is the relationship between medications and esophageal diverticuli. Langdon (13) described three sequelae of retained medications, not an insignificant problem in an elderly population disposed to polypharmacy. First, diverticular pH is usually slightly alkaline. During prolonged stasis, "enteric" coated medications can lose their coatings and subsequently become inactivated by gastric juices. Second, medications retained in the diverticulum do not enter the bloodstream at constant intervals. The levels of such medications could range from subtherapeutic to fatal. The implications for elderly patients on medications for diabetes, cardiac arrhythmias, seizure disorders, etc. could be devastating. Third, if stuck at any level, many medications can ulcerate the esophagus. As the esophagus has no serosa, prolonged stasis of these medications could put the patient at significant risk for perforation, mediastinitis, and death.

PHYSICAL EXAMINATION

Physical examination in ZD is usually unremarkable. Occasionally, manual compression of the neck may elicit a gurgling sensation or crepitus in some patients. Rarely, ZD can present as a compressible neck mass.

One report has discussed the efficacy of flexible laryngoscopy to diagnose ZD (14). The authors describe pooling of secretions in the hypopharynx as a "sign of the rising tide." During videofiberoscopy, swallowed cream appeared to visibly back up in the hypoharynx as a wave after its initial and complete disappearance. Such a finding is not seen in other disorders of the upper esophageal sphincter, and the finding disappears after successful surgical correction of the ZD. However, although flexible

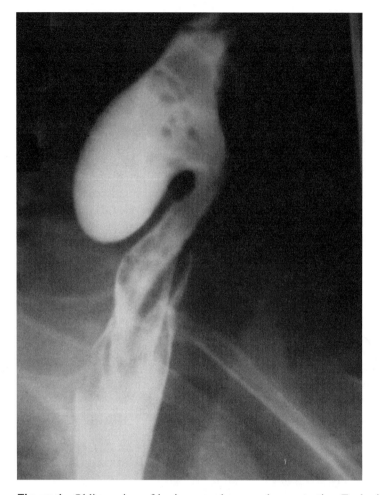

Figure 1 Oblique view of barium esophagram demonstrating Zenker's diverticulum.

laryngoscopy can increase suspicion to the presence of a ZD, a barium swallow is still necessary to confirm the presumptive diagnosis.

TESTING

The diagnosis of ZD is traditionally made by modified barium swallow (Fig. 1). The diverticulum is visible on lateral or oblique projection. The exact appearance of the sac can vary widely in the same patient, depending on the angle and moment of exposure during swallowing. However, nearly all patients with ZD demonstrate a filling deficit, which does not move between films (as a food bolus would).

DIFFERENTIAL DIAGNOSIS

The diagnosis of ZD can frequently be made by history alone. However, the constellation of symptoms seen in the patient with ZD can be seen in any patient with dysphagia. Furthermore, dysphagia occurs in up to 2% of patients over 65 years old. Therefore, the differential diagnosis of dysphagia should be considered in any patient suspected of having ZD (Table 1).

TREATMENT OPTIONS

There is no adequate medical treatment for symptomatic Zenker's diverticuli, and symptomatic patients should undergo surgery. Wheeler (16) performed the first attempted excision of a diverticulum in 1885, and since then several surgical procedures have been described for the treatment of pharyngeal pouches. They include both external and endoscopic approaches.

External

Treatment of ZD has traditionally been accomplished by open surgery, from cricopharyngeus myotomy alone to diverticulectomy, diverticulopexy or diverticular inversion, all with or without cricopharyngeus myotomy.

The first attempts to remove ZD carried a high mortality rate secondary to mediastinitis, and therefore other methods were attempted. After 1910, Lahey and Warren (17) developed a two-stage procedure in which they sutured the dissected

Table 1 Differential Diagnosis of Dysphagia in the Elderly

Critical/life threatening (rule out immediately)
    Anaphylactic reaction
    Stroke
    Tracheoesophageal fistula
    Chest pain—cardiac event
Serious (rule out systematically)
    Esophageal carcinoma—squamous cell or adenocarcinoma
    Gastroesophageal reflux disease (GERD)
    Strictures or webbing—Barrett's esophagitis
    Esophageal diverticula—Zenker's is the most common
    Dysphagia lusoria (retroesophageal right subclavian artery)
    Achalasia
    Esophageal spasm
    Scleroderma
    Myasthenia gravis
    Amytrophic lateral sclerosis
    Parkinson's disease
    Dementia or delirium
    Medication reaction/interaction
    Ludwig's angina (tongue swelling epiloglottis, swelling in suprahyoid area)
Local (rule out systematically)
    Oral candidiasis
    Xerostomia (dry mouth)
    Oral hygiene—poorly fitting dental appliances
    Globus hytericus (something's caught in my throat)
    Cervical spinal deformities

Source: From Ref. 15.

diverticular sac to the skin, with extirpation at a second operation several days later. With increasing use of antibiotics in the earlier 20th century came growing acceptance of single-stage diverticulectomy. Since most major complications associated with open surgical approaches arose from mucosal breeches at the suture line, the majority of these techniques were based on maintaining mucosal integrity.

Cricopharyngeus Myotomy

By 1932, Seiffert (18) had successfully described cricopharyngeus myotomy alone in a patient with a small diverticulum, which was left intact. Postoperatively, the patient no longer suffered from dysphagia, and the diverticulum had disappeared on follow-up radiography. Since then, cricopharyngeus myotomy alone has shown varying results, with better outcomes in patients with smaller diverticuli (19). A 4–5 cm myotomy is made, leaving the diverticulum intact. Postoperative radiographs reveal either significant diminution or complete disappearance of the diverticulum. At the Mayo Clinic, such practice has become the treatment modality of choice for small, symptomatic sacs (3,20). As many surgeons consider cricopharyngeus spasm to be the major contribution for the formation of ZD, cricopharyngeus myotomy is often included in addition to other surgical techniques employed in the treatment or prevention of pharyngeal pouches.

Inversion/Invagination

This technique has been used as early as 1900, and together with a sphincterotomy, can still be considered a safe and effective procedure. In this procedure, the dependent sac can be "eliminated" through placement of a pursestring suture around its neck, inverting the sac through it, and tightening the suture. Bowdler and Stell reported a reduced mortality, complication rate, and hospital stay with inversion surgery over open diverticulectomy (11,21,22).

Diverticulopexy with Sphincterotomy

Diverticulopexy involves surgical fixation of the floor of the diverticulum superiorly to the prevertebral fascia or to the pharyngeal musculature so that it will no longer accumulate foodstuffs. It is usually reserved for the treatment of small- to medium-sized pouches. Patients undergoing diverticulopexy should undergo sphincterotomy with a long myotomy, felt to be essential in avoiding recurrence (23). Lerut et al. (24) reported results of very good to excellent in 92% of 94 patients without any deaths.

Diverticulectomy with or Without Sphincterotomy

Advances in surgical technique have evolved so that the most logical approach to elimination of ZD, removal of the sac, has become associated with fairly low complication rates. Diverticulectomy has the advantage that it completely removes the pouch and theoretically can be used to remove pouches of any size. Diverticulectomy also eliminates the possibility of leaving carcinoma behind in residual mucosa. However, it still carries a higher complication rate than other open procedures (25). Diverticulectomy also requires longer operative time, thus increasing risk to elderly and frail patients.

Interestingly, the Mayo Clinic retrospective showed no improvement in the results following the addition of myotomy to diverticulectomy (3). This would indicate that the CPM is no longer as intimately involved in the ongoing progression of

ZD once it has developed. Nonetheless, most authors believe that CP myotomy should be performed with diverticulectomy.

Postoperatively, all patients undergoing external approaches to ZD are traditionally fed by nasogastric tube for 5–7 days before oral feeding is resumed, resulting in an often lengthy and costly hospitalization.

Endoscopic

Mosher (26) is widely credited as the first to use an endoscopic technique to treat pharyngeal pouches by dividing the common septum between the pouch and esophagus, thereby creating a single lumen by internal cricopharyngeus myotomy. In a 1917 paper of Mosher, the author reported good results with his first four patients, but the death of the seventh patient from mediastinitis caused Mosher to abandon the practice. In 1935 Dohlman (27) redescribed and modified the endscopic technique, reporting the author's successful 13-year experience in 39 patients. By 1960, Dohlman and Mattson's (28) series had risen to 100 cases without any deaths or significant complications, with a recurrence rate of 7%.

The endoscopic method has been further modified to include the use of an operating microscope, KTP lasers, and CO_2 lasers (29–33). A recent report from Italy detailed some early successes with endoscopic injection of Botulinum toxin (34). First described in 1981 by van Overbeek (35), endoscopic laser-assisted diverticulostomy has gained great popularity. Krespi et al. (36) found a greater than 96% patient satisfaction with the procedure, with no significant increase in complication rates compared to other endoscopic methods. However, other reports noted a higher incidence of intraoperative hemorrhage and conversion to an open procedure (37).

Many surgeons considered sutureless laser techniques to have a theoretically high risk of mediastinitis, causing them to limit the length of mucosal incision and myotomy. This was successfully addressed in 1993 when Martin-Hirsch and Newbegin (38) in England and Collard et al. (39) in Belgium simultaneously described endoscopic staple-assisted diverticulostomy (ESAD) using a linear transecting and stapling device. This method ensured a tighter mucosal closure than that of sutureless techniques, thereby reducing the risk of mediastinitis.

Many restrospective studies of ESAD have been published, showing high patient satisfaction and low rate of complications (40). Patients undergoing ESAD often resume oral intake on the same day of surgery. In many centers, ESAD is performed as an outpatient procedure. A recent comparison of patients undergoing ESAD to those undergoing open diverticulectomy revealed that hospital charges were significantly less in the endoscopic group (41). Quality of life studies have also demonstrated very high levels of satisfaction for patients who underwent ESAD, with 96% reporting that they would undergo the procedure again (42). ESAD may not always be appropriate for small diverticulum (< 2 cm), as the limitation of the stapler design may prevent complete engagement of the common wall. The completion of diverticulostomy may be optimized by traction sutures to stabilize the common septum between esophagus and diverticulum. Further modifying can be done by shortening the fixed jaw of the stapler to extend septal transection into the fundus of the diverticulum.

In general, endoscopic methods are equally as effective as external methods for the treatment of ZD. However, external approaches have traditionally been associated with a significantly higher rate of complications when compared to endoscopic methods. These complications include vocal cord paralysis, fistula formation, wound infection, pharyngeal stenosis, pouch perforation, mediastinitis, and death. In addition to a lower rate of serious complications, endoscopy offers certain advantages that prove very important in the elderly patient population. They include shorter anesthetic time, earlier resumption of oral intake, decreased postoperative pain, shorter inpatient stay, and straightforward revision surgery. However, limitations to endoscopy do exist. Positioning of the diverticuloscope can prove to be quite challenging, especially in patients with underlying trismus and/or to cervical spinal disease or kyphosis. In such cases, it may be necessary to convert to an open procedure. As mentioned above, endoscopic staplers may not fit completely around the common septum, resulting in insufficient myotomy. Tissue is not removed in endoscopic diverticulostomies, and therefore histologic analysis cannot be undertaken. This leaves a small, but not negligible, risk of retained carcinoma (43).

ALGORITHM

Management of the patient with ZD can be accomplished in a systematic manner. All patients with suspected ZD must first have a barium swallow, preferably in the presence of a speech pathologist who can identify other swallowing abnormalities that may prevent maximum relief of symptoms postoperatively (44).

Once the barium swallow is performed and the diagnosis confirmed, the surgeon will have to decide if the patient is a potential surgical candidate. Symptomatic candidates who are not surgical candidates may be offered a trial of antireflux medications, although they invariably prove inadequate. Botulinum toxin injection and CP dilation may provide temporary relief in a few patients.

Using the barium swallow the surgeon can gauge the length and location of the diverticulum, and thus better decide which surgical option is best for an individual patient. Attempts have been made to classify ZD based on size. van Overbook and Groote (45) divided ZD into small diverticuli (<1 vertebral body), medium-size diverticuli (between 1 and 3 vertebrae), and large diverticuli (>3 vertebral bodies). Morton and Bartley (46) described small pouches as less than 2 cm, medium pouches as 2–4 cm, and large pouches as greater than 4 cm.

Some may argue that smaller sacs might be better remedied with laser because a stapler cannot completely engage the common wall. Patients with smaller sacs also tend to do well with simple open cricopharyngeus myotomy, with or without diverticulectomy. Larger sacs can be successfully treated by endoscopic stapling techniques, provided the patient can tolerate adequate mouth opening and neck extension. Patients for whom scope placement or positioning is not adequate will require an open procedure with CP myotomy.

Some authors propose that patients less than 65 years should undergo excision of the pouch with a long CP myotomy and pathological examination of the pouch because of risks of missed cancer—which if left in place after endoscopic diverticulostomy would have a theoretically longer latency to presentation (43).

Assessment of treatment should be made clinically. There is no role for postoperative radiography. Barium studies may show lax mucosa that appears as a residual pouch, but this bears no clinical implication in an asymptomatic patient (47). Even in completely successful management, a persistent pouch, although smaller, will remain.

CONCLUSION

Zenker's diverticulum is encountered fairly commonly by the otolaryngologist, among our elderly patients. Diagnosis is traditionally achieved by taking a thorough history, which leads to confirmation by a pathognomonic radiographic finding. Recent advances in surgical technique have made this disorder a relatively easily treatable disorder with remarkably high rates of patient satisfaction.

REFERENCES

1. Zenker FA, von Ziemssen H. Krahnkheiten des Oesophagus. In: von Ziemssen H, ed. Handbuch der Speciellen Pathologie and Therapie. Leipzid: FCW vogel, 1877:1–87.
2. Meehan T, Henein RR. An unusual pharyngeal pouch. J Laryngol 1992; 106:1002–1003.
3. Payne WS. The treatment of pharyngoesophageal divertulum: the simple and complex. Hepatogastroeneterology 1992; 39:109–114.
4. Gage-White L. Incidence of Zenker's diverticulum with Hiatus hernia. Laryngoscope 1988; 98:527–530.
5. Cook IJ, Gabb M, Panagopoulos V, et al. Pharyngeal diverticulum is a disorder of upper esophageal sphincter. Gastroenterology 1992; 103:1229–1235.
6. Paterson WG, Kolyn DM. Esophageal shortening induced by short-term intraluminal acid perfusion in opossum: a cause for hiatus hernia? Gastroenterology 1994; 107: 1736–1740.
7. Shirazi S, Schulze-Delrieu K, Custer-Hagen T, et al. Motility changes in opossum esophagus from experimental esophagitis. Dig Dis Sci 1989; 134:1668–1676.
8. DeMeester SR, Sillin LF, Lin HW, et al. Increasing esophageal length: a comparison of laparoscopic versus transthoracic esophageal mobilization with and without vagal trunk division in pigs. J Am Coll Surg 2003; 197:558–564.
9. Sasaki CT, Ross DA, Hundal J. Association between Zenker diverticulum and gastroesophageal reflux disease: development of a working hypothesis. Am J Med 2003; 115(dA):169S–171S.
10. van Overbeek JJM. Pathogenesis and methods of treatment of Zenker's diverticulum. Ann Otol Rhinol Laryngol 2003; 112:583–593.
11. Liang MR, Murthy P, Ah-See KW, et al. Surgery for pharyngeal ouch: audit of management with short and long-term follow-up. JRC Surg Edinb 1995; 40:315–318.
12. Siddiq MA, Sood S, Strachan D. Pharyngeal pouch (Zenker's diverticulum). Postgrad Med J 2001; 77:506–511.
13. Langdon DE. Medication decision in giant Zenker's and esophageal diverticula. Am J Gastro 2003; 98:943–944.
14. Perie S, Dernis HP, Monceaux G, et al. The "sign of the rising tide" during swallowing fiberoscopy: a specific manifestation of Zenker's diverticulum. Ann Otol Rhinol Laryngol 1999; 108(3):296–299.
15. Amella EJ. Dysphagia: the differential diagnosis in long-term care. Lippincotts Prim Care Prac 1999; 3(2):135–149.
16. Wheeler WI. Pharyngocoele and dilation of the pharynx, with existing diverticulum at lower portion of pharynx lying posterior to the oesophagus cured by pharyngotomy, being the first of the kind recorded. Dublin J Med Sci 1886; 82:349–356.
17. Lahey FH, Warren KW. Esophageal diverticula. Surg Gynecol Obstet 1954; 98:1–28.
18. Seiffert A. Zur Behandlung beginnender Hypopharynxdivertikel. Z Laryngol Rhinol Otol 1932; 23:256–258.
19. Ellis FH. The management of Zenker's diverticulum: cricopharyngeal myotomy. In: Kittle CF, ed. Current Controversies in Thoracic Surgery. Philadelphia, PA: Saunders, 1986:10–14.

20. Payne WS, Pairolero PC, Piehler JM. The management of Zenker's diverticulum: diverticulectomy. In: Kittle CF, ed. Current Controversies in Thoracic Surgery. Philadelphia, PA: Saunders, 1986:3–9.

21. Bowdler DA, Stell PM. Surgical management of posterior pulsion pharyngeal diverticula: inversion versus one-stage excision. Br J Surg 1987; 74:988–990.

22. Feeley MA, Right PD, Wiesberger EC, et al. Zenker's diverticulum: analysis of surgical complications from divertuclectomy and cricopharyngeal myotomy. Laryngoscope 1999; 109:858–861.

23. Belsey R. Functional disease of the esophagus. J Thorac Cardiovasc Surg 1966; 52: 164–188.

24. Lerut T, van Raemdonck D, Guelinchx P, Dom R, Begoes K. Zenker's diverticulum: is a myotomy of the circopharyngeus useful? How long should it be? Hepatogastroenterology 1992; 39:127–131.

25. Zharen P, Schar P, Tschopp L, et al. Surgical treatment of Zenker's diverticulum: transcutaneous diverticulectomy versus microendoscopic myotomy of the cricopharyngeal muscle with CO_2 laser. Otolaryngol Head Neck Surg 1999; 121:482–487.

26. Mosher HP. Webs and pouches of the oesophagus, their diagnosis and treatment. Surg Gynecol Obstet 1917; 25:175–187.

27. Dohlman G. Endoscopic operations for hypopharyngeal diveriticula. Proceedings of the fourth international congress on otolaryngology, London, 1948:715–717.

28. Dohlman G, Mattson O. The endoscopic operation for hypopharyngeal diverticula. Arch Otolaryngol1960; 71:744–752.

29. van Overbeek JJM, Hoeksma PE, Edens ET. Microendoscopic surgery of the hypopharyngeal diverticulum using electrocoagulation or carbon dioxide laser. Ann Otol Rhinol Laryngol 1984; 93:34–36.

30. Kuhn FA, Bent JP III. Zenker's diveriticulostomy using the KTP/532 laser. Laryngoscope 1992; 102:946–950.

31. Benjamin B, Gallagher R. Microendoscopic laser diverticulotomy for hypopharyngeal diverticulum. Ann Otol Rhinol Laryngol 1993; 102:675–679.

32. Holinger LD, Benjamin B. New endoscope for (laser) endoscopic diverticulotomy. Ann Otol Rhinol Laryngol 1987; 96:658–660.

33. Maune S. Carbon dioxide laser diverticulostomy: a new treatment for Zenker diverticulum. Am J Med 2003; 115(3A):172S–174S.

34. Spinelli P, Ballardini G. Botulinum toxin type A (Dysport) for the treatment of Zenker's diverticulum. Surg Endosc 2003; 17(4):660.

35. van Overbeek JJ. Meditation on the pathogenesis of hypopharyngeal (Zenker's) diverticulum and a report of endoscopic treatment in 545 patients. Ann Otol Rhinol Laryngol 1994; 103:178–185.

36. Krespi Y, Kacker A, Remacle M. Endoscopic treatment of Zenker's diverticulum using CO_2 laser. Otol Head Neck Surg 2002; 127:309–314.

37. Mattinger C, Hormann K. Endoscopic treatment of Zenker's diverticulotomy of Zenker's diverticulum: management and complication. Dysphagia 2002; 17:34–39.

38. Martin-Hirsch DP, Newbegin CJ. Autosuture GIA gun: a new application in the treatment of hypopharyngeal diverticula. J Laryngol Otol 1993; 107:723–725.

39. Collard JM, Otte JB, Kestens PJ. Endoscopic stapling technique of esophagodiverticulostomy for Zenker's diverticlum. Ann Thorac Surg 1993; 56:573–576.

40. Richtsmeier WJ. Endoscopic management of Zenker diverticulum: the staple-assisted approach. Am J Med 2003; 115(3A):175S–178S.

41. Urken ML, Smith SR, Genden EM. Endoscopic stapling technique for the treatment of Zenker diverticulum vs. standard open-neck technique: a direct comparison and charge analysis. Arch Otol Head Neck Surg 2002; 128:141–144.

42. Stoeckli SJ, Schmid S. Endoscopic stapler-assisted diverticuloesophagostomy for Zenker's diverticulum: patient satisfaction and subjective relief of symptoms. Surgery 2002; 13:158–162.

43. Bradley PJ, Kochaar A, Quraiski MS. Pharyngeal pouch carcinoma: real or imaginary risks? Ann Otol Rhinol Laryngol 1999; 108:1027–1032.
44. Veenker E, Cohen JI. Current trends in management of Zenker's diverticulum. Curr Opin Otol Head Neck Surg 2003; 11:160–165.
45. van Overbeek JJM, Groote AD. Zenker's diverticulum. Curr Opin Otolaryngol Head Neck Surg 1994; 2:55–58.
46. Morton RP, Bartley JR. Inversion of Zenker's diverticula: the preferred option. Head Neck 1993; 15:253–256.
47. Ong CC, Elton PG, Mitchell D. Pharyngeal pouch endoscopic stapling- are post-operative barium swallow radiographs of any value? J Laryngol Otol 1999; 113:233–236.

BIBLIOGRAPHY

Sasaki CT, Ross DA, Hundal J. Association between Zenker diverticulum and gastroesophageal resflux diasease: development of a working hypothesis. Am J Med 2003; 115(dA):169S–171S.
Siddiq MA, Sood S, Strachan D. Pharyngeal pouch (Zenker's diverticulum). Postgrad Med J 2001; 77:506–511.
van Overbeek JJM. Pathogenesis and methods of treatment of Zenker's diverticulum. Ann Otol Rhinol Laryngol 2003:112.
Veenker E, Cohen JI. Current trends in management of Zenker's diverticulum. Curr Opin Otol Head Neck Surg 2003; 11:160–165.

30

Surgical Management of Aspiration in the Geriatric Patient

David E. Eibling
Department of Otolaryngology—Head and Neck Surgery, University of Pittsburgh School of Medicine, Pittsburgh, Pennsylvania, U.S.A.

INTRODUCTION

Elderly patients with severe neuromuscular diseases, head and neck cancer, or a number of other illnesses who suffer intractable aspiration may occasionally require surgical management. Most aspirating patients can be managed conservatively through dietary manipulation, specific feeding strategies, tracheostomy tube removal or valving, or specific muscle-strengthening therapy and will not require surgical intervention. Dysphagia with aspiration is a common comorbidity in a number of illnesses encountered in the elderly (1). However, in many instances, these diseases are self-limited, and with appropriate temporizing measures the aspiration will resolve without surgery. Specific nonsurgical treatment strategies are discussed in the chapters addressing the evaluation of dysphagia and poststroke swallowing rehabilitation. However, a few patients will continue to demonstrate aspiration with pulmonary sequellae despite conservative therapy. The otolaryngologist—head and neck surgeon—may be consulted for surgical intervention for some of these patients.

ETHICAL DILEMMAS

A number of surgical procedures exist and might benefit aspirating patients by either reducing or eliminating aspiration. In most instances, the performance of the appropriate procedure is straightforward. The decision-making, however, is often difficult. The challenge is in determining (i) whether intervention is warranted, (ii) whether intervention is desired by the patient and the patient's family, and (iii) which procedure(s) are best for the patient in question. These questions typically remain unclarified at the time of consultation; hence, the otolaryngologist must often assume the lead role in addressing treatment goals. Discussion of the various procedures, surgical expectations, and quality of life issues must take place in the context of beneficence and patient autonomy. Adopting a solution that seems obvious to the care team may not be congruent with the goals—and needs—of the patient. Careful

325

and honest presentation of the options to the patient is always required, but is often even more difficult in the frail elderly patient who may have higher priority concerns than prolongation of life. Occasionally, the patient and the patient's family do not share the same goals. These circumstances are even more challenging and require open discussion with all concerned, especially the patients if they are cognitively able to participate. It is not unusual for the time spent discussing the procedure with the patient, the patient's family, and the care team to exceed by severalfold the time required to perform the procedure!

APPROACH TO THE PATIENT

For the purposes of this chapter, we will assume that conservative therapy discussed elsewhere in this text has failed and that the decision to proceed with some surgical intervention has been made. Most aspirating patients would have previously undergone a tracheotomy, and if not this may be an appropriate first step. On the other hand, the presence of a tracheostomy has been shown to disrupt swallow function in some patients (2). A trial of decannulation in a monitored setting may be warranted in those with a tracheostomy. If decannulation is not feasible, restoration of subglottic air pressure by tracheostomy tube valving may occasionally avoid the requirement for further intervention (2,3). Other authors (4,5) have not demonstrated a benefit to valving, plugging, or decannulation, so the effects of tracheostomy tube manipulation for a specific patient must be evaluated in real time. Tracheostomy tube plugging and removal may be problematic in long-term care facilities, particularly in frail, neurologically impaired elderly patients (6).

Identification of the specific defect in swallow function is a critical first step in the evaluation of the patient's swallowing function. Not only must the anatomic integrity of the oral cavity, laryngopharynx, and esophagus be assessed, but also the functional capability must be assessed as well. The reader is referred to the chapter on the evaluation of dysphagia for an in-depth discussion of the evaluative process. In most instances, a modified barium swallow will be required, since endoscopic evaluation [fiberoptic endoscopic examination of swallowing (FEES)] may not provide adequate visualization of the pharyngoesophageal segment or upper esophageal sphincter (UES) (7,8). Newer techniques using transnasal esophagoscopy may permit improved endoscopic valuation of UES function. Evaluation of glottic and UES function may help determine whether a limited procedure such as a cricopharyngeal myotomy or vocal cord medialization would benefit the patient. Sensory loss is a critical contributing factor for aspiration pneumonia in stroke patients with dysphagia, so sensory testing may provide additional predictive information in these patients (9).

TREATMENT OF INTRACTABLE ASPIRATION

A stepwise escalation of therapy is indicated for most patients. As noted above, tracheotomy or (paradoxically) decannulation may benefit some patients. In selected patients with specific impairments, vocal cord medialization or cricopharyngeal myotomy (or Botox® chemodenervation) may provide a benefit. For patients with severe pharyngeal dysfunction, however, particularly when associated with laryngopharyngeal sensory loss, it is unlikely that such intervention will be successful, and the optimal course may be to consider some form of aerodigestive separation.

VOCAL CORD MEDIALIZATION

Aspirating patients who have an incompetent glottis due to unilateral vocal cord paralysis often benefit significantly from vocal cord medialization (10). The reader is referred to the chapter on vocal cord paralysis for further discussion. Even after adequate medialization for speech, however, swallowing function will often remain suboptimal. Nevertheless, medialization is a good initial step in patients with glottic incompetence due to unilateral vocal cord paralysis. Occasionally, bilateral vocal cord augmentation will benefit an aspirating patient, but care must be taken to assure that an adequate airway remains!

CRICOPHARYNGEAL MYOTOMY OR CHEMODENERVATION

Failure of UES dilatation may be noted on modified barium swallow and be associated with significant dysphagia and aspiration due to retained bolus in the hypopharynx following deglutition. It may be difficult to discern whether the primary etiologic process is failure of relaxation of the UES or failure of active dilatation due to weakness in laryngeal elevation. Open myotomy is the procedure of choice for cricopharyngeal achalasia, but verification of the diagnosis may be problematic. Chemodenervation of the cricopharyngeus muscle using Botox administered through either a percutaneous or endoscopic route can often provide significant benefit, confirm the diagnosis, and may obviate the need for open myotomy in some patients (11).

AERODIGESTIVE SEPARATION

Patients with severe, intractable aspiration with severe laryngopharyngeal dysfunction will likely not respond to conservative measures. Ongoing soilage of the tracheobronchial tree leads to recurrent episodes of pneumonia (eventually with resistant organisms), oxygen desaturation, the requirement for frequent tracheal suctioning, and high acuity care. In these patients, the most difficult decision is whether they will benefit from a procedure that eliminates vocalization, requires a life-long tracheostomy, and may not return them to an oral diet. Quality of life issues will play a definitive role in the decision-making for most of these options. Elimination of aspiration may permit the patient to be moved to a lower intensity care setting and permit easier access for family; hence, these procedures warrant consideration even in otherwise hopeless cases. A few patients may be able to resume an oral diet following separation, although these patients are in the minority in patients selected for separation (12).

LARYNGEAL STENTING

Separation via laryngeal stenting is uncommonly employed but is an excellent technique for aspirating patients in whom severe swallowing disability is expected to be limited to several weeks (13). A typical example is an elderly patient with a lateral brainstem and cerebellar stroke who is cognitively intact and in whom there is a possibility of significant functional return. Tracheotomy is required, and the stent is placed into the glottis through the stoma and secured for the duration required. Patients must be maintained in a high acuity care setting since they have no other airway except the tracheostomy tube. This is an excellent first step in the management of a severely aspirating patient for whom decision-making or prognostic determination is problematic. Inflating the tracheostomy tube cuff is an alternative strategy that will reduce—but not eliminate—aspiration. Some have reported that continuous suction of secretions from the subglottic airway above the cuff may further reduce aspirated materiel, but this strategy presents technical difficulties. Others have used foam cuff tubes in an effort to reduce the quantity of secretions "leaking" past the tracheostomy tube cuff.

TOTAL LARYNGECTOMY

Total laryngectomy is an ideal means to separate the respiratory and digestive tracts in a patient with a dysfunctional larynx and life-threatening aspiration. A narrow-field procedure preserving a significant amount of supraglottic and pharyngeal mucosa can be quickly performed. This procedure entails less postoperative morbidity than a standard laryngectomy so is appropriate even in ill patients. In some patients, tracheal–esophageal puncture can be considered, although it is unlikely that most patients for whom this procedure is being considered would be candidates. The emotional impact of total laryngectomy for the patient and the family of the patient is the most difficult-to-manage aspect of this procedure. As a result, other (potentially reversible) procedures may be better choices.

LARYNGEAL CLOSURE

A number of laryngeal closure procedures can be performed (14). These procedures tend to be difficult to perform reliably and require nearly as much time to perform as a narrow-field laryngectomy. Laryngeal closure procedures have largely been supplanted by laryngotracheal separation.

LARYNGOTRACHEAL SEPARATION

Separation of the aerodigestive tract by dividing the trachea below the larynx and creating a permanent stoma effectively eliminates aspiration (15,16). Although theoretically reversible, in reality very few patients ever undergo reanastomosis. Although tracheoesophageal puncture (TEP) (or even tracheal-pouch speech) is feasible, it is rarely performed due to patient characteristics. The procedure is more difficult to perform in the presence of a prior tracheostomy, and a high temporary fistula rate should be anticipated (12). However, it can be rapidly performed, is of very low morbidity, and may be more acceptable to elderly patients and their families than total laryngectomy.

The procedure is performed by dividing the trachea at the site of the tracheostomy, with care being taken to preserve as much proximal trachea as possible. A tracheal ring is removed and the proximal mucosa closed with an inverting suture. The suture line is reinforced with an additional line of sutures. If there is insufficient proximal tracheal, a portion of the cricoid cartilage is removed to provide sufficient mucosa for closure. The distal trachea is brought to the skin and a stoma created as in total laryngectomy.

SUMMARY

Surgical management of aspiration is feasible and is occasionally required when conservative measures to control aspiration fail. Decision-making is difficult, particularly in the elderly, since prolongation of life is often perceived by the patient as less important than quality of life issues. Assessment of the patient's wishes, and those of the patient's family, is key in the process. A stepwise progression of intervention techniques is usually employed, beginning with nonsurgical strategies. A number of surgical procedures are feasible, but aerodigestive tract separation is the most definitive. Elimination of aspiration may dramatically improve the quality of life for some patients by reducing pulmonary soilage with its attendant need for management of recurrent pneumonitis, frequent tracheal suctioning, and the need for skilled nursing care.

REFERENCES

1. Marik PE, Kaplan DMA. Aspiration pneumonia and dysphagia in the elderly. Chest 2003; 124(1):328–336.
2. Eibling DE, Gross RD. Subglottic air pressure: a key component of swallowing efficiency. Ann Otol Rhinol Laryngol 1996; 105:253–258.
3. Dettelbach MA, Gross RD, Mahlmann J, et al. The effect of the Passy–Muir valve on aspiration in patients with tracheostomy. Head Neck 1995; 17:297–302.
4. Leder SB, Ross DA. Investigation of the causal relationship between tracheotomy and aspiration in the acute care setting. Laryngoscope 2000; 110(4):641–644.
5. Leder SB. Incidence and type of aspiration in acute care patients requiring mechanical ventilation via a new tracheotomy. Chest 2002; 122(5):1721–1726.
6. Eibling DE, Carrau RL. Detection, evaluation, and management of aspiration in rehabilitation hospitals: the role of the otolaryngologist—head and neck surgeon. J Otolaryngol 2001; 30(4):235–241.
7. Logemann J. Evaluation and treatment of swallowing disorders. San Diego: College-Hill Press, 1983.
8. Langmore SE, Schatz K, Olson N. Endoscopic and videofluoroscopic evaluations of swallowing and aspiration. Ann Otol Rhinol Laryngol 1991; 100:678–681.
9. Aviv J, Martin JH, Keen MS, et al. Air pulse quantification of supraglottic and pharyngeal sensation: a new technique. Ann Otol 1993; 102:777–780.
10. Pou AM, Carrau RL, Eibling DE. Laryngeal framework surgery for the management of aspiration in high vagal lesions. Am J Otolaryngol 1998; 19:1–7.
11. Shaw GY, Searl JP. Botulinum toxin treatment for cricopharyngeal dysfunction. Dysphagia 2001; 16(3):161–167.
12. Eibling DE, Snyderman CH, Eibling C. Laryngotracheal separation for intractable aspiration: a review of 34 patients. Laryngoscope 1995; 105:83–85.
13. Eliachar I, Roberts JK, Hayes JD, et al. A vented laryngeal stent with phonatory and pressure relief capability. Laryngoscope 1987; 97:1264–1268.
14. Sato K, Nakashima T. Surgical closure of the larynx for intractable aspiration: surgical technique using closure of the posterior glottis. Laryngoscope 2003; 113(1):177–179.
15. Lindeman RC. Diverting the paralyzed larynx: a reversible procedure for intractable aspiration. Laryngoscope 1975; 85:157–180.
16. Lindeman RC, Yarington CT Jr, Sutton D. Clinical experience with the tracheoesophageal anastomosis for intractable aspiration. Ann Otol Rhinol Laryngol 1976; 85:609–612.

31
Sialorrhea in the Geriatric Population

Sam J. Daniel
Saliva Management Clinic, McGill University Health Center, Montreal Children's Hospital, Montreal, Quebec, Canada

GENERAL DESCRIPTION OF THE CLINICAL PROBLEM

Sialorrhea, or drooling, is the unintentional loss of saliva from the mouth. It is a significant disability for a large number of geriatric patients, especially those afflicted with neurologic disorders. The prevalence rate of drooling in the geriatric population is unknown; however, most patients with severe neurological disorders such as Parkinson's have troublesome sialorrhea. Drooling often causes functional, social, and psychological burdens on patients and their caregivers.

WHY IS SIALORRHEA PARTICULARLY IMPORTANT IN THE GERIATRIC POPULATION?

Most drooling in the geriatric population is the result of impaired neuromuscular control leading to incontinence of the oral cavity and overflow of saliva from the mouth. Geriatric patients often have a reduced frequency of swallowing, increased nuchal rigidity, and poor posturing, which worsen the problem. Drooling is particularly troublesome for older persons who feel like a "burden" on their family members or caregivers. This problem can also lead to social embarrassment and contribute to worsening their isolation.

BASIC SCIENCE

The major salivary glands comprising the parotid, submandibular, and sublingual glands, along with the minor salivary glands, secrete 1.5 L of saliva daily. The submandibular glands produce 70% of the saliva, while 20% comes from the parotid glands and 5% from the sublingual glands. While the parotid glands secrete mainly in response to external stimuli, submandibular glands produce most of the resting secretions. Saliva has antibacterial properties, lubricates the oral mucosa, and promotes digestion by breaking down carbohydrate with amylase. The secretory innervation of glands is controlled by the parasympathetic nervous system. Parasympathetic fibers to the submandibular gland originate in the superior salivatory nucleus and travel with the nervus intermedius to the facial nerve. They exit with the chorda tympani and are carried with the lingual nerve to the submandibular ganglion. Parasympathetic fibers to the parotid gland originate in the inferior salivatory nucleus. They leave on the glossopharyngeal nerve and continue on Jacobson's nerve. The lesser superficial petrosal nerve joins the otic ganglion, where postganglionic fibers travel on the auriculotemporal nerve to the parotid. Nerve endings within the parasympathetic postganglionic system secrete acetylcholine, and blocking these receptor sites inhibits nervous stimulation to the salivary glands.

HISTORY

Patients or caregivers report drooling with soiling of clothes and frequent need for bib change. Sialorrhea can be variable in severity throughout the day; therefore, it is important not only to qualify the salivary consistency (thick, watery) but also the peak secretion time and fluctuance with various activities. Drooling severity can range from wet lips only, to soiled clothing, to wet clothing, hands, and environment. Drooling frequency can be classified as occasional, frequent, or constant. Other complaints include maceration and chapping of skin around the mouth, chin, and neck. In very severe cases dehydration can occur.

PHYSICAL EXAMINATION

The examination should be comprehensive and include a biopsychosocial evaluation usually performed by a multidisciplinary team, consisting of an otolaryngologist, a speech therapist, an occupational therapist, and a dentist. The role of the speech pathologist is to assess oral motor skills with the goal of possibly improving them.

Head and neck examination should include the oropharynx, oral cavity, and tongue to identify any lesions. Attention should be paid to tongue size and movement, palate and mandible shape, as well as the gag reflex and oral tactile sensation.

A careful inspection of dentition and/or dentures is warranted. Malocclusion, open bite deformity, should be noted. An anterior rhinoscopy should be performed as patients with nasal obstruction tend to drool more. The quality of the perioral skin should also be noted. The neck should be properly examined and palpated.

Finally, a neurological examination should be performed with attention to head control and position.

DIFFERENTIAL DIAGNOSIS

It is important to differentiate drooling caused by hypersecretion from that secondary to poor neuromuscular control.

Hypersecretion occurs most commonly as a side effect of medications that increase activity at the muscarinic receptors of the secretomotor pathway, such as some antiepileptics and anticholinesterases. Specific drugs known to increase drooling include clozapine, donepezil, and galantamine.

Most drooling is secondary to impairment of the oral phase of deglutition caused by neuromuscular disorders. Predisposing factors are listed in Table 1.

Table 1 Factors Predisposing the Development of Drooling

Cerebrovascular accident
Dementia
Motor neuron diseases
Neurological disorders including Parkinson's, ataxia, and essential tremor
Medication
Improper head posture

TESTING

Imaging

Imaging is rarely indicated in the workup of a drooling patient.

A modified barium swallow could be useful in excluding esophageal motility disorders or esophageal spasm. More importantly, the swallow study can be used to evaluate for aspiration as this would be a contraindication to surgical procedures such as submandibular duct relocation.

Radiosialography may be useful to assess the secretory function of the salivary gland, but is not commonly used in clinical practice.

Audiogram

A hearing test should be performed in candidates for tympanic neurectomy due to the inherent risk of hearing loss associated with this procedure.

TREATMENT OPTIONS

An ideal treatment would succeed in reducing sialorrhea while maintaining a moist oral cavity. A multidisciplinary team approach, including an otolaryngologist, a speech therapist, and an occupational therapist increases the success of treatment.

Treatment options include behavioral therapy and oral motor training, pharmacotherapy, local irradiation, and surgery. Indications for surgery include persistent drooling after at least six months of nonsurgical therapy, or moderate to profuse drooling in a patient with severe deficiency in cognitive function preventing participation in physical therapy.

Conservative Options

Behavioral Therapy

In this technique, auditory and verbal cues are presented to help increase the frequency and efficiency of swallowing. Several methods including positive and negative reinforcement are used. Success of this therapy depends heavily on the patient's cognitive level and function. Furthermore, some authors question the long-term benefits of this therapy as patients tend to regress after completion of the treatment.

Oral Motor Training

Geriatric patients are frequently affected by various physical and neurological conditions that cause inefficient swallowing, including poor muscle coordination and hypotonia. In this therapy, an attempt is made to stabilize head position, strengthen lip closure, and decrease tongue thrust by utilizing various exercises. Unfortunately, oral motor training tends to be time consuming, with a varied response rate.

Pharmacotherapy

Medication can be used to block the nerve impulses before the signal gets to the salivary glands. Anticholinergics that inhibit activation at muscarinic receptors have been widely utilized to decrease the volume of drooling. Some of the medications tried include glycopyrolate, scopolamine, atropine sulfate, trihexyphenidyl, and benztropine.

Glycopyrolate

Glycopyrolate reduces salivary flow by reversibly blocking the cholinergic receptors that control salivary secretion. It has the advantages of long action and not crossing the blood–brain barrier. Glycopyrolate improves drooling in over two-thirds of the patients treated; however, a third will choose to discontinue the treatment due to unacceptable side effects. Common adverse effects include dry mouth, thick secretions, constipation, and irritability, and, less frequently, urinary retention and blurred vision.

Contraindications in the geriatric population include glaucoma, gastrointestinal obstruction, obstructive uropathy, ulcerative colitis, and myasthenia gravis.

Scopalamine

Scopolamine, usually used in the treatment of motion sickness, is one of the families of natural alkaloids. It inhibits competitively the acetylcholine at its muscarinic receptors. Transdermal scopolamine allows the programmed release of scopolamine in a free-base form into the bloodstream. Optimum absorption occurs when the system is applied to the hairless skin patch behind the ear. Side effects include dry mouth (most common adverse effect), decreased appetite, fatigue, and conjunctival irritation. Contraindications in the geriatric population include glaucoma, hypertension, and benign prostate hypertrophy.

Atropine Sulfate

Unlike glycopyrolate, atropine easily penetrates the blood–brain barrier. It is a competitive muscarinic antagonist. It does not prevent the release of acetylcholine but antagonizes the effect of this neurotransmitter on the effector cells.

Atropine sulfate has been shown to reduce the amount of resting salivary accumulation by more than 50%.

Side effects observed in the geriatric population include restlessness, delirium, decreased gastric mobility, decreased bladder and urethral tone, constipation, and urinary retention.

Sublingual Atropine

Sublingually administrated atropine has been tried in a small study. Patients were placed on a drop of sublingual atropine twice-daily regimen. Four of the patients improved significantly on the treatment, while one person experienced delirium and two persons had worsening of their hallucination.

Injection of Botulinum Toxin

Botulinum toxin A reduces sialorrhea by affecting the parasympathetic control of the salivary glands. It inhibits the release of acetylcholine by attaching to acceptor molecules at the presynaptic nerve surface. Despite the fact that the blockade is "irreversible," the effect is temporary as new nerve terminals sprout to create new neural connections.

A number of studies in patients with Parkinson's disease have demonstrated good results with Botox injections. The injection of botulinium toxin into the salivary glands can also be performed with ultrasound guidance. This makes it easier to identify the glands, visualize the needle in the parenchyma, and monitor the spread of the fluid being injected.

Adverse effects include transient slight weakness of the masseter muscle leading to a slight difficulty with chewing and transient weakness of the mouth. One study reported temporomandibular joint dislocation after Botox injection. The author has had extensive experience with Botox injection for sialorrhea, and favors it amongst other medical options as there were no systemic side effects in his patients and the benefits last for an average of six months.

Radiotherapy

Radiation decreases drooling by causing glandular atrophy. Unfortunately, patients may have bothersome xerostomia. Furthermore, the potential risk for development of secondary malignancy can not be overlooked.

Surgical Options

Surgical options include submandibular duct relocation, submandibular gland excision, tympanic neurectomy, and submandibular or parotid duct ligation. The author favors duct ligation as it is the least invasive surgery with minimal side effects, and a low rate of recurrence. The author ligates only 3 out of the 4 major gland ducts to prevent xerostomia.

SUMMARY

Sialorrhea is a prevalent problem in the geriatric population that can become a social and psychological burden. A multidisciplinary individualized approach is warranted, as there is a myriad of treatment choices available. Botox injection of salivary glands appears as a very promising option.

BIBLIOGRAPHY

Blasco PA, Stansbury JC. Glycopyrrolate treatment of chronic drooling. Arch Pediatr Adolesc Med 1996; 150(9):932–935.

Camp-Bruno JA, Winsberg BG, Green-Parsons AR, Abrams JP. Efficacy of benztropine therapy for drooling. Dev Med Child Neurol 1989; 31(3):309.

Crysdale WS. Submandibular duct relocation for drooling. J Otolaryngol 1982; 11: 286–288.

Crysdale WS. The drooling patient. Evaluation and current surgical options. Laryngoscope 1980; 90:775–783.

Crysdale WS, Greenberg J, Koheil R, et al. The drooling patient: team evaluation and management. Int J Pediatr Otorhinolaryngol 1984; 9:241–248.

Dunn KW, Cunningham CE, Baekman JE. Self-control and drooling. Dev Med Child Neurol 1987; 29:305–310.

Hyson HC, Johnson AM, Jog MS. Sublingual atropine for sialorrhea secondary to parkinsonism: a pilot study. Mov Disord 2002; 17(6):1318–1320.

Kunwar AR, Doufekias E, Nihalani N, Iqbal MM. Ipratropium bromide for treatment of bethanechol-induced sialorrhea. Ann Pharmacother 2003; 37(9):1343.

Mancini F, Zangaglia R, Cristina S, et al. Double-blind, placebo-controlled study to evaluate the efficacy and safety of botulinum toxin type A in the treatment of drooling in parkinsonism. Mov Disord 2003; 18(6):685–688.

Racette BA, Good L, Sagitto S, Perlmutter JS. Botulinum toxin B reduces sialorrhea in parkinsonism. Mov Disord 2003; 18(9):1059–1061.

32

Post-Stroke Swallowing Rehabilitation

Stephanie K. Daniels
*Research Service, VA Medical Center, and Department of Psychiatry and Neurology,
Tulane University Health Sciences Center, New Orleans, Louisiana, U.S.A.*

Anne L. Foundas
*Department of Psychiatry and Neurology, Tulane University Health Sciences Center,
and Neurology Section, VA Medical Center, New Orleans, Louisiana, U.S.A.*

INTRODUCTION

Stroke is the leading cause of morbidity and the third leading cause of mortality in adults in the United States. Approximately 700,000 individuals in the United States are affected by stroke annually (1). The incidence of stroke increases with age. For those older than 65 years of age, the rate of stroke is similar for white and African Americans; however, the rate of stroke is notably higher for African American under the age of 65 as compared to whites.

Dysphagia is a major source of disability following stroke, affecting quality of life, nutrition, hydration, and pulmonary status. Dysphagia, as identified by video-fluoroscopic swallow studies (VSS), occurs in approximately 76% of acute stroke patients, with the incidence of aspiration ranging from 43% to 58% in acute dysphagic stroke patients (2–4). One-half of dysphagic stroke patients are more likely to be malnourished than stroke patients with intact swallowing (5). The incidence of pneumonia resulting from aspiration in stroke patients may range from 35% during acute care hospitalization to 12% during stroke rehabilitation (6,7). Length of hospitalization is typically increased for dysphagic stroke patients, and these patients are more likely to be discharged to nursing homes in contrast to stroke patients without dysphagia, who are likely to be discharged to home (8).

LESION LOCALIZATION AND SWALLOWING

Dysphagia is common following acute stroke; therefore, a more precise elucidation of the cortical control and lateralization of swallowing can facilitate earlier detection of stroke patients who may be at greater risk for dysphagia and aspiration. Swallowing involves an afferent system, central control, which includes higher cortical and brainstem centers, and an efferent system. The role of the brainstem in deglutition is well understood, and until recently, it was thought that cortical regions had limited, if any, influence on deglutition. Moreover, it was assumed that cortical lesions must be bilateral to result in dysphagia. However, over the past 15 years, studies using the ablation paradigm and functional neuroimaging methodologies have shown that cortical brain regions do influence swallowing. While there is agreement that cortical and subcortical brain regions contribute to swallowing, controversy remains as to whether the cortical representation of swallowing is predominately lateralized to the left or right cerebral hemisphere. Two competing hypotheses have been proposed: lateralization of function versus bilateral representation of swallowing.

Early studies demonstrated that swallowing behaviors may differ in stroke patients with left hemispheric damage (LHD) and right hemispheric damage (RHD). That is, patients with LHD were more likely to have oral stage dysfunction, while patients with RHD were more likely to have pharyngeal stage dysfunction and aspiration (9,10). Other studies of stroke patients have found that hemisphere did not predict dysphagia characteristics or aspiration (11–13). In a study of 54 consecutive acute stroke patients, Daniels and Foundas (13) found that lesion site was more critical than hemisphere or lesion size in predicting patients with risk of aspiration. Specifically, regions anterior to the central sulcus and subcortical periventricular white matter (PVWM) sites were commonly lesioned in patients with risk of aspiration, whereas patients without risk of aspiration were more likely to have lesions posterior to the central sulcus and to subcortical gray matter structures. Alberts et al. (11) evaluated vascular territory and found that large-vessel strokes were commonly associated with aspiration; however, many patients with small-vessel strokes also aspirated. Robbins et al. (10) found an interaction of anterior–posterior location and lesion size. Anterior lesions were significantly larger and were associated with more severe dysphagia than posterior lesions. Specific lesion sites associated with dysphagia included the anterior insula, premotor cortex [Brodmann's area (BA) 6], and the PVWM (13–15). All of these studies were conducted on acute and subacute stroke patients; therefore, it is unclear whether specific lesion locations or large-size lesions are associated with persistent dysphagia and risk of aspiration in chronic post-stroke patients.

Results from functional imaging studies, including positron emission tomography and functional magnetic resonance imaging, are consistent with lesion studies in demonstrating that some specific brain regions seem to be more critical than others in mediating swallowing (16–18). Cytoarchitectonic sites identified as critical in swallowing include primary and premotor cortices (BA 4, 6), primary somatosensory cortex (BA 3-1-2), and the insula. As with lesion studies, findings concerning swallowing laterality have been inconsistent. Bilateral activation of sensorimotor regions has been identified in some studies (16–18); others have found asymmetric, but not lateralized, activation. That is, swallowing was not lateralized to one specific hemisphere across subjects; however, one hemisphere tended to be more important than the other in mediating swallowing. In addition, Kern et al. (19) identified significantly greater activation of the right sensorimotor regions as compared to the left sensorimotor cortex during volitional swallows, with the converse evident for reflexive swallows. There is also evidence that the right insula may be a critical site, as this region has been consistently activated in functional imaging studies (17,18,20).

In summary, swallowing is mediated by a distributed neural network that includes both cerebral hemispheres and subcortical structures with descending input to the brainstem. This neural network is composed of multiple levels along the neuroaxis (cortical, subcortical, brainstem). Specific neural systems (sensory, motor)

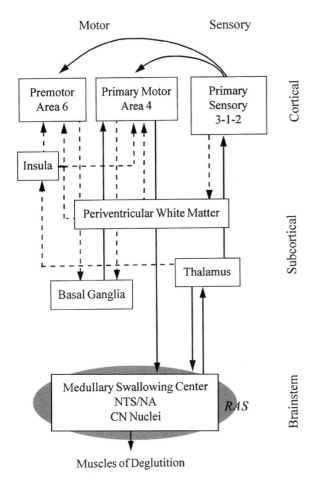

Figure 1 A proposed network for swallowing showing afferent and efferent connectivity of critical cortical, subcortical, and brainstem sites. The solid lines indicate known connections, and the hatched lines indicate proposed connections. *Source*: From Ref. 13.

that cross these levels and interconnect with cortical, subcortical, and brainstem regions are involved in swallowing. Based on the results of lesion and functional neuroimaging studies, Daniels and Foundas (13) have proposed an anatomical model of swallowing that is presented in Figure 1.

SCREENING FOR DYSPHAGIA IN ACUTE STROKE

It is well acknowledged that precise identification of the nature of the deglutitive disorder and determination of specific therapeutic techniques can only be obtained with an instrumental study. However, obtaining an instrumental swallowing evaluation is not warranted in all acute stroke patients and is not cost effective. While a clinical screening examination for dysphagia does not match the sensitivity and specificity of an instrumental study in identifying aspiration, it can be designed to be sensitive enough to identify risk of aspiration in stroke. As aspiration may be silent (no cough evoked with entry of material into the trachea), a screening test must incorporate other clinical features in addition to cough or wet voice after swallowing in order to more accurately identify patients with silent aspiration. Such clinical screening tests have been developed from specific items from the case history, oral mechanism, and clinical swallowing examinations to identify risk of aspiration, both overt and silent, in acute stroke patients.

In studies of acute stroke patients in which VSS was used to confirm dysphagia, Kidd et al. (4) found that decreased pharyngeal sensation, dysphagia on a water swallow test, and stroke severity were associated with aspiration risk. In consecutive stroke patients, Daniels et al. (2) identified six clinical features that were significantly related to risk of aspiration. These features were abnormal volitional cough, abnormal gag reflex, dysphonia, dysarthria, cough after water swallow, and voice change after water swallow. A subsequent study revealed that the presence of any two of these six predictors consistently distinguished patients with moderate to severe dysphagia (laryngeal penetration with stasis or aspiration) from patients with mild dysphagia/normal swallowing (no laryngeal penetration or penetration with clearing) (3). Based on this clinical screening, a clinical pathway was designed and instituted at the New Orleans Veterans Affairs Medical Center in which all acute stroke patients were screened for dysphagia (Fig. 2). Consecutive acute stroke patients presenting during 1½ years with two or more of the six clinical features for risk of aspiration were further evaluated with VSS, and patients with less than two predictors were not evaluated with VSS. This clinical pathway accurately identified patients with dysphagia and aspiration risk. No patients developed pneumonia and most returned to a regular diet (21). McCullough et al. (22) also reported high sensitivity using the presence of two of six of these same clinical features to predict aspiration. However, to achieve high specificity, the presence of four of six clinical features was required.

It is important to note that these screening tools for acute stroke patients have been developed to predict aspiration risk, not dysphagia. Logemann et al. (23) designed a screening tool to predict oral and pharyngeal stage dysfunction, delayed

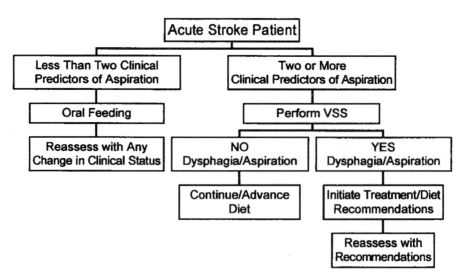

Figure 2 A clinical pathway for dysphagia management of acute stroke patients. *Source*: From Ref. 3.

pharyngeal swallow, and aspiration. A combination of specific features from the history and assessment of the oral mechanism, oral behaviors, gross motor skills, and clinical swallowing were used to identify patients displaying each of these swallowing abnormalities. Both sensitivity and specificity were generally low at approximately 0.70 for each area. Unfortunately, patients were not restricted to a specific clinical diagnosis; therefore, these results cannot be directly related to stroke patients.

INSTRUMENTAL EVALUATION OF OROPHARYNGEAL DYSPHAGIA

The purpose of an instrumental study is to evaluate biomechanic and physiologic function and dysfunction of the oropharyngeal swallowing mechanism, determine swallowing safety, and identify the effects of compensatory strategies, such as posture and bolus consistency, on deglutition. By determining the exact cause of dysfunction, therapeutic intervention can be initiated to address the specific disorder. Recovery of swallowing in acute stroke patients may be rapid, warranting reassessment within a few weeks of the initial swallowing evaluation (24).

The two instrumental tools used to evaluate oropharyngeal dysphagia are VSS and videoendoscopy. While advantages and disadvantages of each have been well documented, no study has been completed to compare the two tests in a homogeneous stroke population; thus, it is difficult to say which instrument is superior in the evaluation of dysphagic stroke patients (25,26). Stroke frequently affects motility in both the oral and pharyngeal stages of swallowing (13); thus, both regions should be assessed. To date, VSS is the only tool that allows for direct assessment of both the oral cavity and pharynx. Disorders occurring before triggering of the swallow, during the actual swallow, and after the swallow can be evaluated with VSS. As esophageal functioning can also be impaired, fluoroscopy can easily be extended to evaluate the esophagus.

While VSS is generally considered the gold standard for oropharyngeal dysphagia evaluation, the videoendoscopic evaluation of swallowing does have certain advantages and may be warranted in place of, or as an adjunct to, VSS. The videoendoscopic evaluation can be completed at bedside and thus may be advantageous for acute stroke patients in the intensive care unit. Laryngeal functioning can be fully evaluated, and the length of the evaluation is not restricted, as there is no radiation involvement. Laryngopharyngeal sensation may also be evaluated with a specially designed videoendoscope that allows for delivery of airpuff stimulation to the medial surface of the pyriform sinuses and aryepiglottic folds in order to evoke a laryngeal adductor reflex (27). While research has suggested that reduced laryngopharyngeal sensation in stroke patients contributes to dysphagia, the association of the laryngeal adductor reflex and the response to airway invasion during swallowing has not been empirically determined (28). Studies have shown that supraglottic penetration can occur in healthy young and older adults without elicitation of a cough (29,30).

The specific needs of each individual stroke patient should determine which instrumental tool is employed. Regardless of the method of evaluation, calibrated volumes of different consistencies should be tested. If possible, sequential swallowing should also be evaluated, as this is the normal mode of liquid ingestion. If dysfunction is evident, therapeutic intervention *must* be attempted during the instrumental evaluation in order to assess the efficacy of the intervention relative to the particular deglutitive dysfunction. The employment of a therapeutic strategy must be specific to the actual biomechanical disorder and not just applied randomly.

TREATMENT OF OROPHARYNGEAL DYSPHAGIA

Unlike the patient with head and neck cancer, a stroke may frequently impair a patient's cognitive, sensory, and motor abilities, all of which can dramatically impact rehabilitation efforts. Thus, it is crucial for the swallowing therapist to have a clear understanding of a stroke patient's elemental neurological and cognitive abilities including language, attention, awareness, memory, visuospatial, and executive functions. For example, if a person is globally aphasic (severe expression and comprehension deficits) and demonstrates reduced supraglottic closure with aspiration on the VSS, use of a chin tuck posture or thickened liquids may be tested on the instrumental examination to determine effectiveness. However, use of a super-supraglottic swallow maneuver may not be feasible due to the patient's reduced comprehension.

Rehabilitation of dysfunction; prevention of aspiration, dehydration and malnutrition; and re-establishment of oral intake are the treatment goals for stroke patients with dysphagia. Selected treatments should have research-based evidence of their effectiveness. While randomized trials using specific therapeutic techniques in the treatment of oropharyngeal dysphagia following stroke have not been completed, numerous Level III studies have been conducted.

In general, swallowing therapy may be defined as compensatory or rehabilitative (31,32). Compensatory therapy does not change the physiology of the swallow; rather, bolus flow is redirected. Compensatory strategies are attempted during the instrumental study to determine their effectiveness. These strategies are generally manipulated by the clinician and require only limited cognitive ability. Benefits are seen immediately but are not permanent. That is, when the compensatory strategy is removed, the previously noted swallowing dysfunction prevails. Alternatively, rehabilitative therapy aims to positively alter swallowing physiology over time, resulting in permanent improvement in deglutitive function. Good attention, comprehension, and memory abilities are critical for the success of swallowing rehabilitation. A brief review of compensatory and rehabilitative treatments and medical and surgical intervention for dysphagia following stroke will be presented.

Compensatory Treatment

Compensatory strategies consist of manipulation of posture, consistency, and sensory input. Facilitory postures that have been studied in dysphagic stroke patients include chin tuck and head rotation to the weak side. The chin tuck posture brings the base of the tongue closer to the posterior pharyngeal wall, widens the valleculae, and narrows the entrance to the airway (33,34). Head rotation to the weaker side of the pharynx facilitates bolus flow and increases deglutitive upper esophageal opening, thereby reducing or eliminating post-deglutitive residuals in the pharynx (35). Other postures are available to improve various aspects of oropharyngeal motility. While not empirically studied in stroke patients, the physiologic disorders for which these postures were designed to lessen or alleviate can be seen in the stroke population.

Research in stroke patients has demonstrated alterations of bolus flow when varying bolus consistency and volume are varied (36,37). Generally, thin liquids are thickened to either a nectar or honey consistency to facilitate swallowing. These liquid consistencies are now premixed, ensuring that the liquid is the prescribed consistency. Liquid barium is also available in nectar and honey consistencies to allow for the evaluation of standardized thickened consistency during VSS. If pharyngeal retention is a problem with increased consistency, cyclic ingestion, which involves alternating a liquid and thick consistency, may be warranted to clear residue.

The use of a sour bolus has also been effective in facilitating oral and pharyngeal motility in stroke patients (38). Studies are now focusing on mixture suppression in order to make a sour bolus more palatable for use in clinical environments (39). Carbonated liquids have also been shown to reduce airway invasion and improve pharyngeal motility in neurologically impaired patients (40).

Rehabilitation Treatment

Rehabilitative therapy includes muscular strengthening and range of motion (ROM) exercises, thermal-tactile application (TTA), and swallowing maneuvers. The effects of muscular strengthening and ROM exercises have been studied primarily in patients with head and neck cancer and in healthy adults. These studies demonstrated increased ROM of the tongue and posterior pharyngeal wall and increased tongue strength (41–43). The Shaker Exercise is designed to strengthen suprahyoid muscles, thereby increasing upper esophageal sphincter opening (44). A randomized trial has been conducted in a heterogeneous group of chronic tube-fed dysphagic patients including post-stroke patients. Results have demonstrated improved physiologic and functional outcomes, including resumption of oral intake after completion of the six week shaker exercise regime (45).

Swallowing maneuvers have also been used in rehabilitative treatment and involve altering the timing, duration, and extent of movement of specific areas of the oropharyngeal swallow (31). Maneuvers include the supraglottic swallow, super supraglottic swallow, effortful swallow, and Mendelsohn maneuver. As with ROM exercises, most of the research has been conducted in populations other than stroke. However, case studies of stroke patients and other neurologically impaired patients have reported improved swallowing and return to oral intake with implementation of these specific maneuvers (46,47).

TTA has been extensively studied in the stroke population. The therapy involves rubbing a cold stimulus (typically a chilled size 00 laryngeal mirror) vertically along the anterior faucial arches to facilitate evocation of the pharyngeal swallow. Results indicate that TTA immediately and temporarily improves speed of swallowing elicitation, but sustained effects are unproven (48–50).

New rehabilitation treatments are emerging, some of which may hold promise in the rehabilitation of swallowing. Before implementation, research must be carefully scrutinized. The research thus far on electrical stimulation (ES) varies in quality and results. ES may involve neuromuscular or sensory stimulation. Direct muscle stimulation of suprahyoid muscles and the thyrohyoid muscles using hooked-wire electrodes has yielded increased laryngeal elevation in healthy adults (51). ES using surface electrodes has also been used to exercise the suprahyoid muscles in dysphagic patients with stroke or other disorders (52,53). Although results are compelling, numerous uncontrolled methodological variables preclude the application of this method to clinical settings at this time. ES provided to the pharynx (via electrodes housed in an intraluminal catheter) is also being employed to provide sensory input to induce reorganization of the motor cortex. Results have revealed increased area of cortical representation of the pharynx in healthy adults and increased contralateral corticobulbar excitability, improved temporal swallow measures, and reduced aspiration on VSS in stroke patients (54,55).

Medical/Surgical Intervention

Medical and surgical approaches to dysphagia, such as vocal fold augmentation, laryngoesophageal separation, cricopharyngeal myotomy, and botulinum toxin injection, may be performed to improve specific swallowing disorders (56). Unfortunately, there are no empirical studies that have been completed to determine the effectiveness of medical and surgical intervention in the rehabilitation of dysphagic stroke patients. Most medical and surgical approaches should be postponed until completion of aggressive behavioral intervention, as swallowing can improve rapidly in the first month following acute stroke (24,31).

For aspiration due to vocal fold paralysis, augmentation may be an option, but it should be completed with an absorbable material such as collagen or fat, as recovery from stroke is expected in a relatively short period of time (56). In a recent study of a heterogeneous population who underwent VSS pre- and post-vocal fold medialization, the incidence of airway invasion did not significantly decrease following surgery (57). A tracheotomy can aid with pulmonary toileting, but it will not prevent aspiration. In fact, it may increase aspiration by restricting laryngeal excursion and reducing laryngeal sensitivity (58). Laryngotracheal separation is a more radical attempt in preventing chronic aspiration. While patients may return to oral diets, the ability to phonate is eliminated. If physiologic aspects of swallowing sufficiently improve, this procedure can be reversed, as the glottis is not affected (59).

Dilation, cricopharyngeal myotomy, and botulinum toxin injection are the medical treatment options for upper esophageal sphincter (UES) dysfunction. Dilation may be the first treatment method prior to surgical or pharmacological intervention. The effects of dilation may be temporary and require repeat procedures (31,60), and may not be beneficial for UES dysfunction related to neurological damage.

Cricopharyngeal myotomy is the most common surgical procedure for oropharyngeal dysphagia (61). Myotomy is most efficacious if the cricopharyngeal dysfunction is due to structural abnormalities; however, evidence is limited supporting the use of cricopharyngeal myotomy for neurogenic dysphagia (61). If reduced UES opening is due to restricted laryngeal elevation, a myotomy will not improve swallowing (31). Before proceeding with the surgery, it is critical that the cause of the dysphagia and UES disorder be determined. Procedures in addition to VSS, such as manometric evaluation, are warranted to determine if UES relaxation and duration of relaxation are impaired.

Botulinum toxin has also been used in the treatment of dysphagia resulting from UES dysfunction. As with other treatment methods, the cause of reduced UES opening must be fully discerned before employing this treatment. While some studies indicate improved swallowing on VSS and by patient report, most of the studies are retrospective, completed in heterogeneous patient populations, and not placebo controlled (62–64).

SUMMARY

Dysphagia is common post-stroke and can significantly increase morbidity and mortality in post-stroke patients. Early screening, instrumental evaluation, and aggressive rehabilitation based on results of the instrumental study can facilitate medical, physiological, and functional outcomes in these patients. Continued research, especially controlled clinical trials, is warranted to further delineate optimal treatment practices for stroke patients with dysphagia.

ACKNOWLEDGMENT

This work was supported by the Department of Veterans Affairs, Rehabilitation Research and Development, through a Career Development Grant (B3019V).

REFERENCES

1. Broderick J, Brott T, Kothari R, et al. The Greater Cincinnati/Northern Kentucky Stroke Study: preliminary first-ever and total incidence rates of stroke among blacks. Stoke 1998; 29:415–421.
2. Daniels SK, Brailey K, Priestly DH, Herrington LR, Weisberg LA, Foundas AL. Aspiration in patients with acute stroke. Arch Phys Med Rehabil 1998; 79:14–19.
3. Daniels SK, McAdam CP, Brailey K, Foundas AL. Clinical assessment of swallowing and prediction of dysphagia severity. Am J Speech Lang Pathol 1997; 6(4):17–24.
4. Kidd D, Lawson L, Nesbitt R, MacMahon J. Aspiration in acute stroke: a clinical study with videofluoroscopy. Q J Med 1993; 86:825–829.
5. Davalos A, Ricart W, Gonzalez-Huix R, et al. Effect of malnutrition after acute stroke on clinical outcome. Stroke 1996; 27:1028–1032.
6. Smithard DG, O'Neill PA, Park C, et al. Complications and outcomes after acute stroke. Does dysphagia matter? Stroke 1996; 27:1200–1204.
7. Teasell RW, McRae M, Marchuk Y, Finestone HM. Pneumonia associated with aspiration following stroke. Arch Phys Med Rehabil 1996; 77:707–709.
8. Odderson IR, Keaton JC, McKenna BS. Swallow management in patients on an acute stroke pathway: quality is cost effective. Arch Phys Med Rehabil 1995; 76:1130–1133.
9. Robbins J, Levine RL. Swallowing after unilateral stroke of the cerebral cortex: preliminary experience. Dysphagia 1988; 3:11–17.
10. Robbins J, Levine RL, Maser A, Rosenbek JC, Kempster GB. Swallowing after unilateral stroke of the cerebral cortex. Arch Phys Med Rehabil 1993; 74:1295–1300.
11. Alberts MJ, Horner J, Gray L, Brazer SR. Aspiration after stroke: lesion analysis by brain MRI. Dysphagia 1992; 7:170–173.
12. Chen MYM, Ott DJ, Peele VN, Gelfand DW. Oropharynx in patients with cerebrovascular disease: evaluation with videofluoroscopy. Radiology 1990; 175:641–643.
13. Daniels SK, Foundas AL. Lesion localization in acute stroke patients with risk of aspiration. J Neuroimaging 1999; 9:91–97.
14. Daniels SK, Foundas AL. The role of the insular cortex in dysphagia. Dysphagia 1997; 12:146–156.
15. Daniels SK, Foundas AL, Iglesia GC, Sullivan MA. Lesion site in unilateral stroke patients with dysphagia. J Stroke Cerebrovas Dis 1996; 6:30–34.
16. Hamdy S, Mikulis DJ, Crawley A, et al. Cortical activation during human volitional swallowing: an event-related fMRI study. Am J Physiol Gastriointest Liver Physiol 1999; 227:G219–G225.
17. Zald DH, Pardo JV. The functional neuroanatomy of voluntary swallowing. Ann Neurol 1999; 46:281–286.
18. Hamdy S, Rothwell JC, Brooks DJ, Bailey D, Aziz Q, Thompson DG. Identification of cerebral loci processing human swallowing with $H_2^{15}O$ PET activation. J Neurophysiol 1999; 81:1917–1926.
19. Kern MK, Jaradeh S, Arndorfer RC, Shaker R. Cerebral cortical representation of reflexive and volitional swallowing in humans. Am J Physiol Gastrointest Liver Physiol 2001; 280:G354–G360.

20. Martin RE, Goodyear BG, Gati JS, Menon RS. Cerebral cortical representation of automatic and volitional swallowing in humans. J Neurophysiol 2001; 85:938–950.

21. Daniels SK, Ballo L, Mahoney MC, Foundas AL. Clinical predictors of dysphagia and aspiration risk: outcome measures in acute stroke patients. Arch Phys Med Rehabil 2000; 81:1030–1033.

22. McCullough GH, Wertz RT, Rosenbek JC. Sensitivity and specificity of clinical/bedside examination signs for detecting aspiration in adults subsequent to stroke. J Comm Dis 2001; 4:55–72.

23. Logemann JA, Veis S, Colangelo L. A screening procedure for oropharyngeal dysphagia. Dysphagia 1999; 14:44–51.

24. Logemann JA, Veis S, Rademaker AW, Huang CW. Early recovery of swallowing post-CVA. Paper presented at the Eighth Annual Meeting of the Dysphagia Research Society, Burlington, Vermont, October 1999.

25. Kidder TM, Langmore SE, Martin BJW. Indication and techniques of endoscopy in evaluation of cervical dysphagia: comparison with radiographic techniques. Dysphagia 1994; 9:256–261.

26. Langmore SE, Logemann JA. After the clinical bedside swallowing examination: what next?. Am J Speech Lang Pathol 1991; 1:13–20.

27. Aviv JE, Martin JH, Kim T, et al. Laryngopharyngeal sensory discrimination testing and laryngeal adductor reflex. Ann Otol Rhinol Laryngol 1999; 108:725–730.

28. Aviv JE, Martin JH, Sacco RL, et al. Supraglottic and pharyngeal sensory abnormalities in stroke patients with dysphagia. Ann Otol Rhinol Laryngol 1996; 105:92–97.

29. Robbins J, Coyle J, Rosenbek J, Roecker E, Wood J. Differentiation of normal and abnormal airway protection during swallowing using the penetration-aspiration scale. Dysphagia 1999; 14:228–232.

30. Daniels SK, Corey DM, Hadskey LD, Legendre C, Rosenbek JC, Foundas AL. Mechanism of sequential swallowing during straw drinking in healthy young and older adults. J Speech Lang Hearing Res 2004; 47:33–45.

31. Logemann JA. Evaluation and treatment of swallowing disorders. 2nd ed. Austin, Tx: Pro-Ed, 1998.

32. Huckabee ML, Pelletier CA. Management of adult neurogenic dysphagia. San Diego, Ca: Singular, 1998.

33. Shanahan TK, Logemann JA, Rademaker AW, Pauloski BR, Kahrilas PJ. Chin-down posture effect on aspiration in dysphagic stroke patients. Arch Phys Med Rehabil 1993; 74:736–739.

34. Welch MV, Logemann JA, Rademaker AW, Kahrilas PJ. Changes in pharyngeal dimensions affected by chin tuck. Arch Phys Med Rehabil 1993; 74:178–181.

35. Logemann JA, Kahrilas PJ, Kobara M, Vakil NB. The benefit of head rotation on pharyngoesophageal dysphagia. Arch Phys Med Rehabil 1989; 70:767–771.

36. Lazarus CL, Logemann JA, Rademaker AW, et al. Effects of bolus volume, viscosity, and repeated swallows in nonstroke subjects and stroke patients. Arch Phys Med Rehabil 1993; 74:1066–70.

37. Bisch EM, Logemann JA, Rademaker AW, Kahrilas PJ, Lazarus CL. Pharyngeal effects of bolus volume, viscosity, and temperature in patients with dysphagia resulting from neurological impairment and in normal subjects. J Speech Hear Res 1994; 37:1041–1049.

38. Logemann JA, Pauloski BR, Colangelo L, Lazarus C, Fujiu M, Kahrilas PJ. Effects of a sour bolus on oropharyngeal swallowing measures in patients with neurogenic dysphagia. J Speech Hear Res 1995; 38:556–563.

39. Pelletier CA, Lawless HT, Horne J. Sweet–sour mixture suppression in older and young adults. Food Qual Pref 2003; 15:105–116.

40. Bulow M, Olsson R, Ekberg O. Videoradiographic analysis of how carbonated thin liquids and thickened liquids affect the physiology of swallowing in subjects with aspiration of thin liquids. Acta Radiol 2003; 44:366–372.

41. Logemann JA, Pauloski BR, Rademaker AW, Colangelo LA. Speech and swallowing rehabilitation for head and neck cancer patients. Oncology 1997; 11:651–656.

42. Fujiu M, Logemann JA. Effect of a tongue holding maneuver on posterior pharyngeal wall movement during deglutition. Am J Speech Lang Pathol 1996; 5:23–30.

43. Lazarus C, Logemann JA, Huang CF, Rademaker AW. Effects of two types of tongue strengthening exercises in young normals. Folia Phoniatr Logop 2003; 55:199–205.

44. Shaker R, Kern M, Bardan E, Taylor A, et al. Augmentation of deglutitive upper esophageal sphincter opening in the elderly by exercise. Am J Physiol Gastrointest Liver Physiol 1997; 272:G1518–G1522.

45. Shaker R, Easterling C, Kern M, et al. Rehabilitation of swallowing by exercise in tube-fed patients with pharyngeal dysphagia secondary to abnormal UES opening. Gastroenterology 2002; 122:1314–1321.

46. Logemann JA, Kahrilas PJ. Relearning to swallow after stroke—application of maneuvers and indirect biofeedback: a case study. Neurology 1990; 40:1136–1138.

47. Kahrilas PJ, Logemann JA, Gibbons P. Food intake by maneuver: an extreme compensation for impaired swallowing. Dysphagia 1992; 7:155–159.

48. Lazarra G, Lazarus C, Logemann JA. Impact of thermal stimulation on the triggering of the swallowing reflex. Dysphagia 1986; 1:73–77.

49. Rosenbek JC, Robbins J, Fishback B, Levine RL. Effect of thermal application on dysphagia after stroke. J Speech Hear Res 1991; 34:1257–1268.

50. Rosenbek JC, Roecker EB, Wood JL, Robbins J. Thermal application reduces the duration of stage transition after stroke. Dysphagia 1996; 11:225–223.

51. Burnett TA, Mann EA, Cornell SA, Ludlow CA. Laryngeal elevation achieved by neuromuscular stimulation at rest. J Appl Physiol 2003; 94:128–134.

52. Freed ML, Freed L, Chatburn RL, Christian M. Electrical stimulation for swallowing disorders caused by stroke. Respir Care 2001; 46:466–474.

53. Leelamanit V, Limsakul C, Geater A. Synchronized electrical stimulation in treating pharyngeal dysphagia. Laryngoscope 2002; 112:2204–2210.

54. Hamdy S, Rothwell JC, Aziz Q, Singh KD, Thompson DG. Long-term reorganization of human motor cortex driven by short-term sensory stimulation. Nat Neurosci 1998; 1:64–68.

55. Fraser C, Power M, Hamdy S, et al. Driving plasticity in human adult motor cortex is associated with improved motor function after brain injury. Neuron 2002; 34:831–840.

56. Ergun, GA, Kahrilas PJ. Medical and surgical treatment interventions in deglutitive dysfunction. In: Perlman AL, Shulze-Delrieu K, eds. Deglutition and its Disorders. San Diego, CA: Singular, 1997:463–490.

57. Bhattacharyya N, Kotz T, Shapiro J. Dysphagia and aspiration with unilateral vocal cord immobility: incidence, characterization, and response to surgical treatment. Ann Otol Rhinol Laryngol 2002; 111:672–679.

58. Nash M. Swallowing problems in the tracheotomized patient. Otolaryngol Clin North Am 1988; 21:701–709.

59. Eisele DW. Surgical approaches to aspiration. Dysphagia 1991; 6:71–78.

60. Calcaterra T, Kadell B, Ward P. Dysphagia secondary to cricopharyngeal muscle dysfunction. Arch Otolaryngol 1975; 101:726–729.

61. Cook IJ, Kahrilas PJ. AGA technical review on management of oropharyngeal dysphagia. Gastroenterology 1999; 116:455–478.

62. Shaw GY, Searl JP. Botulinum toxin treatment for cricopharyngeal dysfunction. Dysphagia 2001; 16:161–167.

63. Parameswaran MS, Soliman AMS. Endoscopic botulinum toxin injection for cricopharyngeal dysphagia. Ann Otol Rhinol Laryngol 2002; 11:871–874.

64. Ravich WJ. Botulinum toxin for UES dysfunction: therapy or poison? Dysphagia 2001; 16:168–170.

33

The Effects of Age on the Voice

Robert Thayer Sataloff
Department of Otolaryngology—Head and Neck Surgery, Thomas Jefferson University and Graduate Hospital, Philadelphia, Pennsylvania, U.S.A.

Sue Ellen Linville
Department of Speech Pathology and Audiology, Marquette University, Milwaukee, Wisconsin, U.S.A.

INTRODUCTION

The normal aging process affects human function profoundly. Some aging effects on the voice are obvious. Hearing even a few words over a telephone usually allows us to know whether we are speaking with a child or an adult. Frequently, we also can identify a speaker as elderly by some of the perceived characteristics of the senescent voice. These include altered pitch, roughness, breathiness, weakness, hoarseness, and tremulousness. Although some of these characteristics associated with advancing age are inevitable, others may be modified through medical or surgical intervention or through voice training. Laryngologists, speech-language pathologists, and voice teachers should be familiar with many of the more important, clinically relevant age-related changes that occur in the human voice.

ANATOMY AND PHYSIOLOGY

Embryologically, the larynx develops most of its anatomical characteristics by the third month of fetal life. At birth, the thyroid cartilage and hyoid bone are attached to each other. The laryngeal skeleton then separates, and the slow process of ossification (cartilages turning to bone) begins (2). Except for the cuneiform and corniculate cartilages, the entire laryngeal skeleton is ossified by approximately age 65. At birth, the larynx is high in the neck, resting at about the level of the third cervical vertebra (C3). It descends to about the level of C5–C6 by the age of five and continues gradual descent, to about the level of C6–C7 between ages 15 and 20. Where does it lie in old age? Descent continues throughout life in both sexes. As the larynx descends, vocal tract length relationships change and average vocal pitch tends to become lower. In infancy, the membranous and cartilaginous portions of the vocal folds are equal in length. By adulthood, the membranous portion accounts for approximately three-fifths of vocal fold length. Total vocal fold length is 6–8 mm in the infant but increases to 12–17 mm in the adult female and to 17–23 mm in the adult male. But then what happens in old age? The dimensions of all other aspects of laryngeal anatomy increase, as well.

The first sound an infant makes usually has a frequency averaging about 500 Hz (one octave above middle C). At this time, laryngeal mobility is limited primarily to vertical movements, and the appearance of the larynx is very similar to that of primates (monkeys). As the child grows, mean fundamental frequency of speech drops gradually, and by eight years of age, it is approximately 275 Hz. Until puberty, male and female fundamental frequencies are about the same.

The vocal tract is altered at many levels during puberty. The tonsil and adenoid tissues atrophy and partially disappear, changing oropharyngeal and nasopharyngeal resonance. The vocal tract continues to grow in length and circumference into adulthood, attaining full by age 20 or 21.

The "power source" of the voice reaches its full potential as the chest enlarges and thoracic and abdominal musculature strengthens. Muscular strength and stamina usually peak during young adulthood.

From young adulthood to old age, the respiratory system undergoes marked anatomic and physiologic changes, including decreased force and rate of contraction of respiratory muscles, stiffening of the thorax, and loss of elasticity of lung tissues (3–6). These changes result in a progressive decline in respiratory function with increasing age after maturation in both men and women. Specific functional losses include decreased elastic recoil of lung tissues, reduced vital capacity, increased residual volume, and decreased expiratory/inspiratory reserve volume. Forced expiratory volume and airflow rate also decline with aging (7). These changes in respiratory function impact speech breathing in both men and women beginning during middle age, although the pattern and extent of those changes vary by gender. For instance, both genders show larger lung volume excursions and higher % vital capacity/syllable measurements with advanced age, although these changes appear to arise from different mechanisms. In men, such changes may be linked with inefficient laryngeal valving resulting from glottal gaps that develop with aging. In women, it is speculated that age-related changes in valving at the level of the velopharynx, tongue, or lips might account for observed changes. Alternatively, declines in laryngeal agility in elderly women as the larynx moves in and out of the airway during speech production may be responsible (8,9).

The larynx also undergoes extensive anatomic and physiologic changes during adulthood and into old age (10). Common laryngoscopic findings include vocal fold atrophy, bowing, edema and a glottic gap. Structurally, cartilages undergo ossification and calcification, intrinsic muscles atrophy, and joints erode (11–16). Age-related changes in the epithelium of the vocal folds are somewhat in dispute. Several investigators report thickening; others have found no evidence of change with aging. It also has been suggested that the epithelium increases in thickness in males up to age 70 and decreases with further aging. In women, the epithelium may progressively increase with aging, particularly after age 70; this would add mass, thereby decreasing fundamental frequency (17). A variety of changes in the lamina propria has been documented, including thickening/edema of the superficial layer, degeneration/atrophy of elastic fibers, and declines in the number of myofibrils (17,18). In elderly men, the mucosa stiffens and increases in viscosity in comparison with women and younger men, resulting in decreased ease of phonation (18,19). The stiffer, thinner vocal folds of older men likely vibrate more rapidly, increasing fundamental frequency. Changes in the larynx from young adulthood to old age are generally more extensive in men than in women, with the possible exception of muscle atrophy, about which there is little information on gender differences (10).

From a vocal fold function perspective, the issue of glottal gaps and aging is interesting to consider. Historically, complete glottal closure has been regarded as a characteristic of normal phonation in young adults. However, based on recent research, it is evident that at high pitch and/or soft loudness levels, glottal gaps of varying configurations are commonplace in young adults of both genders (20–23). With aging, men demonstrate an increased incidence of glottal gaps, presumably as a consequence of vocal fold atrophy. In contrast, young and elderly women do not differ in the overall incidence of glottal gaps. However, they do demonstrate different glottal gap configurations as a function of age. Young women overwhelmingly demonstrate posterior chinks, while elderly women display gaps more anteriorly in the glottis. Stroboscopic studies indicate that vocal fold movement patterns in elderly women are altered. Specifically, greater aperiodicity, reduced amplitude of vibration, and reduced mucosal wave have been observed (24).

Laryngeal muscles appear to undergo atrophy with age. Degenerative changes have been described and correlate histologically with atrophy and loss of internal architecture of muscle fibers. There is also a quantitative increase in connective tissue and fatty infiltration. These degenerative and atrophic changes reduce vocal fold tension and contribute to the development of glottic gaps and breathiness.

Neural changes in the larynx also occur with aging. Degenerative and subsequent regenerative processes have been demonstrated in the recurrent laryngeal nerve, although the total number of nerve fibers remains stable. These changes may partly explain the acoustic characteristics of tremulousness, weakness, and pitch variability in older individuals.

Marked anatomic changes in the supraglottic vocal tract have been reported from young adulthood to old age. Facial bones continue to grow during this period, although the magnitude of that growth (3–5%) is relatively modest (25,26). Changes in facial muscles include decreased elasticity, reduced blood supply, atrophy, and collagen fiber breakdown (27,28). The temporomandibular joint (TMJ) undergoes extensive changes with aging, including thinning of articular discs, reduced blood supply, and regressive remodeling of the mandibular condyle and glenoid fossa (29–32). However, age-related changes in the TMJ can be difficult to distinguish histologically from a TMJ that is involved pathologically (31–34). The oral mucosa loses elasticity with aging and thins, with deterioration of attachments of epithelium and connective tissue to bone (16). However, there is some disagreement as to whether these changes reflect normal aging or result from drugs, disease, or pathological conditions (35–38). Dental structures are also altered with aging, although tooth loss itself is not an inevitable consequence of aging (39). Changes in the tongue's epithelium include thinning and fissuring of the tongue surface (40,41). Pharyngeal and palatal muscles also have been reported to undergo age-related degenerative changes (42–44).

From a functional perspective, loss of salivary function can produce symptoms of oral dryness, dysphagia, and oral discomfort in the elderly; susceptibility of oral infection is also reported to increase (45). The elderly have been reported to experience significant declines in tongue strength, although endurance remains relatively unaffected (46). Lingual pressure reserves during swallowing also decline with aging, although maximum tongue pressures during swallow events remain stable over from young adulthood to old age (47).

CORRELATES OF ANATOMIC CHANGES FROM YOUNG ADULTHOOD TO OLD AGE

Speaking Fundamental Frequency

From young adulthood to old age, the acoustic characteristics of both men's and women's voices are altered as a consequence of age-related changes to the voice production mechanism. In both men and women, speaking fundamental frequency (SF_0) changes, although the pattern of change differs for the two genders (48–56).

In men, SF_0 lowers from young adulthood into middle age (approximately 10 Hz) and then rises approximately 35 Hz to 130–160 Hz after age 65. The reason for the drop in SF_0 is unclear, although subclinical trauma related to normal vocal use has been raised as a possible explanation (51). The rise in SF_0 after middle age in men has been attributed to muscle atrophy or increased stiffness of the vocal folds (57,58).

In women, SF_0 remains fairly constant at 200–260 Hz until menopause, when a lowering of between 10 and 50 Hz occurs, resulting in a drop to 150–190 Hz after age 65 (59). After menopause, SF_0 remains fairly stable in women into old age. There are also indications that professional singers may tend to maintain stable SF_0 levels throughout adulthood (48,49). However, singers and nonsingers need to be compared, with smoking history controlled prior to drawing definitive conclusions as to the effect of professional voice training on SF_0 changes with aging. In terms of pitch range, evidence suggests that older professional singers experience a restriction of pitch range similar to that reported in nonsingers (48,60).

Speech Intensity

In both men and women, age-related changes in speech intensity have been reported, although the genders differ in both the nature and extent of age effects exhibited. Men over the age of 70 use higher conversational speech intensity levels than younger men, even after controlling for hearing acuity. It has been hypothesized that elevated speech intensity levels in elderly men might be an adaptive mechanism related to findings of decreased laryngeal airway resistance in men with aging; however, lower airway resistance values in elderly men (related to incomplete approximation of the vocal folds) presumably would compromise the valving capability of the laryngeal mechanism, making it more difficult for elderly men to sustain higher intensity levels (10,61,62). A definitive explanation for higher conversational speech intensity levels in men with aging awaits further study.

In women, no age-related changes in speech intensity have been found, either in reading or conversational speech (61,63). When compared with elderly men, elderly women demonstrate higher laryngeal airway resistance values across a range of sound pressure levels, with increases particularly steep at high intensity levels (64). It has been speculated that the combination of a physically smaller larynx and higher vibratory rate of the vocal folds could account for higher laryngeal airway resistance values in elderly women (64).

When maximum intensity levels of vowel production are compared, both men and women show reductions with advanced age (65,66). Elderly women also have been found to demonstrate elevated minimum intensity levels, in comparison with young adult women, when producing vowels as softly as possible (66). However, intensity levels of young and elderly women do not differ when producing vowels within a conversational range (61,66).

VARIABILITY IN MEASURES OF VOICE AND SPEECH

The notion that elderly speakers considerably vary in their performance measures of speech and voice has been a consistent finding in many studies (2,24,67–70). This variability results from differences in the rate at which individuals show aging effects as well as differences in variables such as lifestyle, genetics, and environmental factors (10).

Variability among elderly speakers on measures of speech and voice might be increased by compensatory adjustments. For instance, it has been speculated that elderly women employ a wider range of strategies to control laryngeal airway resistance than do elderly men, particularly at high intensity levels when demands on the system are high (64). That is, some older women may increase respiratory drive, whereas others increase airway resistance, and others may combine these strategies. Similarly, findings of increased variability on voice onset time measures in elderly adults have been hypothesized to result from compensatory techniques employed by older adults to maintain perceptual salience (69).

THE ADULT VOICE

It used to be believed that the speaking fundamental frequency of women drops steadily from about 225 Hz in the 20–29-year-old group to about 195 Hz in the 80–90-year-old group (71). More recent data reported by Linville (72) suggest that speaking fundamental frequency is fairly stable after the drop that occurs at the time of menopause. In males, fundamental frequency of the speaking voice drops until roughly the fifth decade, after which it rises gradually, by as much as 35 Hz (51,73). It is important to be aware of normal changes in the speaking voice, because conscious or unconscious unskilled attempts to alter the quality and frequency of the speaking voice often are abusive and may produce problems reflected in the singing voice. Interestingly, although range restrictions in professional singers are similar to those in nonsingers as noted above, it appears as if many of the other age-related changes in the speaking voice may not occur to the same degree in trained voice professionals; additional study is needed.

THE AGING VOICE

There are fundamental changes in the body with aging that often modify the sound of the speaking and singing voice. In older singers, these changes may include breathiness, loss of range, change in the characteristics of vibrato, development of tremolo, loss of breath control, vocal fatigue, pitch inaccuracies, and other undesirable features. Listeners can generally differentiate between young and old speakers because aging affects vocal pitch, loudness, and quality, although the effects may be highly variable (73).

Although some age-related alterations cannot be avoided, it is becoming more apparent that many of these changes can be forestalled or even corrected. Woo et al. (74) reached similar conclusions, recognizing that "presbylarynges is not a common disorder and should be a diagnosis of exclusion made only after careful medical and speech evaluation." As physicians, we need to look closer before concluding: "I can't help your voice; you're just getting older."

AGING

Much of the pioneering work on vocal aging by such scientists as Drs. Robert L. Ringel and Wojtek Chodzko-Zajko of Purdue University (75), as well as the author Sataloff (76), combines general knowledge about the aging process with specific knowledge about laryngeal aging. More recent histologic research has focused on aging changes that occur in the macula flava (77–79). This interdisciplinary approach helps us understand our perceptions of voices over the years and helps explain our recent observations that some "old" voices can be made "young" again.

Aging is a complex conglomeration of biological events that change the structure and function of various parts of the body. Muscle and neural tissues atrophy, and the chemicals responsible for nerve transmission change. Ligaments atrophy and cartilages ossify (including those in the larynx). Joints develop irregularities that interfere with smooth motion. The vocal folds themselves thin and deteriorate, losing their elastic and collagenous fibers. This makes them stiffer and thinner and may correlate with voice changes often noted with aging. The vocal fold edge also becomes less smooth. It appears possible that many of these functions can be maintained at a better level than expected, perhaps allowing a high-quality singing or acting career to extend into or beyond the seventh decade. Although more study is needed, physicians and voice teachers already have some tools for intervention to slow the effects of aging on the voice.

MEDICAL INTERVENTION

Certain aspects of the aging process are relatively easy to control medically. As female singers reach menopause, estrogen deprivation causes substantial changes in the muscles and mucous membranes that line the vocal tract; these changes can be forestalled for many years through hormone replacement therapy. Dosage is best determined by checking estrogen levels prior to menopause. Preparations containing androgens should be avoided because they can cause masculinization of the voice. Expert advice should be sought, particularly in those with possible contraindications to hormone replacement therapy (e.g., history of breast cancer).

Muscle disease causes loss of muscle fibers indistinguishable from that seen with advanced age. Exercise prevents or reverses many of these changes in the young and appears to have the same effect in aging individuals. With aging, respiratory function normally decreases in that residual lung volume increases and vital capacity decreases, with a potential impact on voice. Appropriate exercise, along with proper nutrition and weight control, helps maintain muscle function and coordination, as well as optimal functioning of the respiratory system.

Audiences have established a certain level of performance that is acceptable for a professional singer. At the age of 18, singers with excellent voices may perform at only 50% of their current potential. With increasing age, physical abilities deteriorate, and if singers still perform at only 50% of potential, they will fall below the acceptable performance standard. However, if, through appropriate training, exercise, medication, and other factors, they are able to get to 70%, 80%, or 90% of their potential performance level, they may maintain professionally acceptable performance standards for many decades. For this reason, in treating age-related dysphonia, we combine traditional voice therapy, singing training, acting voice techniques, and aerobic conditioning to optimize neuromuscular performance. In general, rehabilitation is sufficient to restore acceptable voice function and eliminate most of the acoustic information perceived as "old." Occasionally, substantial tissue changes make it impossible for therapy and medical management alone to restore satisfactory voice, and some such patients may benefit from laryngeal surgery.

As lungs and thorax lose their elasticity and distensibility and abdominal muscle mass begins to deteriorate, it becomes increasingly important for a professional voice user to be in peak physical condition. A singer whose respiratory and abdominal conditioning is not good enough to allow him or her to walk up a few flights of stairs without becoming winded will have difficulty maintaining good abdominal support throughout a recital or opera. When the power source of the voice is undermined in this way, excessive muscle use in the neck and tongue usually supervenes. Conditioning muscles gradually under medical supervision restores good support. Regular vocal technical training can eliminate the tremolo and improve agility, accuracy, and endurance in the older speaker or singer just as it can in the beginner.

PSYCHOLOGY AND INTELLECT

Other age-related medical changes may also be significant to vocal function in some people. Personality has been most commonly described in terms of a five-factor mode: extroversion, emotional stability, agreeableness, conscientiousness, and culture. In their 1989 study, Peabody and Goldberg (80) described the five replicable factors, which emerge from factor analysis of a large number of personality traits. In general, personality traits are quite stable after approximately age 30. In IQ testing of the elderly, research indicates that age-related decrements on tests such as the WAIS-R are primarily in the speed tests, measuring perceptual-motor skills. There are more often decrements in *fluid* abilities (such as reaction speed) than in *crystallized* abilities (such as fund of knowledge). Verbal ability is retained until very old age. With renorming of the WAIS-R to age-appropriate populations, IQ changes in the elderly are now clearly seen as functions of educational opportunity and health status (81,82). Alterations in cognition, especially memory, and changes in personality secondary to mood disorders and delusionality may impair a person's ability to concentrate, consistently perform vocal tasks, and cooperate optimally with voice rehabilitation.

ENDOCRINE SYSTEM

Alterations in the hormonal environment may affect vocal function; in males, serum levels of testosterone decline, while in women postmenopausal levels of estrogen are low. These changes impact mucosal structure and secretions, as well as mood. Caution should be exercised in prescribing androgen-containing medications in women, since they may cause irreversible masculinization of the voice. This is of particular concern in professional voice users.

Thyroid disease in the elderly deserves special mention. Both hyperthyroidism and hypothyroidism are notoriously difficult to diagnose during advanced age. The elderly patient with hypothyroidism frequently does not display the "typical" features of mental slowing, loss of energy, neurotic behavior, hearing loss, weight gain, musculoskeletal discomfort, dry skin, and changes in facial appearance. Alterations in thyroid function frequently produce substantial changes in vocal quality, including loss of range, efficiency, and "muffling" of the voice. These vocal derangements generally resolve when the thyroid abnormality is treated.

NEUROLOGIC DISEASES

Neurologic diseases are frequently associated with voice problems. Essential tremor may present as a vocal tremor with a rhythmic, quavering voice. The tremor is present during all phonatory efforts, and increases parallel to vocal intensity. The voice associated with Parkinson's disease is low and monotonic. Many other neurologic conditions may aggravate or mimic age-related dysphagia (83).

HEAD AND NECK

Problems associated with hearing loss have been discussed above and are reviewed in greater detail elsewhere in this book. Oral cavity changes associated with aging may be particularly troublesome to singers. Loss of dentition may alter occlusion and articulation, causing especially disturbing problems for professional voice users and wind instrumentalists. These difficulties may be avoided to some extent by having impressions made while dentition is still normal. Dentures that are more similar to the person's natural teeth can then be fashioned. Although salivary glands lose up to about 30% of their parenchymal tissue over a lifetime, salivary secretion remains adequate in most healthy, nonmedicated people throughout life. However, changes in the oral mucosa are similar to those occurring in the skin (thinning and dehydration). They render oral mucosa in the elderly more susceptible to injury, and the sensation of xerostomia may be especially disturbing to singers. Cancers in the head and neck usually occur in people over 40 years of age and may result in profound voice dysfunction.

OTHER CONDITIONS

Many other factors must also be taken into account in diagnosis and treatment of elderly patients. These include coronary artery disease, cerebrovascular disease, hypertension, obesity, stroke, diabetes, cancer, diet, osteoporosis, hearing loss, vision loss, swallowing dysfunction, anemia, arthritis, neurological dysfunction including tremor, incontinence, gastrointestinal disorders, and other conditions. All of these may have adverse effects on the voice, either through action on the larynx or through impairment of the voice-producing mechanism at another anatomical site.

VOICE THERAPY

Expert voice therapy for presbyphonia can be particularly rewarding. Such therapy is best provided by a team, and it must include attention to the entire body, not just the voice. As discussed above, aerobic conditioning is essential. In our center, voice therapy for presbyphonia begins with general medical evaluation and institution of a medically supervised aerobic conditioning program. This is similar to the cardiac rehabilitation programs instituted after myocardial infarction. It is directed toward restoring the power source of the voice. This is essential for speaking as well as for singing.

The voice therapy team includes a speech-language pathologist, singing voice specialist, and frequently an acting voice specialist. The speech pathologist is responsible for identifying and eliminating voice abuse and misuse, teaching vocal hygiene, and developing an exercise program for the spoken voice that emphasizes appropriate breath and abdominal support, relaxation in the muscles of the head and neck, and appropriate use of resonance to optimize audibility (84).

The singing voice specialist works symbiotically with the speech-language pathologist, caring for both singers and non-singers (85). The purpose of this portion of the therapy program is not to create singers out of every presbyphonic patient we treat. Singing expands an individual's phonatory limits, increasing breath support and phrase length, increasing frequency and intensity ranges, and strengthening the voice beyond the level necessary for even extended speech. The combination of traditional voice therapy and specialized singing exercises expedites and improves outcome.

Since 1995, we have also included an acting voice trainer in our voice team using techniques that are different from, but compatible with, traditional voice therapy (86). Acting voice trainers teach techniques not only for development of speaking voice strength and projection, but also for control of face and body function, phonatory expression of emotion, preparation and interpretation of spoken materials, and other communication skills. Learning these techniques improves not only voice quality and vocal authority, but also gives patients great confidence in their ability to control vocal communication.

SURGERY

In some patients, even the best voice therapy is not sufficient to overcome presbyphonia. When vocal fold thinning or bowing causes failure of glottic closure, hyperfunction (muscular tension dysphonia) develops routinely as the patient tries to compensate in an attempt to eliminate breathiness. This muscle hyperfunction is often responsible for voice fatigue and increased hoarseness, and sometimes for vocal nodules, hemorrhages, or other injuries. As voice therapy eliminates the hyperfunction, breathiness becomes audible again. If the glottal incompetence is minimal, vocal exercises may increase muscle bulk enough to restore glottic closure. At the same time, improved vocal technique will enhance audibility even if slight breathiness remains. However, when glottal incompetence is too great, surgery should be considered.

Thorough evaluation is necessary prior to reaching any surgical decision. Strobovideolaryngoscopy is essential. Frequently, a diagnosis of "bowing" made by mirror examination is refuted during strobovideolaryngoscopy when closer assessment shows that the vocal folds are actually making contact. Such patients usually respond to voice therapy. Omori et al. (87) have recently reported the value of objective assessment of vocal fold atrophy. When stroboscopy confirms a significant glottal gap or when abnormalities or asymmetries of vocal fold motion are detected, laryngeal electromyography should be considered, since superior laryngeal nerve paresis may also be a common cause of "bowing" (88). In unilateral superior laryngeal nerve paralysis, therapy sometimes results in acceptable voice improvement. In unilateral or bilateral superior laryngeal nerve paresis, therapy is most likely to be effective if electromyography reveals no more than a 40–60% decreased recruitment response. Elimination of compensatory hyperfunction and use of stretching exercises (such as pitch changing) often produce surprising improvement. If glottal incompetence is caused by bilateral superior laryngeal nerve paralysis, voice therapy alone is rarely adequate. Surgical results in such patients are also frequently not perfect, although combining surgery and therapy tends to be more helpful than therapy alone.

When surgery is needed in patients with presbyphonia without superior laryngeal nerve paresis or paralysis, medialization procedures in combination with voice therapy usually are effective (89). Operations that alter pitch are indicated occasionally, primarily for females with marked androphonia. When presbyphonia is combined with superior laryngeal nerve paresis or paralysis, treatment becomes more difficult; in most cases, medialization and therapy are adequate. Occasionally, a lengthening procedure (such as cricothyroid approximation or cricothyroid fusion) may be appropriate. Although arytenoid adduction/rotation is an effective procedure for adjusting vocal process height and is an excellent procedure for patients with vocal fold paralysis, this author (Sataloff) does not generally recommend it for presbyphonic patients with mobile vocal folds and intact cricoarytenoid joints.

Specific techniques of phonosurgery, additional references, specific technical information, limits, and complications are available elsewhere (90).

Injection Laryngoplasty

Teflon injection was the standard of care for glottal incompetence for many years. However, occasionally a severe foreign body reaction and granuloma may occur, which are extremely difficult to correct. Because of Teflon's disadvantages and potential complications, it has been largely replaced by better techniques and materials.

Gelfoam Injection

The effects of injection of a more permanent material can be predicted fairly well by prior injection of Gelfoam. This material is injected lateral to the vocal fold in the same position in which Teflon was used. However, Gelfoam is temporary, resorbing in 2–8 weeks. For presbyphonic patients in whom the choice of surgical approach is uncertain, Gelfoam injection may provide a reasonable therapeutic trial.

Collagen Injection

Several other materials are still being injected to treat vocal fold paralysis, especially collagen and fat. Ford and Bless (91–93) have advocated the use of collagen for many conditions, including selected cases of unilateral vocal fold paralysis. Collagen is in liquid form, rather than a thick paste like Teflon. These mechanical differences enhance the ease and accuracy of injection. However, although collagen has proven useful for treatment of vocal fold scar, so far it has been less useful for treatment of vocal fold paralysis because of its tendency to resorb. Early collagen experience was obtained using bovine collagen; now, autologous or allogeneic collagen may be used. The use of human collagen has important advantages. First, it eliminates the risk of serious immune reaction. Second, the collagen can be engineered to different consistencies and biologic properties depending on its intended use. Collagen injection is discussed in the chapter on voice surgery.

Autologous Fat Injection and Fascia Injection

Human autologous fat injection into the larynx was first reported by Mikaelian et al. in 1991 (94) and subsequently by Brandenburg et al. (95). These and subsequent reports dealt with autologous lipoinjection lateral to the vibratory margin, placing fat in the same position in which Teflon was used. The author had continued excellent experience with fat injection, particularly in patients who needed only minimal medialization. For patients with a wide glottic gap, thyroplasty alone or in combination with fat injection has been preferable.

Several technical considerations are important in achieving success with fat injection. The first is patient selection. The patients who do best with autologous fat injection are those who have only a small glottal gap, or those who actually close the glottis during soft phonation but have insufficient resistance on the paralyzed side to permit loud phonation. Such conditions occur after spontaneous compensation for laryngeal paralysis, or occasionally following Type I thyroplasty. Similar situations may be seen in patients with presbyphonia and vocal fold bowing. Second, the fat should be traumatized as little as possible, maintaining large globules. Third, fat should not be injected much more posteriorly than the middle third of the membranous portion of the vocal fold. A properly placed injection at this location provides adequate medial displacement and allows the medialized vocal fold to pull the arytenoid and vocal process into better position. Injecting too far posteriorly creates a mechanical impediment to passive arytenoid motion, often resulting in persistent vertical height disparity at the vocal processes and inferior voice results. Fourth, unlike Teflon, fat requires over-injection by approximately 30%. The vocal fold should be convex at the conclusion of the procedure to account for expected resorption. This over-injection causes moderate dysphonia initially. If the voice is excellent shortly following the surgical procedure, a good final result is unlikely. The amount of over-injection required can be modified by combining fat with fascia, or by using fascia alone. Fascia requires much less over-injection but may have disadvantages, including its viscosity and technical difficulties preparing it for injection.

Thyroplasty

Another excellent approach for medialization to correct glottal incompetence is Type I thyroplasty. This procedure was proposed by Isshiki et al. in 1975 (96). It has been used extensively and modified by many surgeons. At present, the author (Sataloff) uses Gore-Tex almost exclusively for this indication. The surgical techniques for this and the other procedures discussed in this chapter are reviewed elsewhere (90). In some patients, the results of a well-performed thyroplasty (or vocal fold injection) can be predicted preoperatively by external compression of the thyroid laminae during phonation. However, in elderly patients with calcified thyroid cartilages, this test may be difficult or misleading.

Type IV thyroplasty was designed to lengthen the vocal folds and increase their tension in order to raise vocal pitch. The cricoid and thyroid cartilages are approximated anteriorly with nylon sutures. Although this procedure has been used primarily for patients undergoing male to female sex-change surgery, it is also useful in elderly women with excessive vocal masculinization. Unfortunately, the long-term results (beyond 6–12 months) have been disappointing in some cases. Sataloff (90) described an alternative procedure that fuses the cricoid and thyroid, which seems more satisfactory. The position of the cricoid and thyroid cartilage can be held either with sutures or with mini-plates. Surprisingly, these patients have maintained approximately a 1-octave frequency range despite complete cricothyroid fusion and fixation.

Pitch can also be raised by shifting the anterior commissure forward. The procedure is performed by making vertical incisions in the thyroid cartilage similar to those used for Type III thyroplasty. However, the anterior segment is advanced.

The advancement is maintained by interposing silastic blocks in the gaps between the cartilage edges and fixing the cartilage with mini-plates. Care must be taken not to detach the anterior commissure during this procedure and during cosmetic laryngo-plasty used in gender reassignment patients, as discussed in the chapter on voice surgery.

CONCLUSION

Vocal changes associated with aging are common and may be disturbing to patients. In some, the vocal weakness and decreased endurance may even be disabling. Most patients with presbyphonia can be helped. Geriatric voice disorders have traditionally received less attention than they deserve. Intensive management of presbyphonia is encouraged and can be extremely rewarding to both the patient and the voice care team.

Because older singers and actors may have considerably less natural reserve and resilience than youthful performers, it is important to adopt a comprehensive therapeutic approach. With optimal physical and vocal conditioning, proper medical supervision of cardiac and respiratory function, and appropriate medication, weight control, nutrition, and surgery in selected cases, it appears likely that a great many singers, actors, and other voice professionals may enjoy extra years or decades of improved performance.

REFERENCES

1. Sataloff, RT, Linville SL. The effect of age on the voice. In: Sataloff RT, ed. Professional Voice: The Science and Art of Clinical Care. 3rd ed. Chapter 27. San Diego: Plural Publishing Group, 2005:499–511.
2. Kahane J. Age-related histological changes in the human male and female laryngeal cartilages: biological and functional implications. In: Lawrence V, ed. Transcripts of the 9th Symposium: Care of the Professional Voice. New York: The Voice Foundation, 1980: 11–20.
3. Kahane J. Anatomic and physiologic changes in the aging peripheral speech mechanism. In: Beasley DS, Davis GA, eds. Aging Communication Processes and Disorders. New York: Grune and Stratton, 1981:21–45.
4. Dhar S, Shastri S, Lenora R. Aging and the respiratory system. Symposium on geriatric medicine. Med Clin North Am 1976; 60:1112–1139.
5. MCKeown F. Pathology of the Aged. London: Butterworths, 1965.
6. Mahler D. Pulmonary aspects of aging. In: Gambert SR, ed. Contemporary geriatric medicine. Vol. 1. New York: Plenum Publishing Corporation, 1983:45–85.
7. Crapo R. The aging lung. In: Mahler DA, ed. Pulmonary Disease in the Elderly Patients: Lung Biology in Health and Disease. Vol. 63. New York: Marcel Dekker, 1983:1–25.
8. Hoit J, Hixon T. Age and Speech Breathing. J Speech Hear Res 1987; 30:351–366.
9. Hoit J, Hixon T, Altman M, Morgan W. Speech breathing in women. J Speech Hear Res 1989; 32:353–365.
10. Linville SE. Vocal Aging. Albany, NY: Delmar Thomson Learning, 2001.
11. Malinowski A. The shape, dimensions and process of calcification of the cartilaginous framework of the larynx in relation to age and sex in the Polish population. Folia Morphologica (Warsz) 1967; 26:118–128.
12. Roncollo P. Researches about ossification and conformation of the thyroid cartilage in sex and certain other factors. Mayo Clin Proc 1949; 31:47–52.
13. Bach A, Lederer F, Dinolt R. Senile changes in the laryngeal musculature. Arch Otolaryngol 1941; 34:47–56.

14. Ferreri G. Senescence of the larynx. Italian Gen Rev Oto-Rhino-Laryngol 1959; 1: 640–709.

15. Rodeno M, Sanchex-Fernandex J, Rivera-Pomar J. Histochemical and morphometrical ageing changes in human vocal cord muscles. Acta Otolaryngol (Stockholm) 1993; 113: 443–449.

16. Kahane J. Age-related changes in the peripheral speech mechanism: structural and physiological changes. Proceedings of the research symposium on communicative sciences and disorders and aging. ASHA reports. No. 19. Rockville, MD: American Speech Language Hearing Association, 1990:75–87.

17. Hirano M, Kuritat S, Sakaguchi S. Aging of the vibratory tissue of human vocal folds. Acta Otolaryngol 1989; 107:428–433.

18. Ishii K, Zhai W, Akita M, Hirose H. Ultrastructure of the lamina propria of the human vocal fold. Acta Otolaryngol (Stockholm) 1996; 116:778–782.

19. Chan R, Titze I. Viscoelastic shear properties of human vocal fold mucosa: measurement methodology and empirical results. J Acoust Soc Am 1999; 106:2008–2021.

20. Gray S, Titze I, Chan R, Hammond T. Vocal fold proteoglycans and their influence on biomechanics. Laryngoscope 1999; 109:845–854.

21. Murry T, Xu J, Woodson G. Glottal configuration associated with fundamental frequency and vocal register. J Voice 1998; 12:44–49.

22. Pausewang Gelger M, Bultemeyer D. Evaluation of vocal fold vibratory patterns in normal voice. J Voice 1990; 4:335–345.

23. Rammage L, Peppeard R, Bless D. Aerodynamic, laryngoscopic and perceptual acoustic characteristics in dysphonic females with posterior glottal chinks: a retrospective study. J Voice 1992; 6:64–78.

24. Soderson M, Lindestad P. Glottal closure and perceived breathiness during phonation in normally speaking subjects. J Speech Hear Res 1990; 33:604–611.

25. Beiver D, Bless D. Vibratory characteristics of the vocal folds in young adult and geriatric women. J Voice 1989; 3:120–131.

26. Hooton E, Dupertuis C. Age changes and selective survival in Irish males. In: American Association of Physical Anthropology: Studies in Physical Anthropology. No. 2. New York: Wenner-Gren Foundation, 1951.

27. Lasker F. The age factor in bodily measurements of adult male and female Mexicans. Hum Biol 1953; 25:50–63.

28. Levesque J, Coruff P, De Rigal J, Agache P. In vivo studies of the evaluation of physical properties of the human skin and aging. Int J Dermatol 1984; 23:322–329.

29. Pitanguy I. Ancillary procedures in face lifting. Clin Plastic Surg 1978; 5:51–70.

30. Akerman S, Rohlin M, Kopp S. Bilateral degenerative changes and deviation in form of temporomandibular joints: an autopsy study of elderly individuals. Acta Odontol Scand 1984; 42:205–214.

31. Nannmark U, Sennerby L, Haraldson T. Macroscopic, microscopic and radiologic assessment of the condylar part of the TMJ in elderly subjects: an autopsy study. Swedish Dent J 1990; 14:163–169.

32. Pereira F, Lundh H, Westesson P. Age-related changes of the retrodiscal tissues in the temporomandibular joint. J Oral Maxillofac Surg 1996; 54:55–61.

33. Stratmann U, Schaarschmidt K, Santamaria P. Morphometric investigation of condylar cartilage and disc thickness in the human temporomandibular joint: significance for the definition of osteoarthrotic changes. J Oral Pathol Med 1996; 25:200–205.

34. DeBont L, Boering G, Liem R, Eulderink F, Westesson P. Osteoarthritis and internal derangement of the temporomandibular joint: a light microscopic study. J Oral Maxillofac Surg 1986; 44:634–643.

35. Scapino R. Histopathology associated with malposition of the human temporomandibular joint disc. Oral Surg 1983; 55:382–397.

36. Breustedt A. Age induced changes in the oral mucosa and their therapeutic consequences. Int Dent J 1983; 33:272–280.

37. Cruchley A, Williams D, Farthing P, Speight P, Lesch C, Squier C. Langerhans cell density in normal human mucosa and skin: relations to age, smoking and alcohol consumption. J Oral Pathol Med 1994; 23:55–59.

38. Ofstehage J, Magilvy K. Oral health and aging. Geriatr Nurs 1986; 7:238–241.

39. Sonies B. The aging oropharyngeal system. In: Ripich D, ed. Handbook of Geriatric Communication Disorders. Austin, Tx: Pro-ed, 1991:187–203.

40. Adams D. Age changes in oral structures. Dent Update 1991; 18:14–17.

41. Klein D. Oral soft tissue changes in geriatric patients. Bull New York Acad Med 1980; 45:721–727.

42. Sasaki M. Histomorphometric analysis of age-related changes in epithelial thickness and Langerhans cell density of the human tongue. Tohoku J Exp Med 1994; 173: 321–336.

43. Kiuchi S, Sasaki J, Arai T, Suzuki T. Functional disorders of the pharynx and esophagus. Acta Oto-laryngol Suppl 1969; 256:1–30.

44. Tomoda T, Morii S, Yamashita T, Kumazawa T. Histology of human eustacian tube muscles: effect of aging. Ann Otol Rhinol Laryngol 1984; 93:17–24.

45. Zaino C, Benventaon T. Functional, involutional and degenerative disorders. In: Zaino C, Benventano T, eds. Radiographic Examination of the Oropharynx and Esophagus. New York: Springer-Verlag, 1977:141–176.

46. Vissink A, Spijkervet F, Amerongen A. Aging and saliva: a review of the literature. Special Care Dentistry 1996; 16:95–103.

47. Crow H, Ship J. Tongue strength and endurance in different aged individuals. J Gerontol Ser A Biol Sci Med Sci 1996; 51:M247–M250.

48. Brown W, Morris R, Hicks D, Howell E. Phonational profiles of female professional singers and nonsingers. J Voice 1993; 7:219–226.

49. Brown W, Morris R, Hollien H, Howell E. Speaking fundamental frequency characteristics as a function of age and professional singing. J Voice 1991; 5:310–315.

50. Hollien H, Jackson B. Normative data on the speaking fundamental frequency characteristics of young adult males. J Phonetics 1973; 1:117–120.

51. Hollien H, Shipp T. Speaking fundamental frequency and chronologic age in males. J Speech Hear Res 1972; 15:155–159.

52. Honjo I, Isshiki N. Laryngoscopic and voice characteristics of aged persons. Arch Otolaryngol 1980; 106:149–150.

53. Mysak E. Pitch and duration characteristics of older males. J Speech Hear Res 1959; 2:46–54.

54. Peroraro Krook M. Speaking fundamental frequency characteristics of normal Swedish subjects obtained by glottal frequency analysis. Folia Phoniatrica (Basel) 1988; 40: 82–90.

55. Saxman J, Burk K. Speaking fundamental frequency characteristics of middle aged females. Folia Phoniatrica (Basel) 1967; 19:167–172.

56. Stoicheff M. Speaking fundamental characteristics of nonsmoking female adults. J Speech Hear Res 1981; 24:437–441.

57. Kahane J. Connective tissue changes in the larynx and their effects on voice. J Voice 1987; 1:27–30.

58. Segre R. Senescence of the voice. Eye Ear Nose Throat Mon 1971; 50:223–227.

59. De Pinto O, Hollien H. Speaking fundamental frequency characteristics of Australian women: then and now. J Phonetics 1982; 10:367–375.

60. Linville SE. Maximum phonational frequency ranges capabilities of women's voices with advancing age. Folia Phoniatrica (Basel) 1987; 39:297–301.

61. Morris R, Brown W. Age-related differences in speech intensity among adult females. Folia Phoniatrica (Logop) 1994; 46:64–69.

62. Melcon M, Hoit J, Hisxon T. Age and laryngeal airway resistance during vowel production. J Speech Hear Disord 1989; 54:282–286.

63. Ryan W. Acoustic aspects of the aging voice. J Gerontol 1972; 27:265–268.

64. Holmes L, Leeper H, Nicholson I. Laryngeal airway resistance of older men and women as a function of vocal sound pressure level. J Speech Hear Res 1994; 37:789–799.

65. Ptacek P, Sander E, Maloney W, Jackson C. Phonatory and related changes with advanced age. J Speech Hear Res 1966; 9:353–360.

66. Morris R, Brown W. Age-related voice measures among adult women. J Voice 1987; 1:38–43.

67. Linville SE. Glottal gap configurations in two age groups of women. J Speech Hear Res 1992; 35:1209–1215.

68. Linville SE, Fisher H. Acoustic characteristics of perceived versus actual vocal age in controlled phonation by adult females. J Acoust Soc Am 1985; 78:40–48.

69. Petrosino L, Colcord R, Kurcz K, Yonker R. Voice onset time of velar stop productions in aged speakers. Perceptual Motor Skills 1993; 76:83–88.

70. Sinard R, Hall D. The aging voice: how to differentiate disease from normal changes. Geriatrics 1998; 53:79.

71. McGlone R, Hollien H. Vocal pitch characteristics of aged women. J Speech Hear Res 1963; 6:164–170.

72. Linville SE. The sound of senescence. J Voice 1996; 10:190–200.

73. Mueller PB. The aging voice. Semin Speech Lang 1997; 18(2):159–168.

74. Woo P, Casper J, Colton R, Brewer D. Dysphonia in the aging: physiology versus disease. Laryngoscope 1992; 102:139–144.

75. Special issue on vocal aging. J Voice 1987; 1(1):2–67.

76. Sataloff RT, Rosen DC, Hawkshaw M, Spiegel JR. The three ages of voice: the aging adult voice. J Voice 1997; 11(2):138–143.

77. Gray SD, Hirano M, Sato K. Molecular and cellular structure of vocal fold tissue. In: Titze IR, ed. Vocal Fold Physiology. San Diego, CA: Singular Publishing Group, Inc., 1993:1–35.

78. Sato K, Hirano M. Age-related changes of the macula flava of the human vocal fold. Ann Otol Rhinol Laryngol 1995; 104(11):839–844.

79. Campos-Banales ME, Perez Pinero B, Rivero J, Ruiz-Casal E, Lopez-Aguado D. Histological structure of the vocal fold in the human larynx. Acta Otolaryngol (Stockh) 1995; 115(5):701–704.

80. Peabody D, Goldberg LR. Some determinants of factor structures from personality trait descriptors. J Pers Soc Psychol 1989; 57:552–576.

81. Botwinic J. Aging and behavior. New York: Springer-Verlag, 1978:22–30.

82. Anastasi A. Psychological testing. 6th ed. New York: Macmillan Publishing, 1988: 347–351

83. Sataloff RJ. Professional voice: The Science and Art of Clinical Care. 3rd ed. San Diego: Plural Publishing Group, 2005:847–902.

84. Heuer RJ, Rulnick RK, Horman M, Perez KS, Emerich KA, Sataloff RT. Voice therapy. In: Sataloff RT, ed. Professional Voice: The Science and Art of Clinical Care. 3rd ed. San Diego: Plural Publishing Group, Inc., 2005.

85. Sataloff RT, Baroody MM, Emerich KA, Carrol LM. The singing voice specialist. In: Sataloff RT, ed. Professional Voice: The Science and Art of Clinical Care. 3rd ed. San Diego: Plural Publishing Group, Inc., 2005.

86. Freed SL, Raphael BN, Sataloff RT. The role of the acting-voice trainer in medical care of professional voice users. In: Sataloff RT, ed. Professional voice: The Science and Art of Clinical Care. 3rd ed. San Diego: Plural Publishing Group, Inc., 2005.

87. Omori K, Slavit DH, Matos C, Kojima H, Kacker A, Blaugrund SM. Vocal fold atrophy: quantitative glottic measurement and vocal function. Ann Otol Rhinol Laryngol 1997; 106(7 pt 1):544–551.

88. Sataloff RT, Mandel S, Manon-Espaillat R, Heman-Ackah YD, Abaza A. Laryngeal electromyography. San Diego: Plural Publishing Group, 2005.

89. Isshiki N, Shoji K, Kojima H, Hirano S. Vocal fold atrophy and its surgical treatment. Ann Otol Rhinol Laryngol 1996; 105(3):182–188.

90. Sataloff RT. Voice surgery. In: Sataloff RT, ed. Professional Voice: The Science and Art of Clinical Care. 3rd ed. San Diego: Plural Publishing Group, 2005:1137–1211.

91. Ford CN, Bless DM, Loftus JM. The role of injectable collagen in the treatment of glottic insufficiency: a study of 119 patients. Ann Otol Rhinol Laryngol 1973; 101(3): 237–247.

92. Ford CN, Bless DM. Collagen injected in the scarred vocal fold. J Voice 1988; 1: 116–118.

93. Ford CN, Bless DM. Selected problems treated by vocal fold injection of collagen. Am J Otolaryngol 1993; 14(4):257–261.

94. Mikaelian D, Lowry LD, Sataloff RT. Lipoinjection for unilateral vocal cord paralysis. Laryngoscope 1991; 101:465–468.

95. Brandenburg J, Kirkham W, Koschkee D. Vocal cord augmentation with autologous fat. Laryngoscope 1992; 102:495–500.

96. Isshiki N, Okamura H, Ishikawa T. Thyroplasty Type I (lateral compression for dysphonia due to vocal cord paralysis or atrophy). Acta Otolaryngol 1975; 80:465–473.

97. Heuer RJ, Baroody M, Sataloff RT. Management of Gender Reassignment (sex change) Patients. In: Sataloff RT, ed. Professional Voice: The Science and Art of Clinical Care. 3rd ed. San Diego: Plural Publishing Group, 2005:1359–1364.

34

Vocal Fold Paralysis: Surgical Treatment

Steven M. Zeitels

Department of Otology and Laryngology, Harvard Medical School, Boston, Massachusetts, U.S.A.

GENERAL DESCRIPTION OF THE CLINICAL PROBLEM

Vocal fold paralysis (VFP) can be understood as denervation of the intrinsic musculature of the larynx and an associated immobility of the arytenoid. This will lead to
varying degrees of dysfunctional voice, swallowing, airway, and coughing (1). The
severity of these deficits is often related to underlying variants in normal anatomy,
age and compensatory capabilities, synkinetic reinnervation, comorbid diseases
and deficits, and prior aerodigestive tract surgery, as well as needs and expectations
of the patient.

   VFP is primarily the consequence of loss of recurrent laryngeal nerve (RLN)
function. It may occur subsequent to a surgical procedure that requires dissection
in the brain or in the region of the RLN, which includes surgery of the skull base, neck,
and mediastinum. VFP has even been documented from endotracheal intubation. If
an individual has not undergone a procedure, VFP should not be assumed to be idiopathic. Other causes must be ruled out, such as neoplastic compression of the brain or
RLN, a degenerative neuromuscular disorder, or cerebrovascular disease. Idiopathic
RLN paralysis is typically believed to be due to a viral inflammation of that nerve.

   The treatment of unilateral vocal paralysis (UVP) is most commonly a transoral or transcervical medialization since the airway is usually adequate if one cricoarytenoid joint retains abductory and adductory function. Conversely, bilateral VFP
usually requires vocal fold lateralization to widen the glottal airway aperture. This
chapter is confined to UVP.

WHY IS UVP PARTICULARLY IMPORTANT IN THE GERIATRIC POPULATION, INCLUDING RECENT CONCEPTS IN PATHOPHYSIOLOGY?

UVP can be severely disabling and potentially grave in the geriatric population,
whose swallowing mechanisms and airways may harbor subclinical deficits. The
most frequent disabling life-threatening symptom is that of dysphagia with aspiration. This can occur because of a number of interdependent reasons. First, many

older patients have had age-related diminution of sensation in the pharyngeal and laryngeal mucosa. Second, inadequate closure of the larynx can lead to initial aspiration of portions of a swallowing bolus as well as secondary aspiration if the food bolus is not completely stripped from the pharyngeal vestibule. Essentially, the incompetent patent glottis leads to an inadequate trans-pharyngo-esophageal pressure gradient during pharyngeal emptying. Finally, inadequate glottal closure and cough that can result are associated with poor pulmonary toilet. In turn, tracheobronchitis can evolve into pneumonia.

Vocal dysfunction associated with VFP is often more severe in older patients because many have sustained normal age-related reduced pliability of the vocal membranes from years of use. The coupling of denervation-related aerodynamic glottal incompetence with stiff vocal membranes causes extremely severe hoarseness. This will usually be disproportionate to what would be expected based on a nonstroboscopic laryngoscopic examination.

There are also age-related changes of the cricoarytenoid joint, which have yet to be scientifically assessed. What is the normal range of motion of the arytenoid at different ages? If there has been a "normal" gradual decrease in abductory function of the contralateral arytenoid, the ability and degree to which the paralyzed vocal fold can be medialized is diminished while ensuring for a safe airway. This is further complicated by the fact that frequently there is diminished brain-related central nervous system in the elderly. This can impede voice recovery and enhancement associated with surgical reconstruction and/or voice therapy.

A seldom-discussed feature of the dysphonia in the elderly is that their spouse and friends often have hearing deficits. Poor vocal projection coupled to diminished auditory acuity and discrimination in their peers leads to substantial frustration and, on rare occasions, danger.

HISTORY

The most common and universal presentation of all patients with UVP is dysphonia and hoarseness. The voice is typically breathy and strained from aerodynamic incompetence and often diplophonic from differential elasticity since one vocal fold is flaccid. The hyperfunctional hyperadduction of the innervated vocal fold often leads to an inordinately high pitch. The dysphonia associated with UVP in the geriatric patients is also typically worse in those who have sustained work-related phonotrauma as a professional speaker, i.e., educator, clergy, executive, attorney etc. The gradual phonotraumatic reduction of vocal membrane pliability associated with "normal" diminution of vocal function is often under-appreciated until accompanied by impaired glottal closure.

Geriatric patients with UVP do not usually have airway difficulties. Those who do often have a history of obstructive sleep apnea. If there is substantial baseline diminished abduction of the contralateral arytenoid, the patient is likely to develop stridor and airway difficulties. In this scenario, symptoms will be worse with deep inspiration and/or in a sleep state due to the Bernoulli's effect on the flaccid glottal soft tissues.

Patients may present with mild coughing or frank aspiration, which is usually worse with thin liquids. Those with a history of cerebrovascular disease and stroke often have diminished pharyngo-laryngeal sensation and proprioception, and these individuals are at high risk for pulmonary sequelae if they develop a new UVP.

PHYSICAL EXAMINATION

When a patient is suspected of having a UVP, it is critical to perform a complete oto-laryngologic examination including the neck. A careful cranial nerve exam is valuable to assist with the diagnosis, assess the physiological dysfunction, and to prognosticate voice enhancement should the patient undergo surgical intervention. Careful attention should be given to the 5th, 9th, 11th, and 12th nerves to assess deglutition and to rule out a skull-base tumor.

Fiberoptic laryngoscopy should be done to evaluate abductory and adductory glottal function as well as supraglottal compensatory strategies. Ideally, this should be recorded for review with the patient and in slow motion. An optimal way to assess this is through the task of having the patient "sniff" to stimulate the posterior cricoarytenoid muscle followed by an "eee." The examination often reveals that the paralyzed vocal fold is infralaterally displaced at the glottal level and that more cephalad corniculate region is accordingly displaced anteromedially. The degree of abduction and caudal displacement of the paralyzed vocal fold is directly related to the severity of the denervation and/or degree of synkinetic reinnervation (2). These factors are difficult to distinguish, even with laryngeal electromyography due to the imprecision of that technique. Regardless, this information is not critical for clinical management and surgical reconstruction.

Telescopic strobolaryngoscopy has enhanced optical resolution and is the optimal approach for visually assessing membrane pliability and aerodynamic competence. It is common for the vocal folds to oscillate with two different resonant frequencies due to the innervation-related flaccidity of the paralyzed vocal cord. This often appears as a flutter vibration on one side and creates the acoustical perception of diplophonia.

DIFFERENTIAL DIAGNOSIS

The primary diagnosis per which VFP must be differentiated from is that of impaired vocal fold mobility secondary to cricoarytenoid joint restriction. Although there is impaired mobility of the arytenoid in both scenarios, dysphonia associated with paralysis is usually substantially more severe due to flaccidity of the thyroarytenoid muscle associated with the glottal incompetence. The vocal distinction between these diagnoses will usually become even more obvious when the individual is asked to phonate in a range of pitch frequencies. Additionally, those with mechanical cricoarytenoid motion restriction will often have a bilateral problem and will be associated with glottic stenosis and potential airway difficulties.

TESTING

Upon presentation, apart from the head and neck examination, UVP patients should undergo radiographic imaging from the skull base through the entire path of the recurrent nerve to rule out a neoplastic etiology. They should also undergo objective assessment of vocal function, including acoustic and aerodynamic evaluation (3). This should be done at a conversational level and in loud voice to evaluate maximal range tasks. Laryngeal electromyography may also be quite helpful (4). Although it is slightly painful, it is well tolerated if the examiner has reasonable experience. It is especially valuable when differentiating mechanical restriction of the cricoary-tenoid joint from the denervation of the intrinsic musculature. Laryngeal electro-myography may also prognosticate the degree of denervation as well as prognosticate reinnervation. This can be very helpful in deciding when to perform a reconstructive procedure and to select the surgery of choice. These are the primary tests that should be performed; however, in selected scenarios, a variety of blood tests may be obtained depending upon the consideration of a variety of less common medical diagnoses.

TREATMENT OPTIONS

The treatment options that exist for VFP are all in the form of static reconstruction. The denervated vocal fold is repositioned so that the vibratory epithelium is in position to make better contact with the contralateral mobile one. The surgical inter-ventions are comprised of injection medialization, transcervical laryngeal framework surgery, and neural reinnervation. It should be clear that even neural reinnervation is a form of static reconstruction. The surgically induced synkinetic reinnervation does not actually lead to mobility of the arytenoids since fine neural motor pathways are not restored.

INJECTION MEDIALIZATION

Injection medialization can be temporary or permanent and can be done in the clinic or the operating room based upon the injectable material that is selected. Most laryngologists do not use injectable Teflon at this time, although there are selected circumstances that some still do. We rarely perform lipoinjection (5) for paralysis due to the imprecision associated with the procedure. This is in part because of the need to over-inject due to the irregular resorbance of fat. Further-more, it is typically done in the operating room by means of direct laryngoscopy in a scenario where there is little phonatory feedback from the patient to "tune" the result.

Today, the most frequently used office injection material is cymetra (6). It is purchased in the form of a powder and must be reconstituted by the surgeon. It can be injected transorally in the office through a curved injector with a 22-guage needle (7). We typically anesthetize the oropharynx with cetacaine and then nebulize 4% plain lydocaine into the laryngeal introitus. As necessary, 4% lidocaine can be dripped directly to the site of injection. We typically use the Ford Xomed injecting device. Ideally, an initial puncture and injection is done lateral to the pro-cess. Subsequent to that, a more anterior injection can be made on the ventricular surface of the vocal fold in the mid-musculomembraneous region deep to the vocal ligament. The vocal fold should be over-injected since the collagen has been reconstituted in a dissolvable fluid medium and because the collagen mostly reabsorbs over time.

Office injection of cymetra provides an excellent temporizing strategy for those in whom normal reinnervation is still possible, but severe dysphonia is present. Cymetra injections can also be repeated as necessary to re-expand the paraglottic space while awaiting innervation. It is our subjective impression that 70% to 80% of the cymetra will absorb over time.

LARYNGOPLASTIC PHONOSURGERY: BACKGROUND

Laryngoplastic phonosurgery has evolved to be a dominant treatment modality for the dysphonia associated with UVP. There has been a convergence of physiological principles of glottal vibration with surgical technique theory, which has enhanced vocal outcomes. Although medialization of the musculomembranous vocal fold by means of rearranging the laryngeal cartilage framework was described by Payr (8) in 1915, Isshiki et al. (9–11) championed the systemic analysis and laryngoplastic treatment of paralytic dysphonia in the 1970s. Isshiki et al. (9,10) designed the medialization procedure of the musculomembranous vocal fold with the use of a synthetic implant in 1974, and shortly thereafter, the author designed the arytenoid adduction procedure to treat patients with large glottal gaps secondary to a malpositioned arytenoid. Patients who require repositioning of the arytenoid typically have minimal or unfavorable synkinetic reinnervation of the intrinsic laryngeal musculature. Therefore, the arytenoid at the glottal level is infero-laterally displaced, resulting in a flaccid foreshortened vocal fold.

PRINCIPLES AND THEORY OF LARYNGEAL FRAMEWORK SURGERY

The ideal procedure(s) to treat aerodynamic glottal incompetence that is associated with paralytic/paretic dysphonia should attempt to simulate the normal vocal fold position during phonation with regard to the following interdependent parameters: (i) position of the musculomembranous region in the axial plane, (ii) position of the arytenoid in the axial plane, (iii) height of the vocal fold, (iv) length of the vocal fold, (v) contour of the vocal fold edge in the musculomembranous region, (vi) contour of the vocal fold edge in the arytenoid region, and (vii) mass and viscoelasticity of the vocal fold (augmentation vs. medialization) (12). Furthermore, the procedure(s) would ideally be easy to perform, associated with few complications, reliable, reversible, and not threatening to the airway.

Isshiki (11) delineated many of the pertinent cartilaginous relationships for executing laryngeal framework procedures. It is likely that a number of undesirable outcomes from these operations occur as a result of clinically indeterminable variations in anatomy. This clinical scenario is most commonly encountered when there is difficulty closing a wide posterior interarytenoid glottal aperture. The differences in shape, size, and contour of human arytenoid cartilages and their associated cricoarytenoid joints have not been analyzed in large-scale anatomical investigations. Future advances in radiographic imaging will enable us to answer these questions. Understanding these potential anatomical differences may provide fundamental information to improve the results of laryngoplastic phonosurgery. As an initial attempt to examine anatomical laryngeal framework variation, especially with regard to gender, Sprinzi et al. (13) performed a comprehensive analysis of 98 larynges. Further studies are clearly needed.

MEDIALIZATION LARYNGOPLASTY

Silastic medialization has been the mainstay of treatment since Isshiki introduced it over 25 years ago. There have been a number of implant systems described during the 1990s. Most recently, GORE-TEX® was introduced by McCulloch and Hoffman

(14,15) as a medialization implant for the musculomembranous vocal fold, and it has been the mainstay of our approach for six years (16,17).

The primary advantages of GORE-TEX are its ease of handling, placement, and adjustability, all of which enhance the speed and precision in which the operation can be performed. The position of the GORE-TEX can even be adjusted and fine-tuned extensively, while the implant remains within the patient rather than removing it for modification as is done with silastic. This in vivo adjustability is especially valuable in those patients in whom there is other associated vocal-edge pathology and in those who are extremely hyperfunctional during the procedure. The in vivo adjustability of GORE-TEX is unlike virtually all other implant approaches. Furthermore, precise positioning of the thyroid-lamina window is less critical, since GORE-TEX can be placed into an appropriate position despite a slightly malpositioned window.

Because of these characteristics, GORE-TEX is also well suited to restore aerodynamic glottal competence in scenarios where there are complex anatomic defects such as those encountered with trauma and cancer resections (18). Even subtle contour changes from the loss of superficial lamina propria associated with sulcus vergeture can be reconformed to treat a small glottal gap. This is advantageous in the geriatric patient, since it is not uncommon to encounter VFP in an older individual, who has long-term loss of superficial lamina propria.

ARYTENOID PROCEDURES: POSTERIOR GLOTTAL INCOMPETENCE

Since Isshiki introduced the arytenoid adduction procedure in 1978 to enhance posterior glottic closure in those patients with an abducted arytenoid, there have been many investigations confirming its efficacy. Zeitels et al. (12) described a new adduction arytenopexy procedure 20 years later, which was the first modification of Isshiki's arytenoid adduction technique (6,13). The arytenoid adduction procedure only simulates the lateral cricoarytenoid muscle, while the adduction arytenopexy models the synchronous adductor contraction of all of the intrinsic musculature. Repositioning the arytenoid should primarily be done when the malpositioned cartilage leads to phonatory aerodynamic glottal incompetence.

This adduction arytenopexy procedure results in a slightly longer vocal fold, which is appropriately aligned in all three dimensions with a well-conformed medial edge of the glottal aperture. This clinical observation was confirmed in a cadaver study (12). In contradistinction to the classical arytenoid adduction in which an anterolateral directed suture is used, the adduction arytenopexy procedure achieves a longer vocal fold by posteromedially displacing the arytenoid and maintaining its position with a posteriorly based suture. In the same study, the adduction arytenopexy procedure was more effective than was the classical arytenoid adduction in closing interarytenoid gaps because it did not result in excessive hyper-rotation of the vocal process.

During adduction arytenopexy, the body of the arytenoid is medialized to the limit of the medial cricoarytenoid joint capsule in a normal gliding fashion along the cricoid facet. This leads to placement of the arytenoid in a more normal adduction position for effective glottal closure during laryngeal sound production. It is clear from the convex contour of the cricoid facet and the precisely accommodating concave contour of the arytenoid base that hyper-rotation (simulating the lateral cricoarytenoid muscle) based on an axial plane is not indicative of normal arytenoid adduction. Both Koufman and Isaacson's (19) diagrammatic depiction of a typical arytenoid adduction as well as Neuman et al.'s (20) cadaver study reveal an abnormally contoured medial arytenoid that results in an abnormal interarytenoid chink. In many patients, the clinical significance of this chink may be minimized by redundant interarytenoid and periarytenoid soft tissue.

Despite ideal positioning of the arytenoid from the arytenopexy procedure, intraoperative observations revealed that optimal vocal quality required an accompanying medialization laryngoplasty. This is due to the flaccidity of the denervated glottis, which results in severe differential viscoelasticity of the vocal folds and associated valvular incompetence. The denervated glottal tissues have impaired elastic-recoil closing forces due to atrophy and fibrosis. On stroboscopy, this is revealed as an abnormally wide excursion of the vocal edge and as a long open-phase quotient during vibratory cycles.

GORE-TEX is now used exclusively by the author and is placed lateral to the paraglottic muscles (inner thyroid perichondrium) to avoid wide excursion of the glottal tissues during entrained oscillation. The denervated musculature of the paraglottic space is highly susceptible to the potential closing forces secondary to Bernoulli's effect. This fact is utilized to counterbalance the loss in normal elastic-recoil closing forces from the denervation.

A well-positioned arytenoid obviates the need for complex implant shapes that are intended to close the posterior glottis from an anteriorly positioned thyroid-lamina window. Additionally, there are a number of technical advantages to performing medialization laryngoplasty with adduction arytenopexy rather than with arytenoid adduction. Since there is not an anterior thyroid-lamina suture, the implant is unencumbered by the adduction of the arytenoid. Furthermore, the adduction arytenopexy is done prior to the medialization so that the implant can be sized more accurately, with the structural positioning of the posterior glottis already established. Finally, complex implant shapes that violate the thyroid-lamina inner perichondrium are unnecessary.

The adduction arytenopexy, which positions the arytenoid for normal phonation, can allow for a simple smaller implant shape to be placed lateral to the thyroid perichondrium because posterior glottic tissues are already aligned. The primary goal of the implant with arytenopexy is to prevent lateral excursion of the flaccid paraglottic tissue during oscillatory cycles rather than to medialize the vocal edge, which is mostly accomplished by the adduction arytenopexy. The technique for implant medialization becomes similar what is required for patients with vocal-muscle atrophy, which is easy to correct.

CRICOTHYROID SUBLUXATION

Observations made from the vocal-outcome data in those patients, who underwent adduction arytenopexy and medialization laryngoplasty, revealed that fairly normal conversational-level phonation was achieved (12). However, there were remarkable limitations of maximal-range capabilities, especially frequency variation and maximal phonation time. This was thought to be secondary to suboptimal viscoelastic tension in the denervated vocal fold soft tissues despite the aforementioned improvements in three-dimensional repositioning of the vocal edge. Over time, even denervated vocal musculature is not typically electrically silent. Therefore, the ideal resting length for vibration of a paralyzed vocal fold is longer than that of normally innervated vocal muscles. This need to increase viscoelastic tension in the denervated vocal fold and thereby improve aerodynamically efficient entrained oscillation catalyzed the development of the cricothyroid subluxation (C-T sub) procedure (13,21).

The C-T sub procedure has further enhanced postoperative vocal quality in UVP since it is an easily adjustable method of increasing and varying tension and length of the denervated musculomembranous vocal fold (13,21). This is unlike all prior operations, which were designed primarily to treat paralytic dysphonia by repositioning the vocal fold edge (9–12,19,22). Those procedures that alter tension and length of the vocal fold were conceived to modify pitch rather than to treat paralytic dysphonia (23–25). The C-T sub suture (i) models C-T muscle contraction, (ii) produces counter-tension on the thyroarytenoid muscle, and (iii) increases the length of the musculomembranous vocal fold (16). C-T sub is easy to perform, is free from complications, and improves the acoustical outcome of other laryngoplastic phonosurgical procedures.

The modified biomechanical properties of vocal fold vibration that were observed subsequent to C-T sub resulted in improved vocal outcome in all patients and were most remarkable in maximal range capabilities (21). C-T sub enhanced the postoperative voice of patients, regardless of whether they required medialization laryngoplasty alone or with adduction arytenopexy. Unlike stretching/lengthening procedures associated with gender reassignment, voice results in denervated patients have not deteriorated with follow-up >1 year. Due to the decreased elasticity of denervated vocal folds, the optimal length (for vibration) is longer than that of normal vocal folds.

The C-T sub procedure was designed to rectify the mechanical impediments that were partially precipitated by disruption of the C-T joint during cricoarytenoid joint dissection. However, C-T sub also improved the vocal outcome of those patients who did not require an arytenoid procedure (because of somewhat favorable synkinesis). In both scenarios, the objective measures of vocal function reveal that C-T sub improved the aerodynamic efficiency of the glottal valve with a commensurate enhancement of the maximal-range acoustical characteristics of the voice. In the treatment of paralytic dysphonia, the postoperative vocal outcome from the combined use of adduction arytenopexy, GORE-TEX medialization laryngoplasty, and cricothyroid subluxation is such that most patients will have a normal phonation time and >2 octaves of dynamic range with minimal acoustical perturbation. Subjective perceptions revealed that most patients demonstrated a register transition between modal and falsetto, an observation not previously reported.

REFERENCES

1. Solis-Cohen J. Motor paralysis of the larynx. In: Diseases of the Throat: A Guide to the Diagnosis and Treatment. New York: William Wood, 1879:636–659.
2. Crumley RL. Laryngeal synkinesis: its significance to the laryngologist. Ann Otol Rhinol Laryngol 1989; 98:87–92.
3. Hillman RE, Montgomery WW, Zeitels SM. Appropriate use of objective measures of vocal function in the multidisciplinary management of voice disorders. Curr Opin Otolaryngol Head Neck Surg 1997; 5:172–175.
4. Woodson GE. Clinical value of laryngeal EMG is dependent on experience of the clinician. Arch Otolaryngol Head Neck Surg 1998; 124:476.
5. Burns JA, Kobler JB, Zeitels SM. Micro-stereo-laryngoscopic lipoinjection: practical considerations. Laryngoscope, 2004; 114:1864–1867.

6. Pearl AW, WP, Ostrowski R, Mojica J, Mandell DL, Costantino P. A preliminary report on micronized AlloDerm injection laryngoplasty. Laryngoscope 2002; 112:990 996.

7. Ford CN. A multipurpose laryngeal injector device. Otolaryngol Head Neck Surg 1990; 103:135–137.

8. Payr E. Plastik am schildknorpel zur Behebung der Folgen einseitiger Stimmbandlahmung. Dtsch Med Wochensch 1915; 43:1265–1270.

9. Isshiki N, Morita H, Okamura H, Hiramoto M. Thyroplasty as a new phonosurgical technique. Acta Otolaryngol (Stockh) 1974; 78:451–457.

10. Isshiki N, Tanabe M, Sawada M. Arytenoid adduction for unilateral vocal cord paralysis. Arch Otolaryngol 1978; 104:555–558.

11. Isshiki N. Phonosurgery: Theory and Practice. Tokyo: Springer-Verlag, 1989.

12. Zeitels SM, Hochman I, Hillman RE. Adduction arytenopexy: a new procedure for paralytic dysphonia and the implications for medialization laryngoplasty. Ann Otol Rhinol Laryngol 1998; 107(suppl 173):1–24.

13. Sprinzl GM, Eckel HE, Sittel C, Potoschnig C, Koebke J. Morphometric measurements of the cartilaginous larynx: an anatomic correlate of laryngeal surgery. Head Neck Surg 1999; 21(8):743–750.

14. McCulloch TM, Hoffman HH. Medialization laryngoplasty with expanded polytetrafluoroethylene: surgical technique and preliminary results. Ann Otol Rhinol Laryngol 1998; 107:427–432.

15. Hoffman HH, McCulloch TM. Medialization laryngoplasty with Gore-Tex. Oper Tech Otolaryngol Head Neck Surg 1999; 10:6–8.

16. Zeitels SM. Adduction arytenopexy with medialization laryngoplasty and crico-thyroid subluxation: a new approach to paralytic dysphonia. Oper Tech Otolaryngol Head Neck Surg 1999; 10:9–16.

17. Zeitels SM, Mauri M, Dailey SH. Medialization laryngoplasty with Gore-Tex for voice restoration secondary to glottal incompetence: indications and observations. Ann Otol Rhinol Laryngol 2003; 112:180–184.

18. Zeitels SM, Jarboe J, Franco RA. Phonosurgical reconstruction of early glottic cancer. Laryngoscope 2001; 111:1862–1865.

19. Koufman JA, Isaacson GL. Laryngoplastic phonosurgery. Otolaryngol Clin North Am 1991; 24:1151–1177.

20. Neuman TR, Hengesteg A, Lepage MS, Kaufman KR, Woodson GE. Three-dimensional motion of the arytenoid adduction procedure in cadaver larynges. Ann Otol Rhinol Laryngol 1994; 103:265–270.

21. Isshiki N. Recent advances in phonosurgery. Folia Phoniatr 1980; 32:119–154.

22. Koufman JA. Laryngoplasty for vocal cord medialization: an alternative to Teflon. Laryngoscope 1986; 96:726–731.

23. Isshiki N. Surgery to elevate vocal pitch. In: Phonosurgery: Theory and Practice. Tokyo: Springer-Verlag, 1989:141–155.

24. LeJeune FE, Guice CE, Samuels PM. Early experiences with vocal ligament tightening. Ann Otol Rhinol Laryngol 1983; 92:475–477.

25. Tucker HM. Anterior commissure laryngoplasty for adjustment of vocal fold tension. Ann Otol Rhinol Laryngol 1985; 94:547–549.

RECOMMENDED READING

Isshiki N. Phonosurgery: Theory and Practice. Tokyo: Springer-Verlag, 1989.

McCulloch TM, Hoffman HH, Andrews BT, Karnel MP. Arytenoid adduction combined with Gore-Tex medialization thyroplasty. Laryngoscope 2000; 110:1306–1311.

Zeitels SM. Adduction arytenopexy with medialization laryngoplasty and crico-thyroid subluxation: a new approach to paralytic dysphonia. Oper Tech Otolaryngol Head Neck Surg 1999; 10:9–16.

Zeitels SM, Hochman I, Hillman RE. Adduction arytenopexy: a new procedure for paralytic dysphonia and the implications for medialization laryngoplasty. Ann Otol Rhinol Laryngol 1998; 107(suppl 173):1–24.

Zeitels SM, Mauri M, Dailey SH. Medialization laryngoplasty with Gore-Tex for voice restoration secondary to glottal incompetence: indications and observations. Ann Otol Rhinol Laryngol 2003; 112:180–184.

35
Cough

David E. Eibling

Department of Otolaryngology—Head and Neck Surgery, University of Pittsburgh School of Medicine, Pittsburgh, Pennsylvania, U.S.A.

INTRODUCTION

Cough is a vital physiologic maneuver that is critical for airway protection. It is also a common symptom accounting for frequent visits to physicians of many specialties. It may be an indication of significant disease; hence, the symptom of cough should trigger further investigation and treatment. Finally, chronic cough is a bothersome complaint that can independently adversely affect quality of life for those affected. Regardless of the role of cough in the particular patient, it is always necessary that the complaint be addressed by the treating physician.

COUGH AS A PHYSIOLOGIC FUNCTION

Lung function deteriorates rapidly when air exchange epithelium, spaces, and passages are coated or obstructed by retained debris and secretions. Highly specialized functions of respiratory epithelium require appropriate levels and viscosity of surfactant. Physiologic mechanisms maintain the integrity of this material, which is replaced rapidly and moved out of the airway via ciliary function of the cells lining the passages. A wide variety of situations arise in which this function fails to operate efficiently, and cough is one of the key "back-up" processes that move large amounts of mucus and debris out of the airway by creating brief, high-speed airflow through the airway.

Effective cough is dependent on a number of linked functions, including intact airway sensation, adequate lubrication, maintenance of airway patency throughout a wide range of pressure and volume, and the ability to build up pressure and release it suddenly. Adequate muscular strength and the ability to seal the airway by tightly closing the glottis are required to generate this pressure, and intact neurologic function to coordinate the actions is required to release it rapidly to produce high-velocity airflow.

Failure of the system to function effectively may be due to many factors, including those due to primary disease processes as well as interventions undertaken to treat those processes. The most common example of the latter is general anesthesia, during which cough is effectively eliminated, requiring alternative means of addressing physiologic airway secretions that accumulate. Respiratory complications due to ineffective cough often represent a major source of morbidity for patients with spinal cord injury, and devices have been developed (i.e., the Coughalator™) that utilize external power sources to duplicate the airflow characteristics of cough and clear materiel from the airways.

Chronic illness, muscle weakness or atrophy, and even physiologic changes of aging such as reduced laryngopharyngeal sensation or presbylarynx can impair the effectiveness of cough in the elderly. Failure of aspirated materiel to stimulate a cough is a particularly ominous sign in the dysphagic patient and is addressed elsewhere in this text. Ineffective cough, the so-called "death rattle," is a common terminal event and accompanies many different disease processes. Cough is not only an important physiologic process, but also an important symptom, a topic we will address in the remainder of this chapter.

COUGH AS A SYMPTOM

Although physiologic, cough may also indicate an underlying disease process. In most instances, cough is present as a sign of respiratory inflammation. The cough that accompanies an upper respiratory infection may last for several weeks. Cough that is due to infectious agents that lasts longer than three weeks suggests unusual infections such as tuberculosis (TB), pertussis, histoplasmosis, or other chronic granulomatous disease. A recent increase in the incidence of pertussis has been noted, likely due to the lower numbers of immunized children resulting in a community reservoir. Cough in a smoker is a response to increased airway secretions that accumulate as a response to the irritants in tobacco smoke. Cough may also be present for a variety of other reasons, some of which are listed in Table 1. It is critical that serious, potentially life-threatening causes such as pneumonia or lung cancer be ruled out early; hence, any algorithm that addresses cough will necessarily feature chest radiography as an early step. We will address these and other common causes of cough later in this chapter as we discuss the approach to the patient with a cough.

CHRONIC COUGH AS A COMPLAINT

Chronic cough is defined as a cough of more than two months of duration since infectious cough will have resolved by that time. Cough may significantly adversely affect the quality of life for the affected patient, especially if it lasts more than a week or two, and is often perceived by the patient to represent the disease process, not merely a symptom. Cough may result in secondary symptoms as well as fatigue, chest wall or abdominal discomfort, and stress urinary incontinence. Most patients who present to an otolaryngologist with complaints of cough will have chronic cough, and most will have undergone prior evaluation by their primary care physician. At this stage in the process, most patients are more concerned with getting rid of the cough than they are with any potential diagnosis. Despite assumptions that most chronic cough will defy diagnosis and treatment, Irwin and colleagues have pointed out that the etiology of nearly all chronic cough can be diagnosed and most can be successfully treated (1). Therefore, the conscientious physician will seek to diagnose and treat cough, not only to determine and treat the cause but also to eliminate or control the cough, which is adversely affecting the patient's quality of life.

Table 1 Causes of Cough—by Site

Referred
  Cranial nerve inflammation/compression
  Stimulation of ear canal
Sino-nasal
Sinus drainage
  Postnasal drip
Tenacious nasopharyngeal secretions
Thornwaldt's bursa
Laryngeal
  Tumor
  Infectious
    Laryngitis due to URI
    Croup
  Inflammatory
    Gastro-esophageal-laryngeal reflux (LPR)
  Inhaler laryngitis
  Paralysis
Alimentary tract
  GERD
  Zenker's diverticulum
  Aspiration
Large airways
  Infectious
    Pertussis?
  Tumor
  Inflammation
    Smoking
    Aerosol
  Extrinsic compression
Small airways and alveoli
  Infectious
    Pneumonia
    Bronchitis
    TB
    Empyema
  Tumor
    Lung cancer
    Metastases
    Pleural space
Inflammatory/degenerative
  Asthma
    Smoking
    Pulmonary fibrosis
    COPD
  Vasculitis
    Churg–Straus
    Goodpasture's
    Wegner's
Cardiac
  Left heart failure
  Pulmonary hypertension
Medications
  ACE inhibitors
  Chemotherapeutic agents

Abbreviations: COPD, chronic obstructive pulmonory disease; LPR, laryngo-pharyngeal reflux; TB, tuberculosis; URI, upper respiratory infection; ACE, angiotensin-converting enzyme.

CHRONIC COUGH IN THE ELDERLY

Smyrnios, Irwin, and co-workers extensively evaluated 30 patients older than 64 who presented to a pulmonary clinic with chronic cough of at least three weeks duration (2). Forty causes were identified in the 30, and at least one cause was detected for each patient. Among the subset of patients who were nonsmokers and not on angiotensin-converting enzyme (ACE) inhibitors, sinusitis/post-nasal drainage (PND), gastroesophageal reflux disease (GERD), and asthma were responsible for 100% and accounted for 85% of cases in the entire group. In their cohort of patients, directed therapy was effective in all patients. The authors noted that the causes of chronic cough in the geriatric population were similar to those of younger patients they had reviewed in previous series. They emphasized the importance of continuing the evaluation of symptomatic patients until the cause(s) is/are identified and treated in order to improve the quality of life for the affected patient.

APPROACH TO THE PATIENT WITH COUGH

The evaluation of a patient who complains of a cough begins, as does essentially any other complaint, with a focused history and physical examination. Common, treatable causes of cough are often eliminated early in the evaluation. In most instances, common etiologies such as bronchitis, intrathoracic lesions, or cough due to ACE inhibitor usage have already been ruled out by the primary care physician. By the time the otolaryngologist is consulted for cough, most patients will represent challenging diagnostic dilemmas.

HISTORY OF THE PATIENT WITH COUGH

A diagnostic algorithm, such as that presented in Figure 1, will assist in directing the history. It is important that early in the evaluation the current status of the workup be determined. For example, although most patients will arrive having already undergone chest radiography, some may not, and for some the most recent radiograph may have been some months or even years ago. It is critical that the consultant verify the results of a recent prior chest radiograph or repeat the study if verification of the interpretation cannot be secured.

The history should address, as in any other complaint, the duration and character of the complaint. Specific clues to underlying etiology may be identified by asking about timing of the cough. Cough during meals, especially with liquids, suggests aspiration. Cough at night may be due to reflux, but other factors such as an asthma trigger in the bedroom may be responsible. Morning productive cough suggests chronic bronchitis. If the cough results in expectoration of sputum, the amount and character should be addressed in the questioning. The patient should be asked about the presence of "postnasal drip," sinus symptoms, voice changes, reflux symptoms or medication, other respiratory symptoms, and prior respiratory diseases such as asthma, chronic obstructive pulmonary disease (COPD), etc. Questioning directed toward a smoking history as well as a review of the patient's medications should be routine. Specific classes of medications that should be asked about include anticholenergics, inhalers, and diuretics. ACE inhibitors should be noted, with specific questioning as to any potential relationship between timing of

```
┌─────────────────────────────────────────────────────────────┐
│ Acute----→ URI  → wait                                       │
│              Severe with fever → diagnose and treat          │
│ Chronic  →Hx and PE                                          │
│           →Chest radiograph                                  │
│                                                              │
│     Smoker  → Quit                                           │
│     ACE inhibitor → Switch to different antihypertensive     │
│                                                              │
│ Non smoker – No ACE inhibitor                                │
│       → Sinusitis/PND                                        │
│       →  GERD?LPR                                            │
│       →  Asthma                                              │
│                                                              │
│ Empiric therapy for one or more →                            │
│         Cough controlled → continue Rx                       │
│                                                              │
│ Cough not controlled → consider further work-up              │
│             Chest CT                                         │
│             Bronchoscopy with BAL                            │
│             Methacholine challenge test                      │
│                                                              │
│ Cough continues → symptomatic management                     │
└─────────────────────────────────────────────────────────────┘
```

Figure 1   Diagnosis of cough.

medication initiation or change in specific drug or dosage. First-generation ACE inhibitors (lisinopril, enalapril) are well-known causes of cough, and typically the patient's primary care physician has already changed to another medication. Second-generation ACE inhibitors (which selectively inhibit angiotension II receptors) such as losartan (Kozaar^{TM}) are not as notorious but can lead to cough in susceptible individuals. The prevalence of cough due to these agents in any specific practice is a function not only of the medication and the patient population, but also the practice! Only 3–7% of patients on ACE inhibitors seen in an internal medicine practice are likely to complain of cough, whereas the number in a typical otolaryngology practice may be 10 times that number.

It was once thought that chronic cough that disappears during sleep was likely to be of a psychogenic etiology. Later studies, however, have demonstrated that cough due to a number of etiologies, such as GERD or chronic bronchitis, may also diminish or stop at night, negating the value of this observation (3).

PHYSICAL EXAMINATION OF THE PATIENT WITH COUGH

Diagnostic clues are often encountered during the history that make the diagnosis obvious but do not relieve the physician of the necessity of performing an evaluation—specifically an examination of the upper aerodigestive tract. This examination should include an examination of the ears, nasal cavities, pharynx, larynx, and neck. Cerumen or foreign bodies in the ear canal have occasionally been implicated as the cause of chronic cough, and indeed, removal of cerumen often triggers cough in approximately 20% of individuals. However, chronic cough due to cerumen impaction is most likely exceedingly rare, if it occurs at all. Nasal examination should include nasal endoscopy to rule out occult sinusitis. Most otolaryngologists have had the experience of identifying obvious purulent nasal drainage in a patient with postnasal drip and cough but no other indication of sinusits. Laryngo-pharyngeal examination is required as well; hence, many otolaryngologists will typically examine the nose with a flexible nasolaryngoscope and then proceed at the same time to examine the larynx.

Laryngoscopy may demonstrate a variety of pathologic changes. Often the examiner will be unable to determine on the basis of examination whether the findings are the *cause* or the *result* of the chronic cough. For example, vocal process granulomata may be present due to cough due to some other cause rather than accounting for the presence of the cough. Gastro-esophageal-pharyngeal reflux is a common etiology of chronic cough, but diagnosis is often challenging. Criteria for the diagnosis of gastro-esophageal-pharyngolaryngeal reflux [often termed laryngo-pharyngeal reflux (LPR)] via laryngoscopy is controversial and a considerable number of studies have examined the question. There is now consensus that posterior glottic changes (so-called "pachydermia laryngis") are not specific for GERD, and that generalized edema, specifically involving the true cords, subglottis, and supraglottic structures, is more likely to indicate the presence of acid reflux. Neck examination is required as well, with careful attention to palpate for the presence of supraclavicular nodes.

In most instances, the patient would already have undergone chest examination to include auscultation and percussion. As noted above, chest radiographs would most likely have been obtained. Nevertheless, occasionally repeat examination is valuable, particularly if the examiner detects wheezing or other pulmonary findings to suggest a pulmonary etiology.

ADDITIONAL TESTING

Further tests ordered by the otolaryngologist are most likely to be radiographic studies. If the history and examination suggest sinus disease, sinus CT may be indicated. If the history suggests that the cough is possibly due to aspiration, then a modified barium swallow or endoscopic examination of swallowing is indicated. Often a chest CT is warranted, particularly if the examination demonstrates the presence of a paralytic vocal cord, deviation of the trachea or thyroid mass, or a supraclavicular mass. In many instances, a chest CT would already have been obtained. Every effort should be made to obtain the CT for review in order to rule out a substernal thyroid or other superior mediastinal mass.

The diagnosis of many causes of chronic cough is often made by the response to therapy; hence, I am including therapeutic trials in the "testing" category. The most common examples of these are the use of nasal steroids and or nonsedating antihistamines for suspected chronic sinusitis resulting in cough, and empiric proton pump inhibitor (PPI) therapy for suspected acid reflux. Occasionally, a 24-hour dual probe pH study will be required, although this typically is reserved for patients in whom GERD is suspected but who do not respond to therapy. Treatment of xerostomia with fluids, oral therapy, and judicious reduction in diuretic therapy may benefit some patients and provide a clue to the etiology. Empiric therapy with inhaled bronchodilators, occasionally with inhaled topical steroids, is frequently employed by primary care physicians and pulmonary specialists in cases of suspected cough-variant asthma.

Additional testing likely to be requested by a pulmonary specialist includes pulmonary function tests and fiberoptic bronchoscopy with bronchial-alveolar lavage (BAL). Occasional methacholine chloride challenge tests are requested if asthma is suspected, but this test is rarely used in the elderly, and then only after all other diagnoses have been excluded. Expectorated sputum and BAL irrigant is collected for cytology, Gram stain, culture, and evaluation for acid-fast bacilli. Skin tests for TB may be indicated if known to be negative previously and not obtained recently. An erythrocyte sedimentation rate, autoimmune studies, and routine hematologic studies may be indicated in some instances. Specific tests for pertussis may be indicated in selected cases.

TREATMENT OF CHRONIC COUGH

Treatment of cough will be dictated by the diagnosis identified by the evaluation, including the use of empiric pharmacologic measures. Cough due to reflux that responds to empiric PPI therapy may be able to be managed chronically with lifestyle changes and H-2 blockers, reserving PPI therapy for breakthrough. Sinusits/PND-related cough may be able to be managed with chronic nasal hygiene after the active sinus disease is managed. Management of thickened secretions with increased fluids and adjustment of diuretic therapy by the treating physician may provide long-term relief.

Removal of triggering agents, particularly cigarette smoke, is often beneficial in the management of cough as well as the myriad of other health benefits. The bothersome chronic cough in a smoker may constitute an ideal opportunity for the physician to convince the smoker to consider quitting.

Discussion regarding the role of ACE inhibitor therapy in the patient with cough should address the relative risks and benefits. Patients should be warned not to discontinue their ACE inhibitor on their own, but rather to discuss the possibility of alternative antihypertensive treatment with their primary care physician.

Therapy should be etiology-specific whenever feasible. In some instances, treatment of more than one etiology may be required. For example, the occasional patient may require prolonged and simultaneous treatment of chronic sinusitis, asthma, and GERD. In instances in which specific treatment is not successful, then nonspecific treatment with cough-suppressant therapy may be indicated to reduce the adverse effects of cough on the quality of life. It is important that the treating physician maintain vigilance for a potentially unrecognized underlying etiology, particularly when the symptom of cough has been suppressed.

SUMMARY

Most cough is due to acute upper airway infections and resolves within three weeks. Patients with cough that lasts longer than three weeks are considered to have chronic cough. Common causes of chronic cough are smoking and ACE inhibitor usage. Of the remainder, most can be attributed to sinusitis/PND, GERD/LPR, or asthma. The relative contribution of the common etiologies does not differ between younger and geriatric patients. All patients with chronic cough should undergo an evaluation to include a focused history and physical, as well as a chest radiograph. Patients referred to an otolaryngologist should undergo examination of their sino-nasal tract as well as laryngoscopy. Additional testing to include radiographic studies of the sinuses, esophagus, and chest CT may be required. Diagnostic therapeutic trials of treatment for chronic sinusitis, GERD/LPR, and asthma may be helpful in reaching a diagnosis. Long-term management is most effective when directed against specific etiologies; however, nonspecific therapy may be required in some instances for symptom control.

REFERENCES

1. Irwin RS, Madison JM. The persistently troublesome cough. Am J Respir Crit Care Med 2002; 165:1469–1474.
2. Smyrinos NA, Irwin RS, et al. From a prospective study of chronic cough: diagnostic and therapeutic aspects in older adults. Arch Intern Med 1998; 58:1222–1228.
3. Mello CJ, Irwin RS, Curley FJ. The predictive values of the character, timing, and complications of chronic cough in diagnosing its cause. Arch Intern Med 1996; 156:997–1003.

36

Laryngopharyngeal Reflux in the Elderly

Karen M. Kost and Richard J. Payne
Department of Otolaryngology, McGill University, Montreal General Hospital, Montreal, Quebec, Canada

INTRODUCTION

Laryngopharyngeal reflux (LPR) is prevalent in Western society. It is estimated that at least 33% of the American population over the age of 40 suffers from LPR (1). A study involving 100 community volunteers with a mean age of 60 years discovered that 35% of subjects complained of one or more symptoms of LPR and that nearly two-thirds had positive findings on examination (2). LPR affects individuals of all ages; however, as one ages the incidence increases (1,2).

Laryngopharyngeal reflux is most commonly associated with symptoms such as hoarseness, throat clearing, and cough (3). Increasingly worrisome pathologies such as laryngospasm, arytenoid fixation, laryngeal stenosis, and carcinoma have also been described (3–7). Consequently, the early diagnosis of LPR in the geriatric population is important for quality of life issues and to prevent more serious manifestations.

The diagnosis of laryngopharyngeal reflux in elderly patients is a challenge to physicians. Symptoms are often atypical or not apparent, especially when compared to either patients with gastroesophageal reflux or younger patients. Treatment often begins with patient education as to necessary lifestyle changes. Dietary changes such as increasing daily water intake and decreasing caffeine, cigarettes, alcohol, and chocolate are important. Decreasing the amount consumed at meals while increasing the frequency is also warranted. These lifestyle modifications may be difficult for the geriatric population to achieve. Many elderly patients are accustomed to certain routines and habits, while others living within institutions may not have access to dietary modifications or more than three meals per day. Proton-pump inhibitors (PPI) are generally first-line medications for LPR, with H2 inhibitors used in some circumstances. When medical therapy fails in the presence of severe symptoms and/or the development of complications (subglottic stenosis, neoplasia) surgical options may be considered, although they are rarely necessary.

LARYNGOPHARYNGEAL REFLUX

Geriatric Population

LPR in the geriatric population poses unique challenges to health care providers in terms of diagnosis and treatment. Most of the literature dealing with the geriatric population and reflux centers around gastroesophageal reflux disease (GERD) and not LPR. GERD peaks in the seventh decade and occurs more commonly in the elderly population than the general population (8,9). Approximately 33% of the North American adult population experience the classic symptoms of GERD: heartburn and regurgitation (10). The prevalence rises to 59% in patients older than 65 years (11). Elderly patients pose a diagnostic challenge since they rarely complain of classical symptoms related to GERD. The same can be said for symptoms of LPR. In a community-based cohort study by Reulbach et al. (2) in 2001, it was determined that the prevalence of LPR was common in patients with no prior history of reflux disease. Although elderly patients may have physical findings consistent with LPR while remaining asymptomatic, many do have symptoms that can directly impact quality of life.

Hoarseness, throat clearing, and vocal fatigue are all symptoms associated with the majority of cases of LPR and may lead to communication problems for elderly patients. The inability to effectively communicate can lead to the alienation of individuals in our society. The geriatric population is at great risk for this problem since LPR may coexist with other otolaryngologic disorders such as presbycusis that also contribute to interaction difficulties. Alternatively, the individual with hoarseness may have difficulty vocalizing or projecting the voice, while hearing-impaired companions of the same age group have difficulty understanding.

Thick mucous, chronic cough, and dysphagia constitute other symptoms of LPR that may be troublesome in the elderly patient. LPR is frequently a comorbid condition in elderly patients with pre-existing respiratory pathology. Inability to pass thick mucous resulting in cough can add to an already fragile respiratory condition in these patients, who often lack respiratory reserve (1). Dysphagia can increase the likelihood of aspiration, compromise proper nutrition in this patient population, and lead to reduced compliance with daily medications. LPR is associated with laryngospasm, obstructive sleep apnea, chronic rhinitis, and asthma (4,6). While acid reflux is unlikely to be the sole cause of the above disorders, it is likely to play a role in their development and severity (12). It is well known that severe asthmatics have a high incidence of coexistent reflux and that adequate control of the reflux may result in a diminution of asthma-related symptoms and medications.

After examining 228 patients with GERD who were divided into two groups based on age (<60 years, ≥60 years), Zhu et al. (13) concluded that GERD is more severe in the elderly. However, Fass et al. (14) demonstrated that older patients with GERD perceive heartburn and regurgitation less severely than younger patients, despite a trend to increased acid exposure. The reason for this phenomenon has been a source of speculation and discussion, yet no definitive etiology has been uncovered. According to Fass, the underlying mechanism may be related to an age-related reduction in esophageal chemosensitivity. Dysphagia and aspiration occur more frequently in elderly patients as a result of decreased sensory discrimination in the oral cavity. In 1997, Aviv (15) tested for laryngopharyngeal sensory abnormalities in subjects divided into three groups: patients aged 20 to 40 years, 41 to 60 years, and over 61 years. It was concluded that laryngeal sensation decreases in the areas supplied by the superior laryngeal nerve as one gets older. This type of sensory deficit may contribute to the development of dysphagia and aspiration. Saliva helps neutralize and clear acid from the larynx and hypopharynx. Decreased salivary production contributes to the development of LPR and is frequently found in the elderly as a consequence of several factors, such as Sjogren's disease, medications (e.g., diuretics), previous radiotherapy, and tobacco (16).

Pathophysiology

Laryngopharyngeal reflux refers to the backflow of acid from the esophagus into the pharynx. In the past, it was believed that LPR was simply the extraesophageal or laryngopharyngeal extension of GERD. It was hypothesized that as GERD worsened so should the amount of gastric juices passing through the upper esophageal sphincter (UES). Recent studies have deviated from this traditional thinking. The most recent literature favors the theory that the severity of acid reflux in the esophagus is not commonly predictive of LPR (10,12). The rationale is that it is the competence of the UES and its ability to protect the laryngopharynx that determines the amount of gastric juice that will pass into the larynx, not the amount of refluxed acid in the esophagus. Thus, small amounts of acid in an esophagus with an incompetent UES will more commonly lead to LPR than large amounts of gastric juices in the presence of a competent UES (3,4).

The mucosa in the throat is less resistant and therefore more vulnerable than esophageal mucosa to gastric juice such that cell damage occurs after minimal insult (17). It is considered normal to have up to 50 episodes of acid reflux from the stomach to the esophagus per day through the lower esophageal sphincter. On the other hand, even a single episode of reflux of acid through the upper esophageal sphincter can result in significant laryngeal damage (18). The damage to the laryngopharynx is attributed to acid and pepsin exposure (17). The esophagus is able to better protect itself against gastric acid and can therefore withstand a greater exposure than the comparatively defenseless laryngopharynx.

The anatomic mechanisms that protect against GERD and LPR include: lower esophageal sphincter (LES) tone, the crural diaphragm, LES intrathoracic and intra-abdominal length, and sling fibers from the gastric oblique muscle layer (19–21). According to Pengyan, sensory impulses in the pharynx leading to gastroesophageal reflux are more prevalent in people aged 66–78 years than in younger age groups. Furthermore, the decreased length of the intra-abdominal segment of the LES in the elderly contributes to GERD as well (19).

Upper esophageal sphincter dysfunction is significant in laryngopharyngeal reflux but not in GERD (22). It is the competence of the UES, which may account for the differences observed in these two unique entities. UES function changes as one ages as a result of cricopharyngeal and proximal esophageal changes (23). A decreased UES resting tone as well as defective UES opening contribute to the ability of gastric juices to bathe the laryngopharynx (24,25). Moreover, sensory discrimination at the level of the laryngopharynx innervated by the superior laryngeal nerve decreases as one ages (15,26). This phenomenon may prevent protective reflexes in the laryngopharynx from clearing gastric juices. It may also play a role in delayed symptomatology and thus diagnosis of LPR in the elderly. Loss of motor function in the laryngopharynx and oral cavity associated with aging contribute to LPR as well (27).

Many esophageal protective mechanisms against gastric reflux, such as esophageal peristalsis, gastric emptying, bicarbonate secretion, LES tone, and salivary secretion, change as one ages (13,28,29). It has recently been uncovered that gastric acid secretion does not decline with age, but may actually increase (14,29). While primary esophageal peristalsis is preserved in elderly patients, secondary peristalsis is less frequent and sometimes absent (30). Furthermore, several medications that are more commonly taken by the elderly, such as benzodiazepenes, nitrates, and calcium channel blockers, contribute to decreasing LES tone (31,32). As a result, the effects of acid in the esophagus are worsened, and the contribution to LPR may be enhanced.

The mechanisms behind LPR and GERD differ in many ways. Patients suffering from LPR have predominantly upright reflux as opposed to GERD type reflux, which occurs when patients are supine (4). GERD occurs as a result of prolonged exposure to acid, whereas pathology resulting from LPR occurs after only minimal insult (33). Appropriate management of LPR consistently necessitates higher medication dosages for longer periods of time when compared to the treatment of GERD (34,35). A prospective study published by Koufman et al. (36) in 2002 involving 58 patients with documented LPR in which 81% had normal esophagoscopy and biopsy serves to highlight the distinctions between GERD and LPR.

Studies have shown that abrupt distention of a long length of esophagus that occurs during forceful acid reflux into the esophagus leads to UES relaxation (37). The laryngeal inlet remains patent so that gastric juices reflux unimpeded into the laryngopharynx; this event occurs independently of swallowing, so the larynx is not elevated (38).

CLINICAL EVALUATION

History

There are many symptoms associated with LPR ranging from hoarseness to regurgitation. According to studies, extraesophageal otolaryngologic symptoms of GERD are more prevalent in the elderly (39). Symptoms of LPR include dysphonia, persistent throat clearing, vocal fatigue, chronic cough, thick mucus, and dysphagia (40). In 1991 Koufman (3) reported on a series of 225 patients using dual probe pH studies to document LPR and noted that the most common symptoms were dysphonia in over 50% of patients and chronic cough (Table 1). In fact, otherwise unexplained cough or dysphonia may be the sole manifestations of LPR.

The reflux symptom index (RSI) has been helpful in determining the degree of LPR in individual patients (Table 2) (41). It consists of nine symptoms graded from one to five by the patient for a maximum score of 45. A total score of greater than 13 is considered abnormal and suggestive of LPR. The RSI is reproducible and has been validated. Nonetheless, this instrument may be more of a challenge when dealing with the elderly population since the symptoms are less marked or may be the

Table 1 Symptoms of Laryngopharyngeal Reflux

71% dysphonia
51% chronic cough
47% globus pharyngeus
42% chronic throat clearing
35% dysphagia

Source: From Ref. 3.

Table 2 The Reflux Symptom Index

Within the past month, how did the following problems affect you? (0 = not at all, 5 = severe)	
Hoarseness or a problem with your voice	0 1 2 3 4 5
Clearing your throat	0 1 2 3 4 5
Excess throat mucus or postnasal drip	0 1 2 3 4 5
Difficulty swallowing food, liquids, pills	0 1 2 3 4 5
Coughing after you ate or after lying down	0 1 2 3 4 5
Breathing difficulties or choking episodes	0 1 2 3 4 5
Troublesome or annoying cough	0 1 2 3 4 5
Sensations of something sticking in your throat or a lump in your throat	0 1 2 3 4 5
Heartburn, chest pain, indigestion, or stomach acid coming up	0 1 2 3 4 5

Source: From Ref. 41.

result of other conditions. For example, chronic cough may be associated with lung disease, heart failure, or even a dry mouth. Geriatric patients are more likely to have decreased sensation at the level of the laryngopharynx when compared to the rest of the population. Therefore, elderly patients tend to have fewer symptom-related complaints in cases of mild LPR (15,23), leading to challenges in diagnosis unique to this population.

There is clearly an association between GERD and LPR since gastric juices overflowing into the laryngopharynx must first travel through the esophagus. However, the relationship is complex and the presence and severity of one does not always indicate the presence of the other. The most common symptoms of GERD, heartburn and regurgitation, are absent in up to 75% of patients suffering from LPR (42). Further complicating this matter is that elderly patients with GERD complain of heartburn and regurgitation to a lesser degree than younger patients (3,43,44). These studies also indicate that elderly patients with severe esophageal mucosal disease display fewer symptoms than younger patients. In a study from Ossakow et al. (45) in 1987, only 6% of patients suffering from LPR complained of heartburn, while nearly every patient with gastroenterology type reflux complained of this symptom. Interestingly, hoarseness was present in all of the patients with laryngopharyngeal reflux.

Physical Examination

The physical examination for laryngopharyngeal reflux begins when the patients utter their first words. The presence or absence of hoarseness is often initially evident. Vocal fatigue and throat clearing should all be evaluated as the patient is speaking. Examination of the oral cavity and oropharynx for xerostomia, erythema, evidence of postnasal drip, and thick mucus is warranted. Nasal examination looking for evidence of rhinitis is also necessary.

Laryngeal examination using a mirror may be appropriate as a baseline examination for patients in whom LPR is not suspected. However, it is imperative that flexible laryngoscopy be performed in all patients who are suspect for LPR. Examinations should be recorded whenever possible for the following reasons: as a permanent record for review or comparison, for review with the patient, and objective index of treatment success. Standardized scoring systems, such as the reflux finding score (RFS) (Table 3), are very helpful tools for initial diagnosis and evaluation of treatment following therapy. This score is based on eight findings with a maximum score of 26. Any score greater than 7/26 is suggestive of LPR. Of note, the aging

Table 3 The Reflux Finding Score

Sign	Scoring system
Laryngeal erythema/hyperemia	2 = arytenoids
	4 = diffuse
Vocal fold edema	1 = mild
	2 = moderate
	3 = severe
	4 = polypoid
Diffuse laryngeal edema	1 = mild
	2 = moderate
	3 = severe
	4 = obstructing
Ventricular edema	2 = partial
	4 = complete
Subglottic edema/pseudosculcus	0 = absent
	2 = present
Posterior commissure hypertrophy	1 = mild
	2 = moderate
	3 = severe
	4 = obstructing
Granuloma/granulation tissue	0 = absent
	2 = present
Thick mucus	0 = absent
	2 = present

Source: From Ref. 47.

larynx may develop a pseudosulcus unrelated LPR, and this must be taken into account when using the RFS in the geriatric population (12). Therefore, clinical judgment as to the etiology of the pseudosulcus is necessary to score appropriately. When evaluating treatment success, it is important to remember that symptoms of LPR frequently improve after four months of therapy, while improvement in the physical exam may be noted only after six months. Therefore, patients may feel better before they "look" better.

Adjunctive Tests

Ambulatory 24-hour double-probe pH testing is the diagnostic test of choice at this point of time for the general population (1). It is highly sensitive and specific for LPR (46). However, it is not used initially because it is invasive and may be uncomfortable. Despite being considered the "gold standard," dual-probe pH testing suffers from the following limitations: there are no clear-cut criteria as to upper probe placement, and confusion exists as to what constitutes a positive test or pathologic endpoint in terms of pH level. Upper probes are frequently placed 5 cm below the upper esophageal level, although ideally they should be positioned in the hypopharynx or post-cricoid area. Maintaining reliable contact between the probe and mucosal surface is difficult, such that dramatic changes in impedance produce spurious results. Although clear pathologic endpoints have been established for the diagnosis of GERD, there is controversy in LPR as to length of exposure and whether a pH of

4 or 5 is necessary in establishing the diagnosis. Finally, there is a significant incidence of false-negative results in dual-probe pH testing, owing to the likely behavior changes with the probe in place and the fact that reflux may occur inconsistently. Despite these limitations, it should be considered in cases of treatment failure.

As a result of the difficulties and limitations associated with dual probe pH studies, endoscopic examination alone is considered appropriate in the geriatric population. It is simple, rapid, inexpensive, accurate, and well tolerated. Although topical anesthetics and decongestants may be used, they are best avoided when sensory testing is performed. Oral intake is not permitted for up to one hour following use of topical anesthetics in order to prevent inadvertent aspiration. Using a standardized measure such as the RFS allows for the evaluation of the same objective criteria in each patient (Table 3) (47). A reduction in the score may be expected 6 months following initiation of treatment, while symptomatic improvement is usually noted after 3 to 4 months of therapy. It is also becoming increasingly popular to use the responsiveness of symptoms to PPI as a method of indirect diagnosis LPR (48,49). In this situation, improvement in symptoms is interpreted as LPR that is resolving.

Barium swallow, esophagoscopy, and esophageal manometry are of little or no value in the diagnosis of LPR and may be poorly tolerated in elderly patients. This being said, they are each clinically useful when used appropriately. The barium swallow will only demonstrate GERD 50% of the time, but it is useful when there is clinical suspicion of stricture, neoplasm, or fungal infection. In the presence of LPR, esophagoscopy will demonstrate typical GERD findings in only 20–30% of cases. It is very useful when there is concern over esophageal disease, neoplasms, and Barrett's esophagus. Manometry plays an important role in the diagnosis of motility disorders, which may in turn impact the treatment of LPR.

MANAGEMENT OF LPR

LPR results in symptoms that alter the quality of life of many elderly patients. There are a considerable number of otolaryngologic complications of LPR that can seriously impede on the health and welfare of individuals. These include laryngitis, vocal fold nodules, paroxysmal laryngospasm, Reinke's edema, vocal fold granulomas, and globus pharyngeus (40,50,51). Evidence also exists that LPR likely plays a role in "idiopathic" subglottic stenosis and laryngeal carcinoma (4).

Lifestyle Adjustments

Adjustments to lifestyle can be achieved in the geriatric population to improve LPR. Weight loss and avoiding tight-fitting clothing can lessen reflux of gastric juices (52). Decreasing serving sizes at meals while increasing the frequency of meals (six small meals/day) may be beneficial (53). Avoiding oral intake to within three to four hours of bedtime and elevating the head of the bed four to six inches should be encouraged (52). Increasing total water intake throughout the day while avoiding caffeine, cigarettes, alcohol, and chocolate can decrease the frequency of reflux. Changing medications to ones that do not promote LES or UES relaxation can also be beneficial (39).

Such modifications may present unique challenges to geriatric patients. As a result of comorbidities, such as heart failure, these patients are often fluid restricted

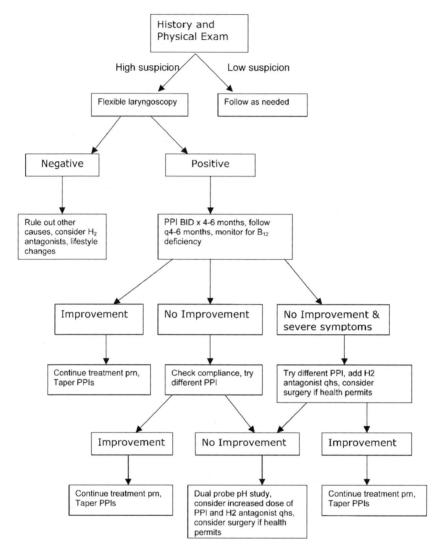

Figure 1 Diagnosis and treatment algorithm for LPR. *Abbreviation*: LPR, laryngopharyngeal reflux; PPI, proton pump inhibitor.

and are therefore unable to increase water intake. Many elderly people live in institutions in which three meals are served daily. The cost and logistics at instituting 4 to 6 meals daily may exceed available resources. Altering medications to ones that do not affect the LES or UES may not be possible. Nonetheless, every effort should be made to institute as many measures as is possible.

Pharmacotherapy

Medications include PPI' (proton pump inhibitors), H_2 antagonists, and antacids. H_2 receptor antagonists are successful in nearly 50% of patients and may be considered for treatment of minor LPR (54). Since the 1980s, proton-pump inhibitors have been first-line therapy for moderate to severe LPR, while H_2 antagonists may still be used in very mild cases. PPIs target the H+–K+ ATPase enzyme, which is the final pathway for acid production in the parietal cell (54). PPIs are most effective when taken twice daily for four to six months (55–57). This regimen is more aggressive and prolonged than the accepted treatment for GERD. In severe cases with complications such as granulomas, a further increase in dose may be necessary. For patients with incomplete improvement, consideration should be given to adding an H_2 antagonist qhs. Polypharmacy and changes in hepatic and renal functions contribute to the complexity of following such a regimen (57). PPIs may affect vitamin B_{12} absorption, and it is therefore recommended to periodically verify B_{12} levels in elderly patients on long-term therapy, particularly those with poor diets (48,49).

Treatment failure is most often due to poor compliance with medications and lifestyle modifications. However, true resistance to PPIs has been documented and may account for some cases.

Surgery

Fundoplication is safe and can be highly effective in elderly patients with very low LES resting pressures (53,58). Patients failing medical management who are developing complications as a result of the acid reflux are potential candidates. Performing the procedure laparoscopically reduces many of the morbidities associated with the open technique (58).

Algorithm

See Figure 1.

SUMMARY

Laryngopharyngeal reflux is distinct from GERD in terms of pathophysiology, diagnosis, and management. LPR may be seen alone or in association with other vocal disorders such as nodules, polyps, cysts, and less commonly, carcinoma. LPR may also coexist with conditions such as obstructive sleep apnea and asthma.

Although the incidence of LPR increases in the elderly, diagnosis may be difficult owing to atypical and/or reduced signs and symptoms. The reflux symptom index and reflux finding score are useful clinical indicators of the presence of LPR. Most frequent symptoms include dysphonia, throat-clearing, vocal fatigue, globus pharyngeus, cough, dysphagia, and thick mucus. Heartburn and dyspepsia are infrequent complaints. Commonly observed signs include edema of the larynx, ventricles, vocal folds and/or subglottis, laryngeal erythema, posterior commissure hypertrophy, thick mucus and granulation tissue. The diagnosis of LPR is clinical, and adjunctive diagnostic measures such as dual/triple pH probe testing are reserved for treatment failures.

The management of LPR consists of appropriate lifestyle and dietary modifications, vocal hygiene and empiric proton pump inhibitor therapy. Response to treatment is judged as a function of symptomatic improvement initially, followed later by an amelioration of the signs. Treatment failure is often related to poor compliance with all or part of the management protocol.

REFERENCES

1. Koufman JA. Laryngopharyngeal reflux 2000: a new paradigm of airway disease. ENT Ear Nose Throat J 2002; 81(suppl 2):2–6.
2. Reulbach TR, Belafsky PC, Blalock PD, et al. Occult laryngeal pathology in a community-based cohort. Otolaryngol Head Neck Surg 2001; 124:448–450.
3. Koufman JA. The otolaryngologic manifestations of gastroesophageal reflux disease (GERD): a clinical investigation of 225 patients using ambulatory 24-hour pH monitoring and an experimental investigation of the role of acid and pepsin in the development of laryngeal injury. Laryngoscope 1991; 101(suppl 53):1–78.
4. Bain WM, Harrington JW, Thomas LE, Schaefer SD. Head and neck manifestations of gastroesophageal reflux. Laryngoscope 1983; 93:175–179.
5. Halstead LA. Gastroesophageal reflux: a critical factor in pediatric subglottic stenosis. Otolaryngol Head Neck Surg 1999; 120:683–688.
6. Ward PH, Hanson DG. Reflux as an etiological factor of carcinoma of the laryngopharynx. Laryngoscope 1988; 98:1195–1199.
7. Freije JE, Beatty TW, Campbell BH, et al. Carcinoma of the larynx in patients with gastroesophageal reflux. Am J Otolaryngol 1996; 17:386–390.
8. Heading R. Epidemiology of oesophageal reflux disease. Scand J Gastroenterol 1989; 24(suppl 168):33–37.
9. Allen R, Rappaport W, Hixson L, et al. Referral patterns and the results of antireflux operations in patients with more than sixty years of age. Surg Gynecol Obstet 1991; 173:359–362.
10. Revicki DA, Wood M, Maton PN, Sorensen S. The impact of gastroesophageal reflux disease on health-related quality of life. Am J Med 1998; 104:252–258.
11. Ouatu-Lascar R, Triadafilopoulos G. Oesophageal mucosal diseases in the elderly. Drugs Aging 1998; 12:261–276.
12. Belafsky PC, Postma GN, Amin MR, Koufman JA. Symptoms and findings of laryngopharyngeal reflux. ENT Ear Nose Throat J 2002; 81(suppl 2):10–13.
13. Zhu H, Pace F, Sangaletti O, et al. Features of symptomatic gastroesophageal reflux in elderly patients. Scand J Gastroenterol 1993; 28:235–238.
14. Fass R, Pulliam G, Johnson C, et al. Symptom severity and oesophageal chemosensitivity to acid in older and young patients with gastro-oesophageal reflux. Age Ageing 2000; 29:125–130.
15. Aviv JE. Effects of aging on sensitivity of the pharyngeal and supraglottic areas. Am J Med 1997; 103(suppl 1):74S–76S.
16. Sonnenberg A, Steinkamp U, Weise A, et al. Salivary secretion in reflux esophagitis. Gastroenterology 1982; 83:889–895.
17. Axford SE, Sharp N, Ross PE, et al. Cell biology of laryngeal epithelial defenses in health and disease: preliminary studies. Ann Otol Rhinol Laryngol 2001; 110:1099–1108.
18. Little FB, Koufman JA, Kohut RI, Marshall RB. Effect of gastric acid on the pathogenesis of subglottic stenosis. Ann Otol Rhinol Laryngol 1985; 94:516–519.
19. Xie P, Ren J, Bardan E, et al. Frequency of gastroesophageal reflux events induced by pharyngeal water stimulation in young and elderly subjects. Am J Physiol 1997; 272:G233–237.
20. DeMeester TR, Wernly JA, Bryant GH, et al. Clinical and in vitro analysis of determinants of gastroesophageal competence. Am J Surg 1979; 137:39–46.
21. Mittal RK, Rochester DF, McCallum WE. Sphincteric action of the diaphragm during a relaxed lower esophageal sphincter in humans. Am J Physiol 1989; 256:G139–144.
22. Helm JF, Dodds WJ, Riedel DR, et al. Determinants of esophageal acid clearance in normal subjects. Gastroenterology 1983; 85:607–612.
23. Schindler JS, Kelly JH. Swallowing disorders in the elderly. Laryngoscope 2002; 112: 589–602.

24. Ekberg O, Feinberg MJ. Altered swallowing function in elderly patients without dysphagia. AJR Am J Roentgenol 1991; 156:1181–1184.

25. Shaker R, Ren J, Zamir Z, et al. Effect of aging, position and temperature on the threshold volume triggering pharyngeal swallows. Gastroenterology 1994; 107:396–402.

26. Calhoun KH, Gibson B, Hartley L, et al. Age-related changes in oral sensation. Laryngoscope 1992; 102:109–116.

27. Ward PH, Colton R, McConnell F, et al. Aging of the voice and swallowing. Otol Head Neck Surg 1989; 100:283–286.

28. Dodds WJ, Hogan WJ, Helm JF, et al. Pathogenesis of reflux esophagitis. Gastroenterology 1981; 81:376–394.

29. Collen MJ, Abdulian JD, Chen YK. Gastroesophageal reflux disease in the elderly: more severe disease that requires aggressive therapy. Am J Gasroenterol 1995; 90:1053–1057.

30. Ren J, Shaker R, Kusano M, et al. Effect of aging on the secondary esophageal peristalsis: presbyesophagus revised. Am J Physiol Gastrointest Liver Physiol 1995; 268:G772–779.

31. Castell DO. The lower esophageal sphincter. Physiologic and clinical aspects. Ann Intern Med 1975; 83:390–401.

32. Castell DO. Esophageal disorders in the elderly. Gastroenterol Clin North Am 1990; 19:235–254.

33. Postma GN, Tomek MS, Belafsky PC, Koufman JA. Esophageal motor function in laryngopharyngeal reflux is superior to that in classic gastroesophageal reflux disease. Ann Otol Rhinol Laryngol 2001; 110:1114–1116.

34. Wiener GJ, Koufman JA, Wu WC, et al. The pharyngo-esophageal dual ambulatory pH probe for evaluation of atypical manifestations of gastroesophageal reflux (GER). Gastroenterology 1987; 92:1694.

35. Wiener GJ, Koufman JA, Wu WC, et al. Chronic hoarseness secondary to gastroesophageal reflux disease: documentation with 24-h ambulatory pH monitoring. Am J Gastroenterol 1989; 84:1503–1508.

36. Koufman JA, Belafsky PC, Daniel E, et al. Prevalence of esophagitis in patients with pH-documented laryngopharyngeal reflux. Laryngoscope 2002; 112:1606–1609.

37. Kahrilas PJ, Dodds WJ, Dent J, et al. Upper esophageal sphincter function during belching. Gastroenterology 1986; 91:133–140.

38. Jacob P, Kahrilas PJ, Herzon G. Proximal esophageal pH-metry in patients with 'reflux laryngitis'. Gastroenterology 1991; 100:305–310.

39. Raiha IJ, Impivaara O, Seppala M, et al. Prevalence and characteristics of symptomatic gastroesophageal reflux in the elderly. J Am Geriatr Soc 1992; 40:1209–1211.

40. Toohill RJ, Kuhn JC. Role of refluxed acid in pathogenesis of laryngeal disorders. Am J Med 1997; 103(suppl 1):100S–106S.

41. Belafsky OC, Postma GN, Koufman JA. Validity and reliability of the reflux symptom index (RSI). J Voice 2002; 16:274–277.

42. Aviv JE, Parides M, Fellowes J, Close LG. Endoscopic evaluation of swallowing as an alternative to 24-hour pH monitoring for diagnosis of extraesophageal reflux. Ann Otol Rhinol Laryngol Suppl 2000; 109(suppl 184):25–27.

43. Triadafilopoulos G, Sharma R. Features of symptomatic gastroesophageal reflux disease in elderly patients. Am J Gastroenterol 1997; 92:2007–2011.

44. Raiha I, Hietanen E, Sourander L. Age Aging 1991; 20:365–370.

45. Ossakow SJ, Elta G, Colturi T, et al. Esophageal reflux and dismotility as the basis for persistent cervical symptoms. Ann Otol Rhinol Larygol 1987; 96:387–392.

46. Richter JE, ed. Ambulatory esophageal pH monitoring: practical approach and clinical applications. 2nd ed. Baltimore: Williams & Wilkins, 1997.

47. Belafsky PC, Postma GN, Koufman JA. Validity and reliability of the reflux finding score (RFS). Laryngoscope 2001; 111:1313–1317.

48. Garnett WR. Consideration for long-term use of proton pump inhibitors. Am J Health-Syst Pharm 1998; 55:2268–2279.

49. Termanini B, Gibril F, Sutliff VE, et al. Effect of long-term gastric acid suppressive therapy on serum vitamin B12 levels in patients with Zollinger–Ellison syndrome. Am J Med 1998; 104:422–430.
50. Ulualp SO, Toohill RJ, Shaker R. Pharyngeal reflux events in patients with single and multiple otolaryngologic disorders. Otolaryngol Head Neck Surg 1999; 121:725–730.
51. Price JC, Jansen CJ, Johns ME. Esophageal reflux and secondary malignant neoplasia at laryngoesophagectomy. Arch Otolaryngol Head Neck Surg 1990; 116:163–164.
52. Long RG. Reflux oesophagitis and its treatment. Br J Clin Pract Symp Suppl 1994; 75:36–40.
53. Ramirez FC. Diagnosis and treatment of gastroesophageal reflux disease in the elderly. Cleveland Clin J Med 2000; 67:755–765.
54. Klinkenberg-Knol EC, Meuwissen SG. Treatment of reflux oesophagitis resistant to H_2-receptor antagonists. Digestion 1989; 44(suppl 1):47–53.
55. Koufman JA. Laryngopharyngeal reflux is different from classic gastroesophageal reflux disease. ENT Ear Nose Throat J 2002; 81(suppl 2):7–9.
56. Koufman JA, Aviv JE, Cusiano RR, Shaw GY. Laryngopharyngeal reflux: position statement of the committee on speech, voice, and swallowing disorders of the American Academy of Otolaryngology—Head and Neck Surgery. Otolaryngol Head Neck Surg 2002; 127:32–35.
57. Leite LP, Johnston BT, Just RJ, Castell DO. Persistent acid secretion during omeprazole therapy: a study of gastric acid profiles in patients demonstrating failure of omeprazole therapy. Am J Gastroenterol 1996; 91:1527–1531.
58. Dallemagne B, Weerts JM, Jeahes C, Markiewicz S. Results of laparoscopic Nissen fundoplication. Hepatogastroenterology 1998; 45:1338–1343.

37

Identifying and Treating Sleep Disorders in the Elderly

Lianqi Liu and Sonia Ancoli-Israel
Department of Psychiatry, University of California–San Diego and VA San Diego Healthcare System, San Diego, California, U.S.A.

Lavinia Fiorentino
Doctoral Progam in Clinical Psychology, San Diego State University and University of California–San Diego, San Diego, California, U.S.A.

GENERAL DESCRIPTION OF THE CLINICAL PROBLEM

Approximately 50% of older adults complain of difficulty sleeping. Both subjective reports and objective measurements have suggested that when compared to younger adults, older adults take longer to fall asleep, have lower sleep efficiency (defined as the amount of sleep given the amount of time in bed), have more nighttime awakenings, wake up earlier than they would like in the morning, and require more daytime naps.

In part, these changes are a result of an older adult's decreased ability to sleep. This decreased ability has been associated with several factors, including medical and psychiatric illness, medication use, changes in the endogenous circadian clock, specific sleep disorders, and behavioral issues. Given the high prevalence of sleep complaints and sleep disorders in this population, there is a clear need for health care professionals to have an increased awareness of these sleep disturbances to better enable them to assess and treat these patients. As part of this understanding, it is also important to have knowledge of normal sleep.

NORMAL SLEEP

Sleep can be broken down into two states, rapid eye movement (REM) sleep and non-rapid eye movement (NREM). NREM sleep is further subdivided into stages 1, 2, 3, and 4, which represent a continuum from light sleep (stage 1) to deep sleep (also called slow wave sleep or stages 3 and 4). Sleep is entered through the transitional stage—stage 1, followed by stages 2,3, and 4, respectively. About 90 minutes after sleep onset, REM sleep begins. REM sleep is characterized by rapid eye movements (thus the name), similar to those seen in the waking state. Muscle atonia is also present.

Typically, this 90–100-minute cycle repeats itself 4–5 times during the night. Healthy adults show stable and distinct patterns of sleep architecture, i.e., cyclic alternations of the different sleep stages. Most deep sleep occurs in the first third of the night and most REM sleep occurs in the morning hours. Although the function of sleep is not totally understood, numerous studies have suggested that different sleep stages serve at least partially different functions. Both REM and NREM sleep are necessary for good health and optimum daytime performance (1).

WHY IS POOR SLEEP PARTICULARLY IMPORTANT IN THE GERIATRIC POPULATION?

Sleep complaints are common in all age groups, but are particularly common in older adults. In a study of more than 9000 adults over the age of 65 years, 28% reported difficulties in falling asleep, while 42% reported difficulties in both falling asleep and staying asleep (2). At follow-up three years later, the sleep complaints had resolved in 15% of those who initially had reported difficulties. Interestingly, the incidence of new insomnia was 5% (i.e., 5% of those without sleep difficulties at baseline had a new sleep complaint at follow-up) (3).

In older adults, chronic insomnia is a significant problem. In a telephone interview with 1000 randomly selected adults, the prevalence of chronic insomnia was highest in those aged 65 years and over (20%) (4). Epidemiologic studies indicate that elderly women are more likely to experience insomnia than men (5). Patients with poor health, longer duration of insomnia, older age, and higher income are more likely to discuss their sleep problems.

Patients with sleep complaints often fail to report them to their physicians (4,6). It is therefore imperative that physicians ask their patients about sleep since the patient often will not initiate the discussion, and sleep disturbances in the older adult can have significant and serious consequences.

In several studies, insomnia was shown to decrease quality of life, decrease performance (particularly slower reaction time and poorer balance), and to be associated with greater symptoms of depression, anxiety, and deficits in attention and memory (7–10). Diminished cognitive function is sometimes secondary to severe insomnia and may be particularly problematic in the elderly, as it may be mistaken for dementia (10).

Insomnia in the elderly is also associated with morbidity. Difficulties with sleep have been associated with poor health status, and long-term persistence of insomnia has been associated with heart disease, diabetes, and respiratory disease (2,3). Slower response times may increase the risk of falls (which are directly related to an increased risk of mortality), while changes in cognition may lead to early institutionalization and loss of the ability to conduct normal daily activities (11–13).

HISTORY

When compared to young and middle-aged adults, older persons report more time spent in bed but more subjective sleep complaints, including difficulty with sleep initiation, decreased total sleep time, increased nighttime awakenings, early-morning awakenings, and daytime napping (2). Despite an increased amount of time spent in bed, elderly persons' total nighttime sleep is markedly reduced. Consequently, many older adults spend a considerable portion of the night awake in bed. This results in a significant decrease in sleep efficiency. Compared to a sleep efficiency of 90% or more in younger adults, older adults' sleep efficiency usually drops to 70–80% (14). However, contrary to common beliefs, healthy older adults do not sleep less than their younger counterparts; in fact, they average about seven hours of sleep a night (15).

With age, sleep architecture changes. These changes include a reduction in or even absence of slow wave or deep sleep (stages 3 and 4) and a slight decrease in REM, proportional to the reduction in the amount of total sleep time. This results in the night being spent in lighter sleep (stages 1 and 2) (16). However, the total amount of sleep needed may not necessarily change. Tests of daytime sleepiness indicate that the elderly often experience significant daytime sleepiness when compared to their younger counterparts (17). Since daytime sleepiness suggests insufficient sleep at night, these data suggest that it is the ability to sleep that is reduced with age and that the elderly may require more sleep than they are able to obtain.

DIFFERENTIAL DIAGNOSIS

There are many factors that decrease the ability to sleep, including medical and psychiatric disorders, medication use, circadian rhythm disorders, specific sleep disorders, and behavioral problems.

Medical and Psychiatric Disorders

Medical and psychiatric illness often causes sleep disruption. Medical conditions that are known to commonly cause sleep difficulties in older persons include disorders causing pain (e.g., fibromyalgia, arthritis, malignancies), neurodegenerative disorders (e.g., Parkinson's disease or Huntington's disease), pulmonary disorders (e.g., asthma or chronic obstructive pulmonary disease), cerebrovascular disease, rheumatological disorders, and dementia (5,18). As an example, more than half of patients with Parkinson's disease complain of sleeping difficulties. These sleep problems arise in part from the disease process itself (e.g., biochemical changes in the brain, dementia, bradykinesia and rigidity, tremor, and respiratory disturbances associated with airway and respiratory movements), and in part as a consequence of the sleep disruptive symptoms of the disease (e.g., pain) or as iatrogenic side effects of the treatment implemented. Parkinson's disease can result in pain in the legs and back, difficulties getting in and out of bed, turning in bed, and vivid dreams and nightmares. Although drug treatment with low to moderate doses of dopamine agonists or antiparkinsonian agents may improve sleep by reducing rigidity and bradykinesia, these same medications may exacerbate or create new sleep disturbances, such as those secondary to visual hallucinations associated with levodopa, nocturnal dystonia, and choreic movements.

Complaints of difficulty sleeping are also often correlated with some kind of psychiatric disorders. Insomnia is particularly common in mood disorders and may be a diagnostic symptom for major depression and generalized anxiety disorder. Some depressed persons complain about insomnia, and insomnia is often the earliest complaint of persons who are at the beginning of the onset of depression (19). Studies have shown that not only can insomnia be a symptom of depression, but that patients with untreated insomnia are three times as likely to develop depression (20).

In a large survey conducted in 2003 by the National Sleep Foundation, sleep problems in older adults were associated with medical illness, rather than aging per se, particularly heart disease, lung disease, stroke, bodily pain, and depression. In each case, significantly more of those with the medical/psychiatric conditions reported sleeping less than six hours a night, more insomnia, and more daytime sleepiness (15). In addition, individuals with multiple medical problems had a particularly high risk of sleep problems.

Medication Use

Many kinds of medications are known to cause complaints of insomnia, daytime sleepiness, or both. Examples of activating and sedating medications often used by older adults are listed in Table 1 (21).

Since elderly persons take proportionally more medications for their medical and/or psychiatric problems, and have slower metabolisms, any complaints associated with sleep must be evaluated as possible side effects of drugs. Oftentimes, these medications are necessary to manage health concerns, and discontinuing a medication that contributes to sleep difficulties is sometimes unrealistic and ill advised. Thus, careful consideration of the dose and timing of such medications can be important in the management of sleep difficulties.

Circadian Rhythms

Circadian rhythms are important biological regulators in all mammals. Hormone secretion, body temperature, and sleep–wake cycles are examples of the many physiological systems that fluctuate routinely within 24-hour intervals. Studies have shown that in humans, the sleep–wake cycle is regulated by the combined effect of an endogenous pacemaker situated in neurons of the suprachiasmatic nucleus (SCN) in the central nervous system, and exogenous and environmental stimuli such as amount of light exposure, food intake, and time spent awake.

As people age, their circadian rhythms tend to desynchronize. The progressive deterioration of the SCN and its subsequent weakened functioning are hypothesized to contribute to the disruption of circadian rhythms in older adults (22). It is hypothesized that the normal sleep–wake cycle deteriorates in part in the elderly secondary to the diminished secretion of nocturnal endogenous melatonin (23). Inconsistency of external cues, also called *zeitgebers*, such as low exposure to light, irregular meal times, and decreased exercise, also contributes to the disruption of sleep–wake patterns.

Table 1 Examples of Activating and Sedating Medications Often Used by Older Adults

Medications with activating effects	Medications with sedating effects
Alcohol	Long-acting hypnotics
CNS stimulants	Antihypertensives
Beta-blockers	Antihistamines
Bronchodilators	Anxiolytics
Calcium channel blockers	Tranquilizers
Decongestants	Antidepressants
Stimulating antidepressants	
Stimulating antihistamines	
Thyroid hormones	

The most common desynchronized pattern noted in older adults is the advanced sleep phase syndrome (ASPS), a condition characterized by an advanced need for sleep that typically causes the person to get sleepy in the early hours of the evening (e.g., 7–9 P.M.) and wake up spontaneously during the early hours of the morning (e.g., 3–5 A.M.). Most older adults fall into one of two patterns. The first pattern is when they force themselves to stay up later into the evening and not go to bed until the more conventional time of 10:00 or 11:00 P.M., but because of their advanced rhythm, still find themselves awake at 4:00 in the morning. These adults are not in bed long enough to get a full night's sleep and find themselves needing to nap the following afternoon. The second scenario finds the older adults falling asleep while watching television or while reading in the early evening, waking up after an unintentional nap of anywhere from 30 to 90 minutes, getting into bed and suddenly experiencing both difficulty falling asleep and early morning awakening.

Specific Sleep Disorders

Sleep Disordered Breathing

Sleep disorder breathing (SDB), commonly known as sleep apnea, is a condition characterized by repeated episodes, lasting 10 seconds or longer, of breathing cessation during sleep. These events can be complete (i.e., apneas) or partial interruptions in breathing (i.e., hypopneas). The respiratory disturbance index (RDI) is the rate of breathing interruptions per hour (number of events/hour of sleep), and represents a measure of severity of SDB. An RDI of 10 or higher is considered clinically relevant and pathological. Sleep disordered breathing is generally diagnosed with an overnight sleep study.

Apneas can be obstructive, central, or mixed. Obstructive apneas are caused by an anatomical collapse (i.e., obstruction) of the upper airway. Patients with obstructive sleep apnea cannot breathe despite the effort to breathe, which often results in choking and panting sounds, and loud snoring (often reported by frustrated bed partners). Central apneas result from failure of the brain to appropriately regulate the breathing process at the central nervous system level. Patients with central type apnea do not even attempt to breath, but simply stop breathing until the apneic event is over. Mixed apneas entail episodes of breathing cessation that have characteristics of both central and obstructive apneas, usually beginning as central and developing into obstructive apneas. The apneic events can occur in any of the sleep stages, but they tend to occur primarily in stage 1, 2, or REM sleep and tend to be longer and more severe in REM. The supine position during sleep can aggravate the apnea (i.e., positional apnea), most likely caused by gravity pulling the tongue back into the oropharynx and hindering the flow of air.

As a result of each apneic episode, patients wake up in order to breathe, and then fall back asleep until the next episode, and so on repeatedly. This results in very fragmented sleep. It is important to note that more often than not, patients with SDB do not remember waking up during the night, most likely because the arousals are very brief. Excessive daytime sleepiness and impaired cognitive and memory functioning are additional consequences of both the sleep fragmentation and the hypoxia associated with SDB (24).

Sleep-disordered breathing is a very common condition in middle-aged and older adults. Ancoli-Israel et al. (25) reported that 70% of elderly men and 56% of elderly women had RDI >10, in comparison to 15% of younger men and 5%

of younger women (13,26). The risk factors for SDB include high body mass index (i.e., obesity), older age, being male, smoking, and hypertension (27).

Periodic Limb Movements in Sleep

Periodic limb movements in sleep (PLMS) is a condition characterized by involuntary jerking or kicking of the limbs, most often the legs, during sleep. The movements are repetitive, typically occurring in clustered episodes that last between 0.5 and five seconds, repeating every 20–40 seconds. PLMS are often associated with arousals. The PLMS index is a measure of the number of jerks per hour of sleep and represents a measure of the severity of the condition. A PLMS index of five or more, with each kick causing an arousal, is considered clinically significant. The presence of PLMS can only be confirmed with an overnight sleep study.

In addition to causing complaints of insomnia, PLMS can cause very disruptive sleep, leaving patients feeling fatigued and sleepy during the day (e.g., excessive daytime sleepiness). The awakenings associated with the periodic leg movements are often, as in patients with SDB, not remembered. Therefore, these patients are frequently unaware of their poor sleep quality. Some patients may also suffer from other sleep disturbances, such as SDB and REM sleep behavior disorder (RBD). Many patients with PLMS also suffer from restless leg syndrome (RLS), characterized by an unpleasant crawling and sometimes painful feeling in the legs during wake time that is associated with uncontrollable leg movements.

The presence of PLMS in the population has been known to increase with age. Research indicates that 45% of elderly adults suffer from PLMS, compared to only 5–6% of the younger population (28,29).

REM Sleep Behavior Disorder

RBD is a condition where the muscle atonia typical of REM stage sleep is absent. Patients with RBD move vigorously during their REM stages and often engage in behaviors that are self-aggressive or violent toward a bed partner. Patients with RBD tend to have clear memories of their dreams and enact their dream contents. However, their aggressive behavior during sleep is often in contrast with the patient's waking personality.

The etiology and prevalence of RBD are not yet clear. However, reports show that older men may be more at risk of developing RBD (30). People who are taking antidepressants or who are withdrawing from alcohol or sedative use may also be more likely to have RBD symptoms. RBD has been associated with neurodegenerative conditions, such as dementia, Parkinson's, Guillain–Barre syndrome, olivo-ponto-cerebellar degeneration, and subarachnoid hemorrhage (31), and other sleep disorders, such as narcolepsy and PLMS.

To accurately diagnose RBD, a complete history of the sleep disorder should be given by both the patient and, if possible, by the patient's bed partner. An overnight sleep study with video recording may also be necessary.

Behavioral Problems

Almost all patients with difficulty sleeping develop poor sleep habits. These might include spending too much time in bed, irregular sleep schedules, excessive napping, inappropriate use of caffeine and alcohol, and engaging in stimulating (rather than relaxing) activities close to bedtime.

In general, the longer one spends in bed, the more fragmented and disturbed sleep becomes while the less time spent in bed results in more consolidated sleep. For example, eight hours of sleep out of 8.5 hours in bed is often more efficient than eight hours of sleep out of nine or 10 hours in bed.

Circadian rhythms are more robust when the sleep schedule is regular. Keeping a regular sleep schedule involves going to bed at the same time each night and, even more importantly, getting up at the same time each day. Since sleep is part of a homeostatic process (i.e., one needs to be awake for a certain amount of time before being sleepy enough to fall asleep), "sleeping in" and excessive napping can both contribute to difficulty falling asleep at night.

Caffeine is known to disrupt sleep. Most adults are unaware, however, that alcohol also disrupts sleep. Although alcohol may cause initial sleepiness, when it leaves the blood stream several hours after ingestion, the individual wakes up.

Dementia

Although dementia is a medical disorder, sleep disturbances in this condition are so widespread that they are described here in detail. Demented patients who wake up during the night in a confused and often agitated state can be difficult to care for, and caregivers often cite poor sleep as one of the primary reasons for institutionalization of these patients (32).

Sleep/wake patterns in dementia are polyphasic, with frequent nighttime awakenings and redistribution of sleep episodes throughout the day (33). Jacobs et al. (34) reported that many institutionalized demented patients were neither awake nor asleep for a full hour in the day or night, and that while the mild to moderately demented and the severely demented patients had extremely fragmented sleep at night, the severely demented patients were sleepier than the others both during the day and night (35).

A number of studies have examined the sleep of demented patients compared to aged controls. Demented patients have consistently been found to have a lower sleep efficiency, increased number of nocturnal awakenings, and an increase in the proportion of the night spent in light stage 1 sleep, with a decrease in the proportion of REM sleep and a decrease in slow wave sleep (stages 3 and 4) (24). The effects of dementia on EEG slow waves can be difficult to detect because of the already low levels of slow wave sleep found in nondemented older adults. The presence of comorbid depression in dementia patients also contributes to the difficulty in characterizing sleep changes attributable to the dementia.

Dementia is also associated with deterioration in circadian rhythms. The beta-amyloid plaques seen in the brains of patients with Alzheimer's disease have been found in the SCN but not other areas of the hypothalamus (36). These results suggest that there is selective cell death in the endogenous circadian pacemaker, which would affect circadian rhythms. Deterioration in circadian rhythmicity is also caused by a decrease in *zeitgebers* for many dementia patients. Older adults with dementia, particularly those in nursing homes, often have few regular entrainment cues to synchronize their rhythms, such as low levels of social interaction, irregular physical activity, chronic bed rest, and low levels of light exposure.

There has also been growing interest in the relationship between SDB and dementia. It is known that SDB can produce cognitive impairment during the day. The high prevalence of SDB in older adults has been hypothesized to exacerbate the cognitive decline in dementia patients (37). Ancoli-Israel et al. (38) found that, among older adults with dementia, those with severe sleep apnea have significantly more cognitive impairment than those with mild or no apnea, particularly in the areas of attention, initiation and perseveration, conceptualization, and memory. The cardiovascular sequelae of SDB may also indirectly cause stroke-related dementia. Consideration of comorbid SDB should be made for patients with dementia.

In patients with dementia, it may be difficult to determine the nature of the sleep disturbance when they are unable to report subjective complaints. These patients may also not be compliant with overnight polysomnogram (PSG). Actigraphy is a useful, noninvasive methodology that can be used to assess sleep and circadian rhythms in these patients (39). Caregivers are also another good source of information. It is important to ask about SDB-related symptoms such as snoring and observation of breathing cessation followed by gasps for air.

TESTING

The diagnosis associated with the complaint of insomnia can often be made based on history alone. Given the increased prevalence of medical conditions in older age, a comprehensive review of medical history and medication intake by the clinician, including prescription medications, over-the-counter drugs, caffeine, alcohol, and nicotine, is especially important when assessing sleep in this population. Diagnosis of a sleep disorder secondary to a medical condition requires that the sleep difficulty be severe enough so that it necessitates separate treatment. However, there are times when it is appropriate to refer a patient to a sleep disorders clinic for an overnight sleep study. There are several ways in which sleep can be measured.

The gold standard is the PSG, which records brain waves, eye movements, submental electromyography (EMG), as well as respiration, oximetry, heart rate, tibialis EMG, and other physiological variables of interest. Patients come to the sleep clinic several hours before bedtime to have the wires attached to their head and body. They then go to sleep in a private bedroom, which is often also equipped with an infra-red video camera. Their physiology is monitored all night and observed by a specially trained sleep technician. In the morning, after the patient awakens and all wires have been removed, the record is scored for sleep stages, amount of sleep, and amount of disturbances. There are many variations of the gold standard, which record fewer channels of information, depending on what disorder is suggested by the patient's history.

Technology is now available to record a full PSG in the patient's home, and some clinical laboratories and many research laboratories now conduct these unattended sleep recordings. However, the American Academy of Sleep Medicine, in conjunction with the American Thoracic Society and the American College of Chest Physicians, recently published a practice parameter report based on the systematic evaluation of data on portable monitoring for diagnosing SDB, which concluded that there is insufficient evidence at this time to recommend portable monitoring using a full PSG (40). Many laboratories have also used devices that monitor only a few channels of information. The report also concluded that monitoring of a minimum of four channels (with at least two channels of respiration) can be used in attended situations, but not unattended, and that devices of only one channel (such as oximetry) should never be used (40).

Another methodology that is used is actigraphy. An actigraph, a small device usually worn on the wrist, records movement that can be used to distinguish between wake and sleep (39). The main advantage of actigraphy is that it is easy to wear and can record information both during the night and day for extended time periods, i.e., multiple days and nights. It can be used to measure sleep and activity rhythms that might not otherwise be available using traditional (e.g., PSG) techniques. Actigraphy is particularly beneficial in the study of insomnia, treatment effects, and circadian rhythms (39).

For the diagnosis of narcolepsy or any disorder of daytime sleepiness, a multiple sleep latency test is often performed the morning after the PSG. This test determines how sleepy patients are during the day by measuring how long it takes them to fall asleep. This involves the patients going back to bed five times at two-hour intervals during the day. They are allowed to stay in bed for a total of 20 minutes. If not asleep in 20 minutes, they get out of bed. If they do fall asleep, they are only allowed to sleep for a few minutes before they are woken up. In this way, one can measure the latency to sleep onset during the five naps throughout the day.

TREATMENT

Medical/Psychiatric Conditions and Medication Use

The ideal approach to treatment of a sleep disorder secondary to a medical illness and/ or substance use is to first address the treatment of the medical condition, manage the pain or discomfort experienced by the patient, and assess possible medication changes. Management of pain and discomfort associated with medical illness can sometimes alleviate insomnia without the need of sedative-hypnotic medications. If, however, sedative hypnotics are required, they should be prescribed in the lowest effective dose and should be short-acting to reduce likelihood of excessive daytime sleepiness (Table 2).

Since the prevalence of depression is higher in older adults than in younger adults, sleep disturbances related to depression are particularly important to consider in this population (41). Older adults with depression have more disturbed sleep than younger adults with depression (42), and symptoms of depression are associated with

Table 2 Pharmacological Interventions for Insomnia

Drug	Onset of action	Half-life (hr)	Geriatric dose (mg)
Benzodiazepines			
Temazepam (Restoril[R])	1–2 hr	10–15	7.5–15
Lorazepam (Ativan[R])	1–2 hr	8–14	0.5–1
Alprazolam (Xanax[R])	<1 hr	10–14	0.25–0.5
Estazolam (Prosom[R])	1–2 hr	15–30	0.5–1
Oxazepam (Doral[R])	2 hr	10–15	10–15
Benzodiazepine Receptor Agonists			
Zolpidem (Ambien[R])	15–30 min	1.5–4	5–10
Zaleplon (Sonata[R])	15–30 min	1	5–10
Eszopiclone (Lunesta[R])	1 hr	6–9	1–2
Melatonin Agonist			
Ramelteon (Rozerem[R])	45 min	2–5	8

an increased likelihood to complain of difficulties with sleep (2). These findings are important for two reasons: first, older adults complaining of insomnia should be asked about other symptoms of depression (e.g., depressed mood, anhedonia), and second, treatment of the depression will likely result in improved sleep quality. Again, thorough assessment is critical. An older adult complaining of difficulties with sleep, who has an underlying depression, will not likely benefit from direct treatment of the insomnia in the long term. Two possibilities are to treat the depression with a therapeutic dose of a sedating antidepressant or to address difficulties with sleep as part of nonpharmacological treatment for depression (e.g., challenge catastrophic thinking about sleeplessness).

When it is suspected that the medication is causing or perpetuating the insomnia, adjustment of the time of day at which an older adult takes his or her medication may improve sleep quality. Generally, sedating medications should be taken at night, and alerting medications should be taken during the day whenever possible. Alternatively, another medication may be found with the same therapeutic benefit without the adverse impact on sleep.

Circadian Rhythm Disturbance

The treatments available for ASPS range from behavioral to pharmacological; however, the most effective is late-afternoon or early-evening bright light exposure. Light is a powerful *zeitgeber* that affects the endogenous pacemaker and helps reset the 24-hour circadian rhythm. Research shows that exposure to bright light in the evening helps patients with ASPS stay alert later into the evening and sleep later in the morning, thus regulating their sleep–wake cycle (43). Body heat regulation is another behavioral treatment that has been found to be effective for patients with ASPS (42). Some research also suggests that exercise helps older as well as younger patients regulate their circadian rhythms (44). Finally, melatonin has been used as a circadian rhythms regulator; however, the research is equivocal on the correct dose, the correct timing, and whether it is a successful treatment (45).

Sleep Disordered Breathing

There are several treatment options available for SDB. The treatment of choice for each patient will depend on the severity of the SDB, the general medical condition, and compliance and tolerance of the various treatments.

Weight loss is very effective for overweight patients who can take off the weight and keep it off (46). For positional apnea, an easy and noninvasive technique is to sew a pocket with a tennis ball inside the back of a pajama shirt, so that the supine position will be avoided (21).

The treatment most widely and effectively used for obstructive apnea is continuous upper airway pressure (CPAP) or bilevel positive airway pressure (BiPAP). Both CPAP and BIPAP blow air in the patient's nose through a mask attached to a hose connected to a machine. The pressure of the air is continuous for the CPAP and alternating during inspiration and expiration for the BiPAP. Both devices need to be correctly titrated during an overnight sleep study for the specific needs of each patient, although newer self-titrating machines are available that can be sent home with the patient. The CPAP and BiPAP have been proven effective in eliminating apneas and hypopneas, normalizing oxygen desaturations, and reducing snoring and daytime sleepiness. However, these machines are not a cure for SDB, and they are often considered burdensome. For some patients, compliance is a problem (47,48). The initial acceptance rate of CPAP is 70–80%, and the long-term compliance rate is 80–90% (49,50). A recent study suggests that individuals who engage in more active copying skills (e.g., planful problem solving) are more likely to use CPAP regularly (48). Surgical interventions for patients with anatomical abnormalities are also available. The type of surgical intervention depends on the location of the anatomical abnormality that is obstructing the airflow. Nasal reconstruction is indicated for nasopharynx abnormalities. Pharyngeal reconstruction (e.g., uvulopalatopharyngoplasty) is sometimes indicated for soft palate, uvula abnormalities, or enlarged tonsils. Laser-assisted uvulopalatoplasty has not been shown to work in patients with sleep apnea of any degree (51). In patients where the base of the tongue is obstructing the airflow, a genioglossus advancement or hyoid laryngoplasty are sometimes performed. These interventions move the tongue forward and free the air passage. However, many patients have multiple anatomical abnormalities that cause SDB. The success rates of the surgical intervention vary. Due to the lack of an ability to exactly define the anatomic location, surgical results can be unpredictable. Surgery is indicated for patients who have a defined anatomic abnormality. When the RDI is less than 20, the response to a uvulopalatopharyngoplasty is excellent. In the elder population, surgery is often contraindicated because of the risk factors due to general medical conditions more common in older age (e.g., heart failure, stroke, degenerative CNS diseases).

Another treatment used to reduce the snoring and decrease the number of respiratory events is the use of oral appliances. Tongue retaining devices and mandibular advancement devices have been developed and are particularly indicated for patients who cannot tolerate CPAP or BiPAP and have mild to moderate SDB. These devices pull the tongue or lower jaw forward, thus enlarging the airway.

Table 3 Pharmacological Treatments for PLMS

Generic name	Trade name	Dose	Intake time (min) (before bedtime)
Benzodiazepines			
Clonazepam	Klonopin	0.25–2 mg	30–60
Tempazepam	Restoril	15–30 mg	30–60
Opiate agents			
Acetaminophen/ codeine	Tylenol #3	30 mg codeine	30–60
Acetaminophen/ codeine	Tylenol #4	60 mg codeine	30–60
Propoxyphene hydrochloride	Darvon	65–135 mg	30–60
Dopaminergic agents			
Carbidopa/levodopa	Sinemet	25/100–25/250 mg	30–60
Pergolide	Permax	0.05–0.25 mg	30–60
Pramipexole	Mirapex	0.25–0.75 mg	30–60
Ropinirole[a]	Requip	0.125–0.5 mg	At bedtime
Anticonvulsant/ antineuralgic			
Gabapentin	Neurontin	600–2400 mg	At bedtime

[a]Only ropinirole has FDA approval for the treatment of RLS; the rest are off-label.

Table 4 Sleep Hygiene Rules for Older Adults

Keep a regular sleep/wake schedule
Avoid caffeine and alcohol after lunch
Avoid naps or limit to 1 nap of <30 min/day
Limit liquids in the evening
Spend time outdoors (without sunglasses), particularly in the late afternoon or early evening
Exercise daily
Check effect of medication on sleep and wakefulness

The effectiveness of oral devices varies from 50% to 100% (52), and they may not work at all with dentures.

Pharmaceutical treatments for SDB are not very effective and are not therefore typically indicated. However, for REM sleep apnea, tricyclic antidepressants that inhibit REM sleep are sometimes prescribed, and respiratory stimulants, such as progesterone and acetazolamide, have been prescribed for central sleep apnea.

PLMS/RLS

The suggested treatments for PLMS are pharmacological. Dopaminergic agents (e.g., levidopa/carbidopa, pergolide, pramipexol, ropinirole, and gabapentine) are the treatment of choice for patients with PLMS and/or RLS (Table 3) (51). These agents generally reduce both the number of limb movements and the associated arousals. However, there is some evidence that levidopa/carbidopa tends to shift the leg movements from nighttime to daytime (53). Benzodiazepines (e.g., temazepam and clonazepam) and opiates (e.g., Tylenol with codeine) are sometimes used. Benzodiazepines do not decrease the number of limb movements per se, but they may help enhance the patient's overall sleep efficacy by diminishing the number of arousals (54). Conversely, opiate agents tend to reduce the number of limb movements, but they are not as effective in reducing arousals (55). However, only ropinirole has received FDA approval for the treatment of RLS; all the other listed medications, including the other dopaminergic agents, the benzodiazepines and the opiates, are used off-label.

RBD

The treatment of RBD is primarily pharmacological and in most cases successful. Clonazepam (0.25–3 mg) is the most prescribed drug for RBD. It reduces the night-time movements without changing muscle tone and is effective in 90% of RBD

Table 5 Instructions for Sleep Restriction Therapy for Older Adults

---

Calculate the average amount of time in bed per night of the prior 2 wks
Stay in bed for this amount of time plus 15 min
Get up at the same time each day
No naps allowed during the day
When sleep efficiency has reached 75% to 85%, allowed to go to bed 15 min earlier
This procedure should be repeated until 8 hr or desired amount of sleep is acquired

---

Table 6 Stimulus-Control Therapy for Older Adults

Go to bed only when sleepy
Use the bed only for sleeping (and sexual activity)
If not asleep within 15–20 min, get out of bed and go to another room, and return to bed only when sleepy
Repeat this pattern throughout the night until you can fall asleep
Get up at the same time each morning (even if you only slept 1 or 2 hrs)
Avoid naps during the day

patients (30). However, clonazepam may cause excessive daytime sleepiness, and it is not indicated for patients with comorbid conditions. In addition, the treatment of RBD includes preventative measures to avoid injury to the patient and the patient's bed partner during the night. Precautions should include sleeping in wide spaces not elevated from the ground, removing sharp objects from around the patient, and locking doors and windows of the bedroom.

Behavioral Treatments

Along with all other treatments, good sleep hygiene rules (i.e., good sleep habits) should be taught and reinforced. Table 4 lists the sleep hygiene rules for older adults (16).

Other behavioral treatments that have been shown to be effective in the older adult include sleep restriction therapy (Table 5) (16), stimulus control therapy (Table 6) (16), and cognitive behavioral therapy (57).

Dementia

Sleep continuity can be enhanced with the use of sedative-hypnotic medications but some unwanted problems due to exacerbation of insomnia and dementia symptoms and side effects often arise. Some nonpharmacological alternatives have proven beneficial to patients with dementia. For many patients, it is important to re-establish entrainment cues to strengthen circadian rhythms. Some studies have found that bright light therapy in the morning and/or evening can consolidate circadian rhythmicity and improve sleep in demented patients (58–60). Maintenance of regular physical activity of some sort and social interaction can also promote robust circadian rhythms. Increased physical activity and improving the environment (i.e., keeping it bright during the day and dark and quiet at night) are optimal treatment approaches as well (61). In cases with comorbid of SDB, it is important to treat the condition. In an ongoing, randomized, double-blind, placebo-controlled study, Ancoli-Israel et al. (62) found that with adequate education and a good caregiver, patients with mild/moderate dementia are able to tolerate CPAP to the same extent as clinic patients with sleep disorders, and the CPAP treatment of SDB may yield improvement or at least slow down the cognitive functioning deterioration in some aspects of cognitive functioning in these patients (63).

CONCLUSION

Symptoms of sleep disorders are very common in the elderly, but diagnosis and treatment are infrequent. In this age group, sleeping difficulties are often secondary to medical problems, psychiatric problems, or medication usage. Specific sleep disorders, such as sleep-disordered breathing, periodic limb movements in sleep, and REM behavior disorders, are very common and need to be ruled out. By properly making the correct diagnosis and then applying the appropriate treatment, older adults should be able to get a better night sleep and thus be more alert during the day.

ACKNOWLEDGMENT

This work was supported by NIA AG08415, NIA AG15301, NCI CA85264, NIH M01 RR00827, the Department of Veterans Affairs VISN-22 Mental Illness Research, Education and Clinical Center (MIRECC), and the Research Service of the Veterans Affairs San Diego Healthcare System.

REFERENCES

1. Rechtschaffen A. Current perspectives on the function of sleep. Perspect Biol Med 2000; 41(3):359–390.
2. Foley DJ, Monjan AA, Brown SL, Simonsick EM, Wallace RB, Blazer DG. Sleep complaints among elderly persons: an epidemiologic study of three communities. Sleep 1995; 18(6):425–432.
3. Foley DJ, Monjan A, Simonsick EM, Wallace RB, Blazer DG. Incidence and remission of insomnia among elderly adults: an epidemiologic study of 6,800 persons over three years. Sleep 1999; 22(suppl 2):S366–S372.
4. Ancoli-Israel S, Roth T. Characteristics of insomnia in the United States: results of the 1991 National Sleep Foundation Survey. I. Sleep 1999; 22(suppl 2):S347–S353.
5. Ancoli-Israel S. Insomnia in the elderly: a review for the primary care practitioner. Sleep 2000; 23(suppl 1):S23–S30.
6. Shochat T, Umphress J, Israel AG, Ancoli-Israel S. Insomnia in primary care patients. Sleep 1999; 22(suppl 2):S359–S365.
7. Zammit GK, Weiner J, Damato N, Sillup GP, McMillan CA. Quality of life in people with insomnia. Sleep 1999; 22(suppl 2):S379–S385.
8. Hauri PJ. Cognitive deficits in insomnia patients. Acta Neurol Belg 1997; 97(2):113–117.
9. Walsh JK, Benca RM, Bonnet M, et al. Insomnia: assessment and management in primary care. Am Fam Phys 1999; 59(11):3029–3037.
10. Crenshaw MC, Edinger JD. Slow-wave sleep and waking cognitive performance among older adults with and without insomnia complaints. Physiol Behav 1999; 66(3):485–492.
11. Armstrong AL, Wallace WA. The epidemiology of hip fracture and methods of prevention. Acta Ortho Belg 1994; 60:85–101.
12. Tinetti ME, Williams CS. Falls, injuries due to falls and the risk of admission to a nursing home. N Engl J Med 1997; 337:1270–1284.
13. Rubenstein LZ, Josephson KR, Robbins AS. Falls in the nursing home. Ann Intern Med 1994; 121:442–451.
14. Bliwise DL. Sleep in normal aging and dementia. Sleep 1993; 16(1):40–81.
15. National Sleep Foundation. Sleep in America Poll. www sleepfoundation org/polls/ 2003SleepPollExecutiveSumm pdf2003.
16. Ancoli-Israel S, Poceta JS, Stepnowsky C, Martin J, Gehrman P. Identification and treatment of sleep problems in the elderly. Sleep Med Rev 1997; 1(1):3–17.
17. Dement WC, Seidel W, Carskadon MA. Daytime alertness, insomnia and benzodiazepines. Sleep 1982; 5:S28–S45.
18. Cohen-Zion M, Gehrman PR, Ancoli-Israel S. Sleep in the elderly. In: Lee-Chiong TL, Carskadon MA, Sateia MJ, eds. Sleep Medicine. Philadelphia: Hanley & Belfus, 2002:115–124.

19. Gillin JC. Psychiatry disorders. In: Kryger M, Roth T, Dement WC, eds. Principles and Practice of Sleep Medicine. Philadelphia: Saunders, 2000:1123–1195.

20. Ford DE, Kamerow DB. Epidemiologic study of sleep disturbances and psychiatric disorders: an opportunity for prevention? JAMA 1989; 262(11):1479–1484.

21. Ancoli-Israel S. Sleep problems in older adults: putting myths to bed. Geriatrics 1997; 52(1):20–30.

22. Lydic R, Schoene WC, Czeisler CA, Moore-Ede MC. Suprachiasmatic region of the human hypothalamus: homolog to the primate circadian pacemaker? Sleep 1980; 2: 355–361.

23. van Coevorden A, Mockel J, Laurent E, et al. Neuroendocrine rhythms and sleep in aging men. Am J Physiol 1991; 260(4):E651–E661.

24. Bliwise DL. Review: Sleep in normal aging and dementia. Sleep 1993; 16:40–81.

25. Ancoli-Israel S, Kripke DF, Klauber MR, Mason WJ, Fell R, Kaplan O. Sleep disordered breathing in community dwelling elderly. Sleep 1991; 14(6):486–495.

26. Young T, Palta M, Dempsey J, Skatrud J, Weber S, Badr S. The occurrence of sleep-disordered breathing among middle-aged adults. N Engl J Med 1993; 328(17):1230–1235.

27. Lavie P, Herer P, Hoffstein V. Obstructive sleep apnoea syndrome as a risk factor for hypertension: population study. BMJ (Clin Res Ed) 2000; 320(7233):479–482.

28. Ancoli-Israel S, Kripke DF, Klauber MR, Mason WJ, Fell R, Kaplan O. Periodic limb movements in sleep in community-dwelling elderly. Sleep 1991; 14(6):496–500.

29. Bixler EO, Kales A, Vela-Bueno A, Jacoby JA, Scarone S, Soldatos CR. Nocturnal myoclonus and nocturnal myoclonic activity in a normal population. Res Commun Psychol Psychiatry 1982; 36:129–140.

30. Schenck CH, Mahowald MW. Polysomnographic, neurologic, psychiatric, and clinical outcome report on 70 consecutive cases with the REM sleep behavior disorder (RBD): sustained clonazepam efficacy in 89.5% of 57 treated patients. Cleveland Clin J Med 1990; 57:S10–S24.

31. Schenck CH, Bundlie SR, Ettinger M, Mahowald MW. Chronic behavioral disorders of human REM sleep: a new category of parasomnia. Sleep 1986; 9(2):293–308.

32. Pollak CP, Perlick D, Linsner JP, Wenston J, Hsieh F. Sleep problems in the community elderly as predictors of death and nursing home placement. J Comm Health 1990; 15(2): 123–135.

33. Prinz PN, Peskind ER, Vitaliano PP, et al. Changes in the sleep and waking EEGs of nondemented and demented elderly subjects. J Am Geriatr Soc 1982; 30:86–92.

34. Jacobs D, Ancoli-Israel S, Parker L, Kripke DF. Twenty-four hour sleep–wake patterns in a nursing home population. Psychol Aging 1989; 4(3):352–356.

35. Pat-Horenczyk R, Klauber MR, Shochat T, Ancoli-Israel S. Hourly profiles of sleep and wakefulness in severely versus mild-moderately demented nursing home patients. Aging Clin Exp Res 1998; 10:308–315.

36. Swaab DF, Fliers E, Partiman TS. The suprachiasmatic nucleus of the human brain in relation to sex, age and senile dementia. Brain Res 1985; 342:37–44.

37. Ancoli-Israel S, Coy TV. Are breathing disturbances in elderly equivalent to sleep apnea syndrome? Sleep 1994; 17:77–83.

38. Ancoli-Israel S, Klauber MR, Butters N, Parker L, Kripke DF. Dementia in institutionalized elderly: relation to sleep apnea. J Am Geriatr Soc 1991; 39(3):258–263.

39. Ancoli-Israel S, Cole R, Alessi CA, Chambers M, Moorcroft WH, Pollak C. The role of actigraphy in the study of sleep and circadian rhythms. Sleep 2003; 26(3):342–392.

40. Chesson A, Berry RB, Pack AI. Practice parameters for the use of portable monitoring devices in the investigation of suspected obstructive sleep apnea in adults. Sleep 2003; 26(7):907–913.

41. Blazer D, Burchett B, Service C, George LK. The association of age and depression among the elderly: an epidemiologic exploration. J Gerontol 1991; 46(6):M210–M215.

42. Gillin JC, Duncan WC, Murphy DL, et al. Age-related changes in sleep in depressed and normal subjects. Psychiatry Res 1981; 4:73–78.

43. Campbell SS, Terman M, Lewy AJ, Dijk DJ, Eastman CI, Boulos Z. Light treatment for sleep disorders: consensus report. V. Age-related disturbances. J Biol Rhythms 1995; 10(2):151–154.
44. Baehr EK, Eastman CI, Revelle W, Losee-Olson S, Wolfe LF, Zee PC. Circadian phase-shifting effects of nocturnal exercise in older compared with young adults. Am J Physiol Regul Integr Comp Physiol 2003; 284(6):R1542–R1550.
45. Haimov I, Lavie P. Potential of melatonin replacement therapy in older patients with sleep disorders. Drugs Aging 1995; 7(2):75–78.
46. Loube DI, Loube AA, Mitler MM. Weight loss for obstructive sleep apnea: the optimal therapy for obese patients. J Am Diet Assoc 1994; 94:1291–1295.
47. Stepnowsky C, Marler MR, Ancoli-Israel S. Determinants of nasal CPAP compliance. Sleep Med 2002; 3(3):239–247.
48. Stepnowsky C, Bardwell WA, Moore P, Ancoli-Israel S, Dimsdale JE. Psychological correlates of CPAP compliance with continuous positive airway pressure. Sleep 2002; 25(7): 758–764.
49. Fleury B, Rakotonanahary D, Tehindrazanarivelo AD, Hausser-Hauw C, Lebeau B. Sleep and breathing: long term compliance to continuous positive airway pressure therapy (nCPAP) set up during a split-night polysomnography. Sleep 1994; 17(6):512–515.
50. Collard P, Pieters T, Aubert P, Delguste P, Rodenstein DO. Compliance with nasal CPAP in obstructive sleep apnea. Sleep Med Rev 1997; 1(1):33–44.
51. Walker RP, Grigg-Damberger M, Gopalsami C. Uvulopalatopharyngoplasty versus laser-assisted uvolopalatoplasty for the treatment of obstructive sleep apnea. Laryngoscope 1997; 107:76–82.
52. Schmidt-Nowara WW, Lowe A, Wiegand L, Cartwright R, Perez-Guerra F, Menn S. Oral appliances for the treatment of snoring and obstructive sleep apnea: a review. Sleep 1995; 18(6):501–510.
53. Shochat T, Loredo JS, Ancoli-Israel S. Sleep disorders in the elderly. Curr Treat Options Neurol 2001; 3(1):19–36.
54. Earley CJ, Allen RP. Pergolide and carbidopa/levodopa treatment of the restless legs syndrome and periodic leg movements in sleep in a consecutive series of patients. Sleep 1996; 19(10):801–810.
55. Mitler MM, Browman CP, Menn SJ, Gujavarty K, Timms RM. Nocturnal myoclonus: treatment efficacy of clonazepam and temazepam. Sleep 1986; 9:385–392.
56. Kavey N, Walters AS, Hening W, Gidro-Frank S. Opioid treatment of periodic movements in sleep in patients without restless legs. Neuropeptides 1988; 11(4):181–184.
57. Edinger JD, Heolscher TJ, Marsh GR, Lipper S, Ionescu-Pioggia M. A cognitive-behavioral therapy for sleep-maintenance insomnia in older adults. Psychol Aging 1992; 7:282–289.
58. Ancoli-Israel S, Gehrman PR, Martin JL, et al. Increased light exposure consolidates sleep and strengthens circadian rhythms in severe Alzheimer's disease patients. Behav Sleep Med 2003; 1(1):22–36.
59. Ancoli-Israel S, Martin JL, Kripke DF, Marler M, Klauber MR. Effect of light treatment on sleep and circadian rhythms in demented nursing home patients. J Am Geriatr Soc 2002; 50(2):282–289.
60. Satlin A, Volicer L, Ross V, Herz L, Campbell SS. Bright light treatment of behavioral and sleep disturbances in patients with Alzheimer's disease. Am J Psychiatry 1992; 149:1028–1032.
61. Alessi CA, Yoon EJ, Schnelle JF, Al-Samarrai NR, Cruise PA. A randomized trial of a combined physical activity and environmental intervention in nursing home residents: do sleep and agitation improve? J Am Geriatr Soc 1999; 47:784–791.
62. Greenfield D, Gehrman P, Linn MS, et al. CPAP compliance in mild–moderate Alzheimer's patients with SDB. Sleep 2003; 26:A154.
63. Ancoli-Israel S, Cohen-Zion M, Palmer BW, et al. Effect of CPAP on cognitive functioning in patients with dementia and SDB: Preliminary results. Sleep 2002; 25:A19–A20.

38

Methodologies in the Diagnosis of Sleep Apnea

Gopal Allada

Division of Pulmonary and Critical Care and Sleep Medicine, Department of Pulmonary and Critical Care, Oregon Health and Science University, Portland, Oregon, U.S.A.

Diagnosing obstructive sleep apnea–hypopnea syndrome (OSAHS) relies on obtaining an appropriate clinical history combined with a diagnostic polysomnogram (PSG). A complete history is essential not only to confirm the symptoms of OSAHS but also to explore other possible causes for the patient's presentation. The physical exam is a necessary part of the evaluation and can give insight into the risk of sleep apnea as well as the potential site of obstruction. Other modalities such as radiologic imaging and portable studies (including pulse oximetry) have been used for screening and diagnostic purposes with varying success. The gold standard, however, remains a full diagnostic polysomnogram. This chapter reviews each of these aspects of diagnosing OSAHS with specific attention to the geriatric patient.

DEFINITIONS OF SLEEP-DISORDERED BREATHING (SDB)

OSAHS is defined by the presence of apneas and hypopneas due to obstruction occurring in the upper airway, usually at the pharyngeal and/or glottic levels. The syndrome also includes the presence of daytime sleepiness as measured by subjective questionnaires or by studies that determine a subject's propensity to sleep during the daytime, such as a multiple sleep latency test (MSLT). The exact cutoff for how many apneas and hypopneas constitute true pathology has been the subject of some debate. Most feel >5–10 apneas and hypopneas per hour contribute to short-term morbidity and longer-standing consequences, such as systemic hypertension and possibly increased mortality.

An *apnea* is defined as the cessation of airflow for a minimum of 10 seconds. There are varying definitions of a *hypopnea*, but it incorporates some reduction in airflow (by 30–50%) for a minimum of 10 seconds combined with an oxygen desaturation of 2% to 4%. The number of apneas and hypopneas per hour is also referred to as the respiratory disturbance index (RDI). SDB also incorporates other criteria, including *respiratory effort-related arousals*, which reflect an *arousal* noted on electrocephalography (a change in sleep architecture for at least three seconds) as a

411

result of increased respiratory efforts as indicated by direct observation and/or the presence of paradoxical breathing during a polysomnogram. Respiratory effort-related arousals also indicate upper airway obstruction, but they do not meet the criteria of either an apnea or hypopnea.

EPIDEMIOLOGY OF SDB IN THE ELDERLY

Studies have conflicted about the relationship between age and sleep-disordered breathing. While the Wisconsin Sleep Cohort Study (WSCS) did not demonstrate an increase in OSAHS with age in subjects between 30 and 60 years old, the prevalence of OSAHS is higher in the elderly in other studies. In WSCS, 24% of men and 9% of women had an RDI >5 (with 4% of men and 2% of women having OSAHS) (1). Depending on the specific population and the definition used for sleep apnea, the prevalence of an RDI >5 in the elderly ranges from 27% to 75%. In a study of 427 community-dwelling elderly aged over 65, 62% (70% in men, 56% in women) had an RDI >10 and 24% had an RDI >40. When subjects were subdivided by age (65–69, 70–79, and 80–89), there was no statistically significant increase in the prevalence of RDI >10 in either older group (2). It is not clear if this represents a true plateau of sleep apnea prevalence or a survival bias, where the more severely affected die before reaching the older age group. Interestingly, the difference in prevalence between men and women decreased with each advancing age cohort and was essentially equal in men and women aged 80–89. The presence of significant sleep apnea is associated with increased mortality. Those patients with an RDI >30 had a statistically shorter survival, although age, pulmonary disease, and cardiovascular disease, rather than RDI, were independent predictors of death (3). The possibility of cardiovascular and/or pulmonary consequences secondary to sleep apnea may explain the shorter survival in patients with a higher RDI. The prevalence of OSAHS is also increased in nursing home and medical inpatients compared to independently living elderly (4). While there is some debate with regards to the clinical significance of sleep apnea in the elderly, most studies indicate that this syndrome has a higher prevalence in this population.

REASONS FOR SLEEP APNEA IN THE ELDERLY

Several factors have been implicated with the increased prevalence of sleep apnea in the elderly. As we age, our weight and body mass index (BMI = weight in kg/height in m^2) increases. In the elderly, body weight predicts sleep apnea as much as age (5). There are also functional changes in the upper airway associated with aging. Age-related declines in both skeletal muscle and the genioglossus strength are noted especially in subjects older than 79 years (6). There is also increased pharyngeal fat deposition and decreased genioglossus response to negative pressure with aging (7). Pharyngeal resistance increases with age in normal men, and supraglottic resistance is higher in men than women (8). There may be hormonal factors in play. Many women with OSAHS are postmenopausal. Genioglossal muscle tone is higher in premenopausal women compared to postmenopausal women. After supplementation with estrogen and progesterone, the muscular tone increased in postmenopausal women (9). Other factors that are age-dependent, such as hypothyroidism, changes in sleep architecture (reduced slow wave sleep and increased sleep fragmentation), declining vital capacity, and altered ventilatory control, may contribute to the increased prevalence of sleep apnea in the elderly (10).

The combination of our aging population with the increased prevalence of OSAHS in the elderly makes recognition of this syndrome an important aspect in caring for the geriatric patient. The diagnosis of OSAHS begins with a complete history and thorough physical examination. The utility of various radiologic methods in diagnosing sleep apnea has been studied more so in recent years, although it has not been routinely incorporated into standard practice. The relative shortage of sleep laboratories and the cost of attended polysomnograms have prompted various methods for screening for OSAHS with the hopes of identifying not only patients with the syndrome, but also those who may be more serious cases. Ultimately, the gold standard for diagnosing sleep apnea is an attended polysomnogram.

TAKING THE HISTORY OF A PATIENT WITH SUSPECTED OSAHS

A complete history for a patient with suspected obstructive sleep apnea helps to identify patients with the syndrome and may also determine whether or not they have another cause for their symptoms. When a bedroom partner is available, one can assess for signs of which the patient may not be aware. In the general adult population, gender plays an important role in the risk of OSAHS. In community-based studies, the ratio of male:female cases is 2–3:1, although this ratio appears to decline with increasing age and postmenopausal women. Given that clinic-based samples have reported up to a 10:1 male:female ratio of cases, sleep apnea is likely underdiagnosed in women in the general population.

Symptoms attributable to obstructive sleep apnea can be divided into daytime and nighttime complaints. Daytime symptoms include sleepiness, morning headaches, fatigue, decreased attention, decreased libido and/or impotence, depression, and personality changes. Nighttime symptoms include snoring, witnessed apneas, dyspnea, restlessness, choking/snorting, nocturia, diaphoresis, drooling, and reflux. Unfortunately, theses symptoms are neither sensitive nor specific for sleep apnea. The differential diagnosis of excessive daytime somnolence in the elderly is extensive (Table 1). Sleep in the elderly tends to be polyphasic, suggesting that the presence of

Table 1 Causes of Excessive Daytime Somnolence in the Elderly

Obstructive sleep apnea
Central sleep apnea
Mixed sleep apnea
Upper airways resistance syndrome
Periodic limb movements of sleep
REM-behavior disorder
Parasomnias (e.g., sleepwalking, night terrors)
Poor sleep hygiene
Insufficient sleep syndrome
Medications
Medication withdrawal
Narcolepsy
Depression

Abbreviation: REM, rapid eye movement.

a daytime nap does not necessarily reflect pathologic sleepiness. Their sleep tends to be *phase advanced*, meaning their circadian rhythm is shifted towards earlier awakening and sleep times over the course of the day. A sleep diary may be helpful in determining a patient's 24-hour sleep–wake cycle. Determining the impact of these symptoms on the patient's daily life and activities is also an important feature of the history. A history of motor vehicle accidents may identify a particularly severe case of sleep apnea if excessive sleepiness were the cause of the accident. Questionnaires such as the Epworth Sleepiness Scale or the Stanford Sleepiness Scale are validated ways to assess for daytime sleepiness.

A thorough review of the past medical history is indicated. This information will identify disorders that are associated with and/or aggravated by sleep apnea, as well as help risk stratify patients who may require surgical intervention for treatment. The relationship between obstructive sleep apnea and systemic hypertension is now strongly supported by large cohort studies. This association trends with increasing RDI and is independent of potentially confounding variables, such as age, race, gender, weight, alcohol use, and tobacco use (11). This association, however, declines with aging. Other conditions associated with obstructive sleep apnea (either as a potential cause or consequence of) include obesity, acromegaly, Down syndrome, cardiovascular disease (ischemic heart disease, congestive heart failure, arrhythmias, strokes), pulmonary hypertension, Parkinson's disease, and glucose intolerance.

The elderly have a higher incidence of hypertension, congestive heart failure, ischemic heart disease, chronic obstructive pulmonary disease, arthritis, gastrointestinal disorders, pain syndromes, cancer, chronic renal failure, diabetes, hypothyroidism, and neurologic disorders. All of these disorders can contribute to disrupted sleep whether it is directly caused by the condition or the medications used to treat them. Some of these disorders are associated with other sleep disorders, such as central sleep apnea (strokes, congestive heart failure), restless legs syndrome/periodic limb movements of sleep (chronic renal failure), and rapid eye movement (REM) disorder (Alzheimer's dementia, Parkinson's disease). Several medications commonly taken by the elderly, such as hypnotics, sedatives, and antidepressants, may contribute to daytime sleepiness and can also worsen pre-existing sleep apnea. Caffeine intake or the use of other stimulants may indicate attempts to compensate for pathologic sleepiness. Alcohol use prior to bedtime is known to relax the genioglossus muscle during sleep and aggravate both snoring and obstructive sleep apnea. Symptoms of depression should also be elicited, as this is associated with early morning awakenings and potentially increased sleepiness. In all comers, a positive family history of sleep apnea increases the risk of both snoring and sleep apnea in first-degree relatives (12). Disproportionate craniofacial anatomy has been noted to be common in familial groups with OSAHS (13). The clinical significance of a positive family history in the geriatrics patient is less clear. A history of a difficult intubation may also correlate with increased risk of sleep apnea.

CLINICAL EXAMINATION OF A PATIENT WITH SUSPECTED OSAHS

A complete physical examination is indicated in the geriatric patient with suspected sleep apnea with attention focused on the body habitus, facial morphology, oropharynx, and nasal examination. Most studies concerning the utility of the physical examination have not focused on elderly patients. In the general adult population, the risk of sleep apnea increases significantly with obesity (1). As we age, however, there is a declining effect of increasing weight on the odds of having sleep apnea. In the Sleep Heart Health Study (a study of 5615 community-dwelling men and women aged 40–98), the odds ratio for an apnea–hypopnea index (AHI) >15 was 35% less for an 80-year old (1.3) compared to a 40-year old (2.0) with respect to incremental increases in BMI (14). Neck circumference (measured at the superior border of the cricothyroid membrane) is a surrogate marker for pharyngeal fat. Greater neck circumference (generally >17 in or 43 cm) correlates with an increased risk of sleep apnea (15). Craniofacial abnormalities, such as a narrow mandible and/or maxilla, dental overbite, dental malocclusion, and retrognathia, are associated with obstructive sleep apnea.

The upper airway exam (with endoscopy) should consist of inspection for hypertrophied tonsils, enlarged adenoids, macroglossia, a high and narrow hard palate, an elongated, edematous uvula (from the repetitive trauma of snoring), a crowded oropharynx, and obstruction at the base of the tongue. Endoscopy can be performed in the seated and supine positions. The upper airway in patients with OSAHS is smaller in the supine position compared to seated position (16). Dynamic endoscopy involves performing Mueller's maneuver. This involves placing the endoscope directly above the segment to be evaluated while the patient inspires against occluded nostrils. The degree of collapsibility is then noted at each level and potentially identifies areas of surgical correction. Anterior rhinoscopy may reveal nasal obstruction from a deviated septum, enlarged nasal turbinates, or polyps, which can affect sleep apnea in multiple ways. Subsequent mouth breathing leads to loss of nasal reflexes that help maintain upper airway muscle tone (17). Mouth breathing also leads to posterior rotation of the mandible and tongue base, which can narrow the airway. Nasal obstruction contributes to "upstream resistance," which increases the collapsibility of the pharynx.

While there is no consensus on which upper airway measures are most predictive of OSAHS, recent studies have tried to determine which aspects of the exam correlate best with the severity sleep apnea. One such study looked at several aspects used by anesthesiologists to identify patients likely to have a difficult intubation. Of the measures assessed [modified Malampati grade (MMP), tonsil size, BMI, thyroidmental distance (TMD), and hyoid-mental distance (HMD)], only MMP, tonsil size, and BMI were reliable in predicting OSA severity (with MMP being most predictive) (18). Another study confirmed the predictive value of BMI and MMP and added pharyngeal abnormalities (e.g., ogivale-palate), while tonsil size was not predictive (though only a small percentage of subjects had hypertrophied tonsils). The study also noted a high prevalence of nasal obstruction in those with sleep apnea, implicating it as a factor for OSAHS (19). Small studies have not validated the use of the Mueller maneuver in predicting either good or poor candidates for surgical outcome of uvulopalatopharyngoplasty (UPPP) (20).

Because these studies have focused mainly on middle-aged adults, caution should be taken if applied to the geriatric population. Obstructive sleep apnea does not usually consist of a single stenotic area of obstruction, but rather multiple levels of a narrowing in addition to an increased propensity for collapsibility. In geriatric patients, functional properties of the upper airway may play a more important role than areas of frank obstruction. This concept is supported by the observation that BMI (a surrogate marker for upper airway fat and narrowing) plays less of a role in the elderly as it does in middle-aged adults. Interestingly, the cross-sectional areas of the naso-, oro-, and hypopharynx were statistically *higher* in apneics ≥65 years old compared to those less than 65 (21). Additional studies that focus on the predictive value of the physical examination in geriatric subjects are needed to determine how practitioners assess these patients.

RADIOLOGIC IMAGING IN THE DIAGNOSIS OF OBSTRUCTIVE
SLEEP APNEA

Although its clinical application is somewhat limited, radiologic imaging has been helpful in providing insight for the biomedical basis of OSAHS (22,23). Techniques such as cephalometry (lateral radiographs of the head and neck), fluoroscopy, computed tomography (CT) scanning, and magnetic resonance imaging (MRI) scanning have been studied in patients with and without sleep apnea. From these studies, we have learned that patients with obstructive sleep apnea are characterized by a small, collapsible oropharyngeal airway and by nasopharyngeal airway narrowing (24). CT scans have also demonstrated that the obstruction occurs at the retropalatal and retroglossal levels and that upper airway configuration in apneics has an anterior–posterior orientation (lateral narrowing), whereas the normal airway has its major axis in the lateral direction (25). There is also greater fat deposition posterolateral to the oropharyngeal airspace at the level of the soft palate in apneics compared to weight-matched controls (26). The upper airway has been studied during both inspiration and expiration in normal subjects. The cross-sectional area of the upper airway initially gets smaller at the onset of inspiration, but then becomes larger as the respiratory cycle approaches end-inspiration. At the onset of expiration, the upper airway reaches its maximum and then progressively declines until end expiration is reached (27). This suggests that the effect of negative inspiratory pressures on the airway is overcome by increased upper airway dilator musculature tone in normal subjects. The upper airway in patients with OSAHS appears to be headed to a closed position at end expiration. This may reflect both a dysfunction of upper airway muscle tone and/or a baseline narrowing of the upper airway itself.

There have been few studies that have evaluated radiologic imaging specifically in the geriatric population. In one study of *normal* subjects (apneics and snorers excluded) aged 20–79, CT scanning actually revealed a greater upper airway cross-sectional area as well as increased upper airway musculature tone in response to applied negative upper airway pressures in older (>60) compared to younger subjects (<40) (28). Another study examined whether older patients differ from younger patients with sleep apnea. There are subtle differences in upper airway dimensions in older patients with OSAHS. When comparing younger and older patients with sleep apnea, those greater than 65 years of age had greater naso-, oro-, and hypopharyngeal cross-sectional areas than their younger counterparts as measured by CT scan. The same group was studied using cephalometry, which revealed a trend in greater distance from the hyoid bone to the mandibular plane (MP–H) as well as a longer soft palate. There were no differences in posterior airway space, soft palate width, or ANB angle [from the subspinale (A) to the nasion (N) and to the supramentale (B)] (21).

A radiologic study comparing upper airway dimensions of geriatric patients with and without sleep would be helpful in potentially pointing out differences that would indicate a higher probability for the existence of OSAHS and its severity. As it stands, even in the general adult population, there is little utility in using radiologic imaging for the *diagnosis* of sleep apnea. Most studies that have attempted to determine its utility have been small and not always yielded consistent results. Newer techniques show promise in uncovering the pathogenesis of OSAHS and predicting its presence and severity. A recent case-control study looked at volumetric MRI to assess which upper airway features play a significant role in determining the presence of sleep apnea. The volume of the tongue and the lateral pharyngeal walls were independently associated with an increased risk of sleep apnea (29). The cost of MRI would make it prohibitive to use for diagnostic reasons.

There may be a greater role for radiologic imaging in patients who are considering treatments other than continuous positive airway pressure (CPAP). Cephalometrics had mixed results in predicting a beneficial response to UPPP. One study demonstrated that the presence of a baseline AHI <38, an MP–H ≤ 20 mm, and the absence of retrognathia are predictors of improvement after UPPP. Age was not predictive of surgical outcome, although the mean age was only 43 years (30). Other studies, however, have not demonstrated the utility of preoperative cepahlometrics in patients undergoing UPPP (31). In patients who underwent multilevel pharyngeal surgery (UPPP, genioglossus advancement, hyoid myotomy with advancement), preoperative cephalometric parameters did not predict which patients responded and which did not (32). CT scanning has been studied in predicting surgical outcome. Using three-dimensional upper airway CT, one group noted that patients with smaller upper airways, particularly relative to tongue and soft palate size, had a good response to UPPP (33). MRI offers the most soft tissue detail of all radiologic imaging. It has been recommended as the most beneficial radiologic modality to obtain before UPPP, although outcome data for its utility in predicting surgical success are lacking (22). MRI may help predict those who will have a successful outcome after placement with a mandibular advancement device (MAD). When undergone with a Mueller maneuver, pharyngeal MRI with a MAD in place helped predict which patients have a beneficial response (34).

In summary, radiologic imaging with cephalometrics, CT, and MRI have provided great insight into the upper airway pathology of OSAHS. Its utility in diagnosis is limited by its overall accuracy and expense. Studies focusing on its use for diagnostic purposes in the geriatric population are lacking. Expanding CT and MRI technology may lead to a role as a diagnostic modality in the future, but we are not there yet. Combining imaging with a good history and physical exam may prove useful in assessing the severity of sleep apnea. Preoperative imaging carries more promise than diagnostic imaging, although results in this regard have been mixed, and studies illustrating accurate prognostication of long-term postsurgical outcomes are lacking.

SPECIFIC METHODOLOGIES IN THE DIAGNOSIS OF OSAHS

The cornerstone in the diagnosis of OSAHS is the detection of apneas and hypopneas. This requires a diagnostic polysomnogram performed with the attendance of a trained sleep technician in a sleep laboratory. The cost of attended studies and the relative shortage of sleep facilities have prompted the use of other methods to screen for and diagnose sleep apnea. Such methods have incorporated only some of the features of a diagnostic polysomnogram with the hopes of saving costs and expediting diagnoses. In 1994, the American Sleep Disorders Association (ASDA) classified the various diagnostic methods into four types (35):

Type I—standardized polysomnography, which is considered the reference gold standard. This incorporates electroencephalography (EEG), electro-oculography (EOG), chin and limb electromyography (EMG), electrocardiography (ECG), measurements of airflow and respiratory movements, snore microphone, body position, and oxygen saturation.

Type II—comprehensive portable polysomnography, which includes a minimum of seven channels and allows for sleep staging.

Type III—modified portable sleep apnea testing, which incorporates a minimum of four monitored channels (at least two channels of respiratory movement, or respiratory movement and airflow), heart rate or ECG, and oxygen saturation.

Type IV—continuous single or dual bioparameters, most commonly oxygen saturation and heart rate.

Type II, III, and IV devices have all been studied with both a sleep technician present and in the home setting. In practice, when an attendant is present, a standardized polysomogram is usually performed. In addition, there are little data regarding type II unattended studies for any conclusions to be made about this modality. For these reasons, this review will focus on the utility of unattended type III and IV studies in the diagnosis of sleep apnea. If such modalities could accurately rule in and/or rule out OSAHS, they could potentially be of some use. Of note, most of these studies have focused on relatively healthy white men referred to a sleep clinic or laboratory. Less is known about the applicability of these diagnostic methods in the general primary care population, especially in the elderly and those with coexisting cardiopulmonary disease.

UNATTENDED MONITORING IN DIAGNOSING OSAHS

Pulse Oximetry

Pulse oximetry operates on the basis of differentiating oxyhemoglobin (arterial blood) from deoxyhemoglobin (venous blood) based on their distinct light absorption properties. A sensor is placed on a digit or earlobe to detect arterial flow and subsequent arterial oxygen saturation (SaO_2). The use of pulse oximetry in diagnosing OSAHS is based on two presumptions: (i) oxygen desaturations are effective surrogate markers for apneas and hypopneas, and (ii) the absence of oxygen desaturations excludes the presence of apneas and hypopneas. Independent of these presumptions, it is important to realize the limitations of pulse oximetry technology. Accurate assessment of SaO_2 requires adequate, pulsatile (arterial) blood flow. In patients with peripheral vascular disease or poor cardiac output (both of which are more common in the elderly), the signal output may not be as clear. Darker skinned individuals have falsely elevated SaO_2 readings, while fingernail discoloration (nail polish, onychomycosis) can falsely lower readings. Motion artifact can be quite common in patients who move around and displace the sensor. This is especially problematic during an unattended study where the sensor may not necessarily be placed back correctly, if at all.

While most oximeters incorporate pulse rate, there is no recording of arousals, sleep stage, body position, airflow, or limb movements. There is no way to tell when patients fall asleep, so the denominator for the AHI (apnea–hypopnea index = apneas + hypopneas per hour of sleep) is time spent in bed as opposed to total sleep time. This would tend to reduce the overall AHI compared to polysomnography. Because body position is not recorded, positional OSAHS (abnormal AHI in a particular position, typically supine) cannot be determined.

There have been many studies published regarding the use of pulse oximetry for the diagnosis of sleep apnea. There is much variability among the studies in terms of the population studied, the criteria used to determine an "event," the number of events/hour considered to be significant, and the specific type of pulse oximeter used.

For this reason, the quoted sensitivities, specificities, positive predictive values, and negative predictive values are quite disparate. In addition, because apneas and hypopneas are not truly measured with pulse oximeters, there is no apnea–hypopnea index per se; instead, a respiratory disturbance index, or RDI, is used to estimate the AHI. No large studies focusing specifically on screening elderly patients suspected of OSAHS have been published.

Pulse oximeters measure SaO_2 levels periodically (every 0.5–12 seconds depending on the technology) throughout the night to give a "running average." Both qualitative and quantitative oximetry criteria have been used to diagnose sleep apnea. Qualitative methods rely on an oximetry print out on a strip. A pattern consistent with OSAHS would be a series of oxygen desaturations of short duration, which is characterized by a "saw-tooth" configuration. The "dip" in the saw-tooth reflects an apnea or hypopnea, while the rise reflects the arousal response with hyperventilation and subsequent elevation in SaO_2. The problem with this method is that there is a large degree of subjective interpretation.

For this reason, quantitative methods have been more commonly studied. The criteria for a respiratory event include some degree of episodic desaturation (2–4%) with or without a measurement of hypoxia, such as time spent below 90% SaO_2. In initial studies using a 4% drop in SaO_2 as the cutoff for an event, the sensitivity and specificity for detecting OSAHS were around 40% and 98%, respectively (36,37). The poor sensitivity illustrated that significant oxygen desaturations were not necessary for OSAHS, especially in patients without underlying pulmonary disorders. In addition, the poor sensitivity underscores the problem with using only pulse oximetry as a screening tool for sleep apnea. It is important to note, however, that both sensitivity and specificity can be manipulated depending on which criteria are used to score an event. For example, if a cutoff of a 2% desaturation were used instead of 4%, sensitivity would improve, but at the expense of decreased specificity. If the goal were to capture most sleep apnea patients (at the expense of including more normal subjects), a lower threshold would be appropriate (higher sensitivity, lower specificity); if the goal were to identify the most severe patients (at the expense of missing more mild cases of sleep apnea), then a higher threshold could be used (lower sensitivity, higher specificity).

Efforts to improve on both specificity and sensitivity have focused on combining pulse oximetry with other sleep parameters or clinical history and by improving pulse oximetry technology. When combining a history of moderate to severe symptoms of sleep apnea, pulse oximetry appears to be excellent at confirming cases of OSAHS (especially severe ones) (38). This may be beneficial in identifying patients who are particularly high-risk who should be fast-tracked to earlier treatment. In patients with suspected sleep apnea but little evidence of daytime somnolence, oximetry does not appear to have much utility for distinguishing patients with and without OSAHS (39). When oximetry was used in conjunction with pulmonary spirometry, the test was quite specific for sleep apnea in patients with normal lung function. When patients with abnormal spirometry (force expiratory volume in the first second <80% predicted) were excluded, the specificity for diagnosis of OSAHS was at least 97%, while the sensitivity ranged from 63% to 80% (more sensitive for milder sleep apnea) (40). Because oximetry concomitantly records pulse rate, this has been an attractive adjuvant to use in diagnosing sleep apnea. During an apneic event, bradycardia is noted, which is then followed by a brief run of tachycardia coinciding with the arousal. Thus, heart variability is linked with OSAHS. Using this method appears to improve on the operating characteristic of oximetry alone (41).

Improving pulse oximetry technology has also opened the door for improvements in OSAHS diagnosis. Oximeters that have a sampling frequency of every 12 seconds have much poorer sensitivity than newer ones that sample every two seconds (42). Altering the sampling frequency even amongst the same group of patients will affect the overall number of events scored and would potentially alter treatment decisions (43). Knowing the sampling frequency of the pulse oximeter is integral to the interpretation of the data obtained. Recently, spectral analysis of oxygen saturation and heart rate has been used to improve the sensitivity and specificity of sleep apnea diagnosis. When there are periodicities in ventilation in sleep apnea, there is a phase-lagged change in oxygen saturation with the same periodicity. One group focused on oxygen desaturations and heart rate variability (bradycardia–tachycardia) that occur every 30–70 seconds, as this was the pattern that was seen in patients with OSAHA but was not present in those without the syndrome. When looked at prospectively in 300 patients with suspected sleep apnea, this method had a sensitivity of 94% and a specificity of 82% (44). Such technology is not readily available at the present time, but it may prove useful in the future.

Studies with pulse oximetry have not solely focused on the elderly. Because the geriatric population is more likely to have lower oxygen saturations independent of sleep apnea (marginal increase in alveolar–arterial gradient with aging, and an increased prevalence of pulmonary disease), the specificity of pulse oximetry may not be as good as the quoted studies, although sensitivity may be better. At present time, preliminary evidence suggests that pulse oximetry may have its best utility in excluding OSAHS in the general adult population. Advancing technology in pulse oximeters and the combination of other clinical and sleep parameters may also aid in its utility, although more studies are needed to verify this in an unattended setting. No studies have shown that pulse oximetry can reliably both rule in *and* rule out the diagnosis of OSAHS.

Modified Portable Sleep Apnea Testing (Type III)

Type III studies consist of a minimum of four monitored parameters, including ventilation, heart rate or ECG, and oxygen saturation. Body position and limb movements could potentially be studied but are not mandatory. Because EEG is not utilized, precise documentation of sleep staging and arousals cannot be recorded. There have been several studies comparing *attended* type III monitoring with polysomnography. In general, these studies have revealed that attended type III studies are very effective at both reducing and increasing the likelihood of OSAHS (45). There have been very few trials studying the utility of unattended type III studies. One Colorado study used a system that recorded eye movement, leg movement, SaO_2, nasal–oral airflow, chest and abdominal wall motion, body position, and heart rate. Interestingly, the investigators estimated sleep stage based on body and eye movements and respiratory assessment. RDI as measured by the portable study correlated well with the AHI as measured by polysomnography. For an AHI >10, the home study had a sensitivity of 91% and a specificity of 70% (46).

A Spanish study looked at a different system, which utilized nasal/oral airflow, chest wall impedance, SaO_2, heart rate, snoring, and body position. For an AHI >18 as a cut-off, the sensitivity was 73% and the specificity was 80%. As with the other study, sensitivity could be improved at the expense of lower specificity if a lower AHI threshold were used. The study did also note a failure rate (need to repeat study) of 10% (47). One home trial studied eight elderly women four times over a four-week period with the goal of determining the variability of various sleep parameters in the elderly. While those with mild sleep apnea had less variability in their apnea index, those with more severe apnea had greater variability, suggesting that a single night study may not be adequate in this population (48).

Overall, based on limited evidence, unattended type III studies do a reasonable job at ruling out OSAHS, but there are little data to support their use in ruling in the diagnosis. As with pulse oximeters, advancing technology may improve the operating characteristics of portable monitoring. Recently, a device that could monitor peripheral arterial tone (PAT) was used in conjunction with heart rate, pulse oximetry, and actigraphy (measure of arm movements) to assess OSAHS (49). The PAT signal measures arterial pulsatile volume changes in the finger, which are regulated by α-adrenergic innervation of the smooth muscle vasculature and reflect sympathetic nervous system activity (50). Because apneas and hypopneas terminate with sympathetic surges, this device can indirectly measure an RDI. Combining this information with pulse oximetry and heart rate, an automated algorithm was used to calculate a PAT RDI (or PRDI). This device demonstrated good correlations with PSG-RDI obtained in the sleep laboratory across a wide range of RDI levels. Whether this device could be applied routinely to the geriatric population whose peripheral circulation may be somewhat compromised by poor cardiovascular function remains to be determined.

POLYSOMNOGRAPHY IN THE EVALUATION OF OSAHS

An attended standard polysomnography in a sleep laboratory consists of EEG, EOG, chin and leg EMG, ECG, measurements of respiratory effort, airflow, body position, and SaO_2. A snore microphone is also often added. Esophageal manometry to record changes in intrathroacic pressure is less commonly used. The addition of EEG monitoring allows for documenting the initiation and termination of sleep, specific sleep stages, and arousals (an abrupt change in lasting at least two seconds, often associated with a body movement or respiratory event). Sleep stages are divided into REM sleep and non-REM (NREM) sleep. NREM sleep is further subdivided into four stages, with stages III and IV considered "deeper" sleep. REM sleep is characterized by rapid eye movements and the generalized loss of skeletal muscle, which can be noted on chin EMG recordings. Rechtschaffen and Kales (51) outline the specific, standardized criteria for each sleep stage. EEG monitoring gives exact sleep times and therefore a more precise AHI. In addition, REM-related OSAHS can be identified. While this disorder is treated similarly to other cases of OSAHS (nasal CPAP), there are medical therapies such as REM-reducing agents and physostigmine that could be useful adjuncts or alternatives (52). There are subtle differences in patients with apneas that predominate in NREM versus REM. NREM-predominant sleep apnea may be associated with more daytime sleepiness than REM-related apnea (53). Identifying arousals is important as disruptions in sleep architecture lead to significant sleep fragmentation and reduced daytime alertness. Positional sleep apnea can be identified with body position recording. If sleep apnea occurs predominantly in the supine position, positional therapy (interventions which discourage patients from sleeping on their backs) could also be tried.

In addition to being the gold standard in diagnosing sleep apnea, diagnostic polysomnography can identify other sleep-related disorders, such as central sleep apnea, nocturnal seizures, periodic leg movements of sleep, REM-behavior disorder, obesity-hypoventilation disorder, and upper airways resistance syndrome. Upper airways resistance syndrome is characterized by arousals from sleep associated with increasing respiratory efforts associated with increased upper airways resistance (54). All of these disorders could produce symptoms that mimic those of OSAHS, yet be missed on a portable study. The addition of a trained sleep technician is very helpful in the evaluation of sleep disorders. They are present for the initial setup and are also available for any technical problems that often occur with any one of the many parameters being used. Unattended home studies have a reported data loss rate of between 4% and 33% (49). Technicians can also monitor abnormal movements of limbs (periodic leg movements of sleep), seizure activity, bruxism, rhythmic movement disorder, REM-behavior disorder, nightmares, sleep terrors, sleepwalking, and confusional arousals. If significant sleep apnea is seen in the first portion of the evening, a sleep tech can institute CPAP treatment for the second half of the evening (55). This is known as a split-night polysomnogram. When this type of study is undertaken, the patient can potentially get diagnosed and titrated to the proper CPAP pressure in the same evening.

While polysomonography is the gold standard for diagnosing OSAHS, it is not without its faults. Cost and availability are big concerns. The cost of a polysomnogram varies across the country, but they generally range from $1500 to $2000. While this may seem like a significant expenditure, it is comparable to other tests we order, such as a full sinus CT scan. The advent of split-night polysomnograms has saved the cost of having to perform an additional sleep study for a CPAP titration. The increasing recognition of sleep apnea has created a backlog of persons waiting to get in for their study, thus creating a long list of untreated persons. With more sleep specialists and laboratory space, this problem will hopefully be improved. Unfortunately, because of our aging population and the increasing prevalence of sleep apnea in the elderly, the waiting lists are likely to get longer before they get shorter. Another issue with laboratory studies is that subjects have to sleep in a new environment, which may not be entirely comfortable for them. Some have difficulty falling asleep with all the monitoring equipment. People may change their sleeping patterns; for example, subjects tend to sleep more in the supine position in sleep labs. In addition, when polysomnograms were performed on consecutive nights, there was a portion of subjects who would not have been diagnosed if only one study had been done: this is known as the first-night effect (56). Despite these issues, polysomnography remains the mainstay in the diagnosis of sleep apnea and several other sleep disorders.

RECENT REVIEWS AND GUIDELINES

The American Academy of Sleep Medicine (AASM), American Thoracic Society, and the American College of Chest Physicians recently cosponsored an evidence-based review on the home diagnosis of sleep apnea (45). They concluded that there is *preliminary* evidence that unattended type III and type IV studies can be utilized to decrease the probability that a subject has OSAHS. While there was evidence that these studies could be useful in increasing the likelihood of a diagnosis of sleep apnea, the support is less convincing. Neither study (unattended) could be exclusively used to both rule out and rule in the diagnosis. They did note that attended type III studies had good evidence to support their use for both diagnosing and excluding sleep apnea.

The authors pointed out several limitations in the literature regarding portable studies. Most of the studies were performed in subjects with a high pretest probability of sleep apnea (referrals to sleep clinics and sleep labs), which would likely increase the quoted false-negative rates. Their conclusions may be less applicable to the general population. Most of the studies were in middle-aged men without significant comorbid disease, so their applicability to other populations should be somewhat questioned. The majority of studies compared attended portable monitoring to polysomnography, so fewer conclusions can be made on unattended studies. Because type III and IV monitoring do not include EEG (and subsequent documentation of sleep time), their use of time in bed as a surrogate marker for sleep makes the RDI lower than the expected AHI. This also limits the documentation of arousals. Finally, because the literature is limited to the available technology at the time, consideration for modifications of portable monitors should be made when interpreting future studies.

In 1994, the AASM published guidelines that outline three circumstances for which portable monitoring might be an acceptable alternative in the absence to available polysomnography (57). These included: (i) for patients with severe clinical symptoms that are indicative of OSAHS, and when initiation of treatment is urgent and standard polysomnography is not readily available; (ii) for patients unable to be studied in the sleep laboratory; and (iii) for follow-up studies where diagnosis has been established by standard polysomnography and therapy has been initiated, and the intent is a comparison to evaluate response to therapy. Recently published practice parameters for the use of portable monitoring devices reaffirmed these indications as well as made recommendations for their overall utility in sleep apnea (58). Here is a summary of their recommendations with respect to diagnosing OSAHS as defined by an AHI >15.

Type II devices: There are not enough published data to support their use in either the attended or unattended setting to evaluate patients with OSAHS.

Type III devices: Attended studies: Some type III devices may have utility in ruling out OSAHS in patients with a low pretest probability of the disorder. They can be used to rule in the diagnosis. They may be able to both rule in and rule out OSAHS provided the raw data are reviewed and that patients do not have significant comorbid diseases. A careful history (including a partner questionnaire) and examination should be performed to assess the patient's pretest probability of having OSAHS.

Unattended studies: Type III studies have insufficient evidence to recommend usage in ruling in and/or ruling out the diagnosis of OSAHS.

Type IV devices: The routine use of these devices in either the attended or unattended setting is not recommended for ruling in and/or ruling out OSAHS based on the available evidence.

Other comments regarding type III and IV devices:

1. Because these studies do not include EEG monitoring, sleep cannot be documented. Under current Medicare guidelines, two hours of sleep must be documented.
2. Symptomatic patients who have a nondiagnostic or negative test should undergo an attended PSG if a sleep disorder remains a clinical consideration.
3. It is important for the interpreter to understand the capabilities and limitations of the specific device used for the study, because many different kinds of devices have been used in the literature.

4. Screening should not be undertaken with portable devices without available knowledge of the patient's sleep history and complaints.

The fairly tepid recommendations for the use of portable devices in the diagnosis of sleep apnea reflects some of the weaknesses in the current literature: patient

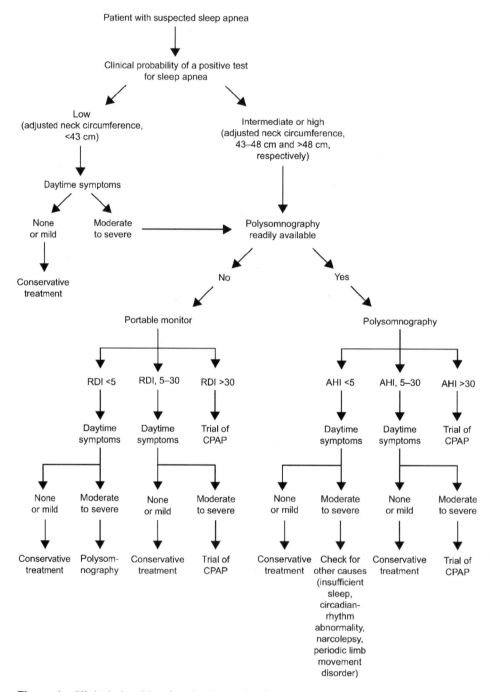

Figure 1   Clinical algorithm for the diagnosis of obstructive sleep apnea.

selection in the studies (referrals to sleep clinics and labs) does not directly apply to the general population, multiple portable devices were used, multiple criteria were used to define an event, multiple criteria were used as a cut-off to define OSAHS, and a paucity of level I and II literature has been published.

CLINICAL DECISION-MAKING ALGORITHM

The use of portable devices will depend on the availability of polysomnography as well as the significance of the patient's symptoms. Estimating a patient's pretest probability of having sleep apnea is important for interpreting the results of any screening test. For example, a negative study in a patient with a low pretest probability of having OSAHS (mildly symptomatic) has different implications than for a patient who snores and reports excessive daytime somnolence. Multiple clinical prediction models of various complexity have been constructed for the diagnosis of OSAHS (59,60). One such model uses neck circumference and the presence or absence of hypertension, snoring, and choking/gasping on most nights (61). The prediction algorithm calls for an "adjusted" neck circumference (ANC) by adding 4 cm for hypertension, 3 cm for habitual snoring, and 3 cm for reporting choking/gasping on most nights. Using this parameter, ANC values of <43 cm, 43–48 cm, and >48 cm correlated with low, intermediate, and high clinical probabilities of having OSAHS. This prediction model has been suggested to be used in a clinical decision algorithm in which intermediate or high clinical probability patients may go on to have portable monitoring for the assessment of OSAHS *if* polysomnography is not readily available (Fig. 1) (62). Whether this could be applied to geriatrics patients who may not report as much snoring or witnessed gasping remains to be seen.

SUMMARY

In conclusion, the diagnosis of OSAHS begins with a detailed history and physical examination to determine the extent of the symptoms and the pretest probability of the diagnosis, and exploration of other possible causes for the patient's presentation. While the elderly are susceptible to a variety of sleep disorders, the prevalence of sleep apnea increases with age for a variety of reasons. Geriatric patients, however, may not present as symptomatic as the typical middle-aged patient. At present time, radiologic evaluation for sleep apnea remains as a research tool only, but with expanding technology may play a role in the future. Ultimately, the diagnosis should be made with an attended polysomnogram. Recently published practice parameters have frowned on the routine use of portable studies in the evaluation for sleep apnea, but they may play a role in patients with a high pretest probability of OSAHS if polysomnography is not readily available.

REFERENCES

1. Young T, Palta M, Dempsey J, Skatrud J, Weber S, Badr S. The occurrence of sleep-disordered breathing among middle-aged adults. N Engl J Med 1993; 328(17):1230–1235.
2. Ancoli-Israel S, Kripke DF, Klauber MR, Mason WJ, Fell R, Kaplan O. Sleep-disordered breathing in community-dwelling elderly. Sleep 1991; 14(6):486–495.

3. Ancoli-Israel S, Kripke DF, Klauber MR, et al. Morbidity, mortality and sleep-disordered breathing in community dwelling elderly. Sleep 1996; 19(4):277–282.

4. Ancoli-Israel S. Epidemiology of sleep disorders. Clin Geriatr Med 1989; 5:347.

5. Bliwise DL, Feldman DE, Bliwise NF, et al. Risk factors for sleep disordered breathing in heterogeneous geriatric populations. J Am Geriatr Soc 1987; 35:132–141.

6. Crow HC, Ship JA. Tongue strength and endurance in different aged individuals. J Gerontol A Biol Sci Med Sci 1996; 51:M247–M250.

7. Malhotra A, Crowley S, Pillar G, et al. Age-related changes in pharyngeal structure and function in normal subjects [abstr]. Sleep 2000; 161(suppl 2):A42.

8. White DP, Lombard RM, Cadieux RJ, Zwillich CW. Pharyngeal resistance in normal humans: influence of gender, age, and obesity. J Appl Physiol 1985; 58(2):365–371.

9. Popovic RM, White DP. Upper airway muscle activity in normal women: influence of hormonal status. J Appl Physiol 1998; 84:104.

10. Bliwise DL. Normal aging. In: Kryger MH, Roth T, Dement WC, eds. Principles and Practice of Sleep Medicine. 3rd ed. Philadelphia, PA: W.B. Saunders, 2000:26–42.

11. Peppard PE, Young T, Palta M, Skatrud J. Prospective study of the association between sleep-disordered breathing and hypertension. N Engl J Med 2000; 342(19):1378–1384.

12. Pillar G, Lavie P. Assessment of the role of inheritance in sleep apnea syndrome. Am J Respir Crit Care Med 1995; 151(3 Pt 1):688–691.

13. Guilleminault C, Partinen M, Hollman K, Powell N, Stoohs R. Familial aggregates in obstructive sleep apnea syndrome. Chest 1995; 107(6):1545–1551.

14. Young T, Shahar E, Nieto FJ, et al. Sleep Heart Health Study Research Group. Predictors of sleep-disordered breathing in community-dwelling adults: the Sleep Heart Health Study. Arch Intern Med 2002; 162(8):893–900.

15. Hoffstein V, Mateika S. Differences in abdominal and neck circumferences in patients with and without obstructive sleep apnoea. Eur Respir J 1992; 5(4):377–381.

16. Andreoli TE, Cecil RL. Cecil Essentials of Medicine. 2nd ed. Vol. XIV. Philadelphia: Saunders, 1990:830.

17. el-Ganzouri AR, McCarthy RJ, Tuman KJ, Tanck EN, Ivankovich AD. Preoperative airway assessment: predictive value of a multivariate risk index. Anesth Analg 1996; 82(6):1197–1204.

18. Friedman M, Tanyeri H, La Rosa M, et al. Clinical predictors of obstructive sleep apnea. Laryngoscope 1999; 109(12):1901–1907.

19. Zonato AI, Bittencourt LR, Martinho FL, Junior JF, Gregorio LC, Tufik S. Association of systematic head and neck physical examination with severity of obstructive sleep apnea–hypopnea syndrome. Laryngoscope 2003; 113(6):973–980.

20. Petri N, Suadicani P, Wildschiodtz G, Bjorn-Jorgensen J. Predictive value of Muller maneuver, cephalometry and clinical features for the outcome of uvulopalatopharyngoplasty. Evaluation of predictive factors using discriminant analysis in 30 sleep apnea patients. Acta Otolaryngol 1994; 114(5):565–571.

21. Levy P, Pepin JL, Malauzat D, Emeriau JP, Leger JM. Is sleep apnea syndrome in the elderly a specific entity? Sleep 1996; 19(suppl 3):S29–S38.

22. Schwab RJ. Imaging for the snoring and sleep apnea patient. Dent Clin North Am 2001; 45(4):759–796.

23. Schwab RJ. Upper airway imaging. Clin Chest Med 1998; 19(1):33–54.

24. Galvin JR, Rooholamini SA, Stanford W. Obstructive sleep apnea: diagnosis with ultra-fast CT. Radiology 1989; 171(3):775–778.

25. Schwab RJ, Gefter WB, Hoffman EA, Gupta KB, Pack AI. Dynamic upper airway imaging during awake respiration in normal subjects and patients with sleep disordered breathing. Am Rev Respir Dis 1993; 148(5):1385–1400.

26. Horner RL, Mohiaddin RH, Lowell DG, et al. Sites and sizes of fat deposits around the pharynx in obese patients with obstructive sleep apnoea and weight matched controls. Eur Respir J 1989; 2(7):613–622.

27. Schwab RJ, Gefter WB, Pack AI, Hoffman EA. Dynamic imaging of the upper airway during respiration in normal subjects. J Appl Physiol 1993; 74(4):1504–1514.

28. Burger CD, Stanson AW, Sheedy PF II, Daniels BK, Shepard JW Jr. Fast-computed tomography evaluation of age-related changes in upper airway structure and function in normal men. Am Rev Respir Dis 1992; 145(4 Pt 1):846–852.

29. Schwab RJ, Pasirstein M, Pierson R, et al. Identification of upper airway anatomic risk factors for obstructive sleep apnea with volumetric magnetic resonance imaging. Am J Respir Crit Care Med 2003; 168(5):522–530.

30. Millman RP, Carlisle CC, Rosenberg C, Kahn D, McRae R, Kramer NR. Simple predictors of uvulopalatopharyngoplasty outcome in the treatment of obstructive sleep apnea. Chest 2000; 118(4):1025–1030.

31. Doghramji K, Jabourian ZH, Pilla M, Farole A, Lindholm RN. Predictors of outcome for uvulopalatopharyngoplasty. Laryngoscope 1995; 105(3 Pt 1):311–314.

32. Yao M, Utley DS, Terris DJ. Cephalometric parameters after multilevel pharyngeal surgery for patients with obstructive sleep apnea. Laryngoscope 1998; 108(6):789–795.

33. Ryan CF, Lowe AA, Li D, Fleetham JA. Three-dimensional upper airway computed tomography in obstructive sleep apnea. A prospective study in patients treated by uvulopalatopharyngoplasty. Am Rev Respir Dis 1991; 144(2):428–432.

34. Sanner BM, Heise M, Knoben B, et al. MRI of the pharynx and treatment efficacy of a mandibular advancement device in obstructive sleep apnoea syndrome. Eur Respir J 2002; 20(1):143–150.

35. Ferber R, Millman R, Coppola M, et al. Portable recording in the assessment of obstructive sleep apnea. ASDA standards of practice. Sleep 1994; 17(4):378–392.

36. Douglas NJ, Thomas S, Jan MA. Clinical value of polysomnography. Lancet 1992; 339(8789):347–350.

37. Gyulay S, Olson LG, Hensley MJ, King MT, Allen KM, Saunders NA. A comparison of clinical assessment and home oximetry in the diagnosis of obstructive sleep apnea. Am Rev Respir Dis 1993; 147(1):50–53.

38. Golpe R, Jimenez A, Carpizo R, Cifrian JM. Utility of home oximetry as a screening test for patients with moderate to severe symptoms of obstructive sleep apnea. Sleep 1999; 22(7):932–937.

39. Hussain SF, Fleetham JA. Overnight home oximetry: can it identify patients with obstructive sleep apnea–hypopnea who have minimal daytime sleepiness? Respir Med 2003; 97(5):537–540.

40. Chiner E, Signes-Costa J, Arriero JM, Marco J, Fuentes I, Sergado A. Nocturnal oximetry for the diagnosis of the sleep apnoea hypopnoea syndrome: a method to reduce the number of polysomnographies? Thorax 1999; 54(11):968–971.

41. Raymond B, Cayton RM, Chappell MJ. Combined index of heart rate variability and oximetry in screening for the sleep apnoea/hypopnoea syndrome. J Sleep Res 2003; 12(1):53–61.

42. Wiltshire N, Kendrick AH, Catterall JR. Home oximetry studies for diagnosis of sleep apnea/hypopnea syndrome: limitation of memory storage capabilities. Chest 2001; 120(2):384–389.

43. Davila DG, Richards KC, Marshall BL, et al. Oximeter's acquisition parameter influences the profile of respiratory disturbances. Sleep 2003; 26(1):91–95.

44. Zamarron C, Gude F, Barcala J, Rodriguez JR, Romero PV. Utility of oxygen saturation and heart rate spectral analysis obtained from pulse oximetric recordings in the diagnosis of sleep apnea syndrome. Chest 2003; 123(5):1567–1576.

45. Flemons WW, Littner MR, Rowley JA, et al. Home diagnosis of sleep apnea: a systematic review of the literature. An evidence review cosponsored by the American Academy of Sleep Medicine, the American College of Chest Physicians, and the American Thoracic Society. Chest 2003; 124(4):1543–1579.

46. White DP, Gibb TJ, Wall JM, Westbrook PR. Assessment of accuracy and analysis time of a novel device to monitor sleep and breathing in the home. Sleep 1995; 18(2):115–126.

47. Parra O, Garcia-Esclasans N, Montserrat JM, et al. Should patients with sleep apnoea/ hypopnoea syndrome be diagnosed and managed on the basis of home sleep studies? Eur Respir J 1997; 10(8):1720–1724.
48. Acebo C, Watson RK, Bakos L, Thoman EB. Sleep and apnea in the elderly: reliability and validity of 24-hour recordings in the home. Sleep 1991; 14(1):56–64.
49. Bar A, Pillar G, Dvir I, Sheffy J, Schnall RP, Lavie P. Evaluation of a portable device based on peripheral arterial tone for unattended home sleep studies. Chest 2003; 123(3):695–703.
50. Grote L, Hedner J, Ding Z. Alteration of digital pulse amplitude reflects α adreno-receptor mediated constriction of the digital vascular bed [abstr]. Sleep 2001; 24(suppl):133R.
51. Rechtschaffen A, Kales A. A Manual of Standardized Technology, Techniques and Scoring System for Sleep Stages of Human Subjects. Los Angeles: Brain Information Service/ Brain Research Institute, UCLA, 1968.
52. Hedner J, Kraiczi H, Peker Y, Murphy P. Reduction of sleep-disordered breathing after physostigmine. Am J Respir Crit Care Med 2003; 168(10):1246–1251.
53. Punjabi NM, Bandeen-Roche K, Marx JJ, Neubauer DN, Smith PL, Schwartz AR. The association between daytime sleepiness and sleep-disordered breathing in NREM and REM sleep. Sleep 2002; 25(3):307–314.
54. Guilleminault C, Stoohs R, Clerk A, Cetel M, Maistros P. A cause of excessive daytime sleepiness. The upper airway resistance syndrome. Chest 1993; 104(3):781–787.
55. Sanders MH, Kern NB, Costantino JP, et al. Adequacy of prescribing positive airway pressure therapy by mask for sleep apnea on the basis of a partial-night trial. Am Rev Respir Dis 1993; 147(5):1169–1174.
56. Chediak AD, Acevedo-Crespo JC, Seiden DJ, Kim HH, Kiel MH. Nightly variability in the indices of sleep-disordered breathing in men being evaluated for impotence with consecutive night polysomnograms. Sleep 1996; 19(7):589–592.
57. Practice parameters for the use of portable recording in the assessment of obstructive sleep apnea. Standards of Practice Committee of the American Sleep Disorders Association. Sleep 1994; 17(4):372–377.
58. Chesson AL Jr, Berry RB, Pack A, American Academy of Sleep Medicine, American Thoracic Society, American College of Chest Physicians. Practice parameters for the use of portable monitoring devices in the investigation of suspected obstructive sleep apnea in adults. Sleep 2003; 26(7):907–913.
59. Flemons WW, McNicholas WT. Clinical prediction of the sleep apnea syndrome. Sleep Med Rev 1997; 1:19–32.
60. Gurubhagavatula I, Maislin G, Pack AI. An algorithm to stratify sleep apnea risk in a sleep disorders clinic population. Am J Respir Crit Care Med 2001; 164(10 Pt 1): 1904–1909.
61. Flemons WW, Whitelaw WA, Brant R, Remmers JE. Likelihood ratios for a sleep apnea clinical prediction rule. Am J Respir Crit Care Med 1994; 150(5 Pt 1):1279–1285.
62. Flemons WW. Clinical practice. Obstructive sleep apnea. N Engl J Med 2002; 347(7):498–504.

39
Snoring: Simple to Obstructive Apnea

Kenny P. Pang
*Department of Otolaryngology, Tan Tock Seng Hospital, Tan Tock Seng, Singapore,
and Department of Otolaryngology—Head and Neck Surgery, Medical College
of Georgia, Augusta, Georgia, U.S.A.*

Amy R. Blanchard
*Section of Pulmonary/Critical Care Medicine, Medical College of Georgia,
Augusta, Georgia, U.S.A.*

David J. Terris
*Department of Otolaryngology—Head and Neck Surgery,
Medical College of Georgia, Augusta, Georgia, U.S.A.*

INTRODUCTION

Sleep is a basic fundamental process that humans appear to need. Yet sleep is a mechanism about which not all is understood. Average humans spend between six and eight hours per day, or about one-third of their lifetime, sleeping. Sleep is a transient state of altered consciousness with perceptual disengagement from one's environment. Contrary to popular belief, sleep is an active process involving complex interactions between cortical, brain stem diencephalic, and forebrain structures (1). There is still significant metabolism and oxygen consumption during this state of "rest," and any disruption of oxygenation or interruption of this physiological process can lead to both night and day manifestations like snoring, choking sensations, apneic episodes, or daytime somnolence.

Snoring, the lay term for noisy breathing during sleep, has historically been believed to be just a nocturnal "nuisance" and an obnoxious human habit. In a 30–35-year old population, 20% of men and 5% of women will snore. By age 60, 60% of men and 40% of women will snore habitually (2). Epidemiological studies have shown that for adults over 65 years old, up to 50% have some form of sleep disruption and poor sleep quality (3). Snoring may be a simple nuisance to the patient or sleep partner when not accompanied by other symptoms or complaints. However, it may be part of a symptom complex indicating sleep-disordered breathing (SDB).

The presence of snoring is a loud "alarm" that alerts one to the possibility of a sleep disorder. Sleep-disordered breathing is a spectrum of diseases related to decreased airflow through the upper airway during sleep, due either to complete or partial upper airway obstruction or increased upper airway resistance. These encompass simple snorers (patients who snore without excessive daytime somnolence and with a normal apnea–hypopnea index), upper airway resistance syndrome (patients with excessive daytime somnolence but who have a normal apnea–hypopnea index), and obstructive sleep apnea (OSA) (patients who snore with both excessive daytime somnolence and an abnormal apnea-hypopnea index). Overall, these sleep disorders result in poor sleep quality, fragmented sleep, intermittent nighttime hypoxemia, reduced percentage of slow wave sleep, and increased sympathetic over-drive. The results are daytime somnolence, morning headaches, poor concentration, loss of memory, frustration, depression, and even marital discord.

EPIDEMIOLOGY

Sleep-disordered breathing is more common and pronounced in older adults than younger adults (4,5). In the largest study of a representative sample of older adults (65–95 years of age), 62% had an RDI >10, and 24% had an AI >5 (6). In this same study, SDB was more common in men than in women and in patients with hypertension than in those without hypertension. In a study of older African Americans and Caucasians, the prevalence was equivalent, but apnea was more severe in the African-American group (7). Foley et al. (3) have also shown that up to 50% of adults over 65 years of age complain of some sort of sleep disruption. Sleep disorders in the elderly are known to be caused by multiple factors, and many of these sleep disturbances may be secondary to medical and psychiatric conditions (8,9). In a study of 1050 individuals with a mean of 74.4 years, 36.7% reported difficulty falling asleep, 28.7% had sleep continuity disturbance, 19.1% had early morning awakening, and 18.9% reported uncontrollable daytime somnolence (10).

PATHOPHYSIOLOGY

The fundamental abnormality in sleep-disordered breathing is in the anatomy and collapsibility of the upper airway. Snoring is caused by a vibration of the structures of the oral cavity/oropharynx: the soft palate, uvula, tonsils, base of tongue, epiglottis, and pharyngeal walls. Partial or complete upper airway obstruction during sleep can lead to excessive soft tissue or abnormal facial skeletal framework. Patients with adenotonsillar hypertrophy have a crowded upper airway with very little space for airflow, while obese patients frequently have soft palate redundancy. It is the vibration of these soft tissues during sleep that results in snoring, when the bulk of this soft tissue exceeds a certain amount. It leads to collapse, partial or complete, of these structures, which then leads to upper airway obstruction during sleep. Patients with retrognathia will have less space available, therefore increasing the like-lihood of airway compromise during sleep. There are some authors who believe that SDB is entirely based on the equilibrium between forces that hold the airway open and forces that tend to collapse the airway (11). The magnitude of the pressures collapsing the airway can be measured, and this measurement can be inferred from the pressure required by continuous positive airway pressure to hold the airway open. This is known as pharyngeal critical pressure (P_{crit}) (12).

   The soft tissues in the upper airway can be divided into the adipose tissues, muscle groups, and lymphoid tissues. The presence of adipose tissues surrounding the airway plays a significant role in SDB. There are fat deposits present under the mucosal membranes as well as surrounding the various muscles in the neck. Adipose tissue is present in the palate, tonsillar fossa, and even in the pharyngeal walls. Oropharyngeal fat deposition reduces airway caliber, thereby worsening upper airway obstruction.

   The muscle groups can be divided into those that are vertical and those that are horizontal. The vertical group includes the palatopharyngeus, salpingopharyngeus, glossopharyngeus, and the levator veli palatini. The constrictor muscles and the tensor veli palatini comprise the horizontal group. The tongue plays a crucial role in the upper airway, not only due to its central location in the oral cavity and oropharynx but also because of its bony attachment. The muscle fibers of the tongue converge and are primarily attached to the posterior surface of the mandible (genial tubercle) in the midline. When the mandible is displaced posteriorly (e.g., retrognathia), airway compromise may occur at the base of the tongue. This anatomical attachment of the tongue forms the basis for the genioglossus advancement procedure, which is done through a mandibulotomy window.

The lymphoid tissues are probably the most amenable to treatment. When there is obvious adenotonsillar hypertrophy, removing the lymphoid tissues may be curative, especially in children (13).

Although mechanically the airway may be visually conceptualized as a simple conduit, it is very dynamic, and airflow is affected by three main variables. Bernoulli's principle states that negative pressure develops at the periphery of fluid flow, and as the flow velocity increases, so does the negative pressure. Therefore, a narrow airway tends to remain narrow. Fluid velocity increases as a given volume moves through a conduit of decreasing size (Venturi effect). If the conduit diameter is reduced, then the velocity and pressure of the fluid or air increases. The final factor is the variable resistor concept, which states that resistance to flow increases with increasing flow. The net effect is that upper airway narrowing perpetuates its own narrowing and the airflow velocity and resistance to flow tend to increase correspondingly.

As with most other tissues in the human body, gravity affects the soft tissues in the upper airway. Lying supine during sleep will cause the soft tissues of the oropharynx to collapse and fall posteriorly, obstructing the airway.

Nasal pathologies have been shown to aggravate and contribute to the severity of SDB, and treatment of the underlying nasal pathology may help, but usually not cure, the disorder. Controlling and relieving nasal obstruction will improve compliance with the use of nasal continuous positive airway pressure. Careful nasal examination is useful to allergic rhinitis, nasal polyposis, or a severely deviated nasal septum.

There is a male predominance in OSA, which in most reports is 2:1. This may be partly a result of hormonal differences since postmenopausal women tend to develop symptoms on average 5 years after menopause, with a prevalence of OSA approaching that of males. There are some reports that progesterone will reduce snoring and sleep apnea in males, while exogenous testosterone can increase upper airway resistance in females (14,15).

DIFFERENTIAL DIAGNOSIS

Most patients with SDB complain of snoring, which may be heroic. Frequently, the sleep partner prompts the patient to see a physician because of concerns over repeated apneas. Patients may complain of frequent awakenings with a choking sensation, nocturia, or nightmares. Patients with severe SDB may be unable to sleep supine. Common patient complaints include early morning tiredness and morning headaches (attributable to the repetitive nocturnal oxygen desaturations). Morning dry mouth and throat are caused by mouth breathing and snoring. Other symptoms include forgetfulness, depression, irritability and, less commonly, impotence.

Excessive daytime sleepiness is very common in patients with SDB and is caused by a combination of frequent arousals, sleep fragmentation, repetitive oxygen desaturations, and reductions in delta and rapid eye movement sleep (16,17).

A thorough sleep history should be obtained to exclude sleep deprivation as a cause of excessive daytime somnolence (EDS). Daytime somnolence refers to a person's propensity to fall asleep in various situations. The international classification of sleep disorders defines sleepiness in subjective terms (18):

Mild sleepiness: Sleep episodes are present only while resting or when little attention is needed. There is only mild impairment of social function.

Moderate sleepiness: Sleep episodes are present daily and occur during very mild physical activities or at times that require a moderate degree of attention. There is moderate impairment of work or social function.

Severe sleepiness: Sleep episodes are present daily or during times requiring mild to moderate attention. There is marked impairment of social or work function.

Most clinicians use standardized scales such as the Epworth Sleepiness Scale, in which the respondent rates the likelihood of sleeping in each of eight situations, with a maximum score of 24 (19). A score of >10 suggests EDS.

CLINICAL EXAMINATION

Clinical evaluation can be divided into general medical, systemic (cardiorespiratory and neurological), and oral examination with an upper airway assessment. All patients should have weight and height, body mass index, blood pressure, and neck circumference (at the level of the hyoid bone) recorded.

Oral anatomy in the elderly differs from that in younger adults. Brown et al. (20), using the acoustic reflection technique, reported that the pharyngeal area in males decreases with age. Other authors have reported that the distance from the hyoid bone to the mandibular plane (MP–H) is longer in the geriatric age group, likely due to increased upper airway fat deposition, resulting in increased tendency for collapse (21). Stanffer et al. (22) showed that older subjects with a significantly high AHI have smaller upper airway areas and increased resistance compared with controls. Tonsil size in the geriatric age group is usually not abnormal but is still graded on a five-point scale (0 = absent, 1+ = small within the tonsillar fossa, 2+ = extends beyond the tonsillar pillar, 3+ = enlarged tonsils but not touching the midline, 4+ = enlarged tonsils touching the midline). The Mallampati classification may also be used to assess upper airway configuration (Fig. 1).

No single classification of pharyngeal and upper airway anatomy for patients with SDB is widely accepted. In 1987, Ikematsu (23) first described the pharyngeal airway anatomy of heavy habitual snorers. He used six features to classify oropharyngeal anatomy: (a) soft palate length (±50 mm), (b) uvula length (±11 mm), (c) uvula width (±10 mm), (d) pillar arch morphology (parallel, webbed, embedded, emerging), (e) oropharyngeal narrowing (anterior arch ±20 mm, posterior arch ±15 mm, shallow oropharynx ±5 mm), and (f) enlarged tongue dorsum (oropharynx not seen with phonation). In 1990, Fujita (24) modified the classification. This classification is probably the most commonly used by clinicians:

Type I: soft palate (velopharyngeal) obstruction

Type II: both soft palate and hypopharyngeal (base of tongue) obstruction

Type III: hypopharyngeal (base of tongue) obstruction

Complementary to Fujita's classification is a dynamic assessment of the upper airway called the Müller maneuver. It consists of a nasopharyngoendoscopic examination of the upper airway during which the patient is performing a reverse Valsava. The site of obstruction is noted, with particular attention to three distinct areas of potential collapse: retropalatal, lateral pharyngeal walls (lateral to medial), and retrolingual. The collapse is quantified on a five-point scale as follows:

(A) **(B)**

(C) **(D)**

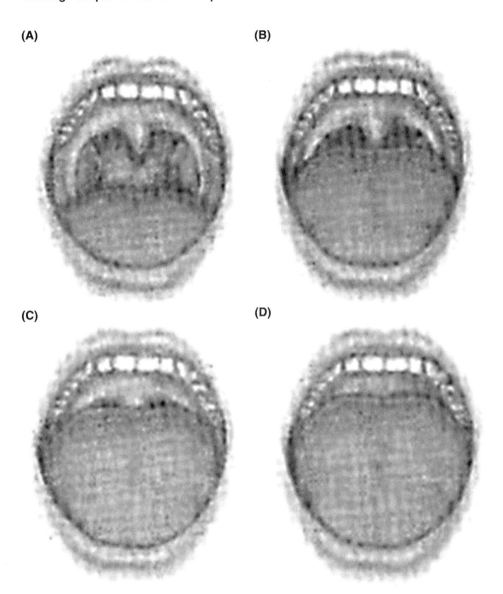

Figure 1 The Friedman classification, which is drawn from the Mallampati classification, is a general way of describing the upper airway configuration.

        0: no collapse
        1+: approximately 25% collapse
        2+: approximately 50% collapse
        3+: approximately 75% collapse
        4+: complete collapse, obliterating the airway

    This dynamic clinical assessment forms the basis for determining the appropriate level for surgical correction.

LATERAL CEPHALOMETRY

Many sleep physicians support the use of lateral cephalograms to estimate the degree of posterior airway space (PAS) narrowing (Fig. 2). Changes in the SNB and SNA angles

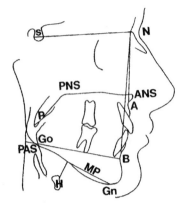

SNA   82
SNB   80
PAS   11
PNS-P 35
MP-H 15

Figure 2 A number of measurements may be identified on cephalometric analysis; the PAS is particularly important in predicting the need for tongue base surgery. *Abbreviation*: PAS, posterior airway space.

are correlated with postoperative changes in AHI. Other studies have also shown that increasing PAS values by a minimum of 10 mm have significantly better surgical outcomes.

DIAGNOSIS OF SDB

The gold standard for differentiating simple snoring from OSA is an attended polysomnogram. It is appropriate to obtain a sleep study for any snoring patient with a history of excessive daytime somnolence, with or without physical findings suggestive of SDB, especially in patients with cardiovascular comorbidities.

Severity of OSA can be classified according to the AHI and lowest oxygen saturation level. The severity is usually graded as the worst of the two (Table 1).

Powell and Riley (25) suggest that any patient with an AHI ≥20 warrants some form of intervention and treatment. Patients with an AHI <20 with EDS, associated desaturation <90%, arrhythmias associated with obstructive events, or complications of SDB also require treatment.

SNORING TREATMENT

Snoring is considered a social disease with no medical significance. Consequently, it is not covered by insurance, and treatment is available but must be paid for out of pocket. This has led to a number of treatment modalities, the efficacies of which are pretty similar but differ mainly in pain outcomes and costs. The majority of benign snoring is secondary to palatal flutter. Thus, treatment is directed at the soft palate. Scarring of the palate has been the objective of all treatments. The theory is that the more collagen deposited into the soft tissues, the stiffer they are and the less likely to flutter. In patients with excessive soft tissues, resection of redundant tissue has also been advocated.

Table 1 Different severity grades of OSA

	AHI	LSAT (%)
Mild	5–19	86–90
Moderate	20–39	70–85
Severe	>40	<70

Abbreviations: AHI, apnea–hypopnea index; LSAT, lowest oxygen saturation level; OSA, obstructive sleep apnea.

Laser-Assisted Uvulopalatopharyngoplasty

This is perhaps the first treatment that was advocated for treatment of benign snoring. In this procedure, a CO_2 laser is used to vaporize the attachment of the uvula to the soft palate. Furrows are made in the soft palate itself. The resultant healing causes a decrease in tissue due to the uvulectomy and stiffening of the soft palate due to the laser-induced thermal effect. Success rates with this procedure have been reported between 80% and 90% in the short term and 60–70% in the long term. The morbidity is minimal, and the drawbacks have to do with the pain of the procedure. Narcotics are usually required for 7–10 days. Occasionally, bleeding and nasopharyngeal incompetence have been reported but are exceedingly rare.

Somnoplasty

The high cost of the laser, along with the pain from the procedure, prompted the development of a microwave-energy delivery system to the soft palate. The Somnus Corporation pioneered this, and the procedure called somnoplasty was developed. In this procedure, energy is delivered to the submucosal surface through a proprietary specialized device. The resultant soft tissue protein coagulation causes a stiffening of the tissue with a decrease in snoring and palatal flutter. Results are similar to all other snoring procedures with successes of 80% and long-term results of 60–70%. The major advantage with this procedure is that pain is minimal with it. Usually, non-narcotics are sufficient for pain control. Multiple treatments are usually required, and the proprietary nature of the device makes its cost high.

Snoroplasty

First pioneered by a number of otolaryngologists at the Walter Reed Medical Center, this procedure involved injection of a sclerotherapy agent into the soft palate. The resultant scarring and soft tissue cauterization effect decreased palatal flutter and led to stiffening of the soft palate with retraction and decrease in volume of noise. Results were reported to be extremely good with single injections, and they seemed to maintain themselves over the long term, as with other procedures. Pain was between that of the laser-assisted procedure and the somnoplasty procedure, with most patients requiring some form of narcotic control. The major drawback is that the drug pioneered in this procedure is no longer manufactured in the United States and must be purchased through a foreign country.

Other Procedures

People have described using electrocautery and coblation techniques for the same desired effects. Results from single-institutional studies and by single authors are similar to those reported above. A relatively new procedure based on implanting poly-Teflon implants to stiffen the palate has recently been described with a high extrusion rate but good success.

SUMMARY

Overall, all of the procedures for snoring have been described as being 70–80% successful in the short term, while decreasing to 60% or so in the long term. No randomized control studies comparing different techniques have been reported.

REFERENCES

1. Goh YH, Lim KA. The physiologic impact of sleep apnoea on wakefulness. Otolaryngol Clin North Am 2003; 36:423–435.
2. Lugaresi E, Cirignotta F, Coccagna G, Baruzzi A. Snoring and the OSA. Electroencephalogr Clin Neurophysiol 1982; 35(S):421–430.
3. Foley DJ, Monjan AA, Brown SL, Simonsick EM, Wallace RB, Blazer DG. Sleep complaints among the elderly: an epidemiological study of 3 communities. Sleep 1995; 18:425–432.
4. Martin J, Shochat T, Gehrman PR, Ancoli-Isreal S. Sleep in the elderly. Respir Care Clin North Am 1995; 5(3):461–472.
5. Reynolds CF. Sleep Disorders. In: Sadaroy J, Lazarus LW, Jarrik LF, eds. Comprehensive review of geriatric psychiatry. Washington, D.C.: American Psychiatric Press, 1991:403–418.
6. Ancoli-Isreal S, Kripke DF, Klauber MR, et al. Sleep disordered breathing in community dwelling elderly. Sleep 1991; 14:486.
7. Ancoli-Isreal S, Klauber YM, Stepnousky C, et al. SDB in Africa-American-elderly. Am J Respir Care Med 1995; 152:1946.
8. Benca RM, Obermeyer WH, Thisted RA, et al. Sleep and psychiatric disorder: a meta-analysis. Arch Gen Psychiatry 1992; 49:651.
9. Monjan A, Foley D. Incidence of chronic insomnia associated with medical & psychosocial factors: an epidemiological study among older persons. Sleep Res 1996; 25:108.
10. Ganguli M, Reynolds CF, Gilby JE. Prevalence and resistance of sleep complaints in rural older community sample: the MOVIES project. J Am Geriatr Soc 1996; 44:778–784.
11. Bliwise DL, Feldman DE, Bliwise NG, et al. Risk factors for SDB in heterogeneous geriatric population. J Am Geriatr Soc 1987; 35:132–141.
12. Coleman JA Jr. Pathophysiology of snoring & OSA. Snoring & OSA. 3rd ed. Chapter 2. Lippincott, Philadelphia: William & Wilkins, 2003:19–24.
13. Pang KP, Bala A. Paediatric obstructive sleep apnea: is a polysomnogram always necessary? J Laryngol otol 2004; 118(4):275–278.
14. Strohl K, Hensley M, Saunders N, et al. Progesterone administration and progressive sleep apneas. JAMA 1981; 245:1230–1235.
15. Johnson M, Anch A, Kemmers J. Induction of sleep apnea syndrome in a woman by exogenous androgen administration. Am Rev Respir Dis 1984; 129:1023–1025.
16. Bonnett MH. Performances & sleepiness as a function of the frequency & placement of sleep disruption. Psychophysiology 1986; 23:263–271.
17. Colt HG, Haas H, Rich GB. Hypoxemia vs sleep fragmentation as a cause of excessive daytime sleepiness in OSA. Chest 1991; 100:1542–1548.
18. International classification of sleep disorders, revised: diagnostic & coding manual. Rochester, Mn.: American Sleep Disorders Association, 1997.
19. Johns MW. A new method for measuring daytime sleepiness: the Epworth's Sleepiness Scale. Sleep 1995; 14:540–545.
20. Brown IG, Zamel N, Hoffstein V. Pharyngeal cross-sectional area in normal men & women. J Appl Physiol 1986; 61:890–895.
21. Maltais F, Carrier G, Cormier Y, Series F. Cephalometric measurement in snorers, non-snorers & patients with sleep apnea. Thorax 1991; 46:419–423.
22. Stanffer JL, Zwillich CW, Cadienx RJ, et al. Pharyngeal size & resistance in OSA. Am Rev Respir Dis 1987; 136:623–627.
23. Ikematsu. A 30-year clinical study in snoring. In: Fairbanks DNL, Fujita S, Ikematsu T, Simmons FB, eds. Snoring & sleep apnea 1st ed. New York: Raven Press, 1987:130–134.
24. Fujita S. Surgical treatment of OSA: UPPP and lingualplasty (laser midline glossectomy). In: Guilleminault C, Partinen M, eds. Obstructive sleep apnea syndrome: clinical research and treatment. New York: Raven Press, 1990:129–151.
25. Powell N, Riley. A surgical protocol for SDB. Oral Maxillofac Surg Clin North Am 1995; 7(2):345–356.

40

Upper Airway Resistance Syndrome

Michel A. Cramer Bornemann
Departments of Neurology and Pulmonary/Critical Care Medicine,
Minnesota Regional Sleep Disorders Center, Hennepin County Medical Center,
Minneapolis, Minnesota, U.S.A.

Vance D. Bachelder
Department of Biomedical Engineering, University of Minnesota Graduate School,
Medical Instrumentation and Device (MIND) Laboratory/Bakken Institute,
Minneapolis, Minnesota, U.S.A.

Robert H. Maisel
Department of Otolaryngology—Head and Neck Surgery, Minnesota Regional Sleep
Disorders Center, Hennepin County Medical Center, Minneapolis,
Minnesota, U.S.A.

INTRODUCTION

Sleep-disordered breathing (SDB) encompasses a broad range of unstable breathing patterns with potentially far-reaching physiologic consequences that occur during sleep. Often underappreciated, sleep-disordered breathing is complex in nature and may be dependent upon a vast and seemingly disparate array of influences. Upper airway resistance syndrome (UARS) is a subset in the general category of disorders that fall under the primary heading of SDB. Unfortunately, SDB is often mistakenly held as being synonymous with obstructive sleep apnea syndrome (OSAS). OSAS is only one such entity in this diverse array of disorders.

It is important to note that not all unstable breathing patterns are necessarily deleterious or clinically significant to the patient. One such example is the serendipitous observation during a routine diagnostic sleep study of a periodic breathing pattern during the transition from restful wakefulness to Stage I sleep. It is not uncommon for periodic breathing of this nature to be of a sizeable duration, particularly if the patient is experiencing difficulty in both initiation and maintenance of sleep. In an otherwise healthy patient, this type of periodic breathing is often devoid of both marked oxygen desaturations and arousals. In developing an effective clinical management strategy for the patient, the technical objective results attained from a formal diagnostic sleep study need to be consistent with the extent of the patient's clinical expression and chief complaints in order to support the medical indication to treat the condition.

The model of SDB is believed to be a continuous spectrum of disorders that begins with a milder form, primary snoring, and progresses through several intermediary forms, including OSAS, before possibly culminating, if the disorder is left unabated, to its most severe form, the Pickwickian syndrome. With ongoing research in the mechanics of breathing and with further characterization of patient population characteristics for each disorder, this model has come under significant scrutiny. In fact, as recently supported by Guilleminault and Chowdhuri (1), UARS appears to be a distinct and separate entity as its physiology and predominant patient population characteristics are not consistent with the current "severity-continuity model" for SDB.

DEFINITIONS IN SLEEP-DISORDERED BREATHING

Technical definitions used for scoring SDB in a polysomnogram (PSG) include discriminating among apnea, hypopnea, and respiratory-effort-related arousals (RERAs). Apneas and hypopneas are further traditionally subdivided into three categories: (i) obstructive, (ii) central, and (iii) mixed respiratory events. *Obstructive* respiratory events are those that are caused by the obstruction of the upper airway. *Central* respiratory events are those that are caused by a decrease, or absolute cessation, in output to the muscles that drive inspiration and are associated with a compromised respiratory control center within the central nervous system. *Mixed* respiratory events have features of both obstructive and central respiratory events. The majority of sleep clinicians consider a mixed event to be predominantly obstructive in nature.

Apnea is defined as the complete cessation of airflow for at least 10 seconds in adults and 3 seconds in infants, regardless of the degree of hemoglobin oxygen desaturation. In adults, hypopnea is defined as a decrease in airflow of at least 30% as compared to baseline with at least a 4% oxygen desaturation. To appropriately score hypopnea, the abnormal respiratory event also needs to be of at least 10 seconds in duration (2). As scoring hypopneas is dependent upon the method of airflow detection, it is thought that this definition of hypopnea would lead to an improvement of intra- and interscoring reliability. Lastly, a RERA refers to a reduction of airflow that does not meet the criteria for apnea or hypopnea but still culminates in an EEG arousal that is either cortical or subcortical in nature (3). The degree of oxygen desaturation, if any, is not a requirement to score a RERA, as the arousal is the most important consequence.

The similarities between apnea and hypopnea are well recognized, as is their essentially indistinguishable impact on the expression of OSAS. The frequency of apneas and hypopneas, and hence the severity of OSAS, is calculated from a formal PSG and reported as an *apnea/hypopnea index*. This index, which is reported as the number of abnormal respiratory events per hour, has a dose-dependent association with both the progression of excessive daytime hypersomnolence and the risk for the development cardiovascular disease.

DETERMINANTS OF UPPER AIRWAY PATENCY DURING SLEEP

Pharyngeal Transmural Pressure and Compliance

Pharyngeal patency is a function of both the transmural pressure across the pharyngeal wall and the compliance of the pharyngeal wall. The generation of diaphragmatic muscle activity initiates the increase in the inspiratory force, thereby resulting in a subatmospheric pharyngeal intraluminal pressure that leads to a propensity for airway collapse (4). Moreover, as predicted by the Bernoulli principle, pharyngeal patency is even more progressively compromised as the inspiratory narrowing results in an increase in airflow velocity that further diminishes intraluminal pressure (4).

Thoracic Caudal Traction

The upper airway is connected through the mediastinum to the thoracic cage by several structures. During wakefulness, inspiratory diaphragmatic activity exerts a caudal traction upon the thoracic cage, which in turn increases the caliber of the upper airway. This mode of improvement in airway caliber is passive in nature. It appears to be independent of the pharyngeal dilating muscles and is thought to be related to the increase in inspiratory transmural pressure as exerted by the transmission of subatmospheric pressure through the trachea and soft tissues surrounding the ventrolateral cervical region (5).

The improvement of airway caliber may also be an active process. During wakefulness, the application of negative pressure to the upper airway elicits a reflexive action upon the genioglossus and tensor palatini muscles. This reflex is thought to contribute to airway patency and is promptly initiated in approximately 50 milliseconds (msec) after the application of thoracic caudal traction (5,6). However, this reflex is absent during sleep, thereby suggesting that sleep eliminates this protective reflex that maintains airway patency in the midst of narrowing or deformation.

Magnetic resonance imaging of the pharynx in patients with OSAS reveals a marked prevalence for abnormally large parapharyngeal fat deposits (7). This deposition in the region of the normally compliant retropalatal region of the upper airway results in further destabilization during sleep by diminishing airway compliance. This fat deposition contributes to an encroachment of the lateral diameter of the airway lumen. This diminution in the caliber of the lateral diameter of the lumen in the retropalatal region is a major contributor, as opposed to the anterior-posterior diameter, to the severity of OSAS.

Finally, clinical studies have supported that nasal obstruction exacerbates the tendency towards OSAS (8). The degree of this influence has been poorly characterized and remains in doubt for cases of moderate to severe OSAS. It is conceivable that a targeted surgical approach, such as septoplasty or turbinoplasty, might prove to be a reasonable treatment option for those with mild SDB.

SLEEP IN THE ELDERLY

Many factors related to sleep undergo an age-dependent change. Aging results in decreases in electroencephalography (EEG) amplitude, alpha wave expression, slow wave sleep (specifically Stages III and IV), REM sleep, and sleep efficiency. There is a significant shift towards an increase in Stage II sleep and the expression of "micro-arousals"—very brief unremembered awakenings lasting less than 3 seconds. In addition, there are age-dependent chronobiological changes, such as the trend towards an advanced sleep cycle as opposed to the delay in sleep that is commonly encountered in adolescents and young adults. As the entrainment of the sleep/wake cycle is heavily influenced by the endogenous circadian rhythm emanating from the suprachiasmatic nucleus of the anterior hypothalamus, chronobiological changes may reflect the deterioration of these brain structures that are known to occur with age.

The prevalence of UARS in various populations has not been defined. If one were to accept the premise that sleep-disordered breathing operates on a continuous spectrum, one might anticipate that the prevalence of UARS might emulate that of OSAS. Conversely, if one accepts Guilleminault's fervent assertion that UARS is a distinct entity and not merely a milder form of OSAS, then the association between UARS and aging is entirely unclear once data regarding this are scarce.

THE FIRST DESCRIPTIONS OF UARS

The term "UARS" was first coined by Guilleminault in 1992 to describe a subgroup of patients with a common constellation of clinical complaints. These patients had been diagnosed as having a narcolepsy-like variant, otherwise designated as idiopathic hypersomnia or CNS hypersomnia (9). These patients initially presented with the chief complaint of excessive daytime sleepiness of unclear etiology. OSAS was not supported as nocturnal PSGs revealed apnea/hypopnea index values that were within normal limits. Narcolepsy was ruled out, since multiple sleep latency tests did not exhibit any episodes of sleep-onset REM. With further careful examination of respiratory waveforms from the PSGs of these patients, Guilleminault was able to discern abnormal repetitive respiratory patterns that were devoid of any significant oxygen desaturation.

Using invasive esophageal manometry (a technique not commonly utilized or accepted in the vast majority of sleep laboratories), these abnormal patterns were accentuated by increases in respiratory effort as distinguished by a progressive escalation in negative inspiratory esophageal pressures (P_{es}). These recurring episodes of increased upper airway resistance (IUAR) were brief in duration, typically only one to three breaths, and were often abruptly terminated after brief EEG arousals of 2–14 seconds in duration. Use of esophageal manometry reflected the swings in intrapleural pressure, thereby providing a more direct and sensitive measure of inspiratory and expiratory airflow patterns, changes often not appreciated by traditional means of airflow monitoring in the sleep or pulmonary physiology laboratory (Fig. 1).

According to Guilleminault et al. (9,11), immediately after each arousal, the unusually elevated P_{es} would suddenly return to baseline and a normal breathing pattern would ensue only to begin the abnormal respiratory cycle once more. Again, it is generally thought that these arousals cause the sequelae associated with UARS. Furthermore, Guilleminault et al. (9) continued to evaluate patients with excessive daytime sleepiness who met their criteria for UARS and found that some had light intermittent snoring while others did not snore. This suggests that the absence of snoring does not necessarily exclude UARS and may additionally distinguish this entity from OSAS (Fig. 2).

The characterization (and research) of UARS is currently limited to only a few investigational centers. Consequently, there is a paucity of information regarding the prevalence and disease outcome data of UARS. The clinical relevance of UARS has become enthusiastically accepted in a few medical circles but widespread acceptance as to its importance and to whether it is a distinct entity separate from OSAS has yet to be attained.

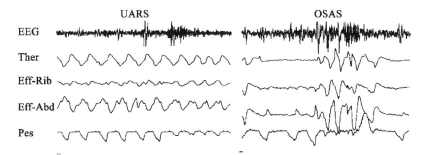

Figure 1 Esophageal manometry (P_{es})—UARS versus OSAS. Reproduction of a RERA in a UARS patient and an apnea in an OSAS patient. Note the similarity in the magnitude of the inspiratory P_{es} nadirs for breaths occurring in both patients prior to an arousal. *Abbreviations*: Ther, oronasal thermistors airflow; Eff-Rib, chest impedance plethysmography; Eff-Abd, abdominal impedance plethysmography; UARS, upper airway resistance syndrome; OSAS, obstructive sleep apnea syndrome; RERA, respiratory-effort-related arousals. *Source*: From Ref. 10.

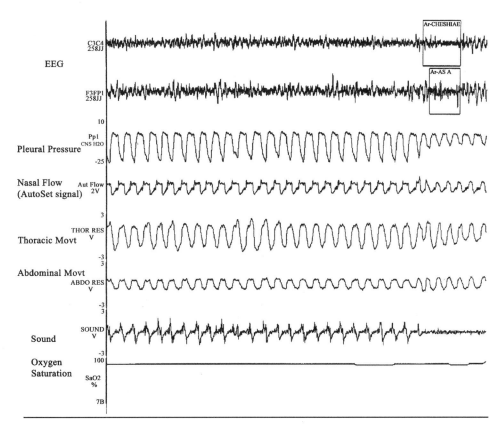

Figure 2 Esophageal manometry—esophageal pressures (P_{es}) and airflow. An example of a resistive event with heavy snoring. The flattened inspiratory flow-time profile is associated with increased pleural pressure (P_{es}) swings. The event is terminated by a cortical arousal (*boxed segments on the EEG*). Pleural pressure swings return to the sleeping baseline, and the inspiratory flow-time profile is once again rounded. *Abbreviation*: EEG, electro encephalography. *Source*: From Ref. 12.

PATHOPHYSIOLOGY OF UARS

The pathologic sequelae of UARS are thought to be secondary to the repetitive arousals. This can be problematic, since there are different arousal types, and their definitions often take into consideration the deviation from the physiologic norm of the monitoring device that was employed. Criteria used to define arousals may relate to changes in the frequencies and amplitudes of EEG activity, EMG activity (i.e., increases in muscle tone in the submental region, inferior intercostal muscles, anterior tibialis, etc.), respiratory rate, and even subtle changes in heart rate variability as detected using a standard lead II electrocardiogram rhythm strip (13). Certainly, in terms of defining subcortical arousals, a consensus definition of such an arousal has yet to be attained. Compared to wakefulness, sleep should be a time of a generalized predominance in parasympathetic tone. As a result, the common thread that binds these definitions of a clinically relevant arousal from sleep is a shift, though it may be intermittent, to a more sympathetic state and adrenergic state.

Not all arousals have the same effect upon the human body. There is evidence to suggest that respiratory-related arousals, in particular, are more likely to cause daytime sleepiness than non-respiratory-related arousals (14). The extent in which they differ, if at all, has yet to be established, but respiratory-related arousals are presumed to promote episodes of sympathetic hyperactivity of various durations. Now that increased sympathetic tone has been associated with the initiation and progression of cardiovascular disease and congestive heart failure along with the deterioration of many other physiologic systems, the importance between the association of increased sympathetic tone and the progression of nonrestorative sleep should not be astonishing.

By definition UARS requires the presence of increased upper airway resistance. The gold standard, and for some clinicians the only currently accepted method, for determining the presence of upper airway resistance is to employ esophageal pressure (P_{es}) manometry.

It appears that upper airway mechanoreceptors are also involved in eliciting a RERA (15). Administration of anesthesia to the upper airway decreases genioglossus activity during apneas, increases apnea duration, and produces more negative P_{es} nadirs (15,16). This supports the premise that the upper airway mechanoreceptor afferent input to the CNS contributes to arousals. It is also possible that chest wall and lower airway mechanoreceptors contribute to arousals in a similar fashion (Fig. 3) (15).

A threshold value in relation to the number of events of IUAR per hour has been proposed as an integral tenet in the development of a formal definition concerning UARS. In the vast majority of UARS cases, the respiratory events will be predominantly of the RERA type. It is important to note that the hallmark of a RERA event is the lack of any significant oxygen desaturation, certainly not greater than a 4% decrease. Most patients with UARS have RDIs that are predominantly RERAs with a bare minimum of frank apneic and hypopneic events. RERA events will need to be better defined and correlated to symptoms and pathologic sequelae before interpreting the meaning of an RDI.

Nasal cannula pressure transducers are a less invasive way of measuring upper airway resistance, and preliminary data suggest that this correlates well with esophageal pressure manometry (17). Nasal cannula pressure transducers are a promising diagnostic tool to assist in the diagnosis of UARS, but the technique still does not have the sensitivity nor specificity of an esophageal manometer. When solely using a nasal pressure transducer to assess inspiratory and expiratory efforts, the numbers

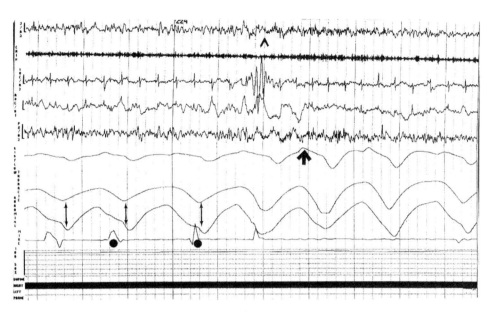

Figure 3 UARS and EEG cortical arousals. A noninvasive PSG from a patient with UARS. An IUAR event is suggested by an EEG arousal preceded by a crescendo snoring and abdominal and thoracic dys-synchrony by plethysmography. Increased airflow by nasal thermistors follows the onset of arousal. Note that the hemoglobin oxygen saturation does not change significantly. The arrowhead indicates an EEG arousal, the thick arrow indicates increased airflow, the thin arrow indicates abdominal and thoracic dyssynchrony, and the closed circles indicate crescendo snoring. *Abbreviations*: UARS, upper airway resistance syndrome; EEG, electroencephalography; PSG, polysomnogram; IVAR, increased upper airway resistance. *Source*: From Ref. 15.

of RERAs in a given nocturnal PSG are often over-reported, and as such UARS can be overdiagnosed. This is problematic when determining an appropriate clinical management strategy, as the clinical relevance of UARS is much in a state of flux.

Another diagnostic technique to assess respiratory patterns and airflow employs monitoring the temperature changes associated with inspiration and expiration. This technique utilizes readily accessible tools such as airflow thermistors or other such thermocoupling devices. Though this technique may be sufficient in diagnosing overt OSAS, it does not correlate well with quantitative airflow and should not be used to detect subtle changes in upper airway resistance (18). It is therefore imperative that when reviewing PSG data or reports, particularly when attempting to discern the presence or absence of IUAR, the conscientious physician should always be aware of the technique utilized to assess airflow (Fig. 4).

CLINICAL FEATURES AND DIAGNOSIS OF UARS

UARS patients must, by definition, have daytime sleepiness and/or fatigue (20). Symptoms may be obvious, but given the indolent nature of the disease process, patients often lack insight concerning the severity of nighttime symptoms or the degree of daytime impairment. It is common for patients to under-report or to not fully appreciate the severity of their daytime sleepiness. It is also common for patients to finally seek a formal consultation based not upon their own concerns

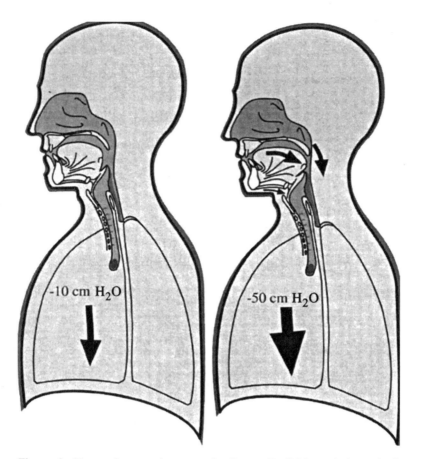

Figure 4 Upper airway resistance and collapse. (*Left*) Normal airway in the presence of normal thoracic pressure. (*Right*) Partial collapse of the upper airway, which produces increased upper airway resistance and results in increasingly negative intrathoracic pressure. *Source*: From Ref. 19.

but upon the insistence of a concerned family member or upon the strong recommendation from their primary care physician. Ideally, it is, thereby, advisable to have the bed partner, or other concerned family members, present along with the patient during the initial evaluation and examination performed by a physician well versed in the subtleties and intricacies of sleep disorders.

Insomnia, sleep fragmentation, and fatigue have all been described as facets associated with UARS (20,21). Gender distribution appears to be equal, unlike OSAS, where men predominate. Patients are usually not obese (mean BMI <25 kg/m^2). Patients with UARS are younger (mean age of 37 years) than their OSAS counterparts (9,15). Snoring is usually present but may be absent. Lastly, it is interesting to note that some patients whose snoring has resolved after undergoing palatal surgery continue to have clinically relevant markers for UARS (22). This observation again underscores the multifactorial nature of sleep-disordered breathing and the expression of its pathology.

Anatomical differences are also beginning to be characterized in groups of patients with UARS. Associated physical features include a high and narrow hard palate, a small intermolar distance, a thin soft palatal mucosa with short uvula, a low soft palate, a long uvula, and the presence of an increased overbite (1). Asian patients may have an increased association with UARS (23). Interestingly, a history of early extraction of wisdom teeth, high anxiety scores, postural hypotension, and a history of fainting have also been associated with this syndrome (1,24).

Interestingly, the respiratory patterns noted in patients with UARS typically are terminated after only attaining a relatively low respiratory effort (P_{es} approx. -6 cm H_2O), whereas OSAS-related arousals typically occur at inspiratory pressures much more negative than normal (P_{es} range -40 to -80 cm H_2O). This suggests that the arousal threshold in UARS is lower than in OSAS (1,25,26). It is possible that patients with UARS have intact, but hypersensitive, upper airway mechanoreceptors, whereas those with OSAS have a blunted mechanoreceptor response (1). This blunted response may result in apneic events of prolonged duration and may consequently contribute to a greater potential for oxygen desaturation, a distinguishing feature of OSAS versus UARS. To further evaluate this premise, one study revealed that sensory examination of the upper airway using a two-point palatal discrimination technique was normal in UARS but impaired in OSAS (27).

SEQUELAE OF UARS

Excessive daytime sleepiness is an essential feature of UARS. The presence of aberrant respiratory patterns alone, noted on a PSG, are not sufficient. Sleepiness may be severe but may be mild as well, suggesting a wide range of symptoms (13,28). Although untreated OSAS does increase the risk of motor vehicle accidents, this has not been established in UARS. However, should a history be elicited that involves the compromise of safety of the patient and/or the general public as a result of the intrusion of sleepiness while operating a motor vehicle or mechanized equipment, UARS patients should be treated with the same precautions as those with OSAS. As primary insomnia is associated with fatigue and not outright excessive daytime sleepiness, sleep-disordered breathing, whether it is UARS or OSAS, should remain in the differential diagnosis of any patient who presents the combination of snoring, insomnia, and daytime sleepiness. One study evaluating a large number of postmenopausal women who presented to a sleep center with the chief complaint of insomnia, not socially disruptive snoring, revealed a surprisingly high prevalence (75%) for SDB (29). This study found an OSA and UARS prevalence of 75% and 8%, respectively.

Sleepiness, regardless of etiology, is often associated with cognitive decline as well as emotional lability. This decline may be disregarded or misdiagnosed in the elderly and may require a PSG that includes a sensitive airflow monitoring device, such as esophageal manometry. The degree of impairment in neuropsychological functioning after formal cognitive studies in patients with SDB appears to be dose related or, simply stated, the higher the RDI, the worse the cognitive impairment (30). However, the clinical significance of these findings when applied to the general population is unclear. It is conceivable that future research in UARS may reveal a subset of patients with cognitive impairment that may benefit from the treatment of UARS.

Elevated nocturnal sympathetic and autonomic responses are thought to be responsible for the significant increases in diurnal blood pressure that have been described in patients with UARS (31,32). Increases in blood pressure are associated with RERAs, while both a pulsus paradoxus and leftward shift of the interventricular septum occurred in conjunction with the most severe decreases in P_{es} (33). It appears that UARS contributes to the development of hypertension in many patients (34).

NONINVASIVE CLINICAL MANAGEMENT

Continuous positive airway pressure (CPAP), typically through a nasal mask interface, is effective treatment for UARS. CPAP is traditionally administered via a fixed pressure setting, expressed in units of cm H_2O, with the patient facing the same positive pressure during both the inspiratory and expiratory limbs of the respiratory cycle. CPAP benefits patients with sleep-disordered breathing by acting as a "pneumatic splint," thereby indiscriminately maintaining the patency of the upper airway. Though it may improve functional residual capacity, CPAP is not considered a true ventilatory mode as it does not support minute ventilation (VE) nor augment tidal volume (V_T). Bi-level positive airway pressure, where the pressure of the inspiratory limb is greater than the expiratory limb by at least a factor of 5 cm H_2O, is a mechanical ventilatory mode, but it is not physiologically indicated in the management of UARS.

CPAP has resulted in fewer cortical arousals, improved multiple sleep latency test scores (an objective measurement of daytime sleepiness), and improved hypertension (9,33,35). However, CPAP compliance in UARS, especially in patients with mild symptoms, is poor (19%). Interestingly, sleepiness improved with CPAP even with only modest nightly use (<3 hr/day) (28). According to the consensus report addressing the appropriate treatment of sleep-disordered breathing as put forth by the American Academy of Sleep Medicine (AASM), the initiation of treatment using nasal intermittent positive pressure ventilation (NIPPV), i.e., CPAP for UARS, should be done as a formal in-lab nocturnal PSG with properly trained technical support well versed in airflow monitoring and NIPPV titration.

UARS should be considered after excluding other causes of daytime sleepiness. Volitional sleep deprivation is common but often overlooked.

The recent variations along the CPAP theme have become legion. All are intended to improve the duration of night-time use of the device for patients having difficulty in tolerating positive pressure ventilation. The use of an autotitrating CPAP device to treat UARS is unclear. Given the subtle or even lack of changes in airflow during RERAs, an autotitrating CPAP device may not be sensitive enough in monitoring airflow restriction to identify clinically significant respiratory events. Despite this, autotitrate CPAP most likely will have a role in treating UARS, but further investigation into its indications and limitations is needed.

Weight loss has the advantage of avoiding surgery and medical devices but is difficult to accomplish. Further, dieting programs and pharmaceutical interventions are not without risk, and their use in UARS has not been studied to any appreciable degree. Lastly, though the state- and positional-dependent nature of OSAS has long been acknowledged; this nature remains uncultivated in terms of further characterization of UARS.

Oral appliances, such as a mandibular advancement device, that are formally fitted by a dental professional have been used to effectively treat mild to moderate OSAS. Regrettably, there are little data available involving their use in UARS. Though these devices are contraindicated in those with temporal mandibular joint disease, they otherwise carry little morbidity and offer an alternative to CPAP.

DIFFICULTIES IN ASSESSING SURGICAL OUTCOMES IN UARS

Surgical intervention for sleep-disordered breathing includes uvulopalatopharyngoplasty, nasal surgery, tongue surgery, and upper airway surgery, including bimaxillary advancement surgery as well as tracheostomy. Tracheostomy is unequivocally successful for OSAS and is typically recommended to the most compromised and debilitated of patients. In the case of primary (or "simple") snoring, the benefits of palatal surgery or UARS remain ambiguous.

Recent articles have suggested that mild apnea symptoms can be relieved by modest upper airway surgery.

Much of the surgical literature addresses the treatment of OSAS. Very little, if any, addresses pure UARS. Given the controversy over the diagnosis and management, and perhaps even the existence, of UARS, one should not extrapolate the results of surgery for OSAS to this patient population. We will have to wait until more objective data are available.

REFERENCES

1. Guilleminault C, Chowdhuri S. Upper airway syndrome is a distinct syndrome. Am J Respir Crit Care Med 2000; 161(5):1412.
2. Clinical Practice Review Committee. Position paper—hypopnea in sleep-disordered breathing in adults. Sleep 2001; 24(4):469–470.
3. Cracowski C, Pepin J, Wuyam B, Levy P. Characterization of obstructive nonapneic respiratory events in moderate sleep apnea syndrome. Am J Respir Crit Care Med 2001; 164(6):944–948.
4. Badr MS. Pathogenesis of obstructive sleep apnea. Prog Cardiovasc Dis 1999; 41:323–330.
5. Wheatley JR, Mezzanotte WS, Tangel DJ. Influence of sleep on genioglossus muscle activation by negative pressure in normal men. Am Rev Respir Dis 1993; 148:597–605.
6. Wheatley JR, Tangel DJ, Mezzanotte WS. Influence of sleep on response to negative airway pressure of tensor palatini muscle and retropalatal airway. J Appl Physiol 1993; 75:2117–2124.
7. Surratt PM, McTier RF, Wilhoit SC. Collapsibility of the nasopharyngeal airway in obstructive sleep apnea. Am Rev Respir Dis 1985; 132:967–971.
8. Sher AE. An overview of sleep disordered breathing for the otolaryngologist. Ear Nose Throat J 1999; 78:694–707.
9. Guilleminault C, Stoohs R, Clerk A, et al. A cause of daytime sleepiness: the upper airway resistance syndrome. Chest 1993; 104:781–787.
10. Loube DI, Andrada TF. Comparison of respiratory polysomnographic parameters in matched cohorts of upper airway resistance and obstructive sleep apnea syndrome patients. Chest 1999; 115(6):1519–1524.
11. Guilleminault C, Stoohs R, Clerk A, et al. From obstructive sleep apnea syndrome to upper airway resistance syndrome: consistency of daytime sleepiness. Sleep 1992; 15(suppl 6):S13–S16.
12. Rees et al. Am J Respir Crit Care Med 162(4):1210–1214.
13. Anders Thomas Frederick, Emde Robert N, Parmeles Arthur H. A manual of standardized terminology, techniques and criteria for scoring at states of sleep and wakefulness in newborn infants. Los Angels: UCLA Brain Information service/BRI publication, 1971.
14. Berg S, Nash S, Cole P, et al. Arousals and nocturnal respiration in symptomatic snorers and nonsnorers. Sleep 1997; 20:1157–1161.
15. Exar EN, Collop NA. The upper airway resistance syndrome. Chest 1999; 115:1127–1139.
16. Berry RB, McNellis MI, Kouchi D, et al. Upper airway anesthesia reduces phasic geioglossus activity during sleep apnea. Am J Respir Crit Care Med 1997; 156:127–132.
17. Hosselet JJ, Norman RG, Ayppa I, et al. Detection of flow limitation with a nasal cannula/pressure transducer system. Am J Respir Crit Care Med 1998; 157:1461–1467.
18. Norman RG, Ahmed MM, Walsleben JA, et al. Detection of respiratory events during npsg: nasal cannula/pressure sensor versus thermistor. Sleep 1997; 20:1175–1184.

19. Newman. Laryngoscope 1996; 106(9):1089–1093.
20. Guilleminault C, Stoohs R, Kim YD, Chervin R, Black J, Clerk A. Upper airway sleep disordered breathing in women. Arch Intern Med 1995; 122:493–501.
21. Guilleminault C, Black JE, Palombini L, Ohayon M. A clinical investigation of obstructive sleep apnea syndrome and upper airway resistance syndrome patients. Sleep Med 2000; 1:1–6.
22. Woodson BT. Upper airway resistance syndrome after uvulopalatopharyngoplasty for obstructive sleep apnea syndrome. Otolaryngol Head Neck Surg 1996; 114:457–461.
23. Ip M, Lam B, Lauder I, et al. A community study of sleep-disordered breathing in middle-aged Chinese men in Hong Kong. Chest 2001; 119:62–69.
24. Kushida CA, Efron B, Guilleminault C. A predictive morphometric model for the obstructive sleep apnea syndrome. Ann Intern Med 1997; 127:581–587.
25. Berry RB, Gleeson K. Respiratory arousal from sleep mechanisms and significance. Sleep 1997; 20:654–675.
26. Kimoff RJ, Cheong TH, Opha AE, et al. Mechanisms of apnea termination in obstructive sleep apnea: role of chemoreceptor and mechanoreceptor stimuli. Am J Respir Crit Care Med 1994; 149:707–714.
27. Guilleminault C, Li K, Chen N, Poyares D. Two-point palatal discrimination in patients with upper airway resistance syndrome, obstructive sleep apnea syndrome, and normal control subjects. Chest 2002; 122:866–870.
28. Rauscher H, Formanek D, Zwick H. Nasal continuous positive airway pressure for non-apneic snoring? Chest 1995; 107:58–61.
29. Guilleminault C, Palombini L, Poyares D, Chowduri S. Chronic insomnia, post-menopausal women, and sleep disordered breathing: Part 1. Frequency of sleep disordered breathing in a cohort. J. Psychosom Res 2002; 53(1):611–615.
30. Adams N, Miltion S, Schluchter M, Redline S. Relation of measures of sleep-disordered breathing to neuropsychological functioning. Am J Respir Crit Care Med 2001; 163:1626–1631.
31. Lofaso F, Coste A, Guilain L, et al. Sleep fragmentation as a risk factor for hypertension in middle-aged nonapneic snorers. Chest 1996; 109:896–900.
32. Lofaso F, Goldenberg F, d'Ortho MP, et al. Arterial blood pressure response to transient arousals from NREM sleep in nonapneic snorers with sleep fragmentation. Chest 1998; 113:985–991.
33. Guilleminault C, Stoohs R, Shiomi T, et al. Upper airway resistance syndrome, nocturnal blood pressure monitoring, and borderline hypertension. Chest 1996; 109:901–908.
34. Silverberg DS, Oksenberg A. Essential hypertension and abnormal upper airway resistance during sleep. Sleep 1997; 20:794–806.
35. Guilleminault C, Stoohs R, Duncan S, Snoring. Daytime sleepiness in regular heavy snorers. Chest 1991; 99:40–48.

41

Surgical Treatment of Sleep-Disordered Breathing

Kenny P. Pang
Department of Otolaryngology, Tan Tock Seng Hospital, Tan Tock Seng, Singapore, and Department of Otolaryngology—Head and Neck Surgery, Medical College of Georgia, Augusta, Georgia, U.S.A.

Amy R. Blanchard
Section of Pulmonary/Critical Care Medicine, Medical College of Georgia, Augusta, Georgia, U.S.A.

David J. Terris
Department of Otolaryngology—Head and Neck Surgery, Medical College of Georgia, Augusta, Georgia, U.S.A.

INTRODUCTION

Sleep-disordered breathing (SDB) is a spectrum of disorders that range from benign snoring to obstructive apnea with cor pulmonale. Patients with SDB can be managed either medically or surgically. Most clinicians begin with lifestyle modifications and behavioral therapy, which can be especially useful in geriatric patients, as many of these patients may not be good surgical candidates. Patients with SDB who are obese are advised to lose weight, pursue an exercise program and a strict diet regime, and are referred to a nutritionist. They are also advised to stop smoking and to avoid sedatives and alcohol. In patients who have increased events in the supine position, positional therapy may be useful. Martin (1) proposed the following regimen of sleep hygiene for older adults:

1. Limit naps to one nap of <30 minutes per day;
2. Take a walk outdoors to increase both exercise and light exposure, particularly in the afternoon;
3. Check the effect of medications on sleep;
4. Avoid caffeine, alcohol, and tobacco, especially after lunch;
5. Limit liquids in the evenings;
6. Keep a regular sleep schedule.

Many geriatric patients with SDB may manifest complications of the disease. These include ischemic heart disease, hypertension, strokes, and cardiac arrhythmias.

The presence of these comorbidities may limit the appropriateness of surgical intervention. Nasal continuous positive airway pressure (CPAP) has a major role in the treatment of SDB. Pressurized air is delivered according to the patient's degree of upper airway obstruction and acts as a pneumatic splint to keep the upper airway patent.

NASAL CPAP

Appropriate CPAP levels can be determined in two ways. The gold standard is attended overnight polysomnography with CPAP titration. During an attended polysomnographic titration, the CPAP pressure is started first at 3–5 cm H_2O, then titrated upward by increments of 1–2 cm H_2O every 15 to 30 minutes until all apneas, hypopneas, snoring, and oxygen desaturations are eliminated. A less-costly alternative is autotitrating CPAP with pulse oximetry. The auto-PAP adjusts and delivers variable levels of CPAP at the initiation of each respiratory cycle by automatically responding to changes that are detected in the airflow resistance, pressure, or intensity of snoring (2). With the availability of the airway pressure data from the auto-PAP, the clinician can obtain the patient's mean pressure, effective 95th percentile required pressure, and the mean treatment AHI. Based on the effective 95th percentile pressure, the clinician may also prescribe a constant CPAP pressure.

The main drawback to the use of nasal CPAP is compliance. With compliance being defined as usage for at least four hours per night, on 70% of the nights, most clinical series quote compliance rates at about 46% to 70% (3). Stradling and Davies (4) found that patients who use nasal CPAP more than five hours per night are more likely to normalize their sleepiness scores than those who use it less.

Common reasons for poor compliance with nasal CPAP include:

1. Nasal problems—nasal stuffiness, irritation, discharge, pain;
2. Mask problems—poor fit, air leak, dry eyes, skin breakdown;
3. Equipment problems—noisy, cumbersome, high air pressure, pressure-related arousals;
4. Concept problems—failure to understand medical benefit.

Aloia et al. (5) found that in geriatric patients, cognitive-behavioral intervention, in the form of support group counseling and supportive phone calls, improved compliance with nasal CPAP. Regular physician follow-up is necessary to document clinical improvement or the need for alternative therapy.

ORAL APPLIANCES

Oral appliances are designed to bring the mandible and the base of tongue forward, either by stabilizing the mandibular position during sleep or by attempting to increase the baseline genioglossus muscle activity, in an effort to increase the posterior airway space (PAS) (6,7). Oral appliances are especially useful in the geriatric age group when the patient is not a candidate for surgical intervention or is unable to tolerate nasal CPAP.

Oral devices can be divided into three basic types:

1. Mandibular repositioning device—these are removable devices worn only at night. They are affixed to the upper and lower teeth and are gradually adjusted to advance the mandible by 5–8 mm.

2. Tongue-retaining device these come in the form of a soft suction cup that is placed in the mouth, creating a negative pressure to hold the tongue in a forward position during sleep.
3. Soft palate lift—this appliance is fitted onto the upper teeth and extends posteriorly to lift up the soft palate.

The American Sleep Disorders Association supports the use of oral appliances as acceptable alternatives to nasal CPAP for patients with primary snoring and mild obstructive sleep apnea (OSA) (8).

SURGICAL TREATMENT

The American Academy of Otolaryngology Head and Neck Surgery, Sleep Disorders Committee 1997 position statement affirmed that surgery for OSA is not "experimental nor investigational, and is considered as part of a comprehensive approach in the medical and surgical management of adults with OSA." These surgical interventions are meant to address either excessive soft tissue obstruction or inadequate facial skeletal framework, and include tracheotomy, nasal airway surgery, uvulopalatoplasty, genioglossus advancement, tongue suspension, hyoid repositioning, midline glossectomy, lingualplasty, and maxillary and mandibular advancement. Patients who cannot tolerate or refuse nasal CPAP should be offered a surgical alternative.

Laser-Assisted Uvulopalatoplasty

The laser-assisted uvulopalatoplasty technique was introduced by Yves-Victor Kamami in 1986 (Fig. 1). A number of other surgeons have popularized and modified the procedure. Kamami's (9) original description of the technique included bilateral vertical transpalatal incisions and partial vaporization of the uvula with the CO_2 laser. Kamami (9) studied 417 snorers who underwent laser-assisted uvulopalatoplasty and found an improvement in 95% of the patients, with 1-year follow-up. Most authors report modest results for patients with mild OSA, although a success rate as high as 75% was reported by Walker et al. (10).

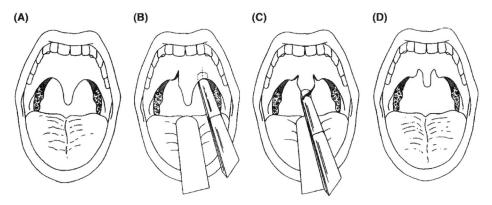

(A) **(B)** **(C)** **(D)**

Figure 1 The laser-assisted uvulopalatoplasty was introduced as a technique for shortening and tightening the uvula and palate in an office setting using a carbon dioxide laser.

Uvulopalatopharyngoplasty

Ikematsu (11) developed uvulopalatopharyngoplasty (UPPP) to treat habitual snorers in the 1950s. Ikematsu (11) achieved this by shortening the soft palate and uvula and removing redundant tissue to tighten the pharynx. The author reported an 80% improvement in a series of over 4000 snorers. Fujita (1979) adapted the UPPP technique for the treatment of patients with OSA. The basic technique involves a palatopharyngeal incision, from the base of tongue bilaterally, across the soft palate horizontally, with removal of the uvula. Redundant soft palatal tissues are resected. The tonsils are removed if present, and the anterior and posterior mucosal edges are apposed with absorbable sutures. Many variations to the original UPPP technique have been described, but the results are similar.

Sher et al. (12) performed a meta-analysis of 37 papers, which included a total of 992 patients who had undergone UPPP for OSA. They found that UPPP was more effective (83% success rate) if used for: (i) OSA patients with Fujita type I retropalatal obstruction and (ii) patients with mild or moderate OSA. The overall response rate in unselected patients, though, was 40.7%. Friedman et al. (13) described a clinical staging for SDB in order to predict the success rate of UPPP (Fig. 2). They described three stages based on Friedman palate position, tonsil size, and BMI:

> *Stage I*: Friedman palate position 1 and 2. Tonsil size 3 and 4. BMI <40.
> *Stage II*: Friedman palate oosition 1, 2, 3, and 4. Tonsil size 1, 2, 3, and 4. BMI <40.
> *Stage III*: Friedman palate position 3 and 4. Tonsil size 1 and 2. BMI (any).

Friedman reported an overall success rate of 80.6% for stage I, 37.9% for stage II, and 8.1% for stage III. Generally, UPPP should be done for patients with retropalatal obstruction, and it can be combined with procedures that address other sites of obstruction.

Genioglossus Advancement and Tongue Suspension

The genioglossus advancement (GA) was conceived as a procedure to address obstruction at the level of the base of tongue (Fig. 3). Other surgical procedures that increase the retrolingual airway space include laser midline glossectomy, lingualplasty, tongue base coblation, hyoid repositioning, tongue suspension (repose), and maxillomandibular advancement (MMA). In Powell and Riley's 306 OSA patients who underwent surgery, 239 patients had GA with or without UPPP. They achieved a success rate of 64% across all severities of OSA. They reported even better success with mild (77%) and moderate (78%) OSA (14). Riley et al. (15) also reported a success rate of 86% for OSA patients who underwent GA and UPPP.

Tongue suspension (repose) was introduced by Woodson et al. (14,16) in 2000 for OSA patients with base of tongue obstruction. The mechanism of action is similar to that for GA in that support for the base of tongue is provided to prevent prolapse during sleep. They reported some benefit for patients with OSA, with low morbidity. This experience was confirmed by Terris et al. (17), and a prospective randomized trial comparing tongue suspension with GA in patients who also underwent UPPP revealed comparable results (18).

Hyoid Repositioning Surgery

Due to the attachment of the muscles of the tongue, muscles of the floor of the mouth, and pharyngeal muscles to the hyoid bone, repositioning the hyoid bone helps increase

(A)   **(B)**

(C)   **(D)**

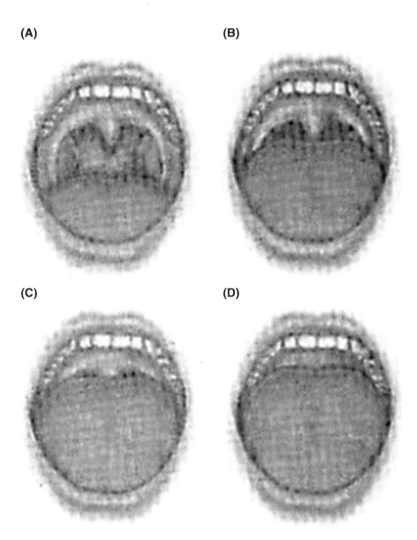

Figure 2 The Friedman classification, which is drawn from the Mallampati classification, is a general way of describing the upper airway configuration.

the PAS and hypopharyngeal area. The hyoid bone may be repositioned either antero-superiorly to the mandible or anteroinferiorly to the thyroid cartilage. Riley et al. (15,19) have found this procedure useful in a select group of patients with BMI less than 30 and mild to moderate OSA, and also in combination with other procedures such as GA.

Tongue Reduction Surgery

Reduction of the base of tongue is an intuitive approach to diminishing obstruction at that level, and there are a number of ways to accomplish this. Fujita (20) reported a series of 22 patients with OSA undergoing laser midline glossectomy and lingual-plasty, in which they achieved an overall success rate of 77%. Chabolle et al. (21) in 1999 described a combination of tongue base reduction and hyoepiglottoplasty in 10 patients with severe OSA. They reported a success rate of 80%, but temporary tracheotomies were required for all of their patients.

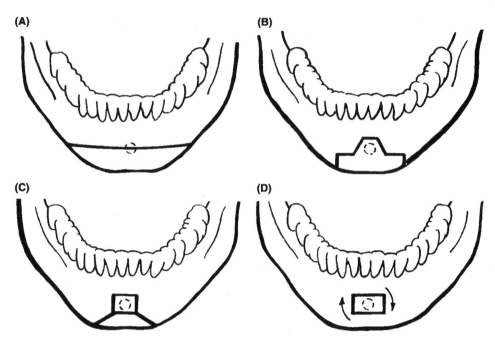

Figure 3 The genioglossus advancement is a procedure designed to enlarge the posterior airway space; a number of techniques have been described to achieve this surgical objective, with the rectangular geniotubricle osteotomy the most widely adopted.

Transpalatal Advancement Pharyngoplasty

Woodson and Toohill (22) reported transpalatal advancement pharyngoplasty in a series of 11 patients with severe OSA who failed UPPP. They underwent advancement of the soft palate to increase the retropalatal space. Woodson and Toohill (22) achieved a success rate of 67% in patients with severe OSA, a BMI >35, predominantly retropalatal obstruction, and failed UPPP. This is a promising technique, but has so far failed to gain widespread acceptance.

Maxillomandibular Advancement

Patients with cephalometrically proven severe mandibular deficiency will benefit from advancement of the maxilla and mandible (Fig. 4). In Riley and Powell's (15) group of 91 OSA patients who underwent MMA after a failed GA ± UPPP, a 97% success rate was achieved. They reported an 81% success rate with MMA even in patients with morbid obesity (BMI >45) (82). They also found that patients with severe mandibular deficiency (SNB <72°) consistently faired poorly with UPPP ± GA and required MMA at a later stage. Therefore, the authors suggested considering MMA as the first surgical option in patients with severe mandibular deficiency. Maxillomandibular advancement may also be combined with other procedures, like GA, to maximize the increase in PAS.

In an analysis of surgical outcomes, Conradt et al. (23) found that MMA compared favorably with nasal CPAP in reducing the severity of OSA in a high percentage of patients selected by cephalometric and polysomnographic studies.

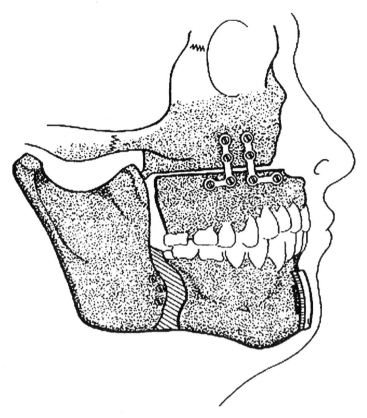

Figure 4 The maxillomandibular advancement involves a sagittal split mandibular osteotomy and a Lefort I maxillary osteotomy to achieve bimaxillary advancement. This approach may be combined with other procedures, including a genioglossus advancement and hyoid myotomy.

Radiofrequency Ablation Technique

Powell et al. (24) first described the use of radiofrequency ablation technique (RFA) in the upper airway. They introduced it as a way of tightening the soft palate to treat primary snoring. It is the use of temperature-controlled radiofrequency volumetric tissue reduction in order to stiffen and scar the soft palate (Fig. 5). The advantages of RFA are that it is minimally invasive, causes little pain, and can be done under local anesthesia as an office procedure. The radiofrequency probe can also be applied to the inferior turbinates for relief of nasal obstruction and to the base of tongue for treatment of OSA.

Subjective results for RFA of the palate based on improvement in snoring have been encouraging, with reports ranging from 67% to 86.6% improvement (25,26). Stuck et al. (27) have the largest series, with 322 snoring patients, and an 84% improvement rate. Caution should be exercised in RFA of the soft palate for mild OSA, as the results are unpredictable and so far disappointing.

Tracheostomy

The most definitive treatment for OSA is a tracheostomy, which completely bypasses any existing upper airway obstruction (28). However, this is not an attractive option

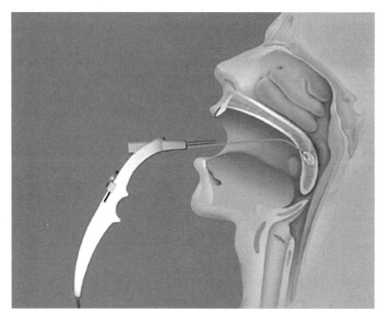

Figure 5 Radiofrequency ablation involves the delivery of radiofrequency energy in a submucosal fashion to the tissues of the palate. This is performed under local anesthesia in the office.

for most patients as it retains a social stigma and obviates the possibility of participating in water sports.

Powell and Riley suggested that patients with OSA be offered surgery based on the level of obstruction as proposed by Fujita:

Type I (*retropalatal*): palatal procedure (e.g., UPPP).
Type II (*both retropalatal and retrolingual*): palatal procedure and a procedure designed to address base of tongue obstruction (e.g., genioglossus advancement, hyoid repositioning procedure, or tongue suspension).
Type III (*retrolingual*): a base of tongue procedure alone.

Patients failing initial reconstructive surgery may be eligible for more aggressive techniques, such as maxillomandibular advancement.

CONCLUSIONS

The geriatric population is prone to sleep disorders. Altered sleeping habits and difficulty in initiating and maintaining sleep, coupled with increased tendency for SDB, predispose geriatric patients to depression. Management of these elderly individuals should therefore be comprehensive, focusing not only on the sleep disorder but also on the psychosocial aspects of the patient's health. Treatment should be customized. Surgical therapy will be appropriate for some patients, but nasal CPAP remains an important first line of treatment in most patients.

REFERENCES

1. Martin J. Assessment and treatment of sleep disturbance in older adults. Clin Psychol Rev 2000; 20(6):783–805.

2. Loube DL. Technologic advances in the treatment of OSAS. Chest 1999; 116:1426–1433.

3. Kribbs NB, Pack AJ, Kline LB, et al. Objective measurement of patterns of nasal CPAP, used by patient with OSA. Am Rev Respir Dis 1993; 147:887–895.

4. Stradling JR, Davies RJO. Is more NCPAP better? [abstr]. Sleep 2000; 23(suppl 4): S150–S153.

5. Aloia MS, Di Diol L, Luiczby IN, Perlis ML, Greenblatt DW, Giles DE. Improving compliance of Nasal CPAP & vigilance in older adults with OSAS. Sleep Breath 2001; 5(1):13–21.

6. Strauss AM. Oral devices for the management of snoring & OSA. In: Fairbanks DNF, Fujita S. eds. Snoring & OSA. 2nd ed. New York: Raven Press, 1994; 229–241.

7. Lowe AA. The tongue & Airway. Otolaryngol Clin North Am 1990; 23:677–698.

8. American Sleep Disorders Association Standards of Practice Committee (Thorpy M. Chair). Practice parameters for the treatment of snoring & OSA with oral appliance. Sleep 1995; 18:511–513.

9. Kamami. Outpatient treatment of sleep apnea syndrome with CO 2 laser, LAUP: laser-assisted UPPP results on 46 patients. J Clin Laser Med Surg 1994; 12(4):215–219.

10. Walker RP, Grigg-Damberger MM, Gopalsami C. Laser-assisted uvulopalatoplasty for the treatment of mild, moderate, and severe obstructive sleep apnea. Laryngoscope 1999; 109(1):79–85.

11. Ikematsu T. A 30-year clinical study in snoring. In: Fairbanks DNL, Fujita S, Ikematsu T, Simmons FB, eds. Snoring & Sleep Apnea. 1st ed. New York: Raven Press, 1987; 130–134.

12. Sher AE, Schechtman KB, Piccirillo JF. The efficiency of surgical modification of the upper airway in adults with OSAS. Sleep 1996; 19(3):156–177.

13. Friedman M, Ibrahim H, Bass L. Clinical staging for sleep-disordered breathing. Otolaryngol Head Neck Surg 2002; 127:13–21.

14. Woodson BT, De Rowe AR, Hawke M, et al. Pharyngeal suspension suture with Repose Bone Screw for OSA. Otolaryngol Head Neck Surg 2001; 122:395–404.

15. Riley RW, Powell NB, Guilleminault C. Obstructive sleep apnea syndrome: a review of 306 conservatively treated surgical patients. Otolaryngol Head Neck Surg 1993; 108:117–125.

16. Woodson BT. A tongue suspension suture for OSA & snorers. Otolaryngol Head Neck Surg 2001; 124:297–303.

17. Terris DJ, Kunda LD, Gonella MC. Minimally invasive tongue base surgery for obstructive sleep apnoea. J Laryngol Otol 2002; 116(9):716–721.

18. Thomas AJ, Chavoya M, Terris DJ. Prospective, randomized trial of tongue base surgery for sleep apnea. Otolaryngol Head Neck Surg 2003; 129(5):539–546.

19. Riley RW, Powell NB, Guilleminault C. OSA & the hyoid: a revised surgical procedure. Otolaryngol Head Neck Surg 1994; 111:717–721.

20. Fujita S. Midline laser glossectomy with lingualplasty: a treatment of OSA. Op Otolaryngol 1991; 2:127–131.

21. Chabolle F, Wagner I, Blumen M, Sequert C, Fhenvy B, De Dienlereult. Tongue base reduction with hyoepiglottoplasty: a treatment for severe OSA. Laryngoscope 1999; 109:1273–1280.

22. Woodson BT, Toohill RJ. Transpalatal Advancement Pharyngoplasty for OSA. Laryngoscope 1993; 103:269–276.

23. Conradt R, Hochban W, Brandenburg V, Heitmann J, Peter JH. Sleep fragmentation & daytime vigilance in patients with OSA treated by surgical maxillomandibular advancement compared to CPAP therapy. J Sleep Res 1998; 7:217–223.

24. Powell NB, Riley RW, Troell RJ, Li KK, Blumen MB, Guilliminault C. Radiofrequency volumetric tissue reduction of the palate in subjects with sleep-disordered breathing. Chest 1998; 113(5):1163–1174.

25. Said B, Strome M. Long-term results of radiofrequency volumetric tissue reduction of the palate for snoring. Ann Otol Rhinol Laryngol 2003; 112(3):276–279.

26. Blumen MB, Dahan S, Wagner I, De Dieuleveult T, Chabolle F. Radiofrequency versus LAUP for the treatment of snoring. Otolaryngol Head Neck Surg 2002; 126(1):67–73.

27. Stuck BA, Starzak K, Verse T, Hormann K, Maurer JT. Complications of temperature-controlled radiofrequency volumetric tissue reduction for sleep-disordered breathing. Acta Otolaryngol 2003; 123(4):532–535.
28. Fee WE Jr, Ward PH. Permanent tracheostomy: a new surgical technique. Ann Otol Rhinol Laryngol 1977; 86(5 Pt 1):635–638.

42

Obstructive Sleep Apnea Epidemiology and Patient-Centered Measures

Eric J. Kezirian
*Department of Otolaryngology—Head and Neck Surgery, University of
California–San Francisco, San Francisco, California, U.S.A.*

Edward M. Weaver
*Department of Otolaryngology—Head and Neck Surgery, University of Washington,
Seattle, Washington, U.S.A.*

INTRODUCTION

Obstructive sleep apnea syndrome ("sleep apnea") is a syndrome of *symptomatic*
recurrent upper airway obstructions during sleep. Increasing awareness about sleep
apnea in the medical community and in the general public has led to increasing study
about this disorder. Sleep apnea results in increased mortality, cardiovascular
disease, quality of life deficits, and performance decrements (1–3). This chapter
addresses the epidemiology of sleep apnea in the elderly, contrasts sleep apnea
between geriatric and middle-aged patients, and discusses patient-centered evaluations of sleep apnea.

DEFINITIONS OF OBSTRUCTIVE SLEEP APNEA SYNDROME

Obstructive sleep apnea syndrome is defined in the International Classification of
Sleep Disorders Diagnostic and Coding Manual as including abnormal physiologic
findings of sleep arousals related to obstructive breathing during sleep as well as
a complaint of excessive sleepiness or insomnia (4). An American Academy of
Sleep Medicine task force recommended the definition be an apnea–hypopnea
index >5 *and* symptoms, where symptoms include either excessive daytime sleepiness not explained otherwise or two of the following symptoms: choking or gasping during sleep, recurrent awakenings from sleep, unrefreshing sleep, daytime
fatigue, or impaired concentration (5). It is important to note that both definitions
include symptoms.

Sleep-disordered breathing refers to the physiologic abnormality of sleep apnea
(e.g., an apnea–hypopnea index >5) measured on a sleep test. The threshold of a
normal versus abnormal apnea–hypopnea index of 5 is arbitrary. An apnea–hypopnea

459

index between 1 and 5 is still associated with medical consequences of sleep apnea (6). In practice, different sleep laboratories use different thresholds to define sleep-disordered breathing and sleep apnea. Furthermore, sleep testing equipment is increasingly sensitive to detect apneas and hypopneas that previously went undetected. Thus, there is significant variation in the literature on sleep apnea prevalence or disease severity.

PREVALENCE OF OBSTRUCTIVE SLEEP APNEA SYNDROME IN GERIATRICS

Several studies have considered the prevalence of sleep apnea through population-based sampling and evaluation. A review of the sleep apnea epidemiology literature discussed many of the methodological challenges inherent to these observational studies (1). For example, most studies rely entirely on laboratory diagnostic criteria (i.e., apnea–hypopnea index) and ignore the symptoms and effects on quality of life. We identified three studies, which utilized laboratory polysomnography (defined as an apnea–hypopnea index $\geq$15) without symptoms; the estimated prevalence of sleep-disordered breathing was 7% to 14% in men and 2% to 7% in women (7–10). These studies primarily included middle-aged adults.

Other studies have focused specifically on the elderly. Ancoli-Israel et al. (11) studied 427 individuals aged 65–95 with a validated in-home study system. Using a definition of sleep-disordered breathing as an apnea–hypopnea index greater than or equal to 20, the prevalence of sleep-disordered breathing was 51% in men and 39% in women. These figures are much higher than estimates for middle-aged adults; it is unclear whether different sampling methods, sleep study techniques, or sleep-disordered breathing definitions may account for some of the difference.

Four cohort studies sampled wide age ranges, allowing side-by-side comparisons of prevalence in broad categories of geriatric and middle-aged adults. Using a home sleep study, Bixler et al. (8,9) found that the prevalence of sleep apnea increased with advancing age through middle age (30–65 years of age) for men and women but showed no significant increases with age for those 65–100 years of age. In contrast, Duran et al. (10) found a higher prevalence of sleep apnea among those aged 70–100 years compared to 30–70 years (49% vs. 7% in women and 57% vs. 14% in men) using a definition of sleep apnea as an apnea–hypopnea index $\geq$15. Tishler et al. (12) identified age as a major sleep apnea risk factor. Similarly, in the Sleep Heart Health Study, the share of people with an apnea–hypopnea index $\geq$15 for age greater than 60 years was 1.7 times higher than that for ages 40–60 years (13).

Overall, the prevalence of sleep apnea appears to be higher in older compared to middle-aged adults. This finding raises the question whether the aging process itself results in the development of sleep apnea. If this were true, one would expect the age-specific prevalence of sleep apnea to increase through adulthood. However, closer examination of the studies reveals that most of the increases in sleep apnea prevalence occur up to 65 years of age and that the prevalence is stable at increasing age after that threshold point (8,9,11,13).

Some alternative potential explanations have been offered for the stable age-specific prevalence at ages above 65 years (1). First is that advancing age is not associated with the development of sleep apnea, at least not for the elderly. If the incidence of new cases of sleep apnea is negligible for this group, the prevalence would remain stable. In fact, the largest study that followed older adults showed that in 18-year follow-up, there was little change in the apnea–hypopnea index associated with aging after adjusting for body mass index (13). However, this single study has not addressed the issue of sleep apnea incidence at advanced age definitively, and several smaller studies provide conflicting evidence on the subject (11,14–16).

A second possible explanation for the stable prevalence is that if the mortality rate associated with sleep apnea increases with age, the overall proportion of people alive in a particular age group with sleep apnea will also remain stable or decrease even in the face of a high incidence of new sleep apnea cases. However, there is no evidence available to support or deny this notion.

IS SLEEP APNEA DIFFERENT IN THE ELDERLY?

A third hypothesis to explain the stable age-specific prevalence in older adults is that sleep apnea in the elderly is a distinct condition from sleep apnea in middle age. If the patients with severe, life-threatening sleep apnea die before age 65 years, then those who live to 65 years are self-selected for having lesser morbidity associated with sleep apnea. This idea may appear far-fetched at first glance, but this hypothesis has some merit on a closer look at the clinical evidence.

The evidence suggests, in fact, that the risk factors for and consequences of sleep apnea in older adults differ from those observed in younger patients. Several studies of sleep apnea in older populations report little or no association of sleep apnea with sleepiness, hypertension, or declines in cognitive function (17–21). The association between sleep apnea and certain risk factors demonstrated for middle-aged persons, such as body mass index, obesity, and disruptive snoring, are weaker in older age groups than in middle-aged individuals (9,12,13,19,22,23). These data suggest a "two-hit" model of sleep apnea: sleep apnea is a slowly progressive disorder that is amplified by certain risk factors like obesity or morbidity vulnerability. Middle-aged sleep apnea patients with risk factors die off, and the rest survive long term. And, in fact, this hypothesis is consistent with the high prevalence but low morbidity of geriatric sleep apnea.

While there is abundant evidence describing the link between sleep apnea and cardiovascular disease as well as mortality in middle-aged adults, the association may be much weaker in older adults. The strongest association between untreated sleep apnea and increased mortality is for individuals in the fourth and fifth decades of life, and the relationship between mortality and untreated sleep apnea (particularly mild and moderate sleep apnea) is weakest in older patients (9). In a cohort of older men, Ancoli-Israel et al. (24) showed that there was no association between the presence of sleep apnea and mortality in older adults, after controlling for the presence of congestive heart failure.

Many questions surrounding age-specific prevalence and differences in sleep-disordered breathing in older adults remain unresolved. While there are limited data on geriatric mortality and cardiovascular disease attributable to sleep apnea, there are even fewer data on geriatric quality of life related to sleep apnea. We will devote the remainder of this chapter to discuss quality of life related to sleep apnea. Clinicians, the public, and policymakers are beginning to recognize the importance of patient-centered assessment of sleep apnea burden and treatment outcome. Quality of life is a prime example of a patient-centered assessment.

SLEEP APNEA AND QUALITY OF LIFE

In a broad sense, quality of life includes myriad features unrelated to a person's health. The economy, for example, affects quality of life. For the remainder of this chapter, "quality of life" refers to health-related quality of life, which can be defined as "the *value* assigned to ... life as modified by the impairments, functional states, perceptions, and social opportunities that are influenced by disease..." (25). There is a distinction between the *components* (e.g., symptoms, functional status, health status, bother) that modify the value of life and the *value* of life (quality of life). The case of violinist Itzhak Perlman illustrates this distinction. The violinist probably has a high quality of life as a world-renowned musician, but has a significantly compromised functional and health status as a paraplegic. These particular component deficits are probably outweighed by Perlman's overall ability to accomplish important goals. For convenience throughout this chapter, we will refer to quality of life somewhat loosely to include health status and health-related quality of life.

In the study of sleep apnea, symptoms and quality of life are of paramount importance for two reasons. First, the definition of sleep apnea explicitly includes symptoms, such as excessive daytime sleepiness. The symptoms produce impairment of quality of life. Second, it is the symptoms and quality of life deficits that motivate patients to seek evaluation and treatment. Patients request reduction in symptoms (e.g., sleepiness, snoring, etc.) and improvement in quality of life far more commonly than they seek reduction in the apnea–hypopnea index per se. An understanding of symptoms, the quality of life impact of disease, and the evaluation of this impact is therefore important for all clinicians who treat patients with sleep apnea. A deep understanding of this patient-centered assessment in geriatric sleep apnea patients, in particular, is lacking.

Quality of life assessment depends on the development and use of instruments that are consistent, valid, reliable, and responsive to treatment (26–28). A discussion of these characteristics is beyond the scope of this chapter, but these requirements help ensure that an instrument has clinical value in measurement of the respective patient outcomes that the instrument was designed to capture.

Guyatt et al. (29) described three types of quality of life measures: specific measures (e.g., age- or disease-specific), general health profiles, and preference-based measures. Specific measures focus on health outcomes specific to an individual disease, condition, or patient population. They usually focus on dimensions of quality of life that are most relevant in the particular disorder or patient population. The major advantage of these specific measures is that they are more focused and therefore more sensitive to quality of life deficits related to the disease. Thus, they are also more responsive to changes in the patient's condition related to the disease. Because they are seen as most relevant to patients, they are most commonly used. The major disadvantage is that because they consider single diseases or populations, they do not allow comparisons of quality of life impact across a spectrum of disorders.

General health profiles, instead, are comprehensive measures of quality of life. Their usefulness is that, in contrast to the specific measures, they can be applied across different disease areas. On the other hand, they are often less sensitive to specific health outcomes relevant to treatment of a certain disease. For example, a health status measure that includes bodily pain will not be impacted by sleep apnea, because bodily pain is not a feature of sleep apnea. It will be greatly impacted by arthritis. On the other hand, one that includes vitality or vigilance may be much more sensitive in sleep apnea patients but not in arthritis patients. For this reason, general health profiles are used largely for research, rather than clinical, purposes. Preference-based measures are used primarily in cost-utility analysis and are also beyond the scope of this chapter.

ASSESSMENT OF SYMPTOMS IN SLEEP APNEA

In the spirit of the sleep apnea-related impact on quality of life, several questionnaires have been developed largely to characterize sleep apnea symptom severity. Assessment of sleep apnea symptoms has proven valuable for two reasons: screening patients for sleep apnea and evaluating the response to treatment. Several instruments have been published and are summarized in Table 1 (26,30–47).

There is a variety of instruments developed either for screening for sleep apnea or measuring symptoms of sleep apnea that either rely entirely on symptoms or include patient-specific factors such as age, gender, and body mass index. Each instrument has important differences in the technique of symptom assessment as well as the demonstrated validity, reliability, and responsiveness to treatment. A complete discussion is beyond the scope of this chapter, but the major features are summarized in Table 1.

ASSESSMENT OF SLEEP APNEA–RELATED QUALITY OF LIFE

Based largely on the importance of quality of life changes in sleep apnea that extend beyond sleep apnea symptoms, several disease-specific instruments to measure sleep apnea quality of life have been developed (Table 2) (26,32,35,48–54) (J. F. Piccirillo, personal communication, 2003). The interested reader is referred to a comprehensive review of sleep apnea quality of life instruments (26).

Just as with symptom assessment, there is a diversity of instruments that can measure disease-specific quality of life. Principally, the measures vary according to the method of assessment (self-administered or administered by trained interviewer), the aspects of quality of life (domains) included, and the established validity, reliability, and responsiveness to treatment. Table 2 describes these key features of the instruments.

GERIATRIC SLEEP APNEA AND QUALITY OF LIFE

There are clearly numerous instruments for assessment of sleep apnea symptoms and quality of life. At this point, the study of the impact of specific treatments and, more importantly, side-by-side comparisons of treatments is in its infancy. In fact, rarely have these instruments been used in comparison of continuous positive airway pressure (CPAP) versus surgical treatment of sleep apnea, and the comparison has never been performed in an exclusively geriatric population (50).

There appears to be significant differences between middle-aged and geriatric adults in not only the physiology of sleep apnea but also the symptomatic and quality of life implications (17–21). If sleep apnea truly has distinct characteristics and implications in the elderly compared to younger age groups, there may be corresponding differences in treatment strategies for both populations. Additional

Table 1 Sleep Apnea Symptom Instruments

Instrument	Symptoms	Uses	Notes	References
Survey screen for sleep apnea	Snoring, snorting, gasping, daytime somnolence	Screening sleep apnea		30
Index of sleep apnea		Screening sleep apnea	Component of the survey screen for sleep apnea. Consistent, valid, reliable, and responsive to treatment	31, 32
Multivariable apnea index	Adds age, gender, body mass index to index of sleep apnea	Screening sleep apnea		30, 32, 33
Berlin questionnaire		Screening sleep apnea		34
Sleep and health questionnaire	Functional impact of sleepiness, breathing disturbances, roommate-observed sleep disturbances, driving impairment, insomnia	Screening sleep apnea	High consistency, low reliability	26, 35
Hawaii sleep questionnaire	Age, gender, sleep patterns, witnessed apneas, loud snoring, gasping arousals	Screening sleep apnea		36
Pittsburgh sleep quality index	Sleep quality, sleep latency, sleep duration, habitual sleep efficiency, meds, sleep disturbance, daytime function.	Symptom measure	Reliable, valid	37–39

Stanford sleepiness scale	Current sleepiness	Sleepiness measure	Correlates with multiple sleep latency test. Responsive to treatment	26, 40–42
Sleep–wake inventory index	Daytime sleepiness	Sleepiness measure	Valid, reliable, responsive to treatment	26, 43–45
Epworth sleepiness scale	General sleepiness	Sleepiness measure	Measures propensity to fall asleep in everyday situations. Valid, reliable, responsive. Not correlated with polysomnogram or multiple sleep latency test	26, 46
Index of daytime sleepiness	Dozing at work or driving, excessive daytime sleepiness	Sleepiness measure	Component of survey screen of sleep apnea. Consistent, valid, reliable, responsive	30, 32
Rotterdam daytime sleepiness scale	Sleepiness: behavioral impact, subjective response, global measure	Sleepiness measure		47

Table 2 Sleep Apnea Quality of Life Instruments

Instrument	Domains	Notes	References
Functional outcomes of sleep questionnaire	Activity level, vigilance, intimacy and sexual relationships, general productivity, and social outcome	Self-administered. Valid, reliable, and responsive to treatment. Moderate correlation with Epworth sleepiness scale	26, 32, 48–50
Sleep apnea quality of life index	Daily functioning, social interactions, emotional functioning, sleepiness	Administered by trained interviewer. Valid, reliable. Responsive to CPAP therapy in patient and bed partner	26, 35, 51–53
Symptoms of nocturnal obstruction and related events	Physical problems, functional limitations, emotional consequences	Self-administered. Valid, responsive to treatment	28, 50, (J.F. Piccirillo, personal communication, 2003)
Snore outcomes survey	General sleep apnea quality of life	Self-administered. Valid, reliable, responsive to treatment	54

Abbreviation: CPAP, continuous positive airway pressure.

research into the differences in sleep apnea among these different age groups must broadly assess physiologic as well as the physical and psychosocial factors that characterize quality of life. With an improved understanding of sleep apnea and the available therapeutic options for all age groups, patients, clinicians, and policymakers will be able to make more informed treatment decisions.

CONCLUSIONS

Sleep apnea has its highest prevalence in geriatric patients, yet it is perhaps least understood in this population. There are data to suggest that sleep apnea has a different physiologic and subjective impact in geriatric patients compared to middle-aged patients. Patient-centered assessment of sleep apnea and treatment outcome are important in all sleep apnea patients. The impact of sleep apnea and its treatment on symptoms and quality of life deserve greater study in geriatric patients.

REFERENCES

1. Young T, Peppard PE, Gottlieb DJ. Epidemiology of obstructive sleep apnea: a population health perspective. Am J Respir Crit Care Med 2002; 165:1217–1239.

2. Shamsuzzaman AS, Gersh BJ, Somers VK. Obstructive sleep apnea: implications for cardiac and vascular disease. JAMA 2003; 290:1906–1914.

3. Sateia MJ. Neuropsychological impairment and quality of life in obstructive sleep apnea. Clin Chest Med 2003; 24:249–259.

4. American Academy of Sleep Medicine. International classification of sleep disorders, revised: diagnostic and coding manual, Westchester, Illinois 2000.

5. Sleep-related breathing disorders in adults: recommendations for syndrome definition and measurement techniques in clinical research. The report of an American Academy of Sleep Medicine Task Force. Sleep 1999; 22:667–689.

6. Peppard PE, Young T, Palta M, Skatrud J. Prospective study of the association between sleep-disordered breathing and hypertension. N Engl J Med 2000; 342:1378–1384.

7. Young T, Palta M, Dempsey J, Skatrud J, Weber S, Badr S. The occurrence of sleep-disordered breathing among middle-aged adults. N Engl J Med 1993; 328:1230–1235.

8. Bixler EO, Vgontzas AN, Lin HM, et al. Prevalence of sleep-disordered breathing in women: effects of gender. Am J Respir Crit Care Med 2001; 163:608–613.

9. Bixler EO, Vgontzas AN, Ten Have T, Tyson K, Kales A. Effects of age on sleep apnea in men: I. Prevalence and severity. Am J Respir Crit Care Med 1998; 157:144–148.

10. Duran J, Esnaola S, Rubio R, Iztueta A. Obstructive sleep apnea–hypopnea and related clinical features in a population-based sample of subjects aged 30 to 70 yr. Am J Respir Crit Care Med 2001; 163:685–689.

11. Ancoli-Israel S, Kripke DF, Klauber MR, Mason WJ, Fell R, Kaplan O. Sleep-disordered breathing in community-dwelling elderly. Sleep 1991; 14:486–495.

12. Tishler PV, Larkin EK, Schluchter MD, Redline S. Incidence of sleep-disordered breathing in an urban adult population: the relative importance of risk factors in the development of sleep-disordered breathing. JAMA 2003; 289:2230–2237.

13. Young T, Shahar E, Nieto FJ, et al. Predictors of sleep-disordered breathing in community-dwelling adults: the Sleep Heart Health Study. Arch Intern Med 2002; 162:893–900.

14. Bliwise D, Carskadon M, Carey E, Dement W. Longitudinal development of sleep-related respiratory disturbance in adult humans. J Gerontol 1984; 39:290–293.

15. Lindberg E, Elmasry A, Gislason T, et al. Evolution of sleep apnea syndrome in sleepy snorers: a population-based prospective study. Am J Respir Crit Care Med 1999; 159:2024–2027.

16. Phoha RL, Dickel MJ, Mosko SS. Preliminary longitudinal assessment of sleep in the elderly. Sleep 1990; 13:425–429.

17. Young T. Sleep-disordered breathing in older adults: is it a condition distinct from that in middle-aged adults? Sleep 1996; 19:529–530.

18. Ancoli-Israel S, Coy T. Are breathing disturbances in elderly equivalent to sleep apnea syndrome? Sleep 1994; 17:77–83.

19. Enright PL, Newman AB, Wahl PW, Manolio TA, Haponik EF, Boyle PJ. Prevalence and correlates of snoring and observed apneas in 5,201 older adults. Sleep 1996; 19:531–538.

20. Ingram F, Henke KG, Levin HS, Ingram PT, Kuna ST. Sleep apnea and vigilance performance in a community-dwelling older sample. Sleep 1994; 17:248–252.

21. Foley DJ, Masaki K, White L, Larkin EK, Monjan A, Redline S. Sleep-disordered breathing and cognitive impairment in elderly Japanese-American men. Sleep 2003; 26:596–599.

22. Ancoli-Israel S, Gehrman P, Kripke DF, et al. Long-term follow-up of sleep disordered breathing in older adults. Sleep Med 2001; 2:511–516.

23. Bliwise DL, Bliwise NG, Partinen M, Pursley AM, Dement WC. Sleep apnea and mortality in an aged cohort. Am J Publ Health 1988; 78:544–547.

24. Ancoli-Israel S, DuHamel ER, Stepnowsky C, Engler R, Cohen-Zion M, Marler M. The relationship between congestive heart failure, sleep apnea, and mortality in older men. Chest 2003; 124:1400–1405.

25. Patrick DL, Erickson P. Health status and health policy: quality of life in health care evaluation and resource allocation. New York: Oxford University Press, 1993.

26. Weaver TE. Outcome measurement in sleep medicine practice and research. Part 1: assessment of symptoms, subjective and objective daytime sleepiness, health-related quality of life and functional status. Sleep Med Rev 2001; 5:103–128.

27. Kirshner B, Guyatt G. A methodological framework for assessing health indices. J Chronic Dis 1985; 38:27–36.

28. Piccirillo JF, Gates GA, White DL, Schectman KB. Obstructive sleep apnea treatment outcomes pilot study. Otolaryngol Head Neck Surg 1998; 118:833–844.

29. Guyatt GH, Feeny DH, Patrick DL. Measuring health-related quality of life. Ann Intern Med 1993; 118:622–629.

30. Maislin G, Pack AI, Kribbs NB, et al. A survey screen for prediction of apnea. Sleep 1995; 18:158–166.

31. Weaver TE, Kribbs NB, Pack AI, et al. Night-to-night variability in CPAP use over the first three months of treatment. Sleep 1997; 20:278–283.

32. Weaver T, Maislin G, Chugh D. Change in OSA symptoms after three months CPAP use: a multisite study. Sleep 1998; 21:94.

33. Gurubhagavatula I, Maislin G, Pack AI. An algorithm to stratify sleep apnea risk in a sleep disorders clinic population. Am J Respir Crit Care Med 2001; 164:1904–1909.

34. Netzer NC, Stoohs RA, Netzer CM, Clark K, Strohl KP. Using the Berlin Questionnaire to identify patients at risk for the sleep apnea syndrome. Ann Intern Med 1999; 131: 485–491. Order.

35. Kump K, Whalen C, Tishler PV, et al. Assessment of the validity and utility of a sleep-symptom questionnaire. Am J Respir Crit Care Med 1994; 150:735–741.

36. Kapuniai LE, Andrew DJ, Crowell DH, Pearce JW. Identifying sleep apnea from self-reports. Sleep 1988; 11:430–436.

37. Buysse DJ, Reynolds CF III, Monk TH, Hoch CC, Yeager AL, Kupfer DJ. Quantification of subjective sleep quality in healthy elderly men and women using the Pittsburgh Sleep Quality Index (PSQI). Sleep 1991; 14:331–338.

38. Buysse DJ, Reynolds CF III, Monk TH, Berman SR, Kupfer DJ. The Pittsburgh sleep quality index: a new instrument for psychiatric practice and research. Psychiatry Res 1989; 28:193–213.

39. Gliklich RE, Taghizadeh F, Winkelman JW. Health status in patients with disturbed sleep and obstructive sleep apnea. Otolaryngol Head Neck Surg 2000; 122:542–546.

40. Hoddes E, Dement W, Zarcone V. The development and use of the Stanford sleepiness scale (SSS). Psychophysiology 1972; 9:150.

41. Hoddes E, Zarcone V, Smythe H, Phillips R, Dement WC. Quantification of sleepiness: a new approach. Psychophysiology 1973; 10:431–436.

42. Sauter C, Asenbaum S, Popovic R, et al. Excessive daytime sleepiness in patients suffering from different levels of obstructive sleep apnea syndrome. J Sleep Res 2000; 9: 293–301.

43. Rosenthal L, Roehrs TA, Roth T. The sleep–wake activity inventory: a self-report measure of daytime sleepiness. Biol Psychiatry 1993; 34:810–820.

44. Gillberg M, Kecklund G, Akerstedt T. Relations between performance and subjective ratings of sleepiness during a night awake. Sleep 1994; 17:236–241.

45. Rosenthal L, Bishop C, Guido P, et al. The sleep/wake habits of patients diagnosed as having obstructive sleep apnea. Chest 1997; 111:1494–1499.

46. Johns MW. A new method for measuring daytime sleepiness: the Epworth sleepiness scale. Sleep 1991; 14:540–545.

47. van Knippenberg FC, Passchier J, Heysteck D, et al. The Rotterdam daytime sleepiness scale: a new daytime sleepiness scale. Psychol Rep 1995; 76:83–87.

48. Weaver TE, Laizner AM, Evans LK, et al. An instrument to measure functional status outcomes for disorders of excessive sleepiness. Sleep 1997; 20:835–843.

49. Gooneratne NS, Weaver TE, Cater JR, et al. Functional outcomes of excessive daytime sleepiness in older adults. J Am Geriatr Soc 2003; 51:642–649.

50. Woodson BT, Steward DL, Weaver EM, Javaheri S. A randomized trial of temperature-controlled radiofrequency, continuous positive airway pressure, and placebo for obstructive sleep apnea syndrome. Otolaryngol Head Neck Surg 2003; 128:848–861.

51. Flemons WW, Tsai W. Quality of life consequences of sleep-disordered breathing. J Allergy Clin Immunol 1997; 99:S750–S756.

52. Hui DS, Chan JK, Choy DK, et al. Effects of augmented continuous positive airway pressure education and support on compliance and outcome in a Chinese population. Chest 2000; 117:1410–1416.

53. Parish JM, Lyng PJ. Quality of life in bed partners of patients with obstructive sleep apnea or hypopnea after treatment with continuous positive airway pressure. Chest 2003; 124:942–947.

54. Gliklich RE, Wang PC. Validation of the snore outcomes survey for patients with sleep-disordered breathing. Arch Otolaryngol Head Neck Surg 2002; 128:819–824.

43

Overview of Head and Neck Cancer

Miriam N. Lango

Department of Surgical Oncology, Fox Chase Cancer Center, Philadelphia, Pennsylvania, U.S.A.

Ara A. Chalian

Geriatric Committee AAO-HNS, Department of Otolaryngology—Head and Neck Surgery, University of Pennsylvania, Philadelphia, Pennsylvania, U.S.A.

INTRODUCTION

By 2030, greater than 20% of the population will be elderly with greater life expectancy than at any other time in history. Over a 50-year period, the proportion of adults greater than 65 years of age will double, and the proportion greater than 85 will almost quadruple. In the early 21st century, a 70-year-old woman has a life expectancy of 15 years, and a male patient 11 years. Therefore, during a period of increasingly limited resources, it will be increasingly less justifiable to withhold definitive care. Historically, treatment of the elderly patient with a head and neck tumor has been heterogeneous, often based on the treating physician's biases regarding patient age and perceived overall health. In spite of past counsel to avoid radical surgical procedures in the elderly, reviews documenting success in performing extensive ablative and reconstructive procedures in this patient population are becoming more common in the surgical literature, but they involve a small and highly selected group. The elderly have frequently been under-represented in retrospective reviews and randomized clinical trials for cancer, making it difficult to generalize findings of these studies to the aging population (1). Systematic clinical studies assessing the impact and treatment of head and neck tumors in the elderly have to date not been done. In the current cost-conscious medical environment, the role of the head and neck surgeon will be to clarify the benefits and risks of surgical as well as nonsurgical treatment options in the elderly patient. Ideally, decisions regarding treatment recommendations will be made in a multidisciplinary setting, which will include surgeons, radiation oncologists, medical geriatric and non-geriatric oncologists, nutritionists, physical therapists, and others. In making treatment recommendations, treating physicians must also integrate the elderly patient's potential life expectancy, the natural history of the disease process, the burden of living with the disease, and patient preference into the decision-making process.

Clinical tools to assess these parameters have been developed and may be utilized to assist the treating physician and patient in decision making, providing the starting point of a rational treatment algorithm for the elderly patient with head and neck tumors. Of note, however, reliable instruments measuring quality of life responsive to changes in patient status have not been validated in elderly patients and are still under investigation.

AGING AND CANCER

Cancer is thought to arise out of a multistep process of genetic changes that depend on many factors including environmental factors, patient factors, and tumor-specific characteristics. The process requires a different number of stages depending on the neoplasm, genetic background of the individual, and other host factors such as immune competence. As such, patients with certain germline mutations may develop tumors early in life, while others develop malignancies only after lifelong exposure to carcinogens. While certain tumor types affect pediatric and young patients, the most common malignancies affect older individuals. The incidence of cancer is 12 to 36 times higher in individuals aged 65 years or more than those between 25 and 44 years, and two to three times greater than in individuals aged 45–65 years (2). According to data collected between 1997 and 2001 through the surveillance, epidemiology, and end results database maintained by the National Cancer Institute, the incidence of most solid malignancies peaks between the ages of 55 and 85 years. Age is considered a risk factor in the development of many malignancies, and the relationship between aging and the development continues to be investigated.

In numerous tumor types, age appears to affect the phenotype of the tumor. For example, well-differentiated thyroid cancers frequently affect younger patients, with the incidence peaking between ages 30 and 50 years. Older patients with well-differentiated thyroid carcinoma, however, have a well-known tendency to harbor more aggressive disease. Certain malignancies such as anaplastic thyroid carcinoma are rarely encountered in patients younger than 65 years. In general, however, aggressive tumor phenotypes are not necessarily confined to older populations, and behavior appears to be highly tumor specific. For example, tongue cancers have been thought to exhibit more aggressive tendencies in young patients. Findings in early studies have however been difficult to reproduce, and more recent reviews have found either no difference or worse outcomes in older patients.

As with many other malignancies, the incidence of upper aerodigestive tract squamous cell carcinoma increases with age. The incidence of laryngeal cancers peaks between the ages of 70 and 74 years (Fig. 1). The incidence of oral cavity and pharyngeal cancer declines finally after the age of 85 years (Fig. 2). The trends apply across multiple ethnic groups. Elderly patients with upper aerodigestive tract cancers are also at increased risk for developing second primary cancers (4–6). In fact, in one study, the incidence of second primary cancers in young patients (<40 years) was seven times less than in middle-aged patients (41–64 years) and eight times less than in elderly patients (>64 years) (4). The second primary tumors may arise both in and out of the aerodigestive tract, suggesting that "field cancerization" from cumulative exposure or intrinsic susceptibility may extend beyond tissues of the aerodigestive tract. The etiology of this increased susceptibility to developing second tumors in the elderly is not well understood, and it should be taken into consideration when making treatment recommendations.

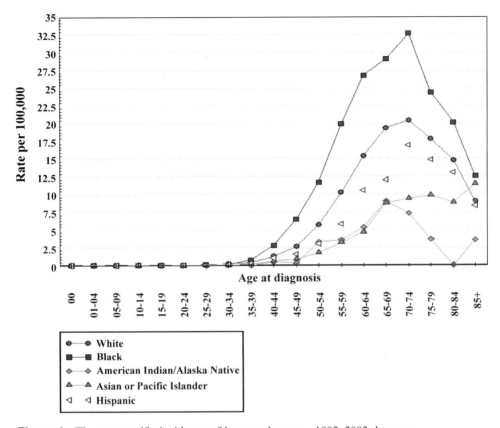

Figure 1   The age-specific incidence of laryngeal cancer, 1992–2002, by race.

BIOLOGY OF AGING AND CANCER

The biologic factors relating aging and malignancy are complex. As elaborated in Chapter 1, the etiology of an age-related predisposition to cancer may arise in the body's inability to accommodate the accumulation of errors at the DNA level. Insight has been gained from studying individuals with one of the described "premature aging syndromes," most of which have been associated with an increased incidence of cancer. Examinations of cells from these patients have revealed an increased level of genomic instability as manifested by unusually high rates of chromosomal translocations and gene mutations. Many of these syndromes, including Werner syndrome, Bloom syndrome, xeroderma pigmentosa, and others, are characterized by mutations in DNA repair genes, which make cells more susceptible to oxidative damage. Whether these genes are also involved in aging and cancer development in the general population is still under investigation.

Noncancerous tissues from aging patients have been found to harbor greater numbers of mutations than matched tissues from noncancer patients. Studies have also consistently shown an age-related increase in the rate of mutations including chromosome breaks and translocations in patients without known cancer. Evidence suggests that the increased rate of mutation is a function of and contributes to the aging process as well as to the development of cancer. The inciting event or events, however, are still unknown.

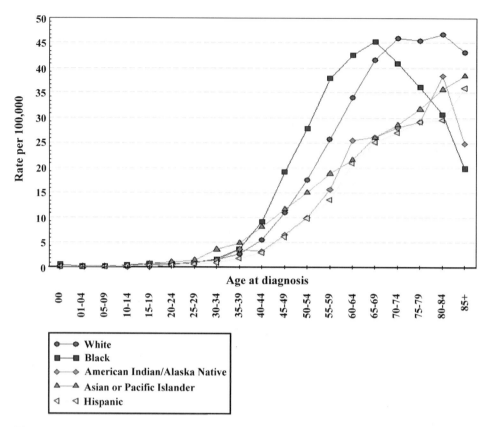

Figure 2 Age-specific incidence of oral cavity and pharyngeal cancer by race. *Source*: From Ref. 3.

In the last decade, attention has turned to cellular structures thought to possibly link cancer and aging. Telomeres are specialized structures on the ends of chromosomes composed of repeating DNA sequences and proteins. They function to stabilize chromosomes during DNA replication and cell division. With each cell division in a human somatic cell, a fraction of the telomere end is lost due to functional limitations in the cell's ability to replicate the chromosomal ends. Telomeres in older people are shorter than those in younger people, suggesting that telomeres function as a type of biologic "clock," shortening over an individual's lifetime. When the telomeres in primary human cultured cells reach a critical length, the cells die. Germ cells, but not somatic cells, contain telomerase, a protein with an RNA template that has the ability to reconstitute telomeres. Introducing telomerase into cultured somatic cells immortalizes them. It is not surprising then that telomerase is reactivated in most types of human cancer, driving unlimited proliferation. Cancer cells subvert cellular senescence programs at the molecular level, enabling them to acquire an unlimited potential for cell division. The extent to which telomere dysfunction contributes to age-related genetic instability and the development of cancer is unknown. Most cells undergo cell death when encountering genetic instability, contributing to manifestations of aging. In the presence of other genetic aberrations, however, the genetic instability caused by telomere dysfunction may generate genetic heterogeneity, providing a substrate for selection, clonal expansion, and the development of cancer. This potential molecular link and others between aging and cancer progression are currently under intense investigation.

TREATMENT OF THE ELDERLY HEAD AND NECK CANCER PATIENT

Information regarding treatment outcomes in elderly cancer patients is scarce. Although greater than 60% of patients with cancer are greater than 65 years of age, they have represented only 25% of patients in randomized clinical trials for cancer. A similar trend is seen in clinical trials for head and neck cancer in which 50% of head and neck cancer patients are greater than 65 years old, representing 24% of those in trials (7). Therefore, conclusions regarding outcomes from these studies may not be generalizable to the elderly, complicating efforts at rational clinical decision making.

Several retrospective studies have examined the results of cancer treatment in elderly head and neck cancer patients. Many of these studies report decreased cancer control and survival relative to younger patients. Bhattacharyya (8) published results of a matched survival analysis comparing head and neck cancer patients aged 70 years and older to a group of patients 50 to 69 years of age. Patients extracted from the surveillance, epidemiology, and end results database were matched for prognostically important factors, including site, extent of disease, nodal involvement, and type of treatment. The overall survival and disease-specific survival were both significantly decreased in elderly patients with tongue and glottic cancers. In another retrospective review examining the impact of age on the prognosis of 1160 patients with newly diagnosed head and neck squamous cell carcinoma (HNSCC), Lacy et al. (5) reported that young patients in general have a better overall prognosis than middle-aged and elderly patients. Elderly patients were found to have a four-fold increased risk of death compared with young patients even when controlling for the impact of prognostically relevant parameters such as TNM nodal stage, and comorbidity. Nevertheless, inherent in all retrospective studies is the reality of bias, particularly regarding treatment selection and intent, making it difficult to draw conclusions from studies such as these. In the retrospective review by Clayman et al. (9), some of these issues are addressed. In this study, the median overall survival of octogenarians undergoing surgery for head and neck cancer was significantly lower than for matched controls, as was the local control and the disease-specific survival. The elderly patient group was also significantly less likely to undergo microvascular reconstruction using free tissue transfer, was more likely to have positive margins, and was nevertheless less likely to undergo adjuvant radio therapy. Therefore, the findings in this study suggests that a factor contributing to the decreased disease control in this population was related to less aggressive treatment, given in an effort to minimize the adverse effects and complications of treatment. The authors point out that despite the decreased disease control in the octogenarian group, their overall survival was comparable to the expected survival based on cohort life statistics derived from U.S. Bureau of the Census data.

AGE, COMORBIDITY, AND FUNCTIONAL STATUS

Allan Greenspan, the chairman of the Federal Reserve Board, has previously noted that the Medicare budget is spent on 5% to 6% of persons who subsequently died within one year, raising speculation regarding the degree to which patients would consent to treatment if they knew the likely outcome (10). The elderly, particularly those with significant functional impairment and comorbidities, are subject to increased treatment-related complications relative to younger patients. Nevertheless, chronologic age often does not reflect the resilience or functional reserve of an individual patient. Aging is a highly individualized process, and the elderly are a heterogeneous group of individuals. Following hospitalization for an acute illness, some patients recover completely, while others suffer a progressive decline and death. When little functional reserve is left, an individual patient is considered frail, and aggressive therapies are often withheld (11–13). The relationships among age, comorbidity, functional status, and predicted life expectancy are complex and inter-related. A decreased physiologic reserve in many organ systems, including cardiovascular, pulmonary, renal, and hepatic, contribute in making a proportion of elderly patients more vulnerable to physiologic stressors, including comorbidities. Functional impairment from a cancer in the aerodigestive tract may further compromise reserve and impact prognosis. In dealing with the elderly patient, disease-specific assessments must be made in a context of global health status, including comorbidity and functional status. Comorbidity, functional status, cognitive impairment, nutritional status, and insufficient social support have all independently been shown to affect survival in elderly cancer patients (14). At this time, the best determinant of functional reserve and life expectancy in the elderly patient is provided by the comprehensive geriatric assessment (CGA) (11–13). This assessment of aging has been formulated as a multidimentional task addressing the multiple domains subject to age-related changes. These domains include health, functional status, nutrition, cognition, socioeconomic, and emotional issues. The CGA includes a measure of comorbidity but additionally appraises other domains facilitating identification of new or overlapping conditions. An evaluation of comorbidity or performance status alone may not be as meaningful a measure of health status as in a younger patient. A comprehensive approach is critical in the elderly who do not infrequently fail to recognize new symptoms, are uniquely vulnerable to adverse drug effects, or may develop atypical or subtle symptoms dismissed as manifestations of pre-existing disorders. CGA therefore assists in the proper determination of comorbidity and the detection and treatment of unsuspected disorders, and it clarifies the degree of functional impairment, which impacts both remaining quality of life and overall prognosis. The setting in which such an assessment is made at this time includes academic oncology programs, multidisciplinary cancer centers, and cooperative group studies. The need for geriatric assessments of elderly cancer patients will likely intensify as the population ages.

COMORBIDITY

The prevalence of underlying medical illnesses or comorbidities increases as a function of age (Fig. 3) but is not limited to the elderly. The presence of comorbidities unequivocally affects the overall survival of head and neck cancer patients (15–19). In fact, the increased burden of comorbid conditions may impact disease control independently of treatment selection. In a study of young (<40) head and neck cancer patients treated with curative intent, the presence of advanced comorbidities increased the relative risk of cancer recurrence and cancer-associated death greater than two-folds relative to matched healthy controls with cancer, suggesting that tumor behavior may be affected by the presence of comorbid conditions (19). The presence of comorbidities is also associated with an increased risk of perioperative medical and surgical complications (20,21).

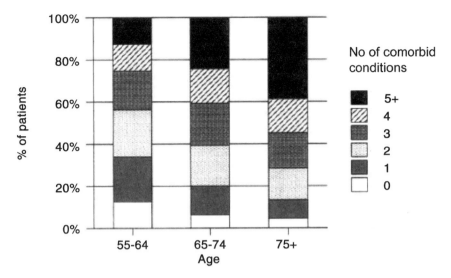

Figure 3 The number of comorbid conditions increases as a function of age. *Source*: From Ref. 14.

Instruments used to gauge the burden of comorbidity in head and neck cancer patients have included the modified Kaplan-Feinstein index, the Charlson comorbidity scale, Adult Comorbidity Evaluation-27 (ACE-27), the Washington University Head and Neck Comorbidity Index, and the American Society of Anesthesiologist (ASA) classification, among others. Indexes require validation in order to determine their power to predict outcome for a selected group of patients. Such an assessment has not been done in the elderly head and neck cancer population. These indicators do not include prognostically significant parameters, such as functional status, nutrition, cognition, socioeconomic factors, and emotional issues, of relatively greater import in the elderly population. Therefore, it is unknown if currently accepted validated indices used to assess head and neck cancer patients may be applied to elderly patients with head and neck cancer.

FUNCTIONAL STATUS

The Eastern Cooperative Oncology Group (ECOG) or World Health Organization (WHO) performance status score and the Karnofsky score are the most widely used scores of functional status in clinical oncology, and they have been shown to effectively predict outcome in multiple oncologic studies. However, in elderly patients, these scores may underestimate the degree of functional impairment. For example, despite a high frequency of comorbidities in the elderly population, 80% nevertheless are scored as 0 or 1 on ECOG performance scoring. A more sensitive screen involves the patients' ability to perform specific tasks including activities of daily living (ADL) and instrumental activities of daily living (IADL). ADLs include feeding, grooming, transferring, toileting, and comprise skills necessary for self-care. IADLs include shopping, managing finances, housekeeping, laundry, meal preparation, ability to take medication, and comprise a set of skills that allow a patient to live independently. Such assessments of functional status may uncover signs of frailty.

The short-term mortality of older persons has been shown to correspond to the degree of functional impairment. The two-year mortality for individuals greater than 70 years old or more who are fully independent is 8%, 14% for those with impaired IADLs, 27% for those with impaired ADLs, and 40% for institutionalized patients (22).

COGNITION/NUTRITION/SOCIAL SUPPORT/POLYPHARMACY

Undiagnosed depression and cognitive dysfunction is common in elderly cancer patients and impacts compliance with planned treatment as well as quality of life. Decline in mental status and depression have both been shown to be independent predictors of mortality in older individuals (22). Screening tools are available including a geriatric depression scale and the mini-mental status exam. Supportive measures may greatly enhance cognitive function. Social support is necessary for continuity of care, emotional support, and compliance with treatment. In addition, elderly patients are at high risk for malnutrition, which is exacerbated by the presence of cancer. Malnutrition has been estimated to occur in 20% of individuals greater than 70 years of age, secondary to poor oral intake, limited access, dementia, or chronic disease (23,24). Malnutrition may contribute to surgical wound complications as well as immune dysfunction, facilitating cancer growth and spread. Finally, a frequent cause of hospitalization includes polypharmacy, which occurs because patients may visit multiple practitioners, suffer complications of drug interactions, and are uniquely vulnerable to drugs at conventional doses, making these patients more vulnerable to drug-related complications.

The value of the CGA has not been evaluated in the setting of elderly patients with head and neck cancer. However, several trials have demonstrated the utility of multidisciplinary CGA in improving functional status, reducing hospitalization, decreasing medical costs, and improving survival of elderly patients (25). Trials have also revealed that CGA has been found effective in prevention of institutionalization, maintenance of independence, prevention of delirium in hospitalized patients, and prevention of falls (12). The effectiveness of such an approach would likely involve incorporating a geriatric physician into the head and neck health care team. This would only be cost effective in a setting with high volume or high-risk procedures.

THERAPEUTIC OPTIONS FOR ELDERLY HEAD AND NECK CANCER PATIENTS

The potential life expectancy of an individual cancer patient is often underestimated, resulting in undertreatment of the cancer. Often, the cancer itself will contribute to functional impairment, exacerbating any comorbidities and worsening the overall prognosis. Historically, there has been a bias against treating elderly patients with surgery, based on the idea that surgery carries a prohibitively high risk. However, older patients are unlikely to receive combined modality therapy with chemotherapy and radiotherapy secondary to justified concerns regarding toxicity. A decline in functional reserve in multiple organ systems alters the pharmacokinetics of many chemotherapeutic agents, increasing the susceptibility of older patients to treatment-related toxicity. The incidence of grade 3 to 5 thrombocytopenia, diarrhea, and renal dysfunction with use of platinum-based chemotherapeutic agents is double that in younger patients and has been associated with a 13% risk of treatment-related mortality (1). Radiotherapy alone appears to be relatively well tolerated in the elderly and has been used for treatment or palliation for many years. Radiation alone may, however, be inadequate treatment for an advanced tumor. With undertreatment, patients are subject to a high rate of treatment failure, which in turn is managed with supportive care and, not infrequently, salvage surgery.

PERIOPERATIVE RISK ASSESSMENT

The risk of perioperative mortality of patients over 65 years of age undergoing major head and neck resections is low relative to that of patients undergoing surgical procedures in other parts of the body (26). Over the last several decades, anesthetic techniques have become safer and have allowed even debilitated elderly patients to undergo surgery safely. Most anesthesiologists use the ASA classification to stratify patients according to their level of risk.

In clinical practice, exercise tolerance in daily life is one of the most important predictors of perioperative outcome in the elderly surgical patient. Poor exercise tolerance may reflect the severity of the underlying disease and is a crude measure of a patient's ability to tolerate general anesthesia.

A head and neck cancer may cause significant functional impairment, relating to its effects on speech and swallowing. Cancer-related symptom severity has been shown to have a major impact on prognosis (27). A patient with a laryngeal cancer may suffer from aspiration, which is poorly tolerated due to the presence of chronic lung disease and diabetes. The treating physicians face a dilemma. The patient may be thought "too sick" to undergo a total laryngectomy. However, treatment with nonsurgical approaches may not alleviate tumor-related symptoms, including life-threatening aspiration, even if the primary tumor is controlled. In cases such as these, the patient's premorbid level of function may be the best indicator regarding whether the patient may be able to tolerate surgical treatment.

INCIDENCE OF SURGICAL AND NONSURGICAL COMPLICATIONS IN THE ELDERLY

The presence of comorbidities predisposes to the development of surgical and non-surgical postoperative complications in patients undergoing major surgical procedures. Since aging is associated with an increased burden of comorbid conditions, surgical procedures in elderly patients have been associated with a higher incidence of postoperative complications. Several studies have suggested that advanced age may be an independent risk factor for postoperative medical complications. However, multiple studies have failed to show an increased rate of surgical complications in elderly patients (8,21,28,29). In fact, some authors have noted a higher rate of surgical complications in younger patients, possibly related to more aggressive resections or more robust immune function in this group. There does not appear to be a higher incidence of flap-related complications or flap failure in elderly patients undergoing microvascular free tissue transfer. Extensive head and neck ablative surgical resections followed by microvascular free tissue transfer are physiologically demanding procedures, which have successfully been performed on octogenarians. Most studies report a significantly higher incidence of postoperative medical complications in this group. Blackwell et al. (29) reported a 62% incidence of medical complications in octogenarians compared with 15% in younger patients. The perioperative mortality rate in most studies is reported between 3.8% and 7% (21,28,30).

In one study, 38% of elderly patients died within one year of treatment, either from recurrent cancer or intercurrent illness (19). The higher rate of medical complications in most studies is attributed to the increased incidence of preoperative comorbidity. These complications result in an increased length of stay and increased cost of treatment for older patients compared with their younger counterparts (29,31). The use of free flap reconstruction in octogenarians continues to be controversial, but it is clearly beneficial in properly selected patients.

THERAPEUTIC MODALITIES: FUNCTIONAL OUTCOMES AND QUALITY OF LIFE

In making treatment recommendations, treating physicians must integrate the elderly patient's potential life expectancy, the natural history of the disease process, the burden of living with the disease, and patient preference into the decision-making process. Most patients with head and neck cancers will, if inadequately treated, not survive their cancers. Since tumors often impair vital functions, including swallowing and speech, the elderly patient's remaining quality of life is adversely affected. Treatment should involve control of cancer coupled with maximal preservation of function. Organ preservation approaches involving chemoradiation may not be appropriate for intermediate laryngeal cancers. However, laser microsurgery of the larynx is often feasible and relatively well tolerated by elderly patients. Given the heterogeneity of the older population, treatment must be individualized.

REFERENCES

1. Argiris A, Li Y, Murphy BA, Langer CJ, Forastiere AA. Outcome of elderly patients with recurrent or metastatic head and neck cancer treated with cisplatin-based chemotherapy. JCO 2004; 22(2):262–268.
2. Parkin DM. Epidemiology of cancer: global patterns and trends. Toxicol Lett 1998; 102–103:227–234.
3. Surveillance, Epidemiology, and End Results (SEER) Program, released in April 2005, http://www.seer.cancer.gov.
4. Koch WM, Patel H, Brennán J, Boyle JO, Sidransky D. Squamous cell carcinoma of the head and neck in the elderly. Arch Otolaryngol Head Neck Surg 1995; 121:262–265.
5. Lacy PD, Piccirillo JF, Merritt MG, Zequeira MR. Head and neck squamous cell carcinoma: better to be young. Otolaryngol Head Neck Surg 2000; 122(2):253–258.
6. Nikolaou AC, et al. Second primary neoplasms in patients with laryngeal carcinoma. Laryngoscope 2000; 110(1):58–64.
7. Hutchins LF, Unger JM, Crowley JJ, Coltman CA Jr, Albain KS. Underrepresentation of patients 65 years of age or older in cancer-treatment trials. NEJM 1999; 341(27):2061–2067.
8. Bhattacharyya N. A matched survival analysis for squamous cell carcinoma of the head and neck in the elderly. Laryngoscope 2003; 113(2):368–372.
9. Clayman GL, Eicher SA, Sicard MW, Razmpa E, Goepfert H. Surgical outcomes in head and neck cancer patients 80 years of age and older. Head Neck 1998; 20(3):216–223.
10. JS. Terminal patients deplete Medicare, Greenspan says. Dallas Morning News 1983:1.

11. Balducci L, Beghe C. The application of the principles of geriatrics to the management of the older person with cancer. Crit Rev Oncol Hematol 2000; 35(3):147–154.

12. Balducci L, Extermann M. Management of cancer in the older person: a practical approach. Oncologist 2000; 5(3):224–237.

13. Balducci L, Yates J. General guidelines for the management of older patients with cancer. Oncology (Huntingt) 2000; 14(11A):221–227.

14. Extermann M, Aapro M. Assessment of the older cancer patient. Hematol Oncol Clin North Am 2000; 14(1):63–77, viii–ix.

15. Piccirillo JF, et al. Development of a new head and neck cancer-specific comorbidity index. Arch Otolaryngol Head Neck Surg 2002; 128(10):1172–1179.

16. Extermann M. Measurement and impact of comorbidity in older cancer patients. Crit Rev Oncol Hematol 2000; 35(3):181–200.

17. Paleri V, Wight RG, Davies GR. Impact of comorbidity on the outcome of laryngeal squamous cancer. Head Neck 2003; 25(12):1019–1026.

18. Hathaway B, Johnson JT, Piccirillo JF, et al. Chemoradiation for metastatic SCCA: role of comorbidity. Laryngoscope 2001; 111(11 Pt 1):1893–1895.

19. Singh B, Bhaya M, Zimbler M, et al. Impact of comorbidity on outcome of young patients with head and neck squamous cell carcinoma. Head Neck 1998; 20(1):1–7.

20. Suh JD, Sercarz JA, Abemayor E, et al. Analysis of outcome and complications in 400 cases of microvascular head and neck reconstruction. Arch Otolaryngol Head Neck Surg 2004; 130(8):962–966.

21. Shestak KC, et al. Effect of advanced age and medical disease on the outcome of microvascular reconstruction for head and neck defects. Head Neck 1992; 14(1):14–18.

22. Balducci L, Stanta G. Cancer in the frail patient. A coming epidemic. Hematol Oncol Clin North Am 2000; 14(1):235–250, xi.

23. Hardy C, Wallace C, Khansur T, Vance RB, Thigpen JT, Balducci L. Nutrition, cancer, and aging: an annotated review. II. Cancer cachexia and aging. J Am Geriatr Soc 1986; 34(3):219–228.

24. Balducci L, Wallace C, Khansur T, Vance RB, Thigpen JT, Hardy C. Nutrition, cancer, and aging: an annotated review. I. Diet, carcinogenesis, and aging. J Am Geriatr Soc 1986; 34(2):127–136.

25. Repetto L, Venturino A, Fratino L, et al. Geriatric oncology: a clinical approach to the older patient with cancer. Eur J Cancer 2003; 39(7):870–880.

26. Morgan RF, Richard M. Hirata, Darrell A. Jaques, John E. Hoopes. Head and neck surgery in the aged. Am J Surg 1982; 144(4):449–451.

27. Pugliano FA, Piccirillo JF, Zequeira MR, et al. New clinical severity staging system for cancer of the larynx. Five-year survival rates. Ann Otol Rhinol Laryngol 1994; 103(2):83–92.

28. Beausang ES, Ang EE, Lipa JE, et al. Microvascular free tissue transfer in elderly patients: the Toronto experience. Head Neck 2003; 25(7):549–553.

29. Blackwell KE, Azizzadeh B, Ayala C, Rawnsley JD. Octogenarian free flap reconstruction: complications and cost of therapy. Otolaryngol Head Neck Surg 2002; 126(3):301–306.

30. Shaari CM, Buchbinder D, Costantino PD, Lawson W, Biller HF, Urken ML. Complications of microvascular head and neck surgery in the elderly. Arch Otolaryngol Head Neck Surg 1998; 124(4):407–411.

31. Kagan SH, Chalian AA, Goldberg AN, et al. Impact of age on clinical care pathway length of stay after complex head and neck resection. Head Neck 2002.

ANNOTATED BIBLIOGRAPHY

Hutchins LF, UJ, Crowley JJ, Coltman CA Jr, Albain KS. Underrepresentation of patients 65 years of age or older in cancer-treatment trials. NEJM 1999; 341(27):2061–2067.

This article highlights the inherent contradiction in many cancer trials: the population at highest risk, the elderly, are often excluded from study.

Piccirillo JF, et al. New clinical severity staging system for cancer of the larynx. Five year survival rates. Ann Otol Rhinol Laryngol 1994; 103(2):83–92.

Piccirillo et al. turned attention away from disease-control to patient survival, relating both clinical variables and tumor staging to overall survival.

44

Head and Neck Cancer in the Geriatric Patient

Jack L. Gluckman and Michael Wolfe

Department of Otolaryngology—Head and Neck Surgery, University of Cincinnati Medical Center, Cincinnati, Ohio, U.S.A.

INTRODUCTION

This chapter is devoted to problems associated with the management of cancers that arise in the mucosa of the upper aerodigestive tract in the geriatric patient. For the purpose of our discussion, we focus on those in the 75-plus age group. In the population as a whole, 60% of all cancers occur in the 12% of patients older than 65 years (1). When combined with the inversed life expectancy, this geriatric population is likely to be the dominant group in any oncologic practice. This undoubtedly holds true in head and neck oncology with a patient cohort that in general has indulged in a lifetime of smoking and drinking.

The incidence of cancer arising in the upper aerodigestive tract seems to increase with age. The reasons for this are unclear but are felt to reflect a prolonged exposure to known carcinogenic agents with an accumulation of genetic defects (2). This explanation may be too simplistic, as some studies have noted that tobacco and alcohol abuse in this geriatric population is significantly less than expected (3–5). Other possibilities include the impaired ability to repair DNA and the impaired immune surveillance found in the elderly (5). Interestingly, some studies found that there was a higher incidence of females in the cohort (6).

It remains unclear as to whether cancers, in general, behave differently in the older patient and, more specifically, whether this holds true for head and neck cancers. Certainly, there is some scientific evidence that cancers are in fact more aggressive in the older age group and that elderly patients have a worse prognosis than a comparable younger group, particularly if the cancer is advanced (7–11). Whether this represents a true increased aggressiveness or is due to the associated debilitating comorbidities, which may prohibit the use of the recommended radical therapeutic modalities necessary to attain cure, is unclear. Further compounding the problem is the fact that older patients tend to present with more advanced disease than younger patients. The reasons for this include a tendency to attribute early symptoms to "the aging process," a dearth of nearby family who would notice any new functional changes, limited access to medical care, and various levels of mental status changes that may camouflage the presenting symptoms. For these reasons, most clinicians believe that if one removes comorbidities from the equation, no difference in tumor behavior truly exists (12,13).

EVALUATION OF THE GERIATRIC PATIENT WITH HEAD AND NECK CANCER

It is an accepted adage that chronological age alone should never dictate the treatment for the patient, and this is confirmed by the experience of many authors (3,14–17). Unfortunately, as much as this concept is preached and understood, advanced age maintains a significant influence on the decision-making process of the physician, patient, and family. Admittedly, this is usually influenced by the perceived presence of comorbidities ("not strong enough to go through the treatment") or life expectancy ("at my age it is just not worth it") rather than chronologic age, but it is a factor nonetheless. It is important, therefore, that the treating physician try and be objective in deciding on the recommended therapeutic regime, and the following factors should be considered during the deliberations.

The Physical Status of the Patient

While many elderly patients are quite robust, in general the older the patient, the greater the infirmity especially if the body has been ravaged by a lifetime of abusive behavior, such as tobacco and alcohol overuse. Frequently found comorbidities, such as atherosclerosis, heart disease, chronic obstructive pulmonary disease, liver disease, diabetes mellitus, and dementia, all may profoundly affect the therapeutic options that can be offered to the patient. Particularly affected is the ability to perform surgery and the type of surgery to be offered. Factors such as duration of anesthesia time, the extent of radical surgery, type of reconstruction to be used, and, of course, the patient's physical and emotional ability to engage in prolonged postoperative rehabilitation all have to be taken into account. The diagnosis of true frailty, i.e., where functional reserve is so limited that the patient is unable to tolerate the stress of any treatment, is a difficult assessment and should only be made in conjunction with the patient's primary care physician or preferably a specialist in geriatric medicine. Careful attention and expert consultation should be obtained in evaluating the presence of low-grade malnutrition and the effects of the multiple drugs that these patients are inevitably on. All these issues may be compounded in patients with cancer of the head and neck where radical therapy may further severely impair precariously balanced bodily functions. If chemotherapy is to be considered, one should remember that the incidence and severity of complications due to this modality are significantly greater in the older patient.

The Emotional Status of the Patient

The emotional reaction of older patients when confronted by a life-threatening disease may be very different from that of a younger patient. The increased awareness of one's own mortality, which comes with age, may lead to greater pragmatism as to what the future holds. Usually, there is a greater concern for quality of life and less for long-term survival. This may frustrate the oncologist who is geared to aggressively pursuing curative therapy. The oncologist must respect the patient's values regarding quality and quantity of survival during and after cancer treatment and be careful not to dismiss these viewpoints. Frequently the patient truly does know best!

Further compounding the situation is the frequently found clinical depression, which may cause or aggravate a fatalistic attitude in the patient. It is difficult for a nonprofessional to understand and recognize this, but if suspected, appropriate treatment should be instituted as soon as possible if it is not to interfere with the therapeutic process. Consultation with the primary care physician and/or a psychiatrist is essential, and the oncologist should avoid the temptation of empirically adding an antidepressant to the already complicated polypharmacy. The problem is that there is usually some urgency to the decision-making process, and very rarely is the patient afforded the luxury of prolonged psychiatric evaluation and the determination of the effect of antidepressant medications before having to decide on therapy. A complex situation indeed!

On the other hand, the burning desire of some patients to see subsequent generations succeed or to participate in future sentinel family events may sometimes serve as a fierce motivation for the patient to live longer under any circumstances and aggressively seek curative therapy.

The Patient's Support System

Strong family support is essential for the successful management of the elderly head and neck cancer patient. Unfortunately, all too often this is absent or woefully inadequate and dysfunctional. Even if there is a caring and supportive family, the patient may aggravate the situation by insisting on not wanting to impose on the family members and directly or indirectly marginalizing their involvement. This can be extremely frustrating to all concerned. Commonly occurring scenarios, which tax the decision-making process include:

A scenario where the spouse may have preceded the patient in death with the patient living alone in less than ideal circumstances, with the children and other relatives scattered geographically and incapable or unwilling to offer the support needed. This leads to each decision being second guessed from afar and constant delays while relatives come and go, frequently at odds with each other.

Another common predicament is the patient being the sole caregiver to an already ailing spouse whose care is now put in jeopardy by the patient's illness. The decision as to which illness takes precedence likewise can now make a difficult decision-making process impossible. If family or friends cannot offer support, local community social services may be needed to educate and assist the patient about possible resources, including home health or temporary nursing care facilities, which may be needed.

On the other hand, occasionally the reverse problem occurs, with family support being overzealous and often misguided, fueled by guilt and/or sibling rivalry. This can render a difficult situation horrendous as dysfunctional family dynamics and personal agendas play out. Ideally, the patient or family should designate one family member as the spokesperson, thereby buffering the physician from the complex family issues and forcing the family to obtain consensus before discussing therapeutic options with the treating physician. Finally, one should appreciate that economic restrictions and lack of transportation to a healthcare facility may further compromise the treatment options.

The Patient's Prognosis

An important question that, as yet, has not been answered is whether the prognosis in older patients is worse than for the younger patient with comparable disease.

The results of studies comparing comparable therapies for comparable disease in the aged and younger population have been equivocal because of the large number of variables, but some have in fact demonstrated a worse local control rate and disease-free survival (3,11,12). Whether this is due to an increased tumor aggressiveness, associated comorbidities compromising the radical nature of the required therapy in order to minimize morbidity is unknown (12,18,19). Whatever the reason, it is the authors' belief that the elderly patient does not do as well as the younger patient; however, in those who do survive, meaningful quality of life is attainable, and these patients are grateful indeed for their survival.

THE DECISION-MAKING PROCESS

Therapeutic decision-making in the head and neck cancer patient is always complicated but, for the reasons already mentioned, can become infinitely more so in the elderly. It is important for the physician to have family participation during the patient–physician encounters in order to ensure that there is agreement regarding the final decisions. We have often found it valuable to have a separate meeting with the family without the patient to permit airing of all the issues. It is also vital that the primary care physician who has taken care of the patient over a long period of time or a geriatric specialist be consulted in particularly complicated cases. Usually, even in the most rational of situations, the frequently stated question "at my age, is it worth it?" hangs over the encounter, and the physician should go the great lengths to directly address this question as appropriate.

Decisions by the physician in managing the geriatric patient should follow the same algorithm that dictates decision-making in all patients, i.e., expressing a realistic opinion regarding treatment morbidity and outcome and yet at the same time never eliminating the hope for a successful outcome.

A reasonable approach is, as for all patients, to decide on the ideal treatment for the tumor and then, taking into consideration all the extenuating circumstances, decide on the correct treatment for the particular patient. Never, ever force patients into any therapeutic decision against their will or where one perceives a reluctance to participate. In the final analysis, it is the patient's decision and the patient's alone, and before signing consent one must be satisfied that the patient understands completely the issues at stake. However, it is good policy to ensure that one of the family sign the consent as a witness.

THERAPEUTIC MODALITIES

It is probably fair to acknowledge that the contemporary management of head and neck cancer has undergone a paradigm shift in recent years, with a tendency to avoid radical mutilating therapies if possible and move toward organ-preservation therapies if feasible. In general, therapeutic decision-making in the geriatric patient should follow this approach. It is generally accepted that elective surgery is reasonably safe through the 9th decade of life and that, more specifically, head and neck surgery has a lower mortality rate in the aged than elective surgery performed in other anatomic regions (20,21). Of even greater significance is that the elderly patient is often able to withstand the combination of conservation surgery and radiation for upper aerodigestive tract cancers, provided the comorbidities, etc. allow it (22). Likewise, radiation administered to older patients in curative doses is regarded as safe (23). It is only the use of chemotherapy where there is a significant higher complication rate (24).

Surgery

In general, as long as the associated comorbidities do not preclude it, there is no reason why standard radical ablative resection and reconstructive surgery cannot be recommended if appropriate. As comorbidities are however likely to be present, it is advisable to perform the ablation and reconstruction as quickly and expeditiously as possible to minimize the anesthesia time. Some may argue that the patient is safest while under anesthesia, but it is our sense that the shorter the surgery the better. Classical conservation surgery, e.g., supraglottic, supracricoid, and vertical partial laryngectomies, is certainly technically feasible in the elderly, but the problem lies postoperatively as the patient may lack the will and strength to be successfully rehabilitated, essentially negating the reason for the conservation surgery, e.g., failed speech and swallowing techniques, or becoming tracheostomy dependent because of poor pulmonary reserve, or gastrostomy dependent. Therefore, if surgery is to be undertaken, patient selection is critical with not only the tumor extent and patient's issues to be considered but also the experience and skill of the surgeon and the entire surgical, nursing, and rehabilitative team. For example, often a simple total laryngectomy for advanced laryngeal cancer may be the ideal operation, even if amenable to conservation procedures, to optimize cure and facilitate rehabilitation in an elderly patient. The experienced clinician must have the courage to recognize this in spite of current trends to organ preservation.

Comorbidities may also influence the type of reconstruction to be used following the ablative surgery. While there is evidence that free revascularized grafts can be successfully used in the elderly (16), one has to also take into consideration the length of time needed to perform such reconstructive procedures and balance the risks of the prolonged operative time with the advantages of the free flap reconstruction. In certain situations, e.g., reconstruction of the anterior mandible, this cannot be avoided, but in others, e.g., following resection of the posterior third of the mandible, a case can be made to avoid bone reconstruction altogether, as particularly the edentulous older patient may do just as well as those who undergo reconstruction.

Irrespective of the surgery used, the immediate postoperative period is the most critical and fraught with hazards for the geriatric patient. If complications do occur, they are not well tolerated by the geriatric population, but as has been repeatedly stated, it is the comorbidities and not chronologic age that increase the risk for these complications.

In general, the older patient is more likely to experience pulmonary and cardiovascular complications as compared to the younger patients who are more likely to experience wound-related problems. Early mobilization and, if possible, early discharge from hospital is key. However, this is unfortunately not always feasible. While the literature evaluating the effect of length of hospital stay on the elderly patient shows mixed outcomes (11,15), there is little doubt in the authors' minds that the longer an elderly patient lingers in the hospital, the greater the risk of complications and depression, with a resultant decrease in successful rehabilitation. The success of this critical postoperative time is directly dependent on having experienced, caring nursing personnel who are able to devote the appropriate amount of time and energy to these patients. Pain management, as an example, is critical, with the ability to control the pain without impairing the mental state of the patient being an art form needing constant surveillance. Likewise, pulmonary toilet and nutritional support performed by experts is an absolute necessity.

Radiation

Radiation is as safe and effective in the elderly patient as in the younger patient. There does, however, appear to be a 10–15% increased incidence of complications due to the radiation effect on normal tissue as compared to younger patients (25). This is particularly a problem in treating cancers of the head and neck where xerostomia, loss of taste, and dental problems can exacerbate an already precarious nutritional status. As the geriatric patient often requires "rest periods" due to inability to tolerate the therapy, the efficacy of the radiation therapy decreases and cure rates fall.

Perhaps the most significant issue related to radiation usage is the inappropriate selection of this modality as a compromise treatment between radical surgery and doing nothing at all, with the idea being that "salvage" surgery can always be performed in case of failure. Experienced surgical oncologists clearly appreciate the naiveté of such an approach and should be careful not to lull the patient and family into a false sense of security with this choice.

Chemotherapy

Most older patients do not do well with chemotherapy. The risk of complications with this modality of treatment increases dramatically after the age of 70 (24). Reasons include changes in the pharmacokinetics and pharmacodynamics of chemotherapeutic drugs in the elderly with increased susceptibility of the normal tissues. This is especially noted in those patients with compromised renal function and poor bone marrow function. Other comorbidities further decrease tolerance and increase the risks of complications. Chemotherapy, therefore, should only be administered cautiously and after consultation with the patient's primary care physician or internist. Care should be taken not to be tempted to use these drugs without clear-cut advantages to the patient. On the other hand, if they are to be used, one must avoid "risk aversion," i.e., blatant underdosing in an attempt to avoid toxicity, which obviates any chance at meaningful efficacy. As it so happens, at the present time, chemotherapy still does not play a clearly defined role in the management of head and neck cancer, and so these issues are less relevant than when treating other cancers.

PATIENT FOLLOW-UP

All oncologists understand clearly the importance of careful follow-up to the success of the cancer treatment. Unfortunately, this is particularly problematic for the geriatric patient. Once the acute phase of the therapy is over and the patient is discharged from the hospital, family support often cannot be sustained at a high level. The ideal discharge is home with strong family support. Until the patient is self-sustaining, this is not often possible, and one must find long-term care, so obtaining a facility that the patient and family find satisfactory becomes a priority. Failure to do so results in a growing sense of despair, often progressing to frank depression, which can make completion of therapy and rehabilitation back into society difficult. Pain management and adequate nutritional support are also difficult.

Likewise, reliable transportation is very important and social services should be recruited early on to help with these issues. It is vital that the treating physician be aware of the fragility of the post-treatment social circumstances and find time to address them. Many a successful therapeutic regimen has been destroyed by the inability to follow through adequately with the crucial post-treatment management plan.

REHABILITATION

Even the most highly motivated geriatric patient will have a significant problem mustering up the physical and emotional strength required to complete a rehabilitation program sufficiently to re-enter society. Some patients manage well but others do not. Becoming tracheostomy and gastrostomy dependent as an example are not desirable, but, if accepted by patient and family, there is no need for the physician to make this the criteria for success. Likewise, speech rehabilitation may not be possible, and all should accept that an electrolarynx is an acceptable means of communication (26).

CONCLUSION

The elderly cancer patient will continue to comprise a large percentage of any head and neck oncologic practice. Age per se should not be a determinant as to the ideal treatment for the patient. Rather, the presence of inevitable comorbidities will ultimately be an important factor in deciding on therapy. Most of these patients are able to withstand contemporary surgical therapeutic options, provided excellent postoperative care is available. An uncomplicated postoperative course is the key to achieving short- and long-term success. Once the therapy is completed, an adequate support system is vital to successful rehabilitation of the patient as a functioning member of society.

REFERENCES

1. Cohen HJ. In: Hazzard WR, Blass JP, Ettinger WH, Halter JB, Ouslander JG, eds. Oncology and Aging: General Principles of Cancer in the Elderly in Principles of Geriatric Medicine and Gerontology. New York: McGraw-Hill, 1999.
2. Hazzard WR, Blass JP, Ettinger WH, Halter JB, Ouslander JG. Principles of Geriatric Medicine and Gerontology. 4th ed. New York: McGraw-Hill, 1999.
3. Koch WM, Patel H, Brennan J, Boyle JO, Sidransky D. Squamous cell carcinoma of the head and neck in the elderly. Arch Otolaryngol Head Neck Surg 1995; 121:262.
4. Nelson JF, Ship I. Intraoral carcinoma. J Am Diet Assoc 1971; 82:564–568.
5. Wolf GT. Aging, the immune system and head and neck cancer. In: Goldstein JC, Kashima FG, Koopman CF, eds. Geriatric Otolaryngology. Philadelphia: BC Decker, 1989.
6. Chin R, Fisher RJ, Smee RI. Oropharyngeal cancer in the elderly. Int J Radiat Oncol Biol Phys 1995; 32:1007–1016.
7. Balducci L, Extermann M. Cancer and aging: an evolving panorama. Hematol Oncol Clin 2000; 14:1.
8. Anisimov I. Age is a risk factor in multistage carcinogenesis. In: Balducci L, Lyman GH, Ershler W, eds. Comprehensive Geriatric Oncology. Amsterdam: Hardwood Academic, 1998.

9. Campisi J. Aging and cancer: the double-edged sword of replicative senescence. J Am Geriatr Soc 1997; 45:482.
10. Preti HA. Prognostic value of serum interleukin-6 in diffuse large-cell lymphoma. Ann Int Med 1997; 127:186.
11. Clayman GL, Eicher SA, Sicard MW, Razmpa E, Goepfert H. Surgical outcomes in head and neck cancer patients 80 years of age and older. Head Neck 1998; 20:216.
12. Barzan L, Veronesi A, Caruso G, et al. Head and neck cancer and aging: a retrospective study in 438 patients. J Laryngol Otol 1990; 104:634.
13. Singh B, Alfonso A, Sabin S, et al. Outcome differences in younger and older patients with laryngeal cancer: a retrospective case-control study. Am J Otolaryngol 2000; 121:92.
14. Rapidis AD, Keramidis T, Panagiotopoulos H, Adressakis D, Angelopoulos AP. Tumours of the head and neck in the elderly: analysis of 190 patients. J Craniomaxillofac Surg 1998; 26:153.
15. McGuirt WF, Davis SP. Demographic portrayal and outcome analysis of head and neck cancer surgery in the elderly. Arch Otolaryngol Head Neck Surg 1995; 121:150.
16. Shaari CM, Buchbinder D, Costantino PD, Lawson W, Biller HF, Urken ML. Complications of microvascular head and neck surgery in the elderly. Arch Otolaryngol Head Neck Surg 1998; 124:407.
17. Sarini J, Fournier C, Lefebvre J, Bonafos G, Van JT, Coche-Dequéant B. Head and neck squamous cell carcinoma in elderly patients: a long-term retrospective review of 273 cases. Arch Otolaryngol Head Neck Surg 2001; 127:1089.
18. Tada T. Nutrition and the immune system in aging: an overview. Nutr Rev 1992; 50:360.
19. Cohen HJ. Biology of aging as related to cancer. Cancer 1994; 74:2092–2100.
20. Kemeny MM. Cancer surgery in the elderly. Hematol Oncol Clin North Am 2000; 14:169.
21. Morgan RF, Hirata RM, Jaques DA, Hoopes JE. Head and neck surgery in the aged. Am J Surg 1982; 144:449–451.
22. Balducci L, Trotti A. Organ preservation: an effective and safe form of cancer treatment. Clin Geriatr Med 1997; 13:185.
23. Zacharia B, Balducci L. Radiation therapy of the older patient. Hemat Oncol Clin North Am 2000; 14:131.
24. Balducci L, Corcoran MB. Cytotoxic chemotherapy in the older cancer patient. Hematol Oncol Clin 2000; 14:196.
25. Pignon T, Horiot JC, Van den Bogaert W. No age limit for radical radiotherapy in lead and neck tumors. Evr J Cancer 1996; 32:2075–2081.
26. Chen AY, Matsen LK, Roberts D, Goepfert H. The significance of comorbidity in advanced laryngeal cancer. Head Neck 2001; 23:556.

ANNOTATED BIBLIOGRAPHY

Clayman GL, Eicher SA, Sicard MW, et al. Surgical outcomes in head and neck cancer patients 80 years of age and older. Head Neck 1998; 20:216–222.

Unlike many other papers, deals with a true geriatric group. Honest and throught provoking.

McGuirt WF, Davis SP. Demographic portrayal and outcome analysis of head and neck cancer surgery in the elderly. Arch Otolaryngol Head Neck Surg 1995; 121:150–154.

Clear analysis. Supporting the role of surgical therapy of these patients if appropriate.

45

Thyroid Diseases in the Elderly

Maisie Shindo and Frances Tanzella
*Division of Otolaryngology—Head and Neck Surgery, Department of Surgery,
State University of New York–Stony Brook, Stony Brook, New York, U.S.A.*

INTRODUCTION

Diseases of the thyroid are commonly seen in the aging population. Clinical manifestations of both benign and malignant thyroid diseases in the elderly are somewhat different than in the young. These differences mandate alternative management strategies when comparing treatment in the elderly and the younger populations. Surgeons who evaluate and manage patients with thyroid disorders need to be familiar with the differences between the young and geriatric populations in the manifestations and management of benign and malignant thyroid diseases. This chapter focuses primarily on the evaluation and management of thyroid diseases in the geriatric population.

HYPOTHYROIDISM

In comparison to the younger age group, hypothyroidism is much more common in the elderly and frequently is subclinical: abnormal thyroid functions test(s) without overt clinical symptoms. The prevalence of overt or subclinical hypothyroidism in the elderly population varies considerably in the literature. This wide variation is in part due to the patient population and criteria used in different surveys, and in part because of variability in dietary intake and ethnicity. In prevalence studies published in the last decade, the incidence of hypothyroidism ranges from 1.6% to 10% (1–6).

The most common causes of hypothyroidism are autoimmune thyroid diseases. Patients with a history of Graves' disease or chronic lymphocytic thyroiditis may develop hypothyroidism years after the diagnosis. This may be a result of the treatment (e.g., radioactive iodine, antithyroid medications) or the natural course of the disorder. Long-term high dietary consumption of iodine has been shown to increase thyroid autoimmunity, which increases the risk of developing hypothyroidism (7,8). Certain drugs may also precipitate the development of hypothyroidism, particularly those containing iodine, such as amiodarone, cough medications, and iodine containing radiographic contrast agents.

Common symptoms of hypothyroidism are cold intolerance, fatigue, dry skin, and constipation. Less common symptoms include paresthesias, ileus, edematous changes, and neurologic manifestations, such as carpal tunnel syndrome, paresthesias, ataxia, and decreased cognitive function. The diagnosis of hypothyroidism is based on laboratory testing. The hallmark is an elevated thyroid-stimulating hormone (TSH) ($>10\,mU/L$). In overt hypothyroidism, the total T4, free T4, and/or total T3 will also be low, while in subclinical hypothyroidism they will be normal. Generally, an elevated TSH with a low T4 is sufficient to make a diagnosis of hypothyroidism. An ultrasensitive TSH is an excellent screening test for hypothyroidism, unless the patient has hypothalamic dysfunction or a TSH producing pituitary tumor, both of which are extremely rare. Low T4 or T3 values alone should not be used to make a diagnosis of hypothyroidism in elderly patients, particularly in the presence of concurrent severe illnesses or in the intensive care setting. In these settings, especially if hypothermia or sepsis is present, the TSH level will actually be normal or low rather than being elevated. Only a small percentage of these patients ($<25\%$) turn out to have hypothyroidism. In others, the abnormality was due to being on other medications, such as steroids, or their nonthyroidal illness. This condition has been termed "euthyroid sick syndrome." Thyroid antibodies are generally not helpful in making a diagnosis of hypothyroidism. However, they may be of prognostic value. In subclinical hypothyroidism with mildly elevated TSH, positive antibodies help predict future thyroidal failure, which helps clinicians plan a management strategy (9).

Surgeons need to be cognizant of the effects of hypothyroidism on various organ systems that can potentially result in perioperative complications. First and foremost are the cardiovascular manifestations. The incidence of hypercholesterolemia and hyperlipidemia in hypothyroid patients is higher than the general population (10). This implies that patients with prolonged hypothyroidism are predisposed to atherosclerotic disease. Hypothyroidism appears to impair myocardial function; thus, patients may present with exertional dyspnea, orthopnea, cardiomegaly, bradycardia, and weak pulse. In severe cases of hypothyroidism, cardiomyopathy with decreased cardiac output and congestive heart failure may be present. Generalized edema may be present as a result of increased capillary permeability and/or congestive heart failure. Echocardiogram changes in hypothyroidism include sinus bradycardia, low voltage, prolonged QT interval, and rarely conduction disturbances. Hyponatremia is usually seen in elderly hypothyroid patients, partly due to excessive secretion of antidiuretic hormone. This condition may be made worse with postoperative pain, a factor that increases antidiuretic hormone secretion. Ventilatory weaning may be prolonged in elderly patients with hypothyroidism due to complex disturbances in respiratory function. These disturbances include impaired chest wall mechanics, decreased ventilatory drive, and possibly diminished diffusion capacity. The hypothyroid state decreases cerebral blood flow; however, the cerebral oxygen consumption remains unchanged, thus increasing the chance of cerebral hypoxia while under general anesthesia. While all of the above alterations in metabolism from hypothyroidism are known, it has not been clearly established that operating on patients in the presence of mild to moderate hypothyroidism increases the occurrence of major complications. In fact, two studies have demonstrated that surgical outcomes in untreated mild to moderately hypothyroid patients are similar to controls with respect to postoperative ventilation, fluid and electrolyte imbalances, frequency of arrhythmias, and incidence of myocardial infarction (11,12). It is difficult to definitely conclude from these studies that there is no increased risk of major complication when operating on hypothyroid patients since the number of subjects were small (59 and 40). In patients who are mildly hypothyroid but need surgical treatment somewhat urgently (for example, cancer, symptomatic tracheal compression), it would not be unreasonable to proceed with surgery with aggressive perioperative monitoring of electrolytes and hemodynamics. For nonurgent elective surgery, it would be prudent to initiate thyroid hormone replacement to correct the hypothyroidism before surgery. Because elderly patients with hypothyroidism may have underlying coronary disease and elderly patients generally require a smaller amount of thyroxine, the initial dose of thyroxine should be lower than the average starting dose in younger patients, which is usually 50–100 µg/day.

HYPERTHYROIDISM

It is important to understand the difference between the terminologies thyrotoxicosis and hyperthyroidism. Thyrotoxicosis means elevated T4 and T3 values, which can be due to thyroidal or nonthyroidal causes. Hyperthyroidism is a sustained hyperfunction of the thyroid gland, which can cause thyrotoxicosis. The risk of hyperthyroidism increases with age. The condition can present in elderly patients with overt clinical symptoms, but more often than not is subclinical. The causes of thyrotoxicosis are listed in Table 1. Contrary to the young population, the most common cause of hyperthyroidism in the elderly is toxic multinodular goiter. In a recent study of 313 patients over 55 years of age with thyrotoxicosis, the etiologies were multinodular goiter in 43%, Graves' disease in 21%, and toxic adenoma in 12%. Overmedication with thyroxine was the cause in 16% of patients. When the patients with hyperthyroidism were subdivided into overt and subclinical hyperthyroidism, the distribution of the etiologies was quite different. In older patients with subclinical hyperthyroidism, the majority of patients (89%) had toxic goiter. Graves' disease (5%) and toxic adenomatous nodule (6%) were seen much less often. The etiologies in elderly patients with overt hyperthyroidism are quite different: 41% have Graves' disease, 38% have toxic multinodular goiter, and 21% have toxic adenomatous nodule. Rarely, immigrants from iodine-deficient goiterous regions may become hyperthyroid when they change to an iodine-rich diet. The mechanism

Table 1 Causes of Thyrotoxicosis

Hyperthyroidism	Thyrotoxicosis without hyperthyroidism
Primary thyroid pathology	Thyroiditis
Graves' disease	Increased TBG or T_4-binding prealbumin
Toxic multinodular goiter	Thyrotoxicosis factitia
Toxic adenomatous nodule	Medications
TSH-secreting pituitary adenoma	Steroids
	Estrogens
	Amiodarone
	Heparin
	Abnormal binding to albumin
	Acute nonthyroidal illness
	Peripheral resistance to thyroid hormone
	Endogenous antibodies to T_4
	Familial dysalbuminemia

Abbreviations: TBG, thyroxine binding globulin; TSH, thyroid-stimulating hormone.

of precipitating the hyperthyroidism is thought to be due to the development of an efficient large goiter in an iodine-deficient region with higher stores of pre-iodinated hormones. The addition of iodine suddenly increases the T4 and T3 production. This results in hyperthyroidism.

Elderly patients may present with either the classic symptoms and signs of hyperthyroidism or with atypical manifestations. One of the consistent findings in hyperthyroidism at any age is that it affects the cardiovascular system, but the presenting clinical signs and symptoms can be quite different between the young and older populations. Unlike the young, who often present with palpitations and tachycardia, the most common cardiovascular manifestation associated with hyperthyroidism in the elderly is congestive heart failure. The second most common is atrial fibrillation. Occasionally, hyperthyroid elderly patients will complain of new or worsening angina. Young persons with hyperthyroidism classically have moist, smooth skin and diaphoresis, whereas elderly hyperthyroid patients' skin tends to be coarse. Neurologically, elderly hyperthyroid patients are less likely to present with the fine tremor that young hyperthyroid patients often have. Young hyperthyroid patients typically have an increase in appetite, and their weight change can vary depending on the types of food that they consume. In contrast, hyperthyroid elderly patients tend to have a reduction in appetite and weight loss with muscle wasting. Myopathy of proximal muscles is a consistent finding in the elderly. Loose bowel movement, which is a frequent complaint in young hyperthyroid patients, is a rare complaint in elderly patients with hyperthyroidism. Rather, those who normally have chronic constipation may note that their bowel movements are more normal. Very rarely, an elderly patient with hyperthyroidism can present with apathetic thyrotoxicosis, where they appear frail, significantly wasted, depressed, and myxedematous. In severe, uncontrolled hyperthyroidism, thyroid storm can precipitate, the manifestations of which are severe arrhythmias, hyperthermia, agitation, pulmonary edema, and cardiovascular collapse.

The hallmark of clinically overt hyperthyroidism is a suppressed low TSH (usually <0.5 mU/L) with elevated T4 and/or T3 levels. Subclinical hyperthyroidism

Table 2 Interpretation of Thyroid Function Tests

	TSH	T4 or FT4	T3
Clinical hyperthyroidism	Low	High	High
Subclinical hyperthyroidism	Low	Normal or upper limit of normal	Normal or upper limit of normal
Medications: estrogens, steroids, heparin, amiodarone Familial dysalbuminemia Peripheral T4 resistance Abnormal binding to albumin	Normal	High	High
Iatrogenic (thyrotoxicosis factitia)	Low or lower limit of normal	High	High
Euthyroid sick syndrome	Low	Low or normal	Low or normal
TSH secreting pituitary tumor	Normal or high	High	High

Abbreviation: TSH, thyroid-stimulating hormone.

is where the TSH level is suppressed but the T4 and T3 values are within normal range, and the patient rarely has any symptoms. Table 2 summarizes the typical laboratory findings that are seen with the different causes of hyperthyroidism. A low TSH value is virtually diagnostic of overt or subclinical hyperthyroidism due to primary thyroid pathology (Graves' disease, toxic goiter, toxic adenoma). One exception to this is euthyroid sick syndrome, as mentioned in the previous section, where the TSH may also be low. T4 and T3 values help differentiate the two entities. T4 and T3 will be normal or elevated in hyperthyroidism, low in euthyroid sick syndrome. The other exception is overmedication with thyroxine replacement (thyrotoxicosis factitia), which is easily diagnosed with the patient's medical history. As shown in Table 2, elevated total T4 and T3 levels alone are not sufficient to make a diagnosis of hyperthyroidism. A suppressed TSH level is required. For example, since T4 and T3 are tightly bound to proteins, medications, such as estrogen replacement, can increase the level of binding proteins and result in elevated total T4 and T3 levels; however, the free T4 and TSH levels are actually normal, and the patient does not have hyperthyroidism. One other cause of elevated T4 and T3 is a TSH-secreting pituitary adenoma, an extremely rare entity, where the TSH is also elevated. In general, similar to screening for hypothyroidism, TSH is also an excellent screening test for hyperthyroidism. It is of utmost importance that surgeons who are evaluating a "hyperthyroid" patient for surgery review the thyroid function tests and confirm that the patient truly has hyperthyroidism and not "thyrotoxicosis" secondary to nonhyperthyroid causes so that the indications for surgery is appropriate. Furthermore, determining the etiology of hyperthyroidism is important in treatment selection and planning.

Untreated hyperthyroidism in the elderly can result in life-threatening complications and therefore deserves prompt management. The treatment of hyperthyroidism depends on the severity of the symptoms and the etiology. Treatment options include medications, radioiodine treatment with ^{131}I, or thyroidectomy, all of which should be discussed with the patient. In general, if the patient has overt hyperthyroidism, antithyroid medications are initiated to decrease the production of thyroid hormones. The two most commonly used antithyroid medications are in the class of thionamides: propylthiouracil (PTU) 100–300 mg/day divided three times daily, and methimazole (Tapazole) 10–40 mg/day divided twice or three times daily. A potentially fatal complication with the use of this class of drugs is agranulocytosis, the incidence of which fortunately is < 0.5%. Other adverse reactions of thionamides are generally minor and include rash, arthralgia, myalgia, neuritis, and hypothyroidism. If the patient has palpitations and tachycardia, a beta-blocker may be added. Inderal is generally the preferred beta-blocker, since unlike other beta-blockers it has some inhibitory effect on peripheral conversion of the inactive thyroid hormone T4 to the active hormone T3. Since Inderal is a nonselective beta-blocker, a contraindication to its use is the presence of restrictive pulmonary disease, e.g., asthma. Once the patient's thyrotoxicosis improves with medications, the decision can be made with regards to what should be the long-term management. Since remission will be achieved in approximately one-third of Graves' disease patients treated with thionamides, continuing the pharmacotherapy with close monitoring for side effects is a reasonable option. Otherwise, ^{131}I is the preferred treatment, since it is quite effective for this disease. Some young patients, especially women of child bearing age, prefer thyroidectomy over [131]I. In the elderly, thyroidectomy is generally performed for failed ^{131}I treatment or the presence of a malignant nodule. The relapse rate for treating toxic multinodular goiters with pharmacotherapy is high. Takats et al. (13) compared the efficacy of antithyroid medications to ^{131}I for treatment of toxic multinodular goiter and reported a 46% relapse rate with methimazole treatment because of noncompliance or dose reduction by the physician. They preferred ^{131}I or thyroidectomy as the definitive treatment for toxic multinodular goiter. While ^{131}I can be effective for treatment of toxic goiters, a larger dose than what is conventionally used to treat Graves' disease is generally necessary. In the same study by Takats et al. (13), 79% of those treated with high doses of ^{131}I achieved euthyroidism, while 21% required re-treatment or continuation of methimazole. Furthermore, when low does of ^{131}I were used, only 29% achieved euthyroidism and 64% required retreatment. The authors also stressed that if ^{131}I is to be used for treatment of toxic goiters, the goal should be to use high doses to achieve hypothyroidism, which can be controlled with thyroxine replacement, rather than trying to achieve euthyroidism, which has a significant risk of relapse. In young patients with low anesthetic risks, excellent results can also be achieved with surgery. Surgery should be recommended as an alterative to ^{131}I, particularly if large or cold nodules are present. In elderly patients, ^{131}I is often used to treat toxic multinodular goiters, since they frequently have comorbidities that increase their risk of perioperative complications. The indications for thyroidectomy in elderly patients with toxic multinodular goiter include very large goiters with significant tracheal compression, presence of a large or cold nodule that may be suspicious for malignancy, failed ^{131}I treatment, and patient preference. Whether the treatment of choice is ^{131}I or thyroidectomy, the patient should be made euthyroid or close to euthyroid with antithyroid medications in order to minimize the risk of developing thyroid storm from the surgery or [131]I. When operating on patients with Graves' disease, an iodine preparation, such as Lugol's solution (5–10 drops tid) or potassium iodide (SSKI) (100–200 mg tid), is started 10 days preoperatively to decrease the vascularity of the gland. Toxic adenomas are less common in the elderly and can be treated with hemithyroidectomy if the patient's anesthetic risks are low. If surgery is contraindicated, they can be treated with [131]I.

There is no general consensus on the treatment of subclinical hyperthyroidism. In a recent survey of 185 endocrinologists on management approaches to subclinical hyperthyroidism, the decision to treat or observe appeared to be influenced by age and level of TSH (14).

NONTOXIC GOITERS

Approaches to management of nontoxic goiters may be different between the young and the old. The management approach to a young patient with a small nontoxic goiter varies considerably among clinicians. While some take a very conservative approach and observe the nodule, others take a more aggressive approach with ultrasound-guided biopsy if the nodule is greater than 1 cm in size. Small nontoxic goiters in the elderly patient can generally be observed with periodic thyroid sonogram and thyroid function tests; nodules are biopsied when growth is observed or if the patient has a history of prior external irradiation.

There is little disagreement that large nodules, particularly if they are hypofunctional, should undergo fine needle aspiration (FNA). Thyroidectomy is recommended if the cytology is suspicious for a malignancy. In young patients with large solid nodules, particularly if they are solid or demonstrate some atypia, surgical excision for definitive diagnosis and long-term treatment may be the preferred management over long-term observation. However, in elderly patients with this scenario, observation with periodic FNAs rather than surgical excision is often recommended.

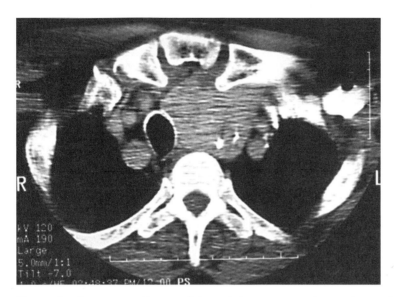

Figure 1   Noncontrast CT scan of the neck demonstrates a large substernal goiter with tracheal deviation to the right in a 70-year-old patient, which was incidentally found on a chest X ray.

Regardless of which approach is taken, the limitations and risks of observation/ FNA should be explained to the patient and the alternative of surgical excision should be considered. Certainly, in a "young" geriatric patient with very little or no comorbidities, surgical excision is a reasonable treatment.

There is little disagreement that thyroidectomy is the preferred treatment modality in young patients with large goiters or nodules causing tracheoesophageal compression. However, the management decision is not as straightforward in the elderly. Certainly, rapidly growing nodules in an elderly patient is worrisome for an aggressive thyroid malignancy (see section on thyroid malignancy below) and therefore requires FNA. Compressive goiters that are known to have been present for years with little change in size in the asymptomatic elderly patient can be observed. However, compressive goiters that are incidentally discovered in elderly patients on a chest X ray or CT scan often pose a management dilemma. If the patient has radiographic evidence of compression, such as a deviated or narrow trachea (Fig. 1) but is asymptomatic, observation with or without FNA of large nodule(s) is a reasonable approach. If the patient is experiencing dysphagia or shortness of breath, it is important to determine if the etiology of the symptoms is due to the goiter or due to some other conditions that frequently coexist in elderly patients, such as congestive heart failure, cricopharyngeal spasm, or esophageal dysmotility. Pulmonary functions tests with flow loops may be helpful if extrathoracic obstruction is seen. However, a normal flow loop does not necessarily exclude symptomatic tracheal compression. An esophagram, if it demonstrates extrinsic compression, may also provide supportive evidence that the goiter is causing dysphagia. However, a normal study does not necessarily mean that the goiter is not the cause of the dysphagia. It is very important to review a noncontrast CT of the chest with lower neck views to determine the extent of tracheal compression or if esophageal compression is truly present to help determine if the patient may actually benefit from thyroidectomy. In the absence of other concurrent conditions that can explain the patient's compressive symptoms, subtotal or near-total thyroidectomy should be recommended.

THYROID MALIGNANCIES

Most thyroid malignancies are well differentiated and occur under age 60, with generally excellent prognosis. The characteristics and behavior of thyroid cancers in the elderly are quite different. The overall distribution of thyroid cancers in the general population is approximately 80% papillary carcinoma, 10% follicular carcinoma, 5% medullary carcinoma, 3.5% Hurthle cell, and approximately 2% aggressive tumors, such as anaplastic cancer and undifferentiated cancers. Lymphoma and sarcomas comprise approximately 1.5% (15). In the elderly population, a lower percentage of papillary carcinoma is seen, and there is a slight preponderance of tumors that tend to be more aggressive. Recent analysis on thyroid cancers in patients over 60 years of age revealed that only 47% to 69% were papillary, approximately 20% were follicular or Hurthle cell, and 6% to 19% were anaplastic or undifferentiated (15,16). Anaplastic thyroid carcinoma is primarily a disease that occurs in patients over 45 years of age, approximately half of the patients being over 60 years of age (17,22).

Unlike young individuals, the geriatric population tend to present with locally aggressive disease and more advanced stage. Lin et al. (16) reported that Tumor, Nodes, Metastases (TNM) staging of the disease [American Joint Committee on Cancer (AJCC) staging] at the time of presentation was stage IV in 49% in patients over 60 years of age in contrast to 11% in those under 60. The incidence of extrathyroidal extension increases with advancing age. Approximately one-half of patients over 70 years of age with well-differentiated thyroid cancer (WDTC) present with T4 stage (AJCC staging) (18). Coburn and Wanebo (19) compared the frequency of high risk factors in three age groups: ages 21–50, 51–70, and over 70. The relative frequencies of extrathyroidal extension in the three groups were 38% in group 1, 49% in group 2, and 79% in group 3, respectively; the incidence of vascular invasion in patients who are over 70 years of age was 78%, also significantly higher than that of the younger population (45% in patients 51–70 years old and 38% in patients younger than 50) (19).

It has been well established that the overall disease-free 10-year survival rate for patients with WDTC is approximately 90% (16,20). However, in the geriatric population, the 10-year survival for WDTC is less than 50% (18,19,21). There appears to be a liner decrement in survival rate with advancing age. In fact, the 10-year survival rate nearly halves with a 10-year difference in age at diagnosis: 10-year disease-specific survival is approximately 50% if diagnosed between age 60 and 70, and < 25% if diagnosed over age 70 (16,18). This has been attributed to several factors. There is a higher preponderance of poor prognostic factors in this population, such as extrathyroidal extension, vascular invasion, and distant metastasis. The radioactive iodine uptake by metastatic disease in follicular-derived thyroid cancers decreases with age (23).

While there is general agreement that WDTC in the young population should be treated first with thyroidectomy, the decision to operate in a geriatric patient who presents with this disease needs to factor in the comorbidities present at the time of diagnosis and extent of the disease. Those whose risk stratification for general anesthesia indicate a low to moderate risk and have localized disease should undergo total thyroidectomy and postoperative [131]I. Those with advanced local disease without distant metastasis, and with low to moderate anesthetic risk, may be considered for surgically "debulking" the gross disease and postoperative irradiation. In patients over 70 years of age, aggressive local resection of the aerodigestive tract, such as laryngotreacheal resection or esophagectomy, is probably not indicated, since the morbidity from this type of aggressive resection is very high in this age group, and one is not likely to alter their disease outcome. Those who have extensive local disease and distant metastasis with coexisting severe comorbidities should in most cases be treated with comfort or palliative measures. External beam irradiation is a reasonable option for treatment of gross residual disease after surgery or for palliation.

REFERENCES

1. Griffin JE. Hypothyroidism in the elderly. AM J Med Sci 1990; 299:334–345.
2. Bemben DA, Winn P, Hamm RM, Morgan L, Davis A, Barton E. Thyroid disease in the elderly. Part I. Prevalence of undiagnosed hypothyroidism. J Fam Pract 1994; 38: 577–582.
3. Parle JV, Franklyn JA, Cross KW, Jones SC, Sheppard MC. Prevalence and follow-up of abnormal thyrotrophin (TSH) concentrations in the elderly in the United Kingdom. Clin Endocrinol 1991; 34:77–83.
4. Chuang CC, Wang ST, Wang PW, Yu ML. Prevalence study of thyroid dysfunction in the elderly of Taiwan. Gerontology 1998; 44:162–167.
5. Muller GM, Levitt NS, Louw SJ. Thyroid dysfunction in the elderly. South African Med J 1997; 87:1119–1123.
6. Samuels MH. Subclinical thyroid disease in the elderly. Thyroid 1998; 8:803–813.
7. Mizukami Y, Michigishi T, Nonomura A, et al. Iodine-induced hypothyroidism: a clinical and histological study of 28 patients. J Clin Endocrinol Metab 1993; 76:466–471.
8. Allen AM, Appel MC, Braverman LE, et al. The effect of iodide ingestion on the development of spontaneous lymphocytic thyroiditis in the diabetes-prone BB/W rat. Endocrinology 1986; 118:1977–1981.
9. Rosental MJ, Hunt WC, Garry PJ, Goodwin JS. Thyroid failure in the elderly. Microsomal antibodies as discriminant for therapy. JAMA 1987; 258:209–213.
10. O'Brien T, Dinneen SF, O'Brien PC, et al. Hyperlipidemia in patients with primary and secondary hypothyroidism. Mayo Clin Proc 1993; 68(9):860–866.
11. Weinberg AD, Brennan MD, Gorman CA, Marsh HM, O'Fallon WM. Outcome of anesthesia and surgery in hypothyroid patients. Arch Intern Med 1983; 143:893–897.
12. Ladenson PW, Levin AA, Ridgway EC. Complications of surgery in hypothyroid patients. Am J Med 1984; 77:261–266.
13. Takats KI, Szaboles I, Foldes J, et al. The efficacy of long term thyrostatic treatment in elderly patients with toxic nodular goiter compared to radioiodine therapy with different doses. Exp Clin Endocrinol Diabetes 1999; 107:70–77.
14. McDermott MT, Wookmansee WW, Haugen BR, Smart A, Ridgway EC. The management of subclinical hyperthyroidism by thyroid specialists. Thyroid 2003; 12:1133–1139.
15. Hundahl SA, Cady B, Cunningham MP, et al. Initial results from a prospective cohort study of 5583 cases of thyroid carcinoma treated in the United States during 1996. Cancer 2000; 89:202–217.
16. Lin JD, Chao TC, Chen ST, Weng HF, Lin KD. Characteristics of thyroid carcinomas in aging patients. Eur J Clin Invest 2000; 30:147–153.
17. Andersen PE, Kinsella J, Loree TR, Shaha AR, Shah JP. Differentiated carcinoma of the thyroid with extrathyroidal extension. Am J Surg 1995; 170:467–470.
18. Vini L, Hyer S, Marshall J, A' Hern R, Harmer C. Long-term results in elderly patients with differentiated thyroid carcinoma. Cancer 2003; 97:2736–2742.
19. Coburn MC, Wanebo HJ. Age correlates with increased frequency of high-risk factors in elderly patients with thyroid cancer. Am J Surg 1995; 170:471–475.
20. Mazzaferri EL, Jhiang SM. Long-term impact of initial surgical and medical therapy of papillary and follicular thyroid cancer. Am J Med 1994; 97:418–428.

21. Girelli ME, Casara D, Rubello D, Mazzarotto R, Saladini, Busnardo B. Differentiated thyroid carcinoma in the elderly: disease outcome, therapeutic approach, and long-term results in a group of 314 patients. J Endocrinol Invest 1999; 22:45–46.
22. Rodriguez JM, Pinero A, Ortiz S, Moreno A, et al. Clinical and histological differences in anaplastic thyroid carcinoma. Eur J Surg 2000; 166:34–38.
23. Schlumberger M, Challeton C, DeVathaire F, et al. Radioactive iodine treatment and external radiotherapy for lung and bone metastasis from thyroid carcinoma. J Nucl Med 1996; 37:598–605.

46
Parathyroid Diseases in the Elderly

Maisie Shindo and Frances Tanzella
Division of Otolaryngology—Head and Neck Surgery, Department of Surgery, State University of New York–Stony Brook, Stony Brook, New York, U.S.A.

Primary hyperparathyroidism predominantly affects individuals between the ages of 55 and 70, with a reported incidence of approximately 2% to 7% in the elderly population (1–3). With the increase in life expectancy in the United States, the prevalence of primary hyperparathyroidism in the geriatric population will likely increase. The clinical presentation of hyperparathyroidism in the elderly is somewhat different from that of the younger population. Management approaches in the two age groups may also differ. This chapter gives a brief overview of primary and secondary hyperparathyroidism and focuses on primary hyperparathyroidism, atypical presentations in the elderly patient population, evaluation of the geriatric patient with hypercalcemia, and the efficacy and safety of parathyroid surgery in the elderly.

PATHOPHYSIOLOGY OF HYPERPARATHYROIDISM

Hyperparathyroidism can be primary, secondary, or tertiary. In primary hyperparathyroidism (PHPT), the parathyroid gland(s) autonomously hypersecretes parathyroid hormone (PTH). The etiology is a single parathyroid adenoma in 80% to 85% of cases, with hyperplasia or multiple adenomas making up the remainder. Secondary hyperparathyroidism occurs when the elevation in parathyroid hormone is a result of chronic renal insufficiency. PTH controls the level of ionized calcium in the extra cellular fluid. When the ionized calcium level falls, PTH secretion is stimulated. In uremia the serum calcium level is severely reduced, which can result in hyperplasia of the parathyroid glands. Vitamin D enhances the intestinal absorption of calcium and may also enhance its renal tubular absorption. It acts with PTH to maintain the level of ionized calcium in the extracellular fluid. Poor calcium intake related to gastrointestinal disorders and vitamin D deficiencies can also cause a compensatory rise in PTH levels. Dietary calcium and vitamin D intake is often marginal in elderly patients. Furthermore, decreased efficiency in absorption of calcium is common in the elderly. All these factors can lead to hypersecretion of PTH to mobilize calcium from the skeleton. In tertiary hyperparathyroidism, which is rarely seen in the elderly, the hyperplastic glands autonomously continue to secrete PTH despite correction of chronic renal failure with successful renal transplantation.

DIAGNOSIS

A diagnosis of PHPT is most often based on an elevated intact PTH with an elevated serum calcium level. However, patients with PHPT may not always exhibit elevated PTH levels on all tests. Some patients may present with high normal PTH levels and an elevated serum calcium level. In the absence of PHPT, an elevated serum calcium should suppress the PTH level. Therefore, a PTH level that is in the upper range of normal with an elevated serum calcium is "inappropriate" and suggests PHPT. In the literature, PHPT is by definition elevated serum calcium in the presence of elevated or inappropriately normal parathyroid hormone. Patients may also not exhibit elevated serum calcium levels on all tests but present with values in the upper normal range. A small group of patients may only exhibit an elevated ionized calcium (4).

It is helpful to look at several sets of calcium and PTH levels as well as 24-hour urine calcium and serum phosphate levels to make the diagnosis of PHPT. Typically in PHPT, the serum phosphate is low, and the 24-hour urine calcium is elevated or in the normal range. Thus, in a patient with only periodic elevations of serum calcium, if the PTH levels are persistently elevated, the serum phosphate is low, and 24-hour urine calcium is high (>350 mg), the diagnosis of PHPT is likely. In an elderly patient with normal or occasional mildly elevated calcium levels, intermittent mild elevation of PTH, normal phosphate, and normal 24-hour urine calcium, the diagnosis of PHPT is somewhat questionable.

Other than PHPT, the differential diagnosis of hypercalcemia in the elderly include thiazide diuretics, renal insufficiency, acute renal failure, chronic vitamin D deficiency, immobilization, hypercalcemia of malignancy, granulomatous disease, and other endocrine disorders (thyrotoxicosis, pheochromocytoma, and adrenal crisis) (5). When the diagnosis is uncertain, it would be prudent to follow the laboratory values. An elevated serum calcium and PTH with a *low* 24-hour urine calcium may be due to familial hypocalciuric hypercalcemia (FHH), which is an autosomal dominant genetic disorder. This condition manifests with hypercalcemia and mildly elevated or inappropriately normal PTH levels. While this condition is usually diagnosed at a younger age, it may manifest for the first time in an elderly patient who has not sought medical attention throughout life. It usually has a benign course and generally is not a surgical disease.

In secondary hyperparathyroidism, the typical laboratory findings are elevated intact PTH, blood urea nitrogen (BUN), and serum creatinine levels. Unlike PHPT, these patients typically have normal or low serum calcium levels and hyperphosphatemia.

MANIFESTATIONS OF PRIMARY HYPERPARATHYROIDISM

Elderly patients with PHPT often present with mildly elevated serum calcium and no other manifestations. They may also present with one or more of the following clinical manifestations: bone disease, neuromuscular symptoms, neuropsychiatric symptoms, cardiovascular manifestations, and hypercalcemic crisis. Rarely do they present with renal calculi, a condition more commonly seen the younger patient (6). The patient may complain of urinary frequency and nocturia, which are common complaints in the elderly, and may not necessarily be secondary to hyperparathyroidism.

Bone Disease

Elderly patients with primary hyperparathyroidism may exhibit variable degrees of bone disease, which may place them at an increase risk of fractures. One effect of PHPT on cortical bone is increased bone turnover with subsequent osteopenia and osteoporosis. While the effects of primary hyperparathyroidism on cortical bone are not completely understood, the resultant bone loss places the elderly patient at an increased susceptibility for serious fractures, disability, and even death. In the young age group, osteoporosis is likely secondary to PHPT. However, PHPT may not be the sole cause of osteopenia in an elderly patient, as other factors, such as menopause, reduced dietary calcium intake, immobilization, smoking, and use of corticosteroids for chronic disease, also contribute to development of cortical bone loss. Elderly patients with PHPT may complain of vague symptoms of bone or joint pain. While these symptoms may be related to PHPT, they may also be related to arthritis, a common condition in the elderly.

Neuromuscular and Psychiatric Manifestations

Classical neuromuscular symptoms in hyperparathyroidism include muscle weakness, atrophy, hyper-reflexia, altered gait, and tongue fasciculations (7). Elderly patients with PHPT have also exhibited a wide spectrum of mental and emotional dysfunction. The neuropsychiatric manifestations may be subtle, with patients experiencing fatigue, lethargy, apathy, or forgetfulness. They may also have been observed to have mood swings, depression, or even paranoia. In elderly patients, these symptoms are often attributed to Alzheimer's or senile dementia, brain atrophy, small vessel disease, or a primary psychiatric disorder. While the exact mechanism responsible for these symptoms remains unknown, mild elevations in serum calcium may produce symptoms; however, the severity of symptoms seems to correlate with the degree of calcium elevation (8). It is important to consider the diagnosis of primary hyperparathyroidism in the setting of new onset psychopathology.

Cardiovascular Effects

PHPT may contribute to left ventricular hypertrophy, dyslipidemia and coronary atherosclerosis, and hypertension. An increased risk of death from cardiovascular disease has been associated with high calcium levels. Asymptomatic PHPT, however, does not appear to be associated with overt cardiovascular abnormalities (1,9,10).

Hypercalcemic Crisis

This condition, where serum calcium levels are persistently higher than 12.5 mg/dL, can occur in the elderly with PHPT, especially in the setting of a concurrent illness that produces dehydration. It is more common in elderly patients, with a 6% incidence as compared to 3% in the younger patient (6). These patients may present with a severely altered mental status and may need hospitalization for hydration. Rehydration should be done judiciously in the elderly patient because of the risk of developing hypokalemia, hypophosphatemia, hypomagnesemia, and cardiac failure from rapid hydration. Hydration increases calcium excretion and will lower the serum level, but it rarely normalizes the serum calcium. If hydration does not effectively lower the calcium level, medications such as calcitonin can be used. Loop diuretics may be required once the patient is adequately hydrated to increase urinary calcium excretion (5,9).

EVALUATION

The surgeon's initial assessment of elderly patients referred for surgical treatment of PHPT should include a history and review of key laboratory tests to confirm the diagnosis, and determine what manifestations of the disease the patient has. Information on medication use, such as the use of thiazide diuretics and lithium, as well as dietary or supplemental calcium intake, should be elicited. A family history of hypercalcemia should raise the possibility of FHH. The key laboratory tests for establishing the diagnosis of PHPT are multiple serum calcium (corrected for albumin levels), the intact PTH level, and a 24-hour urine for calcium. Additional diagnostic tests that can also be helpful include 25-hydroxy vitamin D level to exclude vitamin D deficiency, and serum creatinine with 24-hour urine creatinine. The serum and urine creatinine levels are used to calculate the creatinine clearance ratio using the following formula:

$$\frac{\text{24-hour urine calcium}}{\text{Serum calcium}} \times \frac{\text{Serum creatinine}}{\text{24-hour urine creatinine}}$$

A ratio that is greater than 0.01 is consistent with PHPT and less than 0.01 is suggestive of FHH or may represent inadequate urine volume collection.

[99]Technesium Sestamibi parathyroid (MIBI) scan is generally obtained for preoperative localization if surgery is being contemplated. However, it may also be helpful in establishing the diagnosis of PHPT when the diagnosis is based on equivocal laboratory values. In elderly patients, BUN and creatinine levels may reveal the degree of renal insufficiency that may be associated with hyperparathyroidism. Often, it is difficult to differentiate if the renal insufficiency is a cause or a result of the hyperparathyroidism. If the patient has been known to have long-standing renal insufficiency and subsequently develops hyperparathyroidism, the condition may be secondary hyperparathyroidism rather than primary, and the surgeon should be prepared to perform subtotal/total parathyroidectomy and reimplantation. In patients with a long-standing history of renal calculi and renal insufficiency, renal imaging studies may reveal stones and/or hydronephrosis.

Bone densitometry can be obtained to evaluate the patient for osteopenia or osteoporosis. Serial bone densitometries can then be used to monitor subsequent changes in bone mineralization. An alkaline phosphatase level can also be obtained to assess the severity of bone disease.

SURGICAL TREATMENT

Historically, the traditional approach in parathyroid surgery has been to perform bilateral exploration and examine all four parathyroid glands. With bilateral exploration, multiglandular disease would not be missed; however, there is a greater risk of hypocalcemia and a potential risk of bilateral recurrent laryngeal nerve injury. With the ability to preoperatively localize an adenoma with imaging modalities (e.g., Sestamibi scan, ultrasound), unilateral exploration became popular and acceptable, with low complication and recurrence rates. With unilateral exploration, identification of a normal gland on the same side is required to make sure that the patient does not have four-gland hyperplasia. Nevertheless, if the patient has a second adenoma (double adenoma) on the contralateral side, this approach will miss it. Multiglandular disease is a facet of parathyroid surgery that continues to plague parathyroid surgeons. However, major advances in recent years, such as preoperative localization, radio-guided surgical excision, and intraoperative rapid measurement of PTH, have reduced the risk of missing multiglandular disease.

MIBI scan can localize an adenoma in 75% to 90% of cases, depending on the experience of the nuclear medicine physicians. Those with a positive scan are candidates for unilateral exploration or focused parathyroidectomy.

Intact parathyroid hormone (iPTH) has a very short half-life of approximately three minutes. Because of this very short half-life, the iPTH level should fall rapidly following successful removal of a single functioning parathyroid adenoma. Therefore, measurement of iPTH level in the patient after removal of an identified adenoma would theoretically predict the success of surgery. In 1991, Irvin et al. (11) introduced the concept of using the intraoperative measurement of PTH level to predict the postoperative calcium level. Since then its accuracy and utility have been confirmed by many authors (12–28), and it has become an important tool in parathyroid surgery. Various criteria have been published for intraoperative rapid PTH (IRPTH) levels that predict successful parathyroidectomy. The most commonly used criterion for predicting success is that first described by Irvin and Deriso (12): the IRPTH level falls below 50% of the highest pre-excision level within five minutes of excising the adenoma. Some use the IRPTH level at 10 minutes after excision rather than the five minutes postexcision value. Others also use more stringent criteria, such as the postexcision IRPTH level must fall at least 50% of baseline and must be below the upper limit of normal.

In 1994, Irvin et al. (12,13) published their early experience with a small number of patients demonstrating the feasibility of using IRPTH. They used a "focused" approach to excise an adenoma based on preoperative localization studies and using the IRPTH to determine if the procedure had been successful or needed to be converted to bilateral exploration. They showed that the sensitivity of IRPTH was 94% and that the operative times were significantly shorter. Subsequent to Irvin et al. reports, several authors evaluated the validity of IRPTH by measuring iPTH levels pre- and post-excision of abnormal gland(s) during conventional bilateral exploration. In these studies, the following parameters were evaluated: (i) accuracy in predicting uniglandular versus multiglandular disease, (ii) false positive, defined as IRPTH falls below 50% of baseline when one or more enlarged gland still remains, and (iii) false negative, defined as IRPTH failing to fall below 50% when no additional enlarged glands remain. The accuracy rates in the above studies ranged from 84% to 89%, with long-term chemical cure rates of 98% to 100%. The overall false positive rates were 2% to 13%. Twelve percent to 60% of patients with multiglandular disease will exhibit at least a 50% drop in the IRPTH following excision of only one enlarged gland (false positive). The overall false negative rates were 3% to 8% (18–21).

Subsequent to these initial validation studies, parathyroid surgeons began to use a focused "minimally invasive" approach. With this focused approach, in those with a positive preoperative localization study (MIBI parathyroid scan, and/or ultrasound), a small incision is made in the area of a suspected adenoma. Identification and removal of the adenoma is accomplished through standard open dissection or endoscopically. Others use radioguidance, where MIBI is injected approximately one hour prior to surgery, and a gamma probe is used to assist in the search for the adenoma. Following excision of the adenoma, the radioactive counts are measured with the probe. If the ex vivo count on the adenoma is greater than 20% of background count, the patient is considered to have only one adenoma, and surgery is deemed successful. This minimally invasive radioguided parathyroidectomy is referred to as MIRP. Some surgeons also combine MIRP with the use of IRPTH to confirm biochemical cure. A number of series have reported cure rates of at least 98% using this approach.

Several studies have compared the outcome of parathyroid surgery using a focused approach with intraoperative IRPTH to that of conventional bilateral exploration. The results of these studies indicate that when the focused approach is used, the success rates of the operation are similar to or better than that of bilateral exploration, and furthermore complication rates tend to be lower. Carneiro and Irvin (25) reported that in patients undergoing parathyroidectomy, the long-term postoperative calcium and iPTH levels were normal in 98% ($n = 144$) in those who had a focused approach versus 85% ($n = 176$) in those who underwent conventional bilateral exploration. Burkey et al. (26) compared the outcome of parathyroidectomy using three different approaches: (1) gamma probe ($n = 50$), (2) IRPTH ($n = 50$), (3) bilateral exploration ($n = 50$). The cure rates were 98%, 100%, and 96%, respectively, and the complication rate was higher in the bilateral exploration group compared to the other two. Similarly, Boggs et al. (24) reported a failure rate of 1.5% when Sestamibi and IRPTH were used versus 5% when bilateral exploration was performed without IRPTH. In a study to evaluate whether or not IRPTH improves the results of parathyroidectomy, Miura et al. (21) showed that by adding IRPTH to the operation, the accuracy of Sestamibi scan improved from 83% to 92%, and the accuracy of ultrasound improved from 71% to 86%.

While IRPTH significantly reduces the chances of missing multiglandular disease, operative morbidity, and length of hospital stay, it can still potentially miss multiple gland pathology, which may result in a need for reoperation. Hallfeldt et al. (27) reported that in 2 of 36 patients who met Irwin's criteria (50% IRPTH), but whose absolute IRPTH value remained above normal range, the iPTH levels began to elevate again postoperatively. One of these two patients was re-explored and found to have hyperplasia. Gauger et al. (29) reported changes in IRPTH values in 20 patients who were found to have double adenomas during conventional bilateral exploration. In 11 of the 20 patients, the IRPTH levels were ≤50% of baseline following excision of first adenoma. In these 11 patients, a second adenoma was found during the planned bilateral exploration. Thus, the false positive rate of IRPTH was 55% in this group of patients. In the remaining nine patients, the IRPTH values remained above 50% after excision of the first adenoma, giving a true negative rate of 45%. Similarly, Jaskowiak et al. (22) reported 50% false positive and 50% true negative rates for IRPTH when double adenomas are present. To explain this false positive phenomenon with double adenomas, some hypothesize that the second adenoma, which is usually the smaller one, may be suppressed or may not be hypersecretory. Therefore, if the second gland is not biochemically significant, the IRPTH value will actually drop below 50% after excision of the "active" one (29). Even with four-gland hyperplasia, IRPTH may exhibit kinetics similar to that of single adenomas. For example, one study reported that in 12.5% of patients who were undergoing surgery for known hyperplasia from MEN1 syndrome, the kinetics of IRPTH was similar to that seen with a single adenoma, e.g., <50% of baseline after excision of the first enlarged gland (30). Interestingly, the false positive rates with hyperplasia appear to be lower than that of double adenomas. Gordon et al. (18) reported that in their patients with multiglandular disease, IRPTH had a false positive rate of 24%. Furthermore, all of their false positives were double adenomas, and the first removed adenoma was generally larger than the second. In a retrospectives analysis of sequential changes in IRPTH during conventional bilateral exploration, Weber and Ritchie (20) reported a false positive rate of 37% when multiglandular disease is present; within this group the false positive rate was 67% for double adenomas and 31% for hyperplasia.

In a small percentage of patients, the postexcision intraoperative IRPTH may remain above 50% of baseline, yet their subsequent postoperative calcium and iPTH levels will return to normal, e.g., false negative IRPTH. The significance of a false negative value is that it results in unnecessary further exploration. One possible mechanism for such false negative values is that there can be a sudden rise in circulating PTH during manipulation of the adenoma; therefore, if the postexcision value is compared to a baseline drawn before manipulation, it may not be significantly lower than baseline or sometimes can actually be higher than the baseline. Therefore, some surgeons draw two baseline levels, one either prior to or after incision and one just before excision of the adenoma, and use the higher of the two for the true baseline level (4,12). Another option would be to repeat the IRPTH at either 10 or 15 minutes after excision, at which time the values may be close to 50% of baseline. Alternatively, the surgeon can choose to perform bilateral exploration, which may or may not be necessary.

Parathyroidectomy is indicated in patients who have complications of PHPT, such as nephrolithiasis, deterioration in renal function, acceleration of bone loss and fractures, and recurrent potentially life-threatening hypercalcemic crisis. In those who have not developed complications of the disease, surgical consideration should also be given to those with symptoms of bone and muscle pain, neuropsychological dysfunction, and onset of menopause. However, since the gamut of muscular and neuropsychological symptoms in the elderly is broad, the challenge for the practitioner is to determine which symptoms are truly due to PHPT. The indications for surgery in an asymptomatic patient have also been established. In 1990, an NIH-sponsored consensus panel recommended that parathyroidectomy is indicated in the asymptomatic patient if there are risk factors for progression of the disease. These guidelines are listed in Table 1 (31). In 2002, another concensus panel recommended modification of some of these 1990 guidelines (4). The recommended changes were: (i) calcium concentration 1.0 mg/dL above normal reference range, rather than 1.0–1.6 above normal; and (ii) bone density at the lumbar spine, hip, or distal radius that is more than 2.5 SD below peak bone mass (*t*-score <2.5), rather than age-, sex- and race-matched bone density that is less than 2.0 SD (*z*-score <2.0).

Table 1 Indications for Parathyroidectomy in an Asymptomatic Patient

Serum Ca^{2+} consistently >1–1.6 mg/dL above accepted normal range
Creatinine clearance reduced by 30% (age-matched)
24-hr urine Ca^{2+} >400
Reduction in bone density >2 SD (age-, gender-, and race-matched)
Under 50 years of age
Medical surveillance not suitable
Positive parathyroid Sestamibi scan

While it seems clear that parathyroidectomy should be recommended for those under 50 years of age with asymptomatic hyperparathyroidism, what to do with an elderly asymptomatic patient is not as well defined. Since parathyroidectomy traditionally has been performed under general anesthesia and required bilateral exploration, which has potential significant risks, many asymptomatic elderly patients have often been observed rather than treated surgically. However, in recent years, parathyroid surgery has evolved into minimally invasive focused exploration under local anesthesia, which has significantly lowered the risks and complications associated with surgery, if performed by an experienced surgeon. Minimally invasive focused parathyroidectomy certainly has a greater appeal in the elderly patient, since it can be performed under local anesthesia. Therefore, surgical consideration should be given to asymptomatic healthy elderly patients with a reasonably long life expectancy if they are appropriate candidates for minimally invasive parathyroidectomy (i.e., positive preoperative localization study).

NONSURGICAL MANAGEMENT

Patients who are not medically fit to undergo surgery or refuse surgery are observed or may be managed medically. Medical therapy targets two areas: to lower the serum calcium and to prevent progression of osteopenia or osteoporosis. Truly asymptomatic patients may be managed by reduction in calcium intake (<1000 mg/day), maintenance of hydration, and the avoidance of certain medications, which may precipitate hypercalcemia. Bisphosphonates are often used in patients with hyperparathyroidism and osteoporosis. They may also have a role in lowering the calcium level in acute hypercalcemic crisis, although rebound hypercalcemia may occur with long-term use (9). Estrogen hormone therapy has been shown to increase bone density, but there have been recent concerns regarding their safety. The risk of fractures in the elderly, however, may outweigh the potential risk of hormone therapy. There are trials in progress evaluating the benefits of Raloxifene, originally used in the treatment of breast cancer. This drug may be beneficial in the prevention of osteoporosis (9). Since asymptomatic patients may or may not develop progression of disease and there are no reliable predictors of bone loss, patients who opt for observation should have regular bone densitometry. In those with vitamin D deficiency, supplementation may have significant benefits, including a beneficial effect on the diastolic blood pressure (9). Vitamin D supplementation may initially worsen hypercalcemia; therefore, close monitoring of calcium is essential.

OUTCOME OF TREATMENT

A study by Rao et al. (32) evaluated the long-term effects on cortical bone in patients having undergone parathyroidectomy as compared to nonsurgically treated patients. The study showed that z-scores declined with age in both groups; however, the mean values became significantly less negative over time in the surgically treated group as compared to the z-scores of the nontreated patients. The authors concluded that surgery reduced further bone loss, and the benefit was dependant on the remaining life expectancy of the patient. In another study by Horiuchi et al. (33), the authors compared the use of Etidronate versus parathyroidectomy in the management of primary hyperparathyroidism in elderly women. The results showed an increase in lumbar spine bone mineral density in both groups after one year. The surgically treated group had an increase in lumbar spine bone density of 20%, compared to 10% in the group treated with Etidronate. The authors concluded that bisphosphonates were helpful in treating hypercalcemia and parathyroid hormone induced bone resorption in patients who were not surgical candidates; however, elderly patients should be considered for surgery when their medical condition does not pose an increased risk. There have been conflicting results from studies on the effects of parathyroidectomy on the cardiovascular system. In a study by Hagstrom et al. (34), lipid abnormalities were shown to be corrected by parathyroidectomy. A regression of left ventricular hypertrophy by echo was also noted. However, other studies showed no benefit in cardiovascular outcomes, including no change in hypertension in patients undergoing parathyroidectomy (1,6). Many studies have shown that parathyroidectomy improves neuropsychiatric and neuromuscular symptoms in some elderly patients, thereby improving the quality of life (1,3–7,9,32,33,35). However, it is not possible at this time to predict which patients will actually benefit from improvement of symptoms.

CONCLUSIONS

Primary hyperparathyroidism is a condition found more frequently in the elderly. As the life expectancy increases, there will be a greater number of elderly patients referred for evaluation and possible treatment. Parathyroidectomy is clearly indicated for elderly patients who have complications or symptoms from the disease. It has also been shown to improve the quality of life in patients previously thought to be asymptomatic. A thorough history as well as a comprehensive clinical and laboratory evaluation is essential to determine the course of treatment. Since parathyroidectomy can be performed minimally invasively, and has been shown to be safe, curative, and possibly improve the quality of life in the elderly patient, surgical treatment should be offered to those who are medically fit to undergo surgery and are expected to have a reasonable life expectancy. Those who do not want or are not medically fit to undergo surgery need to be monitored over time. Some elderly patients may not submit to long-term follow-up due to the expense and time commitment. The decision for the type of treatment is best made jointly by the patient, the endocrinologist, the primary care provider, and the surgeon.

REFERENCES

1. Roche NA, Young AE. Role of surgery in mild hyperparathyroidism in the elderly. Br J Surg 2000; 87:1640–1649.
2. Irvin GL III, Carneiro DM. "Limited" parathyroidectomy in geriatric patients. Ann Surg 2001; 233(5):612–616.
3. Kebebew E, Duh Q-Y, Clark OH. Parathyroidectomy for primary hyperparathyroidism in octogenarians and nonagenarians. Arch Surg 2003; 138(8):867–871.
4. Bilizikian JP, Potts JT Jr, Fuleihan GE-H, Kleerekoper M, Neer R, Wells SA. Summary statement from a workshop on asymptomatic primary hyperparathyroidism: a perspective for the 21st century. J Clin Endocrinol Metab 2002; 87(12):5353–5361.
5. Mihai R, Farndon JR. Parathyroid disease and calcium metabolism. Br J Anaesth 2000; 85(1):29–43.

6. Chen H, Parkerson S, Udelsman R. Parathyroidectomy in the elderly: do the benefits outweigh the risks? World J Surg 1998; 22:531–536.

7. Silverberg SJ, Shane E, Jacobs TP, Siris E, Bilezikian JP. A 10-year prospective study of primary hyperparathyroidism with or without parathyroid surgery. N Engl J Med 1999; 341(17):571–578.

8. Watson LC, Marx CE. New onset of neuropsychiatric symptoms in the elderly: possible primary hyperparathyroidism. Psychosomatics 2002; 43(5):413–417.

9. Conroy S, Moulias S, Wassif W. Primary hyperparathyroidism the older person. Age Aging 2003; 32(6):571–578.

10. Almqvist EG, Bondeson A-G, Bondeson L, Nissborg A, Smedgard P, Svennnsson S-E. Cardiac dysfunction in mild primary hyperparathyroidism assessed by radionuclide angiography and echocardiography before and after parathyroidectomy. Surgery 2002; 132(6):1126–1132.

11. Irvin GL, Dembrow VD, Prudhomme DL. Operative monitoring of parathyroid gland function. Am J Surg 1991; 162:299–302.

12. Irvin GL, Deriso GT. A new practical intraoperative parathyroid hormone assay. Am J Surg 1994; 168:466–468.

13. Irvin GL, Prudhomme DL, Deriso GT, Stakianakis G, Chandarlapathy SK. A new approach to parathyroidectomy. Ann Surg 1994; 219:574–581.

14. Irvin GL, Sfakianakis G, Yeung L, et al. Ambulatory parathyroidectomy for hyperparathyroidism. Arch Surg 1996; 131:1074–1077.

15. Chen H, Sokoll LJ, Udelsman R. Outpatient minimally invasive parathyroidectomy: a combination of Sestamibi SPECT localization, cervical block anesthesia, and intraoperative parathyroid hormone assay. Surgery 1999; 126:1016–1022.

16. Carty SE, Worsey J, Virji M, Brown M, Watson C. Concise parathyroidectomy: the impact of preoperative SPECT [99m]Tc Sestamibi scanning and intraoperative quick parathormone assay. Surgery 1997; 122:1107–1116.

17. Patel PC, Pellitteri P, Patel N, Fleetwood M. Use of a rapid intraoperative parathyroid hormone assay in the surgical management of parathyroid disease. Arch Otolaryngol Head Neck Surg 1998; 124:559–562.

18. Gordon LL, Snyder WH, Wians F Jr, Nwariaku F, Kim L. The validity of quick intraoperative parathyroid hormone assay: an evaluation in 72 patients based on gross morphologic criteria. Surgery 1999; 126:1030–1035.

19. Garner SC, Leight GS Jr. Initial experience with intraoperative PTH determinations in the surgical management of 130 consecutive cases of primary hyperparathyroidism. Surgery 1999; 126:1032–1038.

20. Weber CJ, Ritchie JC. Retrospective analysis of sequential changes in serum intact parathyroid hormone levels during conventional parathyroid exploration. Surgery 1999; 126:1139–1143.

21. Miura D, Wada N, Arici C, Morita E, Duh Q-Y, Clark OH. Does intraoperative quick parathyroid hormone assay improve the results of parathyroidectomy? World J Surg 2002; 26:926–930.

22. Jaskowiak NT, Sugg SL, Helke J, Koka MR, Kaplan EL. Pitfalls of intraoperative quick parathyroid hormone. Arch Surg 2002; 137:659–669.

23. Aggarwal G, Barakate MS, Robinson B, et al. Intraoperative quick parathyroid hormone versus same-day parathyroid hormone testing for minimally invasive parathyroidectomy: a cost effectiveness study. Surgery 2001; 130:963–970.

24. Boggs JE, Irvin GL, Carneiro DM, Molinari AS. The evolution of parathyroidectomy failures. Surgery 1999; 126:998–1002.

25. Carneiro DM, Irvin GL. Late parathyroid function after successful parathyroidectomy guided by intraoperative hormone assay (QPTH) compared with the standard bilateral neck exploration. Surgery 2000; 128:925–929.

26. Burkey SH, Heerden JA, Farley DR, Thompson GB, Grant CS, Curlee KJ. Will directed parathyroidectomy utilizing the gamma probe or intraoperative parathyroid hormone

assay replace bilateral cervical exploration as the preferred operation for primary hyperparathyroidism? World J Surg 2002; 26:914–920.

27. Hallfeldt KKJ, Trupka A, Gallwas J, Schmidbauer S. Minimally invasive video-assisted parathyroidectomy and intraoperative parathyroid hormone monitoring. Surg Endosc 2002; 16:1759–1763.

28. Inebet WB, Dakin GF, Haber RS, et al. Targeted parathyroidectomy in the era of intra-operative parathormone monitoring. World J Surg 2002; 26:921–925.

29. Gauger PG, Agarwal G, England BG, et al. Intraoperative parathyroid hormone monitoring fails to detect double parathyroid adenomas: A 2-institution experience. Surgery 2001; 130:1005–1010.

30. Tonelli F, Spini S, Tommasi M, et al. Intraoperative parathormone measurement in patients with multiple endocrine neoplasia type I syndrome and hyperparathyroidism. World J Surg 2000; 24:556–562.

31. Sywak MS, Knowlton ST, Pasieka JL, Parsons LL, Jones J. So the National Institute of Health consensus guidelines for parathyroidectomy predict symptom severity and surgical outcome in patients with primary hyperparathyroidism? Surgery 2002; 132(6): 1013–1020.

32. Rao DS, Wallace EA, Antonelli RF, et al. Forearm bone density in primary hyperparathyroidism: long term follow-up with and without parathyroidectomy. Clin Endocrinol 2003; 58:348–354.

33. Horiuchi T, Onouchi T, Inoue J, Shionoiri A, Hosoi T, Orimo H. A strategy for the management of elderly women with primary hyperparathyroidism: a comparison of Etidronate therapy with parathyroidectomy. Gerontology 2002; 48:103–108.

34. Hagestrom E, Lundgren E, Lithell H, et al. Normalized dyslipidaemia after parathyroidectomy in mild primary hyperparathyroidism: population-based study over five years. Clin Endocrinol 2002; 56(2):253–260.

35. Sheldon DG, Lee FT, Neil NJ, Ryan JA Jr. Surgical treatment of hyperparathyroidism improves health-related quality of life. Arch Surg 2002; 137:1022–1028.

47

Facial Nerve Dysfunction: Etiology and Incidence in the Elderly—Acute Management

Catherine P. Winslow and Mark K. Wax
Department of Otolaryngology/Head and Neck Surgery, Oregon Health and Science University, Portland, Oregon, U.S.A.

INTRODUCTION

Facial nerve dysfunction is a relatively common disorder that imparts great morbidity. The facial nerve (CN VII) provides movement to the ipsilateral half of the face, and functional problems have an extraordinary psychosocial impact on a patient. In the geriatric population, it is common to have ptosis of facial muscles and skin. Loss of sensation can occur through numerous medical problems and the aging process itself. Dry eyes can be caused from medication or disease processes. The aging process by itself imparts morbidity to visual acuity, visual fields, nasal respiration, oral deglutition, lacrimal and salivary flow, and cosmetic appearance of the face. Facial nerve palsy will exacerbate these problems.

ANATOMY

To understand the diverse etiology of facial nerve dysfunction, a brief description of the anatomy is needed. Facial nerve fibers originate in the facial nucleus. These fibers coalesce to form the facial nerve. The nerve exits the cranial vault through the internal auditory canal accompanying the eighth cranial nerve (vestibulocochlear nerve). Within the narrow fallopian canal, in the temporal bone, it is subject to compression from trauma, edema, or a tumor mass. The canal is divided into three segments: the labyrinthine, tympanic, and mastoid. The labyrinthine is the narrowest segment, and it contains the geniculate ganglion. The ganglion receives afferent input from the anterior two-thirds of the tongue. The greater petrosal nerve is the first branch of the nerve after the ganglion. This provides visceral efferent innervation to the lacrimal gland and nasal and palatine glands. Stimulation of this nerve results in secretion from the gland. The stapedius nerve is innervated by a small branch of the nerve. Shortly thereafter, the chorda tympani nerves branches off to supply visceral efferent innervation to the tongue and submandibular and sublingual glands.

513

The nerve leaves the confines of the temporal bone through the stylomastoid foramen and quickly ascends to the anterior face. The main trunk of the nerve branches in a variable pattern, but ultimately five separate branches emerge. The temporal branch provides muscular innervation to the frontalis muscle of the forehead. The zygomatic branch innervates the orbicular oculi, which allows eye closure. The buccal branch provides mimetic function of the midface. The marginal mandibular branch innervates the depressor anguli oris, and the cervical branch innervates the platysma.

ETIOLOGY

Facial paralysis can occur for a number of reasons. The symptoms are unilateral in >98% of cases. Few studies isolate the elderly population with regards to etiology and incidence. Generalized reasons for unilateral paralysis include congenital, traumatic, idiopathic, neurologic, infectious, metabolic, neoplastic, and iatrogenic. An estimated 76,000 Americans are affected by facial paralysis (1). The most common cause of paralysis is idiopathic, or Bell's palsy. A virus is suspected to be responsible for this disorder. It has been estimated to affect 20 people in every 100,000 annually (2). While the vast majority of those afflicted with Bell's palsy experience complete or near-complete recovery, an estimated 10,120 Americans have persistent problems that do not resolve (3). Infection with the Zoster virus (Ramsey–Hunt syndrome), Lyme disease, or otologic sources is the next most common etiology. Ramsey–Hunt syndrome may present as pain, facial paralysis, herpetic eruptions on the face or in the ear canal, and hearing loss. Steroids and antivirals agents are utilized. Lyme disease was diagnosed in 2% of patients with idiopathic facial paralysis in one series (4).

Neoplasms, either benign or malignant, result in approximately 5% of facial paralysis cases, or approximately 17,200 new cases yearly (2,5). Of the benign tumors, acoustic neuromas are the predominant etiology. Central CNS disorders include stroke and other neurological disorders, accounting for approximately 5% of cases. The majority of traumatic causes involve a temporal bone fracture. Peripheral injury can occur from lacerations or compression over the distal branches. Metabolic causes include diabetes, hypertension, and thyroid disorders. Such sources are less commonly found in the United States. Peripheral injury can also occur following facial surgery, such as parotidectomy, face-lifting, or brow-lifting.

CLASSIFICATION

The appearance of facial paralysis is unmistakable. The side of the face that is involved is immobile and ptotic. Varying degrees of dysfunction are possible, and many scales have been devised to document function. The most commonly used is the House–Brackmann Scale (Table 1). Different systems have been devised to account for partial palsy and for palsy that affects only isolated branches of the nerve (5).

INVESTIGATION

The workup for a given patient depends on the suspected etiology. Iatrogenic palsy is easy since there has been a known cause. Idiopathic palsy (Bell's palsy) is a diagnosis

Table 1 House–Brackmann Scale for Facial Palsy

Grade	Clinical findings
I	Normal function
II	Slight weakness
III	Obvious weakness, symmetry at rest, eye closure
IV	Obvious weakness, symmetry at rest, incomplete eye closure
V	Barely perceptible motion, asymmetry at rest
VI	Complete paralysis, no movement

of exclusion and can only be diagnosed when all other pathology has been ruled out. A complete physical examination to include all of the cranial nerves should be performed. Appropriate blood work depends upon the presentation. An audiogram should be obtained due to the proximity of the cochlear nerve to the facial nerve in the internal auditory canal.

Postoperative facial paralysis that involves surgical damage to the seventh nerve generally does not require further workup. Functional testing can be done to attempt to predict the return of function. The most commonly used test is an evoked nerve conduction study, or EnoG.

Topographic testing was heavily used in the past to determine the site of lesion. With the advent of computed tomography (CT) and magnetic resonance imaging (MRI) scans, it has largely fallen by the wayside, and more reliance has been placed on scanning to determine the etiology of the palsy. Generation of tears, presence of a stapedial reflex (tested with an audiogram), and salivary inducement of the submandibular and sublingual glands can identify sites of lesions within the temporal bone. Mimetic function can help determine if all branches or only a selected few are involved.

The patient who presents with a gradual onset of facial paresis must be evaluated for tumors along the course of the facial nerve. Most commonly these are extratemporal, originating in the parotid gland. Scanning of the brain, internal auditory canal, temporal bone, face, and neck can be done with CT or MRI. Traumatic injury can also be evaluated by scanning. The CT is more appropriate for temporal bone etiologies such as trauma, while an MRI will pick up subtle soft tissue changes.

MANAGEMENT

Timing for medical and surgical management is determined on an individual basis. Desire to help the patient with appearance and function is tempered with the knowledge that the nerve may return to normal function, particularly in cases of idiopathic palsy. Surgical intervention that is imparted soon in the disease course can adversely affect the recovery and in many cases is unnecessary.

One exception for acute surgical management of facial palsy is facial nerve repair, or grafting. Surgical repair of a damaged facial nerve is occasionally necessary. This is particularly true if the nerve is injured during the course of a procedure. Otologic surgery, parotid surgery, and face-lifting procedures are most commonly to blame. Patients who suffer blunt trauma and have a significant (>90%) degeneration of facial nerve function may undergo exploration, with possible grafting if a damaged or severed segment is identified. Patients who are victims of penetrating trauma and have immediate complete paralysis also require exploration with possible grafting. The results for immediate repair or nerve grafting are superior to those of other reanimation procedures and provide the patient the opportunity to retain voluntary and symmetric movement.

In patients requiring surgical exploration and manipulation of the nerve, prognosis for facial nerve recovery is dependent upon many factors. The length of paralysis, etiology of paralysis, presence of preoperative paralysis, and need for grafting all impact the final function the patient will be able to attain. Primary repair of the nerve yields the best results. If a facial nerve is interrupted during the course of surgery, an attempt is made to approximate it. This involves several sutures of 9-0 or 10-0 nylon with microscopic assistance. Fewer sutures lead to less reaction and a better prognosis. The sutures are placed in the epineurium. A House-Brackmann grade of III is considered the best attainable recovery following any repair process, due to complete or near-complete interruption of the nerve fibers.

If a gap exists between the fresh ends of a nerve, an interposition graft is required. A nerve from a different location is required to perform this. If a small segment of nerve is necessary, the greater auricular nerve is usually used. This is easily found in the neck, crossing the sternocleidomastoid muscle. It provides sensation to parts of the ear, and there is minimal morbidity associated with harvest. It is usually in the field of dissection if a parotidectomy is being performed. A longer piece of nerve can be obtained from the sural nerve in the leg. This sensory nerve lies on the lateral aspect of the leg and has a large diameter. Some loss of sensation to the lateral ankle and foot will result from its harvest. The nerve graft is then sewn to both fresh edges of the facial nerve with microscopic visualization, as noted above. The anastomosis should be tension-free.

It has long been felt that immediate grafting yields superior results. This has also been shown in several series (6,7). Malignancy involved with the paralysis also imparts a poorer prognosis for recovery. Early grafting can repair the nerve when it has less fibrosis and scarring and is easier to identify. Less atrophy of the muscles is found early in the course of paralysis. Preoperative imaging can be employed to assess the degree of symmetry between the affected muscles and the unaffected side. This has been shown to correlate with significantly improved prognosis with nerve grafting (8).

Mimetic function may not return for 12 to 18 months following repair or grafting. Patients are followed closely and continued on eye precautions until the final result is known. Return of facial tone is a good sign and can herald return of function. Synkinesis, or facial mass movement, is relatively common after nerve transsection. This can be treated with isolated Botulinum toxin (Botox®) injections into the affected muscles to minimize the facial distortion. With good but incomplete recovery and no synkinesis, Botox may also be carefully used on the contralateral side to provide more facial symmetry. Upon complete recovery after nerve repair, further reanimation procedures may be required.

Immediate concerns of facial nerve paresis or paralysis relate not only to the aesthetic and social compromise the disorder imparts but also more importantly on the functional disabilities that might cause permanent impairment. The eye has long been a focus of critical evaluation in the quest to prevent sequelae of facial paralysis. Although the opening of the eye is controlled by the oculomotor nerve (levator muscle), the lid is closed by the action of the orbicularis oculi, controlled by the facial nerve. Lack of closure can lead to minute abrasions of the cornea. When left untreated, they can progress to corneal scarring and blindness. Dry eyes can occur from lack of innervation via the greater petrosal nerve. Conversely, tearing can also be problematic, due to loss of the "pump" mechanism that evacuates tears via the lacrimal system. The pump is dependent on the function of the orbicularis muscle. The tears are not "pumped" into the medial canthus of the eye where normally they are drained by the lacrimal duct into the nose. Instead, they collect in the lateral canthus; since the lower lid is also adynamic, these tears will overflow and run down the cheek. Eye protection is begun immediately upon diagnosis. Eye drops and night-time lubrication and taping can help prevent corneal injury. Eye shields may be necessary, particularly in windy or dusty environments. Ophthalmologic consultation is helpful (9).

We have found that immediate rehabilitation of the upper and lower eyelid maximizes patient comfort and function while minimizing long-term disability. Immediate medical management, such as eye shields and ointments, are necessary prior to surgical intervention. These medical interventions require complex management by an individual who is already caring for a complex medical/surgical problem. These interventions also inhibit ocular vision by causing visual blurring.

There are a number of approaches to facilitate upper eyelid closure. Gold weight implantation was first popularized in the late 1970s. It is a technically simple yet effective technique. In patients who can be evaluated in the preoperative period, determination of the proper weight is important. Using tincture of benzoine, a gold weight can be cemented to the patient's upper lid for a short period of time to ensure the correct prosthetic weight. We have found in patients who are being reconstructed in the intraoperative or immediate postoperative phase that preoperative determination of the weight is not practical. In this setting a 1.2-g weight is used. In order to achieve optimal closure of the eyelid, placement of the prosthesis in the proper anatomic location is important. The majority of complications that were described with its early use can be prevented by meticulous attention to prosthetic placement. These complications, such as extrusion through the thin eyelid skin, distortion of the lid shape, redness of the upper eyelid skin, or unsightliness due to bulging of the lid or angling of the gold weight, have all been reported and are preventable in the majority of cases. The weight should be placed medial to the midline to facilitate closure of the upper lid. It is attached with one to three sutures through fenestrations in the plate to the tarsal plate. This will prevent extrusion of the gold through the lid. Suturing of the prosthesis will also prevent migration in the short term. The weight works by allowing gravity to draw the upper lid inferiorly over the globe. Large series have reported success rates of over 90%. Common causes for removal are inadequate upper lid closure due to too light a weight, extrusion, or a chronic skin inflammation secondary to sensitivity to the gold or a cosmetic deformity.

One advantage of the gold weight implantation is that it is completely reversible. If upper eyelid function returns, then the gold weight can be removed with minimal morbidity (10).

The second component of eyelid rehabilitation that must be addressed is the lower eyelid. Ectropion, a malfunction of the tear drainage and distribution system, is quite bothersome to the patient. Scleral show with redness and tears running down the cheek can be quite debilitating. A goal of lower lid reanimation is to approximate the lower eyelid to the globe. Many procedures have been utilized to correct the lower eyelid. These include plication involving some form of lateral tarsorrhaphy, lower lid tightening procedures, implants to elevate the lower eyelid combined with lid tightening procedures, or suspension. We have found that a modification of the Bick procedure known as the lateral tarsal strip is easily performed and allows for adequate reconstruction of the lower eyelid. The first step in this procedure is performing a lateral canthopexy. The tarsal plate is identified and isolated. A small strip of conjunctiva and mucosa are than removed. This leaves a bare strip of the tarsal plate, and a nonabsorbable suture such as 5-0 nylon is placed through the tarsal plate. This is then anchored to the lateral orbital rim near Whitnell's tubercle. The result is a shortening and tightening of the lower lid. The risk of this procedure is that the lower lid will be foreshortened. We have not found this to be much of a problem, as the eyelid will change over time and the functional and cosmetic results are acceptable.

The mouth is also of great concern to both patient and physician. The orbicularis oris muscle is responsible for much of the preparation of the food bolus, and impairment can result in drooling and dribbling of food. Socially, it can lead to isolation and possibly weight loss.

Dynamic Mouth and Lower Lip Reconstruction

Loss of the facial nerve will have a dramatic effect on the function of the mouth and lower lip. Drooping of the lower lip, drooling of secretions, loss of control of the food bolus while eating, and a crooked smile are all problems encountered by patients. Asymmetry of the lower lip, most evident on smiling, is very noticeable and may prove to be quite debilitating. Dynamic and adynamic measures have all been used to re-animate the lower face and palliate these problems (11). Temporalis muscle transposition is the most useful regional muscle transfer used to restore a voluntary lateral smile in these patients. It should be remembered that a lateral smile, which is the most common type of human smile, is different than a canine smile, which is a full denture smile. The full dentate smile is much more difficult to rehabilitate. Modifications of the temporalis sling have included extensions involving pericranium superiorly that are attached to the fascia overlying the temporalis muscle. Taking only the center slip of the temporalis muscle eliminates some of the cosmetic problems associated with hollowness at the donor site defect. The muscle is harvested and attached to the orbicularis oculi muscle of the upper and lower lip. With this procedure, 95% of the patients will achieve fair to excellent results. Complications with this technique are uncommon except when an alloplastic implant is involved at the distal end to obtain further reach of the temporalis to the lower lip. When periosteum or allogenic dermis is utilized, the complication rate is much less.

Another method of rehabilitating the facial nerve in the lower face is to use static slings. At the time of the initial procedure or postoperatively, a piece of allogenic dermis can be used to suspend the lateral orbicularis and the lateral commissure to the zygomatic process (12). Tunneling from the zygomatic process through the subcutaneous tissue superficial to the superficial musculoaponeuretic system (SMAS) layer is performed. The allogenic dermis can be anchored to the nasolabial fold, upper lip, and lower lip. Excellent static results can be obtained. One must overcorrect the lower lip, as all of the material used to "sling" the lower face will stretch over time. Correction of drooling and bolus control while chewing are all immediately noticeable. Patients can achieve relatively normal looks and function at rest. With dynamic movement of the face, such as smiling, the lack of movement will be noticeable. Complications with this technique include sutures rupturing at the oral commissure and loss of function of the sling, as well as infection. The use of allogenic dermis has greatly decreased the infection rate and morbidity with this procedure.

Nasal breathing can be affected by loss of the nasal dilator muscles, causing collapse of the nasal sidewall.

Nasal Reconstruction

The ability to breath through the nose is very important to the well being of individuals. Many factors can affect this ability. One such event is loss of facial nerve function. When the facila nerve does not function, there is collapse of the lateral nasal wall. This is secondary to failure of the elevators of the external nasal valve to function. Since the contralateral nasal valve functions, the patient has unilateral nasal collapse. Unfortunately, patients rarely complain about the nasal obstruction on the operated side. However, if one inquires then the obstruction is evident. There is little associated cosmetic impact. Perhaps this is why so few patients or physicians recognize the problem.

The ability to open the nasal valve with a rigid or static procedure has been well described in both the facial plastic and general otolaryngology literature for many years. There are many techniques available to accomplish this. One of the simplest that we have utilized has been the "nasal stitch." With this technique, the nasal valve is suspended dynamically with a nonabsorbable 0-nylon suture. The technique involves anchoring the suture to the infraorbital rim lateral to the infraorbital foramen. The suture is then passed in a subcutaneous fashion through the nasal valve (above and below the valve) and tied to the periosteum in a hole drilled in the orbital rim. The suture is tightened to the point where the nasal valve is propped open. Over the long term, airway and nasal patency is maintained. The cosmetic down side of this approach is a slight bulging of the lateral nasal complex that can be appreciated but is of no significance to the patient. Other intranasal techniques, such as butterfly grafting, have been utilized, all with excellent results.

Management of the paralytic face is complex and generally addressed in stages. The reason for paralysis will dictate treatment to a certain extent. If the loss of the nerve is complete and surgical, rehabilitation will be more aggressive than that caused by Bell's palsy. With Bell's palsy, watchful waiting and an appropriate evaluation to determine the etiology of paralysis can treat most patients. Bell's palsy has a greater recovery rate if treated immediately (within 48 hours) with a steroid taper. Antiviral medications have been tried with no significant success. It is felt that the geriatric population has a poorer outcome with idiopathic paralysis. Post-traumatic facial paralysis is also observed, unless EnoG studies show a degeneration of 90% or more. In those patients, exploration of the nerve with possible grafting may improve recovery.

Most surgical reanimation procedures are delayed for 12 to 18 months to determine if spontaneous recovery will occur, and to what extent. One exception is the potential for an adverse effect on vision. The eye is treated immediately with conservative measures. Lubricating drops during the daytime, lubricating ointment at night, and an eye patch or taping at night can help. Closure of the eye can be improved with a gold weight placement or a spring. Early gold weight placement (within 30 days of onset of paralysis) has been shown to be an effective means of preventing visual disturbances, with no higher a complication rate than delayed placement (10).

REFERENCES

1. United State National Center for Health Statistics. Prevalence of selected impairments: United States, 1977. Washington, D.C.: Government Printing Office, 1981. (DHHS Pub. No. PHS 81–1562. Vital and Health Statistics Series 10: Data from the National Health Survey No. 134.).

2. Katusick SK, Beard CM, Wiederholt WC, et al. Incidence, clinical features, and prognosis in Bell's palsy. Ann Neurol 1986; 20(5):622–627.

3. Bleicher JN, Hamiel S, Gengler JS, Antimarino J. A survey of facial paralysis: etiology and incidence. Ear Nose Throat J 1996; 75:355–358.

4. Peltomaa M, Pyykko I, Seppala I, Viljanen M. Lyme borreliosis and facial paralysis—a prospective analysis of risk factors and outcomes. Am J Otolaryngol 2002; 23(3):125–132.

5. May M. Facial paralysis, peripheral type: a proposed method of reporting. Laryngoscope 1970; 80:331–390.

6. Bascom DA, Schaitkin BM, May M, Klein S. Facial nerve repair: a retrospective review. Facial Plast Surg 2000; 16(4):309–313.

7. Falcioni M, Taibah A, Russo A, Piccirillo E, Sanna M. Facial nerve grafting. Otol Neurotol 2003; 24(3):486–489.

8. Kaylie DM, Wax MK, Weissman JL. Preoperative facial muscle imaging predicts final facial function after facial nerve grafting. Am J Neuroradiol 2003; 24(3):326–330.

9. Jackson CG, von Doersten PG. The facial nerve; current trends in diagnosis, treatment, and rehabilitation. Medial Clin Norht Am 1999; 83(1):179–195.

10. Snyder MC, Johnson PJ, Moore GF, Ogren FP. Early versus late gold weight implantation for rehabilitation of the paralyzed eyelid. Laryngoscope 2001; 111:2109–2113.

11. Jobe RP. A technique for lid loading in the management of the lagophthalmos of facial palsy. Plast Reconstr Surg 1974; 53:29–31.

12. Winslow CP, Wang TD, Wax MK. Static reanimation of the paralyzed face with an acellular dermal allograft sling. Arch Facial Plast Surg 2001; 3(1):5507.

48

Disorders of the Salivary Glands

Karen T. Pitman

Department of Otolaryngology and Communicative Sciences, University of Mississippi Medical School, Jackson, Mississippi, U.S.A.

Jonas T. Johnson

Department of Otolaryngology and Radiation Oncology, University of Pittsburgh School of Medicine, Pittsburgh, Pennsylvania, U.S.A.

INTRODUCTION

Saliva is an important element in the maintenance of normal oral health and function. It has many roles and purposes. Saliva provides lubrication of the upper aerodigestive tract, which is essential for both speech and swallowing. Constituents of saliva include immunoglobulins, electrolytes, antimicrobial substances, and bicarbonate and digestive enzymes, all of which further contribute to normal oral health and maintenance. Infection, neoplasia, and degenerative disorders of the salivary apparatus will have a detrimental effect on the production of saliva. While these disorders may affect individuals of any age, they are more common in the geriatric population.

The salivary apparatus is generally described as the paired parotid, submandibular, and sublingual glands. In addition, there are 700–1000 minor salivary glands located in the submucosa of the upper aerodigestive tract between the lips and the larynx. Together, the salivary apparatus normally produces 1000–1500 mL of saliva per day.

BASIC SCIENCE

The parotid gland is dumbbell in shape and predominantly located in the preauricular soft tissues. The so-called deep lobe of the parotid gland extends into the retromandibular space. It is traversed by the facial nerve, which passes through the substance of the gland. Stenson's duct drains the parotid gland and enters the cheek mucosa adjacent to the maxillary second molar. The submandibular gland is located entirely within the submandibular triangle defined by the mandible above and the sling of the digastric muscle below. Wharton's duct runs superiorly from the gland to enter the oral cavity in a small papilla adjacent to the lingual frenulum. The sublingual glands are located in submucosa of the posterior floor of mouth and drain through several small ducts directly into the oral cavity. Within the parynchema of the parotid gland there are also lymph nodes; hence, neoplastic and non-neoplastic lymphatic processes occur within the parotid gland.

The rate and character of salivary production is controlled by the coordinated action of the parasympathetic and sympathetic innervation. Taste and mastication are potent stimuli under normal conditions. Smell and anticipation of oral stimulation is also important. Normal saliva is about 90% water, but salivary consistency varies by the gland of origin and the balance of autonomic input.

The histology of the salivary glands includes specialized ductal, serous, and mucinous secretory and myoepithelial cells. A variety of neoplasms can arise from the salivary glands. These correspond to the cell types present within the glands.

Saliva has many protective functions. Approximately 40% of the amylase secreted in the body derives from the salivary glands. One of its functions is to remove residual carbohydrates from the oral cavity and reduce the formation of caries. Saliva also contains bicarbonate for buffering of oral secretions. This helps to minimize pH fluctuations and serves to protect tooth enamel. The principal immunoglobin found in saliva is IgA. This immunoglobulin is felt to participate in the body's resistance to ingested pathogens. Finally, saliva contains numerous antimicrobial substances that modulate the bacterial, fungal, and viral microflora of the oral cavity. Several growth factors present in saliva facilitate regeneration of the mucosa.

HISTORY

Patients presenting with disorders of the salivary apparatus characteristically complain of one of three symptoms: xerostomia, pain localized to the gland, or swelling or a mass.

Complaints of xerostomia or oral dryness are common in the older patient. Other symptoms related to reduced salivary flow include soreness or a burning sensation in the mouth, thick saliva, dysphagia, or a taste disturbance. Xerostomia is most commonly a consequence of medication. Salivary flow rates are decreased by anticholinergics, some antihypertensives, and the tricyclic antidepressants. Other drugs, such as diuretics, may indirectly contribute to oral dryness. In the geriatric population, salivary flow may be physiologically decreased. In their normal homeostatic state, the decreased flow may not be noticed. The addition of a medication that slightly changes the character of the saliva, whether it be consistency or flow rate, may produce symptoms of xerostomia.

Connective tissue disorders frequently produce the Sicca syndrome (dry eyes and mouth). This is most commonly associated with Sjogren's syndrome. Opthalmologic, serologic, and histologic confirmation is necessary. Most commonly minor salivary glands from the lower lip are biopsied.

Irradiation to the head and neck is another prominent cause of permanent salivary flow impairment. This effect is profound and permanent after as little as 25 Gy. Radioactive iodine treatment may cause transient sialoadenitis with resultant dry mouth. This usually resolves over time.

Pain localized to a salivary gland is most commonly an indication of infection and/or obstruction. Elderly people tend to have an increased incidence of focal obstruction and inspissation of secretions. As people age, the density of the saliva increases due to a decrease in the water content of saliva. This thickened saliva is more prone to become sludge that may plug the duct, resulting in pain and swelling. In general, the pain is localized to the involved gland; however, parotid pain may be referred to the ear. Characteristically, pain due to obstruction is worse with salivary stimulation (eating) and is usually associated with concurrent swelling. Less commonly pain is associated with malignant neoplasia.

Salivary gland enlargement involving the entire gland suggests an inflammatory or infiltrative process. Diffuse enlargement may be due to infection with HIV, autoimmune (Sjogren's), or infiltration (Sarcoid). Sialosis describes the glandular hypertrophy (primarily parotid) that is attributed to fatty infiltration.

A discrete nodule or mass within the substance of the gland is far more likely to represent a neoplasm. The association of facial nerve weakness with a salivary mass is highly suspicious for malignancy. On rare occasions, the first evidence of a malignancy may be neuropathy with an undetected mass. This possibility should be considered in cases of atypical facial paralysis.

PHYSICAL EXAMINATION

Patients who present with dysfunction, pain, or swelling in a salivary gland should be carefully examined. The adequacy of saliva is often apparent on visual inspection of the papillae of the Wharton's and Stenson's ducts while palpating the respective gland.

Palpation of the involved gland allows the examiner to determine if a solitary mass is present. Whether the mass is a discrete module or represents diffuse infiltration of the entire gland is then ascertained. Sometimes a stone can be identified in the duct.

The integrity of the nerves that are near the gland, or pass through it, should be evaluated, including the facial, hypoglossal, and lingual nerves. The marginal branch of the facial nerve overlies the submandibular gland on its way to innervate the lower lip. Deep to the submandibular gland is the lingual nerve, which supplies sensation to the tongue. Also deep but inferior to the submandibular gland is the hypoglossal nerve, which supplies motor innervation to the tongue. The facial nerve travels through the parenchyma of the parotid gland.

The neck is also an important part of the assessment. The presence of a mass in a salivary gland with associated enlargement of the cervical lymph node(s) suggests malignancy. Multiple parotid cysts and extensive cervical adenopathy in at-risk patients may be the herald of HIV infection.

Diffuse and painful swelling is usually an indication of either obstruction or infection. Characteristically, the pain is associated with obstruction and is exacerbated by eating. Infection is frequently associated with overlying cutaneous erythmia. Gentle massage of the involved gland often will express purulent debris from the involved duct. The overwhelming majority of acute bacterial infections in the salivary glands are due to dehydration and staphylococci.

The presence of a discrete painless mass in a salivary gland suggests a neoplasm. Parotid neoplasms are most commonly encountered; however, the potential for a tumor exists in all of the major and minor salivary glands. Approximately 80% of parotid neoplasia are benign. In contrast, 50% of submandibular neoplasia are malignant, and as many as 70% or more of sublingual and minor salivary gland tumors are malignant.

Processes affecting the minor salivary glands of the upper aerodigestive tract will produce localized symptoms (pain or mass) of the affected structure. For example, a mucocele (serous salivary collection in a minor salivary gland) in the lower lip will present as a well-circumscribed mass in the lip.

DIAGNOSTIC TESTING

The choice of whether to pursue further investigation depends upon the clinician's differential diagnosis. In the face of acute bacterial sialoadenitis, culture of the purulent drainage expressed from the duct is appropriate. Imaging may be useful in distinguishing infiltrative processes from salivary masses. Computed tomography (CT) and magnetic resonance imaging (MRI) cannot, however, establish a histologic diagnosis. They merely allow the clinician to further refine the differential diagnosis.

Fine needle aspiration (FNA) biopsy is commonly employed in evaluation of salivary neoplasms. Increasing experience with cytopathology and the advent of immunochemistry have allowed increasing sophistication with FNA. Nevertheless, many authors have reported occasional false positive reports with FNA, which suggests that FNA results should be interpreted with caution and correlated carefully with the rest of the clinical picture.

Biopsy is the gold standard for parotid lesions. It has long been held that the minimal biopsy for a benign parotid tumor is a parotidectomy with facial nerve dissection. Because of the intimate relationship of the parotid and the facial nerve, this approach affords the surgeon the opportunity to completely remove the tumor without endangering the facial nerve. Some benign tumors, such as pleomorphic adenoma, should not be partially removed because of the high probability of multifocal recurrences. When Sicca syndrome is encountered, histologic changes may be diffusely found throughout the salivary apparatus. Accordingly, biopsies of minor salivary glands present under the mucosa of the lower lip are the standard for diagnosing Sjogren's syndrome and can be performed as an office procedure. Serologic tests, (SSA and SSB) may be helpful in the diagnosis as well, but if they are negative they are not useful since these tests too do not have high sensitivity.

Biopsy of infiltrative malignancies and other difficult-to-diagnose processes is frequently required. For example, the association of lymphoma with both Sjogren's syndrome and HIV-associated parotitis may require biopsy when a dominant solid nodule is found within the glands. CT or MRI helps to distinguish the lymphoepithelial cysts associated with these diseases from lymphoma. Biopsy puts the facial nerve at risk, which is minimized when an experienced surgeon performs the biopsy. The emerging availability of fine needle aspiration in the diagnosis of lymphoma is changing clinical practice.

COMMON SALIVARY DISORDERS

Acute suppurative sialadenitis presents as painful inflammation of the affected gland with associated erythema, tenderness, swelling, and purulent drainage. Fever and leukocytosis may be present, and there may be progression to abscess formation. Common etiologies include dehydration and debilitation, especially after major surgery or trauma.

Approximately 40% to 50% of patients with acute bacterial infections involving a salivary gland have an associated stone. Patients with salivary stones typically present with a history of chronic recurrent sialoadenitis. Greater than 90% of all salivary stones are found in the submandibular glands. This is probably reflective of the fact that the submandibular duct runs against gravity into the mouth and the submandibular secretions have higher viscosity and higher concentration of calcium. Since the punctum or drainage site of the duct is smaller than the duct itself, a stone will be able to move in the duct but will impact and block the duct orifice. This leads to intermittent swelling and inflammation. Successful therapy usually requires stone extraction. For small mobile stones opening the duct orifice, an office procedure is the treatment of choice. Large staghorn calculi embedded in the duct cannot be extracted and require excision of the entire gland. Recent introduction of sialoendoscopic instrumentation may change the treatment paradigm for salivary stones in the coming years.

Sialosis describes painless swelling of the salivary apparatus. It is most commonly apparent in the parotid glands. Most cases of sialosis are attributable to nutritional deficiencies and chronic wasting diseases. Histologically, sialosis is characterized by diffuse fatty infiltration of the gland. Accordingly, this can often be recognized on MRI scan. Sialosis may be encountered with such entities as anorexia, bulimia, and chronic conditions such as advanced alcoholic cirrhosis and bronchiectasis. No treatment of sialosis is necessary.

The salivary enlargement associated with Sjogren's syndrome has the histologic appearance of a benign lymphoepithelial infiltration. Ductal destruction leads to sialoectasia. The subsequent lymphoepithelial cysts are characteristic on MRI scan. Diagnosis is made on histologic examination of a minor salivary gland obtained from lip biopsy, since the disease process is systemic and affects all salivary glands.

The most common neoplasms of the parotid are benign. These include the pleomorphic adenoma (mixed tumor) and Warthin's tumor. Both can present as a discrete nodule within the substance of the gland. Untreated pleomorphic adenomas tend to progress and have a potential for malignant transformation or involvement of the facial nerve, hence should be excised, even in the elderly patient. Warthin's tumor may be indistinguishable from lymphoma on FNA or imaging. For these reasons, all parotid lesions should be excised for both pathologic confirmation and care.

A wide variety of primary and metastatic malignancies may involve the salivary glands. Of all the head and neck salivary glands, the parotid is the most common site. Yet remember that 80% of parotid lesions are benign, while 80% of minor salivary gland tumors are malignant. Mucoepidermoid and adenoid cystic carcinoma are the most common histologic tumors found in primary parotid malignancy. These tumors are usually radioresistant. The best cure rates are achieved with total excision. Adjuvant radiation may be required in specific instances or with specific pathologies. Metastatic disease involving the parotid represents metastasis to intraglandular lymph nodes. The most common primary sites that metastasize to the parotid are facial and skin cancers, the majority of which are squamous cell carcinoma. Rarely melanoma or basal cell carcinoma will metastasize to this area.

In as much as the submandibular glands contain no lymph nodes, metastasis into the gland does not occur. However, metastasis to the Zone I (submandibular) lymph nodes can occur, usually a tumor situated in the oral cavity. The close proximity of the gland to lymph nodes in the area makes differentiating the two processes difficult. FNA is often necessary.

TREATMENT OPTIONS

Infection

Patients with acute bacterial parotitis require antibiotics and hydration. Gentle massage may assist in expressing the purulence from the ducts. Sialogogues (salivary stimulants, such as lemon drops, etc.) and warm compresses are also beneficial. The bacteria most commonly associated with parotitis are staphylococcus. Accordingly, an antibiotic effective against staphylococcus is essential. Most patients can be treated on an outpatient basis. Dicloxacillin 500 mg, four times a day, is highly effective.

In most circumstances, patients can be managed in the outpatient setting. Patients with dehydration and severe swelling and pain may require intravenous therapy. Progression to an abscess is unusual, but when it occurs, it generally requires surgery and drainage. Knowledge regarding the anatomic course of the facial nerve is important since most abscesses are loculated and treatment requires breakdown of multiple abscess cavities and extensive interglandular dissection.

Infiltrative Processes

Under most circumstances, the decision to treat an infiltrative process reflects the severity of the parotid involvement and may also be guided by other systemic problems. For instance, the lymphoepithelial infiltration of Sjogren's syndrome will respond to steroid therapy. Most patients with Sicca syndrome secondary to Sjogren's suffer from xerostomia. Many patients benefit from increased hydration and use of artificial saliva. Patients with Sjogren's may benefit from administration of salivary stimulants such as Salogen or Evoxac. When patients with Sjogren's syndrome develop obstruction and infection, administration of antibiotics and increased fluid intake is frequently therapeutic. Massive enlargement of the salivary glands is sometimes associated with Sjogren's syndrome. This may respond to high doses of steroid administration. It is essential, however, for the clinician to remain aware of the fact that patients with Sjogren's are at increased risk to develop lymphoma sometime during their life. Accordingly, MRI imaging may help diagnose

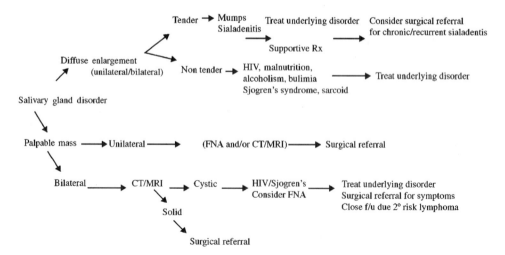

Figure   Algorithm for evaluation of salivary gland disorder.

a solid nodule that requires further diagnostic intervention. Cosmetic parotidectomy is rarely indicated due to the risk to the facial nerve, which is increased in the face of chronic inflammatory changes. Removal of the parotid may further exacerbate xerostomia.

Infiltration of the parotid gland by sarcoid may occasionally be associated with involvement of the facial nerve. Most patients respond to high-dose steroid therapy.

Fatty infiltration and parotid enlargement (sialosis) due to malnutrition and debilitating diseases does not require treatment.

SUMMARY

Infections, infiltrative processes, and neoplasia commonly affect the salivary glands of the geriatric patient. Evaluation begins by determining if the patient's complaints are related to diffuse enlargement of one or more glands or a discreet neoplasm. Neoplasia can be evaluated with imaging and/or fine needle aspiration. For patients with neoplastic processes, advanced patient age is not in and of itself a contraindication to surgery. Not all salivary neoplasms require surgery, but referral to a surgeon familiar with facial nerve anatomy for definitive diagnosis and treatment is appropriate. Functional disorders of the salivary glands are usually manifested as xerostomia and are due to side effects of medications. Discussion with the patient's primary physician may assist in identifying alternative medications aimed at reducing decreased salivary production.

REFERENCES

1. Atkinson JC, Fox PC. Salivary gland dysfunction. Clin Geriatr Med 1992; 8(3):499–511.
2. Fox PC. Management of dry mouth. Dent Clin North Am 1997; 41(4):863–875.
3. Bradley PJ. Benign salivary gland disease. Hosp Med (London) 2001; 62(7):392–395.
4. Davies AN, Broadley K, Beighton D. Salivary gland hypofunction in patients with advanced cancer. Oral Oncol 2002; 38(7):680–685.

49

Reconstructive Issues in the Elderly Patient with Head and Neck Cancer

Eric Genden
Department of Otolaryngology, Mount Sinai Medical Center, New York, New York, U.S.A.

Mark K. Wax
Department of Otolaryngology/Head and Neck Surgery, Oregon Health and Science University, Portland, Oregon, U.S.A.

INTRODUCTION

Cancer of the head and neck is primarily a disease of the elderly. The synergistic effect of alcohol and tobacco in promoting carcinogenesis of these mucosal surfaces has been well documented. The surge in the prevalence of head and neck cancer presenting to the otolaryngologist is coincident with the increased usage of these two substances after a 20–30-year lag period [1]. While the incidence of head and neck cancer that is seen in many major referral centers in certain parts of the United States is decreasing, in other areas it continues to explode. This, of course, is all related to the incidence of tobacco smoking and alcohol exposure in that community. The latency of effect is responsible for the median age of most patients, with head and neck cancer being between 60 and 70 years of age. As life expectancy has increased, so has the incidence of cancer in patients in their 70s, 80s, 90s, and even the centurions [1,2].

It has been shown that prognosis is directly related to disease stage. Advanced age and concomitant medical conditions are not predictors of failure [1–3]. However, complications are more frequently encountered in the geriatic population. There has been no study or report that has analyzed in stepwise regression fashion the effect of age on prognosis or complications. One issue is the definition of what a geriatric population is. Some literature describes it as individuals over 50 years of age. Most people would agree that over 65 is what should be used. Fortunately, a number of articles have examined population groups in the over 80 range, or even over 90 [2,3]. These studies have documented that adequate oncologic treatment involving surgery regardless of patients' age results in equivalent disease-free survival rates compared to a younger population. What is important to note is that the overall survival rate is lower, but when plotted against an actuarial survival for the

529

general octagenarian population, it is equivalent. Thus, the over-riding conclusion is that age should have no relationship to the determination of treatment (1–3).

Measurements of complications have been related to age in some reports and unrelated in others. The frequency of preoperative comorbidities is significantly higher as the population ages. The relationship of this to complications after major head and neck oncologic ablative procedures is indeterminate. It would appear that there is a higher rate of medical complications in this older patient population (1–6). Studies that break out the surgical complications from the medical complications show that the medical complications are significantly higher when the comorbidities are higher (1–3). These complications are equally divided between bronchopulmonary and cardiovascular. In one study, patients with a higher ASA experienced more medical complications ($P = 0.03$) but not surgical complications (4). Another evaluation that compared patients above 65 years of age to patients below 65 showed a higher complication rate (65% versus 49%) in older patients (5). Premorbid conditions were more prevalent in the older patient group (87% versus 72%). The medically related complications were significantly higher (35% versus 10%) in the elder group. Wound healing complications were equivalent. Another study that looked at 13 octogenarians showed a significant increase in the incidence of medical complications (62% versus 15%) when compared to a younger patient population (6).

TYPES OF FLAPS

The basic tenets of reconstruction in the head and neck are to replace composite tissue defects with composite tissue. These composite tissues may contain skin, subcutaneous tissue, muscle, or bone. A large number of body donor sites have been described that have various combinations of these tissue types. It is possible to tailor the type of tissue that will be harvested to replace the defect that is very similar in composition and texture to the resected tissue. What is important to realize is that the restoration of normal function is more problematic. Sensation, as well as muscular control, are important areas that are currently under an intense amount of investigation. We will attempt here to define the most common tissue types that are used in the current milieu. Our understanding of the effect of these various donor sites, both on morbidity that they induce and their ability to functionally rehabilitate the patient, continues to advance.

Pedicled Flap Reconstruction in the Elderly

Treating the geriatric population requires an appreciation for the risks and the benefits of both ablative therapy and reconstructive surgery. While the extent of ablative surgery for head and neck malignancies is often determined by the nature of the primary lesion, the method of reconstruction is usually left to the discretion of the surgeon. Smaller defects are usually managed with local tissue flaps and skin grafts. Comorbidities such as tobacco use, diabetes, and malnutrition may compromise healing. By itself, age is not a contraindication to local flap reconstruction. Extensive defects that are not amenable to local flap reconstruction can be managed with either regional pedicled flaps or microvascular free tissue transfer. Regional pedicled flaps offer a time-efficient reconstructive alternative to free tissue transfer in select cases; however, the surgeon should be aware of the age-specific risks and attendant morbidity associated with regional pedicled flaps (7).

The pectoralis major (PMC) and the latissimus dorsi flaps are the two most common regional pedicled flaps used in contemporary head and neck reconstruction. The complications associated with these flaps include soft tissue necrosis of the flap, hematoma, wound dehiscence, fistula, and infection; however, there is a paucity of literature examining age-specific complications of pedicled flaps. It is clear that patients with concomitant medical problems, which occur more commonly in the geriatric population, pose a higher risk of complications, longer hospital stays, and adverse outcomes (1–6). Additionally, because a vast majority of head and neck cancer patients have a history of tobacco use, respiratory complications following surgery are not uncommon. Early experience with the PMC flap did not suggest that the harvest of this flap may adversely affect pulmonary function; however, Schuller et al. (8) and others found that patients with pre-existing pulmonary disease may be at higher risk for pulmonary complications, including pulmonary atelectasis and restrictive lung disease, following PMC harvest (9–12). Recently, Talmi et al. (13) prospectively evaluated the effect of PMC harvest on pulmonary function and found that while patients with normal preoperative pulmonary function performed well postoperatively, patients with severe pre-existing pulmonary disorders had a decrease in forced vital capacity. Talmi et al. (13) suggested that the pectoralis muscle may play a role in respiration, and although they found that these patients did not clinically manifest evidence of pulmonary insufficiency, they did not specifically examine the age of the affected population. Schuller et al. (8) found that the degree of pulmonary dysfunction was related to the size of the skin paddle and that pulmonary restriction seldom occurred when the skin paddle was less than $40\,\text{cm}^2$. While the degree of pulmonary restriction may be negligible in a younger patient, elderly patients who are more commonly afflicted with chronic obstructive and restrictive pulmonary diseases may be more significantly effected by a tight donor site closure.

Similar principles hold true for the latissimus dorsi flap. Wax et al. (14) reviewed two groups of patients matched for age, sex, length of operation, site of primary, and stage of disease. One group underwent latissimus dorsi myocutaneous flap reconstruction following major ablative procedures and the other group was not reconstructed with a regional pedicled flap. They found that patients with larger skin paddles had a significantly higher rate of pulmonary atelectasis and speculated that the skin paddle size and the patient positioning during harvest may have contributed to the pulmonary dysfunction. These findings and the similar results found after PMC harvest suggest that a large skin paddle may represent a risk factor for postoperative atelectasis in patients with pre-existing pulmonary dysfunction.

Early ambulation following surgery is important in preventing postoperative deep vein thrombosis and pulmonary embolism. This is particularly important in the elderly, who often require assistance during ambulation. While lower extremity donor sites obviously delay ambulation, less obvious is the impact of a pectoralis or latissimus dorsi donor harvest on a patient's ability to ambulate. It has been our experience that both the pectoralis and latissimus harvest temporarily impair an elderly patient's ability to use a walker or a cane for support during ambulation. While this is only a temporary deficit, it should be considered in patients that rely on an aid for ambulation. Early physical therapy can be very effective in strengthening the shoulder and upper extremity to over come such deficits.

While microvascular surgery is not contraindicated in the elderly (4,5,15–17), regional pedicled flaps may offer an efficient method for head and neck reconstruction. It is important, however, to consider the potential morbidity associated with regional pedicled flap reconstruction and carefully evaluate each patient for pre-existing comorbidities that may contribute to postoperative complications.

FASCIOCUTANEOUS FREE TISSUE

Fasciocutaneous free flaps are tissues that have a single identified vascular supply and contain fascia and variable amounts of subcutaneous tissue, as well as skin. The most common donor sites for these flaps are the radial forearm, the lateral arm, scapula, and anterolateral thigh. Each one of these donor flaps has large vessels with relatively consistent anatomy and long pedicles. Survival rate with these flaps is above 95%.

Radial Forearm Flap

The radial forearm flap is based on the radial artery. It contains a significant amount of supple skin with little subcutaneous tissue. This makes it easily moldable in three dimensions for reconstruction of palate, tonsil, and tongue base defects. It has variable amounts of subcutaneous tissue, but in the majority of cases this is very limited. Taking large flaps and de-epithelializing them may allow for some bulk, but it is not a good flap for large volume defects. Because it involves harvesting the radial artery, the hand becomes dependent on the ulnar artery. There have been sporadic and anecdotal stories of hand problems. In the vast majority of cases, there is minimal morbidity associated with removal of the radial artery (18). Reconstruction of the arm following harvest of this flap requires skin grafting and placing the arm in a splint for up to one month to allow the skin graft to heal. Using a circumferential closure, loss of portions of the skin graft has decreased (19). Morbidity at the donor site is minimal in the majority of cases. Occasionally, when some of the skin graft is lost, conservative management is all that is needed. In a series of over 300 radial forearm flaps, less than 2% have required a return to the operating room for a second surgical procedure to repair the donor defect.

The major morbidity of this flap has to do with the functional loss of the hand while the splint is on (18). For this reason, the nondominant hand is used, and physiotherapy is started immediately following removal of the splint. Function of the arm is weak for a number of weeks but almost always returns back to the normal preoperative status. Because this flap could be harvested with a nerve, restoration of sensation to structures in the oral cavity or the head and neck is oftentimes possible.

Lateral Arm Flap

The lateral arm fasciocutaneous flap yields a greater amount of subcutaneous tissue. This makes it a thicker flap with more bulk than the radial forearm flap. The tradeoff for the greater bulk is less suppleness. In hemiglossectomy defects, the bulk may be helpful; however, the lack of suppleness results in an inability to three-dimensionally mold the tissue. For palate or tonsil defects, it yields a suboptimal result. The vessels are smaller, the pedicle length is shorter, and thus the success rate with this flap—other than in expert hands—is slightly less than that for the radial forearm flap (20). The morbidity of this flap is less than for the radial forearm. A smaller numbness over the lateral aspect of the forearm and elbow is the major morbidity.

Scapular Flap

The skin of the back is much thicker than the skin of the arm. On the back, the subcutaneous tissue bulk is relatively consistent. Being the back, large areas of skin can be harvested with this flap (21). The trade-off here is the lack of suppleness and three-dimensional conformability. A major disadvantage of this flap is that the patient needs to be turned on their side. The inability to harvest this flap with two teams increases the surgical time by at least two hours. If not harvesting bone, then no muscles of the back are disrupted and the morbidity is minimal.

Anterolateral Thigh Flap

This flap has recently come into vogue in North America. There exists a vast experience in Asia (22). Morbidity of this flap is minimal. The scar on the anterolateral thigh and the area of numbness associated with it are minimal. There is no requirement for a split thickness skin graft, so there is no morbidity associated with that. The tissue on the thigh can be quite thin and supple, or it can be quite thick. Recent studies have documented that the flap is thicker in the Caucasian population than in the Asian population because of the higher content of body fat. This makes the flap good for larger defects or defects that require more soft tissue bulk. The anatomy is variable, and success rates are not nearly as good as with the other fasciocutaneous flaps. The same issues with three-dimensional conformability exist. Its exact role in head and neck reconstruction is not well defined.

Myocutaneous Flap

The latissimus dorsi and rectus abdominis myocutaneous flaps are the most frequently transferred soft tissue muscle flaps used for head and neck reconstruction. These flaps provide a large amount of skin, subcutaneous tissue, and underlying muscle. These flaps are used where large soft tissue defects are created, for salvage of failed free tissue, or pedicle tissue transfer. They are supplied by a dominant vascular pedicle with usually one artery and two veins that come together. The vessels are of large size and the success rate with this flap is >97%. The pedicle is short, and that can sometimes limit the arc of rotation that one can obtain. Both of these flaps, while good at supplying large volumes of tissue, do so at the cost of a nonmalleable or moldable soft tissue component. The skin is often tethered through large subcutaneous tissue to the underlying muscle and its vascular supply. Consequently, it is difficult to mold this in three-dimensional shape as can be done with some of the fasciocutaneous flaps.

Rectus Abdominis Flap

Removing one rectus abdominis muscle with a piece of the overlying skin and subcutaneous tissue results in very little morbidity. Large amounts of soft tissue can be harvested, and the whole muscle can be taken (23). The major drawbacks to this flap are that most elderly individuals have a significant amount of subcutaneous tissue. In women who have had many children, the perforators to the skin have been stretched, and the anatomy may be unclear. It is possible to raise this flap and find that the skin paddle is nonviable. Even when large soft tissue segments have been removed, it is almost always possible to close this donor site primarily. Proper positioning of the belly button is a prerequisite for a better cosmetic outcome. There have been problems with tightness of the abdominal wall and a high incidence of hernia, but this has been resolved with increased use of mesh and nontight closures of the fascia. Surgical intervention of the abdominal wall increases the likelihood of atelectasis (23). In patients with predisposing chronic obstructive pulmonary disease, this can have a quite significant morbidity. Although this has not been studied in a geriatric population, the data can be extrapolated from across-the-board studies of the rectus abdominis flaps.

Latissimus Dorsi Flap

The latissimus dorsi myocutaneous flap supplies the greatest volume of tissue available for free tissue transfer. It is an extremely reliable flap that can be transferred both as a free tissue transfer and a pedicled flap. The advantages to a free tissue transfer are that the vascular pedicle and muscle are not tethered by the tunnel through the axilla and can be positioned in a more favorable location. The skin of the back is usually thicker, but the subcutaneous tissue is relatively constant. Large muscle bulk can be harvested, and split thickness skin grafting is often necessary at the recipient site. The donor site on the back can inevitably be closed primarily (24). As with other myocutaneous flaps, the skin is often of excellent quality but lacks the multidimensional molding necessary and available from other soft tissue flaps. The major morbidity associated with this flap is the inability to harvest with a two-team approach. There is a 2–3 hour time addition to the overall surgery. Other disadvantages include the amount of tissue that must be harvested, as well as the frequent occurrence of atelectasis (14). While head-to-head comparisons with the rectus abdominis have not been done, the incidence of atelectasis with this flap is quite high, and in patients with chronic obstructive pulmonary disease this must be a consideration in their reconstruction.

Osteocutaneous Flaps

Fibula

Reconstruction of the mandible and the midface structures often mandates use of a bone-containing flap. This is an area where rehabilitation and reconstruction has been most revolutionized by the introduction of free tissue transfer. The ability to harvest bone from a distal site that has not seen prior treatment and comes with a vascularized blood supply has allowed for immediate reconstruction and rehabilitation of patients who have suffered loss of a bony segment. The bone is important in maintaining the shape of the mandible. This is imperative in allowing for dental rehabilitation and adequate cosmesis. Not having bone present allows the jaw to drift to one side (25). Patients will be unable to wear dentures or chew any kind of solid food. The fibula, being at a distal site, can be harvested with a two-team approach and is a relatively straightforward flap to elevate. In the elderly patient, investigation of the vascular supply to the foot is of paramount importance. While there are three arteries (anterior and posterior tibial and peroneal) that supply the foot and lower leg, harvesting of the peroneal artery can lead to vascular insufficiency of the distal extremity. Plaques leading to outflow irregularities in the thigh or groin region can lead to low-flow states that result in wound healing problems in elderly patients. We have had patients with normal or "flappable" bones from their lower extremity, and it has taken a long time to heal their lower legs because of higher inflow obstruction. Consequently, all patients who are to undergo a fibular osteocutaneous free tissue transfer require investigation of the vascular supply to the lower leg and foot. This may take the form of an angiogram, colorflow Doppler, or MRA. All of these have been shown to be efficacious in various centers. Once the vascular supply has been deemed adequate (such that sacrifice of the peroneal artery does not endager the foot), the flap can be harvested as only a bony flap or with variable amounts of soft tissue. There is a small (<5%) chance that the skin paddle will not be viable and an alternative will need to be chosen. Because of the way the skin receives its blood supply from the perineal artery, it is the least malleable of all the soft tissue reconstructions. The necessity of putting the bone in a fixed position further hinders the ability to manipulate the skin into an optimal position. Thus, the bony reconstruction is often done at the price of a suboptimal soft tissue reconstruction. Any length of the mandible and midface can be reconstructed with this simple bone flap (26).

The morbidity from the fibula flap is quite high. Younger patients adapt to it quite well. However, the older population may have quite a bit of trouble healing the large leg wound it incites. Furthermore, taking the deep venous structure predisposes the patient to vascular venous stasis in the lower leg. It is not uncommon for patients to end up with walkers or canes for a number of months before they are rehabilitated. Patients who are marginal in their functional status, as far as their lower limbs go, may not be rehabilitated back to their preoperative functional mobility. This should always be considered in the preoperative evaluation.

Scapula

The lateral border of the scapula is supplied by the circumflex scapular artery, which is a branch of the subscapular artery. The artery then goes on to supply the skin of the back. Thus, a composite tissue flap with soft tissue of skin and subcutaneous tissue, as well as a bony-containing flap supplied by the same vascular pedicle, is possible. This bone is of good stock but of limited length. It can be used to reconstruct the mandible, as well as the midface (21).

Because of the necessity to roll the patient onto their side, this flap has not been utilized as much as the other bony flaps. The small amount of bone that is available also limits its use. The distinct and separate vascular supply to the skin and the bone makes this a unique flap. The skin can be hinged and rotatable in a complex three-dimensional manner through 360°. Furthermore, because of the vascular supply having two branches at 90°, separate skin paddles can also be taken. As mentioned with the latissiumus dorsi myocutaneous flap, this flap can be harvested with the muscle and transferred as a "megaflap." This flap is best used for through-and-through cheek defects that involve the mandible.

The morbidity associated with harvesting the bone is considerable. The muscular attachments of the lateral scapular cage and the humerus must be separated and then reattached. This results in quite a degree of shoulder dysfunction. Intensive physiotherapy under a specialized regime can result in regaining normal preoperative status. However, in an elderly disabled population that may be dependent on their upper extremity for use of a walker or a cane, this can prove to be quite debilitating and doom them to a wheelchair existence.

Radial Forearm Osteocutaneous Flap

This is a unique soft tissue bony flap that fell into disrespect a decade ago. A piece of the radius can be harvested because it is fed through the same vascular perforators as the overlying skin. Unfortunately, when it was first described, the radial bone was harvested in such a manner that the remaining radius fractured in up to 40% of patients. This made most free-tissue-transfer surgeons unwilling to deal with that type of morbidity. As the technique was improved and plating systems were used because of improvements in their mechanical properties, the flap has resurfaced. This flap provides up to 12 cm of bone that is cortical in nature and small. It is attached to the skin of the radial forearm flap, which allows for some of the soft tissue reconstructive characteristics of that flap. The vascular pedicle is tethered by the bone, and consequently the skin cannot be moldable in three dimensions when it is transferred with the bone. Due to the thin nature of the bone, this flap is used in midface reconstruction and for small lateral mandibular defects.

This flap, when harvested with technical modifications and reconstructed with a plate, has been found to have similar morbidity to just harvesting the soft tissue alone. A nondominant arm should be used so that the patients can write while a splint is applied, and split thickness skin grafting over the remaining muscles in the arm has been quite successful. Other than this, the morbidity is minimal (27).

SUMMARY

Free tissue transfer has been used in elderly patients in multiple centers for more than a decade. There is very little literature that compares elderly patients head-to-head with less elderly patients. However, in the studies that do, the survival rate of the free tissue transfer is identical in all age groups. Furthermore, surgical complications are the same between the two age groups, whereas the medical complications are related to the pre-existing functional status and comorbidities. Pulmonary and cardiovascular complications are higher in the elderly population, but this does not impact free tissue transfer. The potential improvement in rehabilitation in terms of swallowing, deglutition, and speech far offsets any possibility of morbidity associated with the flap transfer. However, elderly patients are more prone to be debilitated by minor decreases in function of an extremity than their younger counterparts. This is an area that has not been examined in the head and neck reconstruction literature. Much of the data surrounding morbidity from free tissue transfer is drawn from a younger population group. Whether it is transferable to an older population group is unknown.

Certainly, the elderly have the same disease-free survival rate after being adequately treated for their head and neck cancer. The ability to rehabilitate them with free tissue transfer does improve their rehabilitation and should not be a limitation.

Functional Rehabilitation of the Elderly Following Head and Neck Reconstruction

The goal of reconstruction of the head and neck is to restore speech and swallowing as close to the preoperative state as possible. When faced with a modest defect, this goal is best accomplished with local tissue flaps because the adjacent tissue is commonly sensate and similar with regard to texture and thickness (28). However, extensive defects represent a reconstructive challenge, particularly in elderly patients. As individuals age, they experience a progressive age-related demyelination process that may affect functional performance by decreasing sensation and muscular coordination (29). This decline predisposes the elderly to a greater degree of functional morbidity when they undergo surgery and reconstruction. For these reasons, it is imperative to restore the native anatomy and re-establish sensation. Only by doing so can we achieve optimal functional rehabilitation.

Swallowing and protection of the airway are dependant not only on the patient's ability to manipulate and transport a food bolus, but also on the ability to sense the bolus. The complex interactions between sensation and function have been demonstrated by many authors. These studies have revealed that oral mucosal anesthesia not only leads to oropharyngeal dysphagia, but may also result in aspiration (30). These findings highlight the importance of sensory restoration and the complex interaction between sensation and function. The inherent age-related changes in sensation and muscular coordination may be further compounded following surgical reconstruction in which a nonsensate skin flap is used to reconstruct an area of the oral cavity, oropharynx, or larynx. A general understanding of the age-related changes in sensation and function, as it relates to speech and swallowing, and a thoughtful approach to reconstruction of the head and neck can optimize functional rehabilitation in the elderly patient population.

Unlike regional pedicled flaps, free flaps offer the potential to restore sensation to the skin paddle. Proponents of sensory reinnervation contend that re-anastomosis of the sensory nerves associated with the free flap confers a functional advantage over nonsensate tissue (30,31). However, others believe that random peripheral nerve reinnervation occurs at the recipient site, providing the reconstructed patient with sensation and a functional outcome that is equivalent to direct reinnervation (32). The decision to reinnervate free flaps remains heavily debated. However, because the time and effort required to perform a neuroraphy is negligible, we favor sensory reinnervation when appropriate. The perceived advantage of reinnervation in an elderly patient is complicated by experimental and clinical evidence that demonstrates that the aging process leads to a reduction in terminal and collateral sprouting of regenerated fibers, theoretically limiting the capabilities for target reinnervation and functional restitution (33). Irrespective of these findings, there is no clinical evidence to suggest that elderly patients experience a lesser degree of sensory recovery when compared with their younger counterparts. It has been our experience that even a limited return of sensation of the free flap skin paddle is helpful in achieving improved functional results following oral cavity and oropharyngeal reconstruction.

Anytime an elderly patient is faced with a deficit in oral cavity or oropharyngeal sensation, function may be impaired. Sensation of the lower lip provides cues that are essential in the initial phase of mastication and deglutition. Reconstruction of the inferior alveolar nerve following lateral composite resection can improve oral sensation and therefore improve function (34). An interposition nerve graft is a simple method for inferior alveolar nerve reconstruction, and we have found that the return of lip sensation has a significant impact on functional rehabilitation, particularly in the elderly. Nerve grafting the inferior alveolar nerve can be accomplished by harvesting nerve from either the sural nerve or the antebrachial cutaneous donor site. It is not uncommon that elderly patients suffer from a mild gait disturbance. A sensory deficit resulting from a sural nerve harvest may only worsen a pre-existing gait deficit. As a result, we prefer to harvest from the antebrachial cutaneous donor site where the sensory deficit is better tolerated.

The goal of achieving optimal functional rehabilitation in the elderly is dependant on numerous factors. While speech, mastication, and swallowing are common parameters used to assess functional rehabilitation, quality of life and the ability to perform activities of daily living are essential components of rehabilitation. Following a maxillectomy or partial palatectomy, patients are often rehabilitated with a prosthetic obturator. While prosthetic obturation represents a simple and effective choice for the management of limited defects of the palate, the management of a prosthetic obturator can represent a difficult problem for the elderly. Such patients frequently suffer from a compromise in manual dexterity and/or poor eyesight, making it difficult to manage placement of a prosthesis. Furthermore, it is often difficult to maintain vigilant daily prosthetic hygiene, and as a result patients often experience crusting and malodor. Not uncommonly, elderly patients complain of the social stigma associated with a prosthesis and express frustration with having to wear a prosthesis to perform such simple tasks as answering the phone or drinking a glass of water. Such limitations can negatively impact on a patient's quality of life. In these patients, we have found that local palatal flaps, soft tissue free flaps, and bone-containing free flaps provide elderly patients with a permanent closure of the oro-nasal fistula and an improvement in function and quality of life (34,35).

The palatal island flap is an excellent source of donor tissue for defects of less than one-third of the hard palate. This technique provides a permanent closure of the palatal-nasal defect obviating the need for a palatal obturator. Similarly, the radial forearm free flap provides a larger source of donor tissue for defects that are greater than one-third of the hard palate. The tissue associated with both of these donor sites is thin and pliable and therefore does not interfere with the retention of a denture. We have found that patients with postablative palatal defects that are restored with either surgical technique enjoy a superior quality of life when compared with defect-matched patients who are dependant on a palatal obturator.

Achieving functional rehabilitation in an elderly patient is a challenging goal that requires a reconstructive approach focused not only on restoring mastication, deglutition, and speech but also on quality of life. While younger patients may compensate for postoperative muscular and sensory deficits, the elderly are less able to adapt and therefore require a thoughtful approach to reconstruction and functional rehabilitation.

REFERENCES

1. Sarini J, Fournier C, Lefelorre JL, et al. Head and neck squamous cell carcinoma in elderly patients: a long-term retrospective review of 273 cases. Arch Otolaryngol Head Neck Surg 2001; 127(9):1089–1092.
2. McGuirt WF, Davis SP III. Demographic portrayal and outcome analysis of head and neck cancer surgery in the elderly. Arch Otolaryngol Head Neck Surg 1995; 121(2):150–154.
3. Clayman GL, Eicher SA, Sicard MW, Razmpa E, Goepfert H. Surgical outcomes in head and neck cancer patients 80 years of age and older. Head Neck 1998; 20(3):216–223.
4. Serletti JM, et al. Factors affecting outcome in free-tissue transfer in the elderly. Plast Reconstr Surg 2000; 106(1):66–70.
5. Chick LR, et al. Free flaps in the elderly. Plast Reconstr Surg 1992; 90(1):87–94.
6. Blackwell KE, et al. Octogenarian free flap reconstruction: complications and cost of therapy. Otolaryngol Head Neck Surg 2002; 126(3):301–306.
7. Weiss MF, Lesnick GJ. Surgery in the elderly: attitudes and facts. Mt Sinai J Med 1980; 47(2):208–214.
8. Schuller DE, et al. Analysis of frequency of pulmonary atelectasis in patients undergoing pectoralis major musculocutaneous flap reconstruction. Head Neck 1994; 16(1):25–29.
9. Keidan RD, Kusiak JF. Complications following reconstruction with the pectoralis major myocutaneous flap: the effect of prior radiation therapy. Laryngoscope 1992; 102(5):521–524.
10. Huang RD, et al. Pectoralis major myocutaneous flap: analysis of complications in a VA population. Head Neck 1992; 14(2):102–106.

11. Seikaly H, et al. Pulmonary atelectasis after reconstruction with pectoralis major flaps. Arch Otolaryngol Head Neck Surg 1990; 116(5):575–577.

12. Peh WC, Ho CM, Ngan H. Chest radiograph appearances after head and neck flap reconstructive surgery. Australas Radiol 1993; 37(1):54–56.

13. Talmi YP, et al. Pulmonary function after pectoralis major myocutaneous flap harvest. Laryngoscope 2002; 112(3):467–471.

14. Wax MK, Hurst J. Pulmonary atelectasis after reconstruction with a latissimus dorsi myocutaneous flap. Laryngoscope 1996; 106(3 Pt 1):268–272.

15. Beausang ES, et al. Microvascular free tissue transfer in elderly patients: the Toronto experience. Head Neck 2003; 25(7):549–553.

16. Shaari CM, et al. Complications of microvascular head and neck surgery in the elderly. Arch Otolaryngol Head Neck Surg 1998; 124(4):407–411.

17. Bridger AG, O'Brien CJ, Lee KK. Advanced patient age should not preclude the use of free flap reconstruction for head and neck cancer. Am J Surg 1994; 168(5):425–428.

18. Skoner JM, et al. Short-term functional donor site morbidity after radial forearm fasciocutaneous free flap harvest. Laryngoscope 2003; 113(12):2091–2094.

19. Winslow CP, et al. Pursestring closure of radial forearm fasciocutaneous donor sites. Laryngoscope 2000; 110(11):1815–1818.

20. Wax MK, Briant TD, Mahoney JL. Lateral-arm free flap for reconstruction in the head and neck. J Otolaryngol 1996; 25(3):140–144.

21. Coleman SC, et al. Increasing use of the scapula osteocutaneous free flap. Laryngoscope 2000; 110(9):1419–1424.

22. Wei FC, et al. Have we found an ideal soft-tissue flap? An experience with 672 anterolateral thigh flaps. Plast Reconstr Surg 2003; 111(7):2481.

23. Wax MK, et al. Pulmonary atelectasis after reconstruction with a rectus abdominis free tissue transfer. Arch Otolaryngol Head Neck Surg 2002; 128(3):249–252.

24. Hayden RE, Kirby SD, Deschler DG. Technical modifications of the latissimus dorsi pedicled flap to increase versatility and viability. Laryngoscope 2000; 110(3 Pt 1): 352–357.

25. Wax MK, et al. A retrospective analysis of temporomandibular joint reconstruction with free fibula microvascular flap. Laryngoscope 2000; 110(6):977–981.

26. Urken ML, Sullivan MJ. Free flaps – composite free flaps: fibular osteocutaneous. In: Urken, Cheney, Sullivan, Biller, eds. Atlas of Regional and Free Flaps for Head and Neck Reconstruction. New York: Raven Press, 1995:291–307.

27. Werle AH, et al. Osteocutaneous radial forearm free flap: its use without significant donor site morbidity. Otolaryngol Head Neck Surg 2000; 123(6):711–717.

28. McConnel FM, et al. Functional results of primary closure vs flaps in oropharyngeal reconstruction: a prospective study of speech and swallowing, Arch Otolaryngol Head Neck Surg 1998; 124(6):625–630.

29. Peters A. The effects of normal aging on myelin and nerve fibers: a review. J Neurocytol 2002; 31(8–9):581–593.

30. Kimata Y, et al. Comparison of innervated and noninnervated free flaps in oral reconstruction. Plast Reconstr Surg 1999; 104(5):1307–1313.

31. Netscher D, et al. Sensory recovery of innervated and non-innervated radial forearm free flaps: functional implications. J Reconstr Microsurg 2000; 16(3):179–185.

32. Close LG, et al. Sensory recovery in noninnervated flaps used for oral cavity and oropharyngeal reconstruction. Arch Otolaryngol Head Neck Surg 1995; 121(9):967–972.

33. Verdu E, et al. Influence of aging on peripheral nerve function and regeneration. J Peripher Nerv Syst 2000; 5(4):191–208.

34. Urken ML, et al. Oromandibular reconstruction using microvascular composite free flaps. Report of 71 cases and a new classification scheme for bony, soft-tissue, and neurologic defects. Arch Otolaryngol Head Neck Surg 1991; 117(7):733–744.

35. Genden EM, et al. Comparison of functional and quality-of-life outcomes in patients with and without palatomaxillary reconstruction: a preliminary report. Arch Otolaryngol Head Neck Surg 2003; 129(7):775–780.

50

Appearance Changes with Aging

Donna J. Millay
Division of OtoHNS, Department of Surgery, University of Vermont, Burlington, Vermont, U.S.A.

INTRODUCTION

When encountering another individual, a first impression is often largely dependent on facial appearance (Fig. 1). With variable accuracy, that appearance is a mirror of an individual's age. There are many changes that occur over time which are evident with facial examination. Some of these changes are intrinsic and related to heredity while others are extrinsic and related to external factors, most prominently sun exposure. Although not everyone can accurately articulate the specific changes with aging, all people are aware of them to some degree. Probably the biggest changes are in the skin itself, which exhibits wrinkling, color and texture changes, as well as the acquisition of different types of lesions. The skin also becomes thinner and loses elasticity, creating sagging of the soft tissues. There is overall loss of boney tissue and subcutaneous fat, both of which contribute to an aged appearance. This chapter discusses specific aging changes related to the skin both at a macroscopic and microscopic level as well as changes in the different regions of the head and neck.

SKIN CHANGES

The skin undergoes many changes with advancing age. These changes are a result of a combination of extrinsic and intrinsic factors. Intrinsic changes are inevitable changes that occur as a result of aging regardless of external factors. In other words, intrinsic changes are those that might be seen in areas of the body that are shielded from any sun exposure, the most powerful extrinsic factor. In general, intrinsic changes of the skin include atrophy and loss of substance. The intrinsic aging that occurs in an individual has a definite hereditary component. For example, inherited skin type, such as thick and oily skin, will tend to age more slowly than thinner and drier skin (1). In contrast, extrinsic changes are those that come about by exposure to external factors, with sun exposure being by far the most important. Cigarette smoking is another extrinsic factor, which is thought to produce dermal changes by causing an alteration in cutaneous blood flow. The types of changes that are thought to be a result of extrinsic aging include dysplasia and alteration of the skin structure.

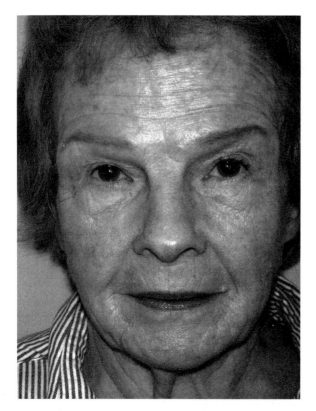

Figure 1   Attractive older woman exhibiting typical aging changes.

To better understand the changes in the skin with aging, it is important to first understand the underlying histologic changes (Fig. 2A) (2). Briefly, the skin is composed of three layers, with the epidermis being the most superficial layer, the dermis lying underneath it, and the subcutaneous tissue being the deepest layer. Within the

(A)   **(B)**

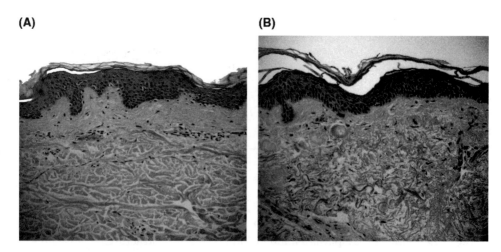

Figure 2   (**A**) Normal skin. (**B**) Aging, photodamaged skin exhibiting changes, including flattening of the dermoepidermal junction and significant elastosis.

epidermal layer the cells go through a series of maturational stages in layers that include the basal layer, the spinous layer, and the granular layer. The most superficial layer is the stratum corneum, which is composed of non-nucleated cells and provides a protection against outside substances and internal evaporation. The epidermis also contains melanocytes and Langerhans' cells. The dermis is composed primarily of collagen and elastin, which provide the skin with strength and elasticity. The dermis is divided into the more superficial papillary dermis and the deeper reticular dermis. The junction of the epidermis and dermis is serpiginous, with projections of the epidermis down into the dermis to form the rete pegs. The subcutaneous layer is composed of fatty tissue, which serves as insulation and cushioning (2).

With aging, the epidermis exhibits fewer changes than the underlying dermis (Fig. 2B). A very prominent feature in the aging epidermis is the retraction of the rete pegs along the dermoepidermal junction at the inferior border of the epidermis. This produces a flattening of the junction and an apparent thinning of the epidermal layer, although there are conflicting reports as to whether there is real significant thinning of the epidermis with aging. The flattening of the dermoepidermal junction decreases the adhesion of the two layers, which physiologically can lead to an increase shearing of the epidermal and dermal layers of the skin. This can predispose to erosion or bullae formation with forces such as those produced by the removal of tapes and bandages. Within the aging epidermis, there is also noted to be an overall decrease in the number of melanocytes and Langerhans cells. The remaining melanocytes tend to proliferate focally and bunch together to form lentigines (3). As the skin ages, there is noted to be a diminished control of proliferation of cells, which may result in excess cutaneous growths such as seborrheic keratosis and skin tags. Dysplasia and cytologic atypia of the epidermis are noted in the aging skin, which appears to be a result of sun exposure.

The dermis shows much more dramatic changes with aging. An overall notable finding is a significant thinning of the dermal layer that occurs through the years. The dermal structure becomes less organized and also becomes less vascular and less cellular. Collagen, which provides tensile strength to the skin, comprises the bulk of the dermis. The overall amount of collagen decreases by approximately 1% per year, and the remaining collagen fibers become thicker and less organized. This loss of structure of the collagen may account for increased fragility of the skin in the elderly. Elastin is another important component of the dermis, giving skin its elasticity. Aging changes of the elastin, or elastosis, can be noted over the age of 30 and become progressive with advancing age. Elastosis consists of thickening and disorganization of the elastic fibers and is particularly prominent in photodamaged skin. It results in a loss of elasticity of the skin and leads to sagging. There is also noted to be a general loss of the vasculature of the dermis as well as thinning of the vascular walls. This results in an increasing pallor of the skin and an increased tendency for bruising. Although there is noted to be an increase in the size of the sebaceous glands in the skin, there is a 40–50% decrease in sebum formation, which contributes to dry skin (4). Hair follicles in the dermis decrease with age, and graying occurs as a result of loss of melanin.

As noted previously, the subcutaneous layer is comprised primarily of fat. The overall change noted in the subcutaneous layer is a gradual atrophy. Due to other factors, there is also a redistribution of fat as it tends to settle inferiorly and become more prominent in the lower face and neck.

The above findings result in the macroscopic changes in the skin, which are observed as one grows older. Wrinkling is the earliest and most noticeable sign of

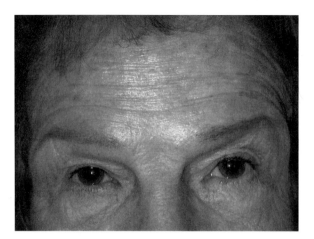

Figure 3 Fine rhytids are evident in the infraorbital region with coarse rhytids seen in the forehead.

aging. Wrinkles are classified as fine, medium, and coarse (5). Fine wrinkles are those that disappear with stretching of the skin and are more evident with the face at rest and less so with facial movement (Fig. 3). These often occur in the cheeks and periorbital areas of the face and probably arise from a combination of extrinsic and intrinsic aging. Medium wrinkles are difficult to see with rest but become readily visible with facial movement, whereas coarse wrinkles do not disappear with stretching and are usually seen at rest and become more evident with facial movement. Coarse wrinkles are frequently seen in the forehead and perioral area with smiling. It has been noted that hereditary factors play a role in wrinkling of the skin. Thicker, oilier skin has less wrinkling, while thin and fair skin becomes wrinkled more easily (1).

A second, very prominent sign of aging is laxity and sagging of the skin. As mentioned previously, the aging elastic fibers of the dermis are responsible for the progressive laxity of the skin with time. As gravity acts upon this lax tissue, it produces the sagging of the skin, which is very characteristic of the aging face. This may begin as very subtle changes and progress with time. Like many other changes, it is more prominent in photodamaged skin. Another change in the appearance of the aging skin is a roughness or lack of smoothness of the skin (2). This change is noted both by appearance and to palpation. The skin may appear uneven and irregular and may be rough to the touch. The previously mentioned changes of the stratum corneum are a major cause of these changes. Also the frequent occurrence of actinic keratoses in the aging skin may contribute to a rough appearance as well.

The skin undergoes various color changes, which are identified with aging. There is a tendency for the skin to lose some of its rosy color, becoming more dull and yellow in appearance. It is thought that this may be due to a loss of cutaneous vasculature. A second change is the gradual formation of telangiectasia with increasing age. These usually first appear on the nose and are also common on the cheeks. A third change is the alteration that occurs with melanin. The overall level of melanin decreases with age, making the aging skin more susceptible to photo damage. Additionally, the pigmentation of the skin may become splotchy secondary to the clumping of melanocytes, producing freckling and lentigines. This is particularly pronounced in sun-exposed skin.

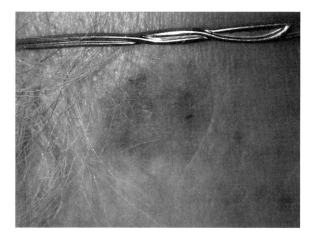

Figure 4 Typical appearance of a seborrheic keratosis.

SKIN LESIONS

There are many skin lesions that are acquired with age that affect the appearance of the head and neck. These include both benign and malignant lesions and can be singular or multiple. They may also be pigmented or nonpigmented, flat or raised.

Seborrheic keratoses are extremely common lesions associated with the aging population (Fig. 4). The etiology of these lesions is unknown. They appear brown to black in color and frequently have a verrucous quality. A "stuck on" appearance is a common and apt description of a seborrheic keratosis. Often multiple lesions are seen throughout the head and neck area, with the size varying from a few millimeters to 2–3 cm. Treatment is superficial removal with paring or cautery and is done for cosmetic reasons only.

Another common lesion in the aging head and neck is the skin tag, or fibro-epitheleal polyp. These are usually seen as small pedunculated lesions found in areas of frequent contact from skin folds or clothes. Common areas where they are seen in the head and neck include the upper eyelids and the neck. Again, these lesions need only be excised for cosmetic reasons, with removal usually being easily accomplished by snipping with a scissors.

Sebaceous hyperplasia is a frequently seen lesion in the elderly population. Microscopically, the sebaceous glands become large and multilobulated, and macroscopically, they appear as papules, which are soft and yellow. The usual size is 1–3 mm, and the papules are often multiple.

A very bothersome condition that is seen in the elderly population is chondrodermatitis nodularis helices (Fig. 5). These are lesions that typically present as a solitary nodule along the helical rim and are caused by inflammation of the perichondrial layer. They are usually erythematous and often have a crust over the central portion. They are very tender to the touch and patients typically complain of difficulty lying on that side when sleeping at night. Occasionally, an intralesional steroid injection may be successful, but most of the time local excision is required for resolution of the lesion.

Xanthalasma is a yellowish lesion seen in the upper or lower eyelids. These lesions are usually flat or minimally raised and may be solitary or multiple. Again, these need only be treated for cosmetic reasons.

Actinic keratosis is a frequent lesion of the aging skin that is related to sun exposure. This lesion tends to have a scaley appearance and a rough feel

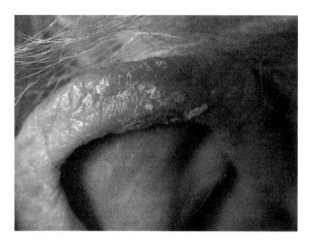

Figure 5 Chondrodermatitis nodularis helicis on the helical rim.

to palpation. It usually lacks a distinct border. Although these lesions are commonly thought to be precursors for squamous cell carcinoma, in fact less than 1% will actually progress to a carcinoma (4). These lesions are commonly treated with a superficial treatment, such as curettage or chemical treatment.

Malignant cutaneous lesions also occur in the head and neck with increasing frequency with aging and account for half of all new malignancies (4). Basal cell carcinoma accounts for 60% to 70% of these malignancies, squamous cell carcinoma for 20% to 30%, and melanoma for 5% to 10%. Sun exposure is the primary predisposing factor for all of these lesions.

Ninety percent of basal cell carcinoma occurs in the head and neck, and while these lesions may be locally aggressive, they rarely metastasize. Basal cell carcinoma classically presents as a solitary nodule with distinct rolled borders but may occasionally be more flat and sometimes ulcerated. It is common that these lesions are chronically crusted. The majority of squamous cell carcinoma (75%) also occurs in the head and neck region. These lesions have a 5% to 10% rate of metastasis, and the frequency increases with increasing size of the primary lesion. These lesions present more frequently as crusted or ulcerated lesions, and a history of bleeding is much more common (Fig. 6). The head and neck is the second most common site for melanoma, occurring here 20% to 35% of the time. These lesions most commonly have dark pigmentation but may be nonpigmented as well. They tend to have an irregular border and can be nodular or ulcerative. Metastases are related to the thickness of these lesions. Surgery is the treatment of choice for all of these malignant lesions. Further treatment is dependent on the type and extent of the lesion.

APPEARANCE CHANGES OF THE HEAD AND NECK

As we have discussed, the skin is a major determinant in the changes in facial appearance with aging. For the remainder of this chapter, we will explore how other factors combine with these changes to produce the characteristic alterations of the aging face and neck. The discussion will include an examination of the area as a whole followed by each individual region.

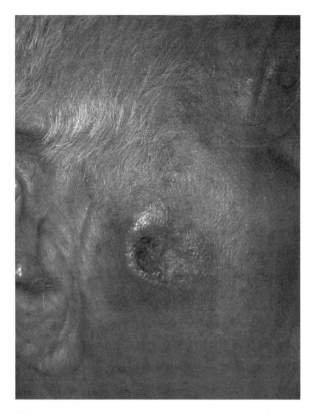

Figure 6 Ulcerated squamous cell carcinoma of the cheek.

There are many changes in the cutaneous, subcutaneous, and boney tissues that contribute to the overall alterations seen in the aging face and neck. The fatty tissue undergoes several changes that result in a characteristic appearance in the elderly population. First, there is a general decrease in subcutaneous fat with aging. Second, gravity, a major external factor that contributes to the aging process, produces a redistribution of subcutaneous fat in the aging face and neck with a gradual descent of fatty tissue from the upper and midface to the lower face and neck. Third, there is a recession of the orbital, temporal, and buccal fat pads, which tend to produce the thinned or gaunt appearance typically seen in the geriatric population (6). There are also changes in the boney tissue of the head and neck that affect the facial appearance. With time, there is an overall loss of boney mass, and in particular there is a loss of facial height from a decrease in the height of the mandible (7,8). This additionally produces a disproportion between the boney and soft tissues, which contributes to the appearance of soft tissue redundancy. This also contributes to a distortion of the classic horizontal thirds of the face, with the upper third becoming more prominent due to a receding hairline, the middle third increasing with increasing nasal tip ptosis, and the lower third diminishing with the decreased height of the mandible.

FOREHEAD

Starting with an analysis of the separate regions of the face is a discussion of the forehead. The primary aging changes seen in this region include brow ptosis and hyperdynamic facial lines (9). In the youthful forehead, there is an absence of rhytids, and the eyebrow is positioned at the level of the superior orbital rim in males and superior to this in females. The earliest aging changes in the forehead are usually the appearance of horizontal forehead rhytids often seen in the fourth decade of life (10). During the next decade, these lines are seen to deepen and vertical glabellar lines may appear (Fig. 7A). At the same time, the brows are seen to descend and flatten as a result of gravity and the loss of elastic tissue support of the skin. The descent of the brows can contribute to redundant upper eyelid tissue. This can also produce an angry, sad, or tired appearance as well as make the eye appear narrower or more closed (1).

The rhytids that appear in the forehead region are hyperdynamic lines, which occur secondary to muscular action. The frontalis is the largest muscle in the forehead and traverses it in a vertical fashion. Its function is to elevate the eyebrows. The consequence of this constant muscular pull is the production of horizontal forehead rhytids (Fig. 7B). As the eyebrows descend with age, this muscular activity becomes more pronounced in a chronic attempt to elevate the brows and results in more prominent rhytid formation. A second muscle in the forehead is the corrugator supercilii muscle. This muscle lies horizontally in the inferior forehead and acts to pull the eyebrows medially and downward. Overuse of this muscle produces vertical glabellar wrinkles, which give the appearance of being angry or chronically frowning (Fig. 7C). A third muscle in the forehead is the procerus muscle. This is a vertically

(A)   **(B)**

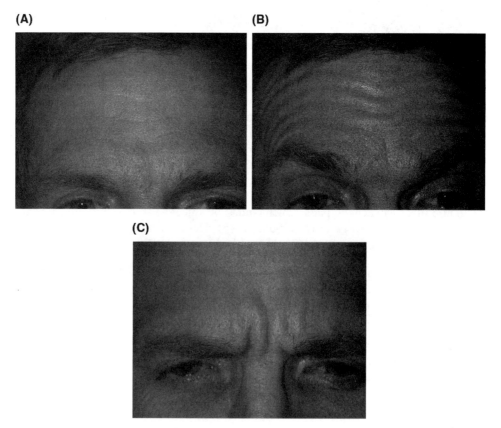

(C)

Figure 7 (**A**) Forehead at rest with horizontal rhytids and vertical glabellar rhytid. (**B**) Dynamic horizontal forehead rhytids. (**C**) Dynamic glabellar rhytids.

oriented muscle over the glabella whose muscular action produces a descent of the medial brows. Overuse of this muscle produces horizontal rhytids at the root of the nose. The orbicularis oculi muscle is the last muscle that affects the forehead area. It acts to depress the medial brow and contributes to lines in the glabellar region. An interesting study, performed by Drs. Ellis and Masri (1), found that patterns of facial expression were formed at a very early age and fit into a few specific patterns. In 48% of patients, they found that a predominant tendency was eyebrow raising, producing characteristic horizontal forehead rhytids. A second group, consisting of 35% of the patients, was prone to chronic frowning, which resulted in vertical glabellar folds. The last group, comprising 17% of the patients, had a pattern of squinting. These patients often had predisposing factors, which included a history of uncorrected vision, stress, or prolonged exposure to light. This group demonstrated the typical lateral canthal lines of crow's feet.

There are a number of options that are available to address and diminish the aging changes that occur in the forehead. Various types of brow lifts can be preformed that can not only elevate the brow position but may also be able to diminish some of the rhytids. Botox has been proven to be very effective in quieting the muscles that produce the characteristic forehead rhytids.

PERIORBITAL REGION

The next region to consider is the periorbital region, which includes the upper and lower eyelids and the medial and lateral canthal areas. An early and familiar sign of aging here is the acquisition of fine wrinkling in the lateral canthal area known as crow's feet. These fine rhytids are produced by the orbicularis oculi muscle, which surrounds the eye circumferentially and acts as a sphincter to close the eye. Probably the earliest aging changes are seen in the eyelids themselves and may be some of the earliest changes seen in the entire face. The upper eyelid most notably develops redundant soft tissue, or dermatochalasis, from an increase in skin laxity. The skin becomes progressively more redundant and may descend down to the eyelid margin or sometimes may even drape over the lashes. This tends to be more pronounced laterally and can at times produce a lateral visual field deficit. As noted above, brow ptosis also contributes to this process. Secondly, the upper eyelids may also develop fat pseudoherniation or prominent fat pads. All of these changes produce a tired appearance, which can be greatly improved with upper lid blepharoplasty and/or brow lift (Fig. 8).

The lower eyelids undergo many changes with aging. As with the upper eyelids, dermatochalasis may develop in the lower eyelids but is not as prominent or problematic. Pseudoherniation of the orbital fat is much more marked in the lower eyelid and produces a series of changes. First, it gives a full or puffy appearance to the eyelids. Second, shadowing occurs underneath the bagging of the lower lids, accentuating the appearance. Third, a depressed area or trough appears beneath the eyelid over the inferior orbital rim. Other changes are noted as well. Relaxation of the orbicularis oculi muscle occurs and, along with the effects of gravity, produces a pouch or fullness in the malar area. Again, the overall effect of these changes results in a more tired appearance. There are many surgical procedures that address these changes. These can include lower lid blepharoplasty with skin and fat removal or repositioning procedures, which elevate sagging tissue. These procedures can be very successful in restoring a more energetic and youthful appearance.

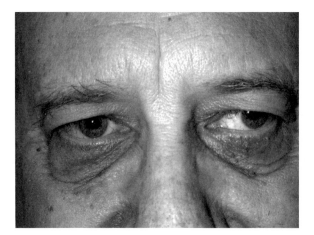

Figure 8 Aging changes in the periorbital area. Note the brow ptosis, upper lid redundancy, and characteristic changes of the lower eyelids.

There are many other changes that can be seen in the eyelids and globe. Upper eyelid ptosis occurs in the aging population, usually from disinsertion of the levator aponeurosis from the tarsal plate. This drooping eyelid can accentuate the tired appearance of the eyes. Lower eyelid laxity commonly occurs with aging and can produce lid malpositions, including ectropion and entropion. The lacrimal gland may also become ptotic, adding a full appearance to the lateral upper eyelid. Proptosis and exophthalmos can also be seen in the aging population (9).

MIDFACE REGION

The midface is a region that encompasses the area laterally from the preauricular crease to the nasolabial fold medially, and from the inferior orbital rim superiorly down to the inferior border of the mandible (9). The most prominent sign of aging in this region is the nasolabial crease and the adjacent nasolabial fold. The nasolabial crease is firmly positioned by attachments to the superficial underlying muscles and the superficial musculoaponeurotic system. With time, the nasolabial fold becomes more prominent as a result of the gravity-related downward redistribution of fat and the gradual sagging of the cutaneous soft tissue. This secondarily causes the nasolabial crease to deepen. Other changes are noted as well. There is a general atrophy of the cutaneous fat as well as more specific atrophy of the buccal fat pad, producing a submalar concavity that is characteristic of the aging face. The malar eminence itself becomes less prominent with a descent of the malar fat pad. Ptosis of the buccal fat contributes to jowling, which forms in the lower face along the mandible. The overall effect in this region is of a general downward drifting of the tissues. Many lifting procedures are available to counteract these changes.

NOSE

The nose undergoes subtle changes throughout a lifetime that produce gradual alterations in its appearance and function. These changes primarily occur from a weakening or stretching of internal structures of the nose. There is seen to be a general weakening of the cartilaginous structures of the nasal tip with a notable softening of the alar cartilages (10). Another change occurs in the attachment of the upper and lower lateral cartilages. These cartilages of the nose are usually tightly adherent, often in a scroll-like fashion, with the edges of the cartilages curling around each other. Over time, this attachment stretches and relaxes, with a resultant inferior displacement of the lower lateral cartilages. As in other regions of the face, fat atrophy is noted, and this is particularly important over the anterior nasal spine, where it can produce a decrease in tip support.

All of these changes combine to produce the characteristic alterations seen in the aging nose. The most notable finding is of an inferior and posterior displacement of the nasal tip from loss of tip support. This produces tip ptosis, which in turn gives the appearance of lengthening of the nose. As the tip becomes more posteriorly displaced, it may accentuate the nasal dorsum and either make a pre-existing nasal hump appear more prominent or create the effect of a new dorsal hump (12). With the softening of the alar cartilages, the lower nose can lose support, producing a broadening of the nasal tip and alar collapse with a diminished airway. In addition to these structural changes, externally the skin may develop fine wrinkles and telangiectasias, two more common signs of aging. In summary, the aging nose may develop tip ptosis with a secondary lengthening of the nose and accentuation of the nasal dorsum while the alar cartilages weaken, resulting in collapse and broadening of the nasal tip.

PERIORAL REGION

As in other regions of the face, aging changes are noticeable in the perioral region as well. As is seen elsewhere, there is a gradual atrophy of the soft tissues. Boney resorption of the mandible occurs, which is worsened with the loss of dentition. A direct result of this can be a loss of prominence of the mentum. The lips undergo specific characteristic changes with aging. Thinning of the red portion of the lips is a common finding in the elderly population. There is also noted to be a gradual lengthening of the upper lip, which gradually covers the upper dentition, particularly noticeable with smiling. Perioral rhytids are very common and are particularly pronounced in people with significant actinic changes or a history of cigarette smoking. Another change in the perioral region is the formation and gradual deepening of the marionette lines. These lines extend inferiorly from the lower end of the nasolabial crease down close to the inferior border of the mandible. Rejuvenation procedures in this area focus on increasing lip fullness and diminishing rhytids in the area (Fig. 9).

NECK

From previous descriptions of the changes that occur with aging in the head and neck, one can surmise the changes that appear in the neck itself. The overall changes in the neck are a result of the constant effects of gravity in combination with the progressive laxity of the skin and muscle in the area. As noted previously, fat tends to settle inferiorly in the region resulting in fat accumulation in the neck, particularly in overweight patients. The submandibular glands may become ptotic, which can add

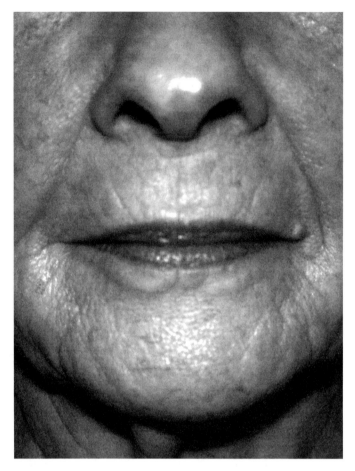

Figure 9 Typical perioral changes are seen with thinning of the lips and perioral rhytids.

to an apparent fullness in the area. Additionally, there is seen to be both a laxity of the cervical skin as well as the supporting platysmal muscles. The medial borders of the platysmal muscles become more prominent, producing platysmal banding. In the early stages, the banding may be seen only with movement, but as it becomes more pronounced it becomes visible at rest as well. All of these changes contribute to the loss of definition of the normal landmarks of the neck. The mandibular border in youth is a very characteristic feature of the neck, but this becomes less defined with aging. Similarly, the cervical mental angle loses its sharp angulation and becomes obscured. Approaches to correcting the aging changes of the neck include procedures to remove excess fat and tighten the sagging skin and muscle (Fig. 10).

EAR

Lastly, there are also noted to be some subtle changes in the ears over time. The size of the ear lobe may be noted to increase with advancing age. Also, the ears may become more prominent as the conchal-scaphoid angle widens.

(A) **(B)**

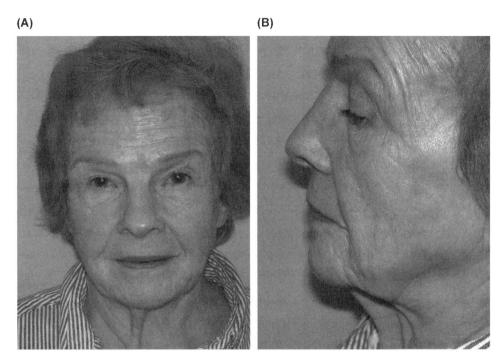

Figure 10 Aging changes of the neck. **(A)** The frontal view reveals moderate jowling and a significant platysmal band. **(B)** The lateral view demonstrates blunting of the cervical mental angle and loss of definition of the mandibular line.

SUMMARY

In summary, gradual changes occur in the appearance of the head and neck through-out a lifetime. Some of these changes are inevitable as part of the physiologic process of aging, while external factors such as sun exposure and tobacco may also play a role. Primary factors that lead to the alteration in appearance include cutaneous changes with loss of elasticity and rhytid formation. The downward drifting of soft tissues from the effects of gravity also produces characteristic changes. All of us are accustomed to judging another person's age with a quick overview of their face, but we as otolaryngologists should also be able identify the specific changes seen in each region of the face and neck and be knowledgeable of the underlying factors that pro-duce these changes. Hopefully, this chapter has given the reader further insight into the appearance changes that occur with aging.

REFERENCES

1. Ellis DAF, Masri H. The effect of facial animation on the aging upper half of the face. Arch Otolaryngol Head Neck Surg 1989; 115:710.
2. Weiss JS, Swanson NA, Baker S. Anatomy and physiology of aging skin. In: Krause CJ, Pastorek NJ, Mangat DS, eds. Aesthetic Facial Surgery. Philadelphia: Lippincott, 1991:461.
3. West MD. The cellular and molecular biology of skin aging. Arch Dermatol 1994; 130:87.

4. Ries WR, Aly A, Vrabec J. Common skin lesions of the elderly. Otolaryngol Clin North Am 1990; 23:1121.

5. Powell N, Humphreys B. Proportions of the aesthetic face. New York: Thieme-Stratton Inc, 1984:1.

6. Prystowsky JH, Siegel DM. Anatomy of facial lines and wrinkles. In: Blitzer A, Binder WJ, Boyd BJ, Carruthers A, eds. Management of Facial Lines and Wrinkles. Philadelphia: Lippincott, Williams and Wilkins, 2000:1.

7. Tardy ME. Rhinoplasty the art and the science. Philadelphia: W.B. Saunders Co., 1997:243.

8. Konior RJ, Kerth JD. Selected approaches to the aging face. Otolaryngol Clin North Am 1990; 23:1083.

9. Koch RJ, Hanasono MM. Aesthetic facial analysis. In: Krause CJ, Pastorek NJ, Mangat DS, eds. Aesthetic Facial Surgery. Philadelphia: Lippincott, 1991:135.

10. Goodwin WJ, Balkany T, Casiano RR. Special considerations in managing geriatric patients. In: Cummings CW, Fredrickson JM, Harker LA, Krause CJ, Richardson MA, Schuller DE, eds. Otolaryngology Head Neck Surgery. 3rd ed. St. Louis: Mosby, 1998:319.

11. Maloney BP. Forehead rejuvenation techniques. Fac Plas Surg Clin North Am 2000; 8:329.

12. Bailey BJ. Geriatric otolaryngology. In: Bailey BJ, Calhoun KH, Deskin RW, et al., eds. Head and Neck Surgery—Otolaryngology. 2nd ed. Philadelphia: Lippincott-Raven, 1998:284.

51

Reconstruction in the Elderly Patient

Adam T. Ross

Division of Facial Plastic and Reconstructive Surgery, Department of Otolaryngology, Medical University of South Carolina, Charleston, South Carolina, U.S.A.

Tom D. Wang

Department of Otolaryngology—Head and Neck Surgery, Oregon Health and Science University, Portland, Oregon, U.S.A.

INTRODUCTION

The need for functional and aesthetic reconstruction of the head and neck will increase dramatically as our population ages. The number of centenarians alone in the United States is projected to increase to over 5 million by 2046 (1). Necessarily, the complexities of reconstruction will require mastery by the facial plastic and reconstructive surgeon, microvascular surgeon, and general otolaryngologist.

It has become clear that chronologic age is less important than clinical age in the treatment of our patients. Nonetheless, no matter how healthy a patient appears, there are certain inevitable physiologic changes to which all patients will succumb over time. This overall decline in physiologic speed and the processes required to repair tissue damage, even at a cellular level, will vary significantly from person to person depending on a combination of environmental insults as well as hard-wired genetics. Astute clinicians possess the ability to keep certain predispositions in mind while assessing a patient and, at the same time, formulate a plan in concert with the findings on physical examination. This is particularly important when assessing each patient for head and neck reconstruction.

While each lesion requiring reconstruction presents a unique challenge, the reconstructive goal remains the same for all lesions: to restore function as well as former appearance. The literature contains excellent descriptions of reconstructive techniques for each type of head and neck defect, although there is no one single text that focuses on the elderly patient and the specific reconstructive needs of this population. Therefore, the constructs discussed in this chapter are not intended to provide technical details for each procedure, but rather to provide situational guidance from both our experience and others in order to aid surgeons in the reconstruction of defects in the elderly population.

RECONSTRUCTION AND DEPRESSION

Before delving into the logistics and techniques of reconstruction, one must remember that patients are infrequently prepared emotionally for many of the issues presented. Issues of the potential effects of cancer, functional deficiencies, and cosmetic deformities weigh heavily in the minds of those we treat.

With head and neck resections often being overtly disfiguring, it is not surprising that many patients develop situational depression. As depression is extremely common in the elderly population, ranging from less than 1% to over 15% depending on the study, one must pay attention to warning signs and refer for medical support if necessary (2). Underdiagnosis of depression is common, and intervention will be beneficial.

Although there is no substitute for personal interaction and the development of a sound relationship, there are certain techniques that may be used to guide patients through the process of reconstruction. It is important to keep expectations at or below those of the surgeon to avoid ultimate disappointment. Realistic goals must be set from the beginning of process. We find it important to discuss these issues with patients, and we usually find it extremely useful to show patients (if possible) the extent of each defect prior to reconstruction. This dramatically improves their understanding of the reconstructive dilemma, as well as increases their postoperative satisfaction.

ANESTHESIA

While systemic and local anesthetics are clearly a risk at all ages, the elderly patient has a decreased ability to respond to stress for many reasons. This population often has a reduced ability to respond to autonomic stimulation and stressors such as surgery due to physiologic changes in their cardiovascular system. Decreased cardiac output and stroke volume, reduced arterial elasticity and peripheral sclerosis, decreased size of sinoatrial and atrioventricular nodes, and sclerosis of the coronary arteries all act in concert to reduce the physiologic reserve of the elderly patient. Decreases in pulmonary function and an inability to mount an adequate cough postoperatively result in increased postoperative pulmonary infections. Diminishing renal blood flow may increase the clearance times of medication, including systemic and local anesthetics (3).

The most common local anesthetics (lidocaine or bupivicaine) exert their effects by blocking sodium channels, an effect that works almost immediately. However, these anesthetics have vasodilatory effects, and therefore a vasoconstrictor (usually epinephrine) is added to the solution prior to injection. Depending on the surgical plan, large quantities of local anesthesia may be necessary if the surgical field is large. It is therefore imperative to work together with the anesthesia team in such patients to minimize perioperative risks. We have found that a final concentration of 0.25% lidocaine and 0.125% bupivicaine is adequate for anesthesia, and epinephrine of 1:200,000 is effective for vasoconstriction.

The elderly population also has a higher incidence of chronic obstructive pulmonary disease and emphysema, and therefore often will present a challenge to the anesthesia team during recovery from general anesthesia. If possible, local anesthesia should be considered with sedation if suitable for the individual patient. However, larger repairs are often easier to manage under general anesthesia, which may therefore be more appropriate. Efforts to minimize irritation from the endotracheal tube at the termination of the case will be helpful, as will the placement of pressure dressings similar to that used after rhytidectomy.

EFFECTS OF AGING

Objective measurements and assessment of anatomic structures vary between the young and old. Changes in the skin with age show characteristic patterns that must be recognized prior to surgical planning of any reconstruction. When assessing reconstruction of the face, the most obvious and quantifiable changes are in the skin and subdermal components, as well as in the bony structures that support it.

The loss of dermal elastin in combination with laxity of facial ligaments leads to a sagging of tissue and the resultant deepening of grooves and folds (i.e., nasolabial and nasojugal folds). As skin ages, it looses its elasticity and stretches, resulting in more tissue to mobilize for reconstruction. This can be of benefit in filling defects, but it must be stressed that this skin is less resilient to insult and tension and must be managed accordingly.

Poor wound healing is more frequent in the elderly, although once again this association has less to do with chronology than associated comorbid conditions (4). Malnutrition and immunodeficiency, two common culprits in the elderly, may result in slower re-epithelialization, inflammation, and general healing and may result in a less optimal functional and aesthetic result. Diabetes and chronic steroid use may also have similar effects, and patients with these conditions should be identified and closely monitored in the postoperative period.

ETIOLOGY

Trauma and cutaneous neoplasms cause most of the defects encountered in reconstruction in the elderly. Congenital lesions are most often repaired when patients are younger, and infections are fortunately more rare in the head and neck than other regions of the body.

Long-term exposure to ultraviolet radiation results in cumulative damage to the skin and may result in precancerous lesions, such as actinic keratoses, or malignancies, such as basal cell carcinoma, the most common cutaneous malignancy. In fact, one out of every five people will develop a skin cancer during their lifetime (5). It has also been shown that individuals who develop a skin cancer are more likely to develop not only additional skin cancers but also other internal malignancies, such as lung cancer (6,7). The increasing incidence of skin cancers may also be related to the depletion of the ozone layer (8).

Basal cell carcinoma and squamous cell carcinoma are both linked in causality with ultraviolet radiation and immunosuppression, and squamous cell carcinoma is more common in the patient with fair skin. Basal cell carcinoma, followed by squamous cell carcinoma and finally melanoma, is the most common cutaneous malignancy in elderly patients (Fig. 1).

Traumatic injuries to the head and neck are mostly from falls or other blunt injury. As will be discussed in detail later in this chapter, special techniques must be kept in mind when treating fractures in the elderly patient.

(A)   **(B)**

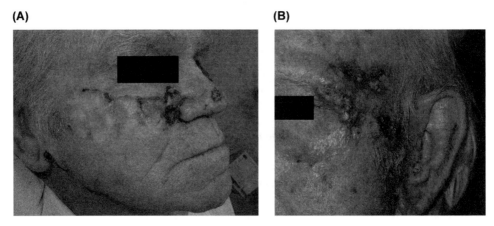

Figure 1   Sclerosing basal cell carcinoma (**A**) and squamous cell carcinoma (**B**) of the skin.

PREOPERATIVE ASSESSMENT

As with any patient, but especially in the elderly, a careful preoperative assessment must be performed. A consultation with an internist is often appropriate, as all efforts must be made to optimize a patient's cardiovascular status and minimize untoward anesthetic effects. Note should be made of patients with hypertension, diabetes, and of smoking history, as these conditions decrease both arterial and immune supply to the skin, therefore promoting poor wound healing. Dehydration, a common problem in the elderly, must also be corrected. The ability to optimize the patient will allow one to maximize surgical intervention.

A list of medications must be obtained, and any medications with anticoagulant effects should be discontinued two weeks prior to surgery, or managed appropriately. Patients should also be asked about their use of alternative treatments or supplements, such as Vitamin E or Gingko Biloba. Patients will often neglect to report their use of these anticoagulants unless they are prompted. There will usually be the need to prescribe medications for each patient, and if a patient's medication list is complicated, clearance for the administration of new medications should be obtained through an internist prior to treatment.

A preoperative consultation should always include assessment by the anesthesia team. Appropriate laboratory tests should be sent to assess surgical risk. An appropriate work-up may identify potential contraindications to anesthesia or limit one's ability to perform a lengthy reconstruction. Surgical goals will then need to be reassessed and discussed with the patient. Although this occurrence is infrequent, it may become more of an issue as the population ages.

GENERAL RECONSTRUCTIVE CONCEPTS

Assessing the Defect

One must always first begin with a careful and systematic assessment of each defect. We believe that it is extremely useful to assess defects of any region from the outside to inside, and then plan the surgical repair from inside to outside.

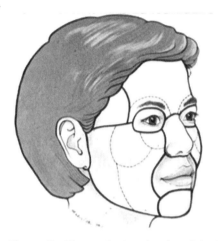

Figure 2   The aesthetic subunits of the face. *Source*: From Ref. 9.

Starting on the "outside," the skin defect must be assessed in terms of aesthetic subunits (Fig. 2). Skin defects crossing the borders of subunits will often require more than one surgical technique to maintain an aesthetically pleasing separation between each subunit. One common example of this concept is that of a nasal lesion that extends into the cheek subunit, where a facial advancement must be performed in combination with an appropriate nasal reconstruction (Fig. 3).

Attention should then be paid to the depth of any defect, identifying the depth of skin involvement, involvement of nerves and blood supply, a deficiency of supporting structure (bone and cartilage), and finally inner mucosal lining. All of these components should be addressed and replaced at the same sitting to achieve a satisfactory outcome.

Finally, the functional implications of such a defect must be assessed. Eye closure and oral competency are the two most important functional issues that require immediate attention. Facial nerve involvement may affect both functions, and one should consider adjunctive eyelid protection, such as a gold weight in patients with poor eye closure. Lip defects should be addressed to facilitate oral nutritional intake. Once functional issues are satisfied, the other aspects of the reconstruction may be considered.

Inner Lining

Lesions that invade into the inner lining of the mouth or nose require internal mucosal replacement to minimize contraction, and/or provide extra blood supply for reconstruction.

Free flap reconstruction often is an excellent option for large mucosal defects to provide both mucosal replacement and blood supply. If the defect is smaller, local advancement or rotation flaps may be used to cover the defect, leaving the donor site to heal secondarily. Pedicled myocutaneous flaps, such as pectoralis or deltopectoral flaps, may also be harvested for this purpose.

Through-and-through intranasal defects may be reconstructed with local flap reconstruction techniques as well. Septal flaps, inferior turbinate flaps, and buccal mucosal flaps may all be used for inner nasal lining. A careful assessment of each defect will allow one to utilize available tissue.

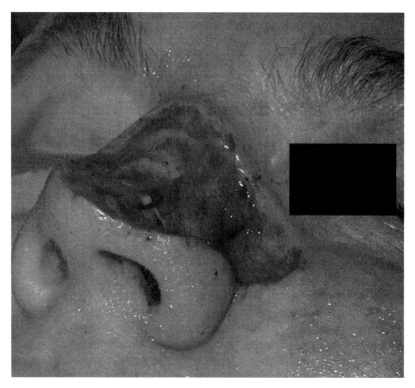

Figure 3 A recurrent basal cell carcinoma has been removed from this patient by Mohs micrographic surgery. Note that the defect crosses the border of the lateral nasal subunit into the medial cheek and is a full-thickness defect involving nasal mucosa.

Structural Support

Replacement of bone can be performed using one of several techniques. Free flap reconstruction can provide a large amount of vascularized bone as well as an epithelial component that is often useful for either skin or internal lining. Bone grafts, such as calvarial bone or iliac crest, may be used as well. Costal cartilage may also be harvested for use in nasal reconstruction.

Structural support may also be provided by allografts, such as irradiated rib cartilage. These allografts are particularly useful in establishing nasal support for large defects. Conchal cartilage is often used to restore support to the nasal valve and alae.

Alloplastic materials are often necessary for certain defects. Titanium mesh is extremely adaptable for many defects, including frontal sinus, orbital floor, and nasal reconstruction. Medpor synthetic implants may also be used for orbital reconstruction, auricular deformities, and nasal alar defects. Hydroxyapatite or other bone cements may be used alone or in concert with other materials to fill bony defects.

Skin Reconstruction

The reconstructive goal in replacing lost skin coverage is to replace the lost tissue with that of similar color and texture. This is best accomplished by covering a defect with adjacent tissue, as it often has a similar texture and has suffered similar environmental insults over the course of time. Conversely, skin adjacent to an excised lesion may be prone to develop cancerous lesions that are as yet undetected. In this case, adjacent (unhealthy) tissue may not be the best option. Also, anatomic landmarks and structures on the face may limit the ability to advance or rotate adjacent skin without undue deformity to local structures (such as the eyelids). If adjacent skin is not appropriate or available, skin from the melolabial, postauricular, preauricular, or supraclavicular regions (in order of preference) may be used as free full-thickness skin grafts to provide a close match to the skin of the face.

If at all possible, scars should lie in the "relaxed skin tension lines," or RSTLs, of the face (Fig. 4) (10). These lines reflect the intrinsic properties of relaxed skin, correspond to the alignment of elastin and collagen in the dermis, and therefore influence wound healing. It should be noted that although wrinkles and RSTLs are usually parallel, wrinkles are a reflection of active muscle contraction and in certain regions of the face (i.e., lateral canthus and glabella) are not aligned. Placement of scars within the RSLTs will achieve the best long-term result. As well, scars placed within the lines separating aesthetic facial subunits will also allow for camouflage. RSTLs become more apparent with aging, and surgeons will often be able to achieve a more acceptable result in this population.

Another principle of scar design is to align the line of greatest tension perpendicular to the RSTLs, along the "lines of maximal extensibility" of the face. Therefore, a scar lying within the RSTL will not only camouflage well, but the tension across its closure (usually the direction of highest tension) will be minimized as a result of the skin's natural elasticity. Widened scars will therefore

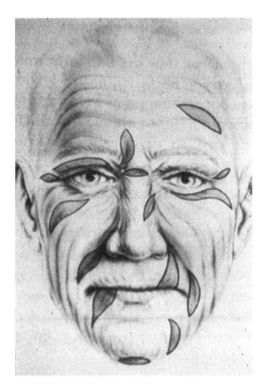

Figure 4 The relaxed skin tension lines of the face, with examples of excised lesions placed within these lines.

be kept to a minimum. Plication of the superficial musculoaponeurotic system may also help both to reduce skin tension as well as to reduce the size of a defect prior to reconstruction.

Rotational flaps in the head and neck are extremely well vascularized and therefore show more rapid healing and make the head and neck less susceptible to infection. Due to the increased vascularity, these flaps are also prone to prolonged edema, and an inferiorly based design should be utilized whenever possible to reduce lymphedema resultant from disruption of venous and lymphatic channels (11).

The general medical condition of the elderly patient, as mentioned earlier, may have a negative impact on wound healing. Therefore, one should consider a delayed approach to local flap reconstruction for wounds. By creating incisions with or without elevating the flap itself, and delaying its transposition, one can condition tissue to survive hypoxia by breaking arteriovenous shunts and reorienting lymphatic drainage. The incisions and elevation also transect the sympathetic input to the skin, causing vasodilatation. Although there are advantages to delay, the clinician must weigh these potential advantages with the disadvantages of prolonged wound care and the effects of second intention healing. In many situations, the surgical option that requires less time, less tissue manipulation, and therefore confers less risk to the patient will in fact be equally successful.

TYPES OF RECONSTRUCTION

Primary Closure

A first consideration of any defect is whether primary closure of the wound may be accomplished. This is the most straightforward method of reconstruction, and often small lesions are amenable to closure at the same sitting as the resection (Fig. 5). Extremely large lesions are obviously not amenable to primary closure. In between these extremes lie the lesions that require clinical judgment. Primary closure should only be performed if there is minimal tension on the wound or other local structures. If performed, meticulous techniques must be used on the skin edges, and wide undermining should be performed to reduce tension and allow for skin edge eversion. Wound closure should always be aligned in relaxed skin tension lines, and this is

(A)   **(B)**

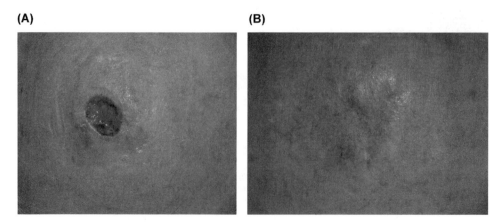

Figure 5 (**A**) A scalp defect created by Mohs resection of a basal cell carcinoma. (**B**) This was repaired with primary closure after wide undermining and is shown after one month.

facilitated by appropriate orientation of the excision. Angles of less than 30° at the apices of the wound will minimize standing cone deformities.

Second Intention Healing

Second intention healing is an often-underutilized option for many wounds. As the elderly population is more susceptible to perioperative surgical risks, a surgeon must understand when this viable option will have acceptable results.

Wounds, if left to heal secondarily, will follow predictable stages of healing. First, as a result of the initiation of the coagulation cascade, a fibrin gel forms with the subsequent appearance of granulation tissue. The inflammatory reaction and macrophage influx allows for wound debridement, and chemotactic factors attract the cells necessary for growth and repair. Neovascularization, collagen deposition, and re-epithelialization occur, followed by wound contraction. Over the longer term, remodeling of the wound allows for a more mature and softer scar (12).

This most conservative form of wound management is best on concave surfaces (not near mobile structures), such as the medial canthus, nose, ear, and temple, and good on flat surfaces, such as the forehead (13,14). These wounds are usually not painful, and no other defect is created to provide donor tissue. As a result, less tension is applied to adjacent structures, although contraction of the wound may alter local tissue over time. Second intention healing is often a better option than skin grafting in patients with compromised vasculature (previous radiation therapy or smokers) and may be used in contaminated wounds with too much debris to allow for immediate reconstruction.

The disadvantages of second intention healing should be recognized as well. There is the need for prolonged wound care, with frequent dressing changes and application of lubrication to keep the wound moist. In the scalp, regions that heal secondarily will not regenerate hair follicles, resulting in alopecia, and there is a propensity for hypertrophic scarring. Wound contraction may adversely affect local structures.

Second intention can also be used in conjunction with other techniques of reconstruction. If tissue is in short supply, some parts of the wound may be left to heal secondarily, with coverage provided for areas not amenable to second intention healing. As well, deeper wounds may be left to heal secondarily for some time, thus filling the wound with granulation tissue to the desired thickness prior to skin grafting. This is often a reasonable option for deep defects of the scalp in areas of alopecia.

Second intention healing is dependent on the effects of the coagulation cascade and inflammation. Without a viable blood supply, neither will occur. Therefore, wounds without periosteum or perichondrium will not heal by second intention. Exposed bone may either be drilled to expose bleeding from the diploic layer or covered with local tissue (15). Epithelialization occurs more slowly over necrotic and dry tissue, and therefore wounds must be kept moist with bacitracin ointment or other moisturizer.

Skin Grafts

If neither primary closure nor second intention fit the bill for a defect, free tissue transfer offers us solutions. Skin grafts may be used on wounds that have a generous blood supply and therefore may have a variable survival rate in the elderly population, especially in the face of prior radiation or vascular compromise.

All flaps are dependent on diffusion of nutrients in the first 3–4 days (plasmatic imbibition) until blood vessels reconnect (inosculation) (16). During this crucial stage (first 5–7 days), movement of the graft will shear the fragile vascular supply. We prefer either bolster placement or tacking sutures to prevent movement and pie crusting of the graft to prevent fluid accumulation (hematoma or seroma) between the tissue bed and the graft. Skin grafts should not be placed over exposed bone or cartilage, as they are devoid of blood supply.

Skin grafts may be either split thickness (Fig. 6) or full thickness. The advantages of split thickness grafts are that survival is higher than full thickness grafts and may be more easily harvested in greater quantity. However, wound contraction is greater with split thickness grafts, and skin color and thickness match is often suboptimal. Full thickness grafts provide a better color and thickness match for most defects and contract less (although some contraction is inevitable). Also, FTSGs can

(A)   **(B)**

(C)

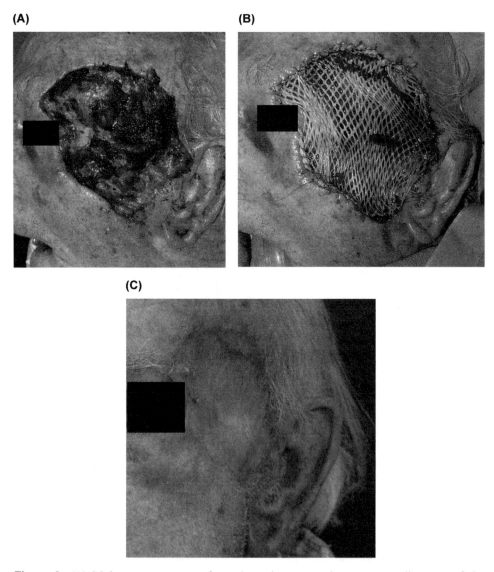

Figure 6 (**A**) Mohs surgery was performed on the temporal squamous cell cancer of the patient in Figure 1B. (**B**) The defect was covered with a left thigh meshed split thickness graft, and (**C**) is shown at 10 weeks follow-up.

be modified somewhat to account for the depth of each defect, and over-thinning the graft will leave a poor contour and obvious scar.

Another free-graft option is the composite graft, which can be obtained from the superior helical root or conchal bowl of the ear. These procedures are ideal for certain defects, especially nasal alar defects, because they supply both skin and underlying support (Fig. 7). However, it is difficult to predict the take rate with defects larger than 1 cm, and these grafts should be used cautiously in the elderly population with vascular compromise.

Local Flaps

Advancement and/or rotation flaps are often utilized if adjacent tissue is available. These local flaps are random in blood supply and are dependent on the subdermal plexus. Due to the high vascularity of the head and neck, the usual limitations on length to width do not usually apply. Individual techniques are well described in other texts, but commonly used flaps are worth mentioning, including tips in elderly patients that will avoid unforeseen complications.

True rotation flaps are best for triangular defects. Planning out the arc of rotation is important, and in reality, due to the limitations of facial anatomy and the desire to place incisions between subunits or RSTLs, most rotation flaps utilize advancement techniques as well. True advancement flaps include the V to Y advancement flap, which is useful when advancing skin towards the border of an aesthetic subunit, such as the upper lip. The Reiger flap (Fig. 8), a modification of the V to Y, is an excellent flap for nasal dorsal defects as a result of the ability to place the incisions in glabellar folds as well as the borders of nasal aesthetic subunits.

The cervicofacial advancement-rotation flap (Fig. 9) is the workhorse for lesions of the cheek and face. The general rule is that the arc of rotation should be four times the diameter of the defect to prevent standing cones, and the incisions should be placed in the subciliary line, preauricular crease (facelift-type incision), and then carried down into the neck inferiorly and then anteriorly in a neck crease to allow for extra rotation if necessary. This flap has a higher incidence of failure or flap loss in smokers and those with a history of preoperative radiation therapy. If the defect is large, the postauricular skin can also be included for more area (bilobed cervicofacial flap) (17). Care must be taken to extend the lateral incision superiorly and laterally before turning inferiorly in the preauricular crease to prevent a downward pull on the lower lid and subsequent ectropion (Fig. 9). Other keys to preventing ectropion are to keep in mind the predisposition in this patient population to senile ectropion, perform a snap test preoperatively, and if there is any question of lid laxity, perform a lid shortening procedure at the same sitting. Even with appropriate precautions, there is still a tendency toward cicatricial ectropion (Fig. 10), and patients should be followed closely to identify ectropion prior to irreversible corneal damage.

Transposition flaps allow the surgeon the flexibility to align scars with RSTLs, lengthen contracting scars, adjust the axis of scars into RSTLs, and control the tension on adjacent structures. The rhombic flap (utilized for square defects), when designed properly, allows for the placement of its flap along the lines of maximum extensibility and scars within the RSTLs (Fig. 11). Another transposition flap, the bilobed flap, is utilized for circular defects, and it can be modified with an arc of rotation of 90° instead of the originally described 180°. This Zitelli (18) modification reduces the incidence of standing cones as well as the total area of adjacent skin

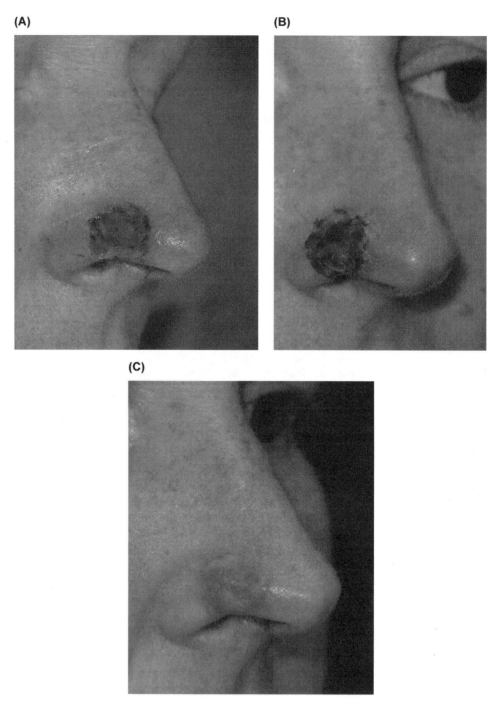

Figure 7 (**A**) Nasal alar basal cell carcinoma resected by Mohs surgery. (**B**) A composite graft from the superior helical root was utilized to replace lost skin and cartilage. The result is shown at three weeks and (**C**) at three months postoperatively.

(A)

(B)

(C)

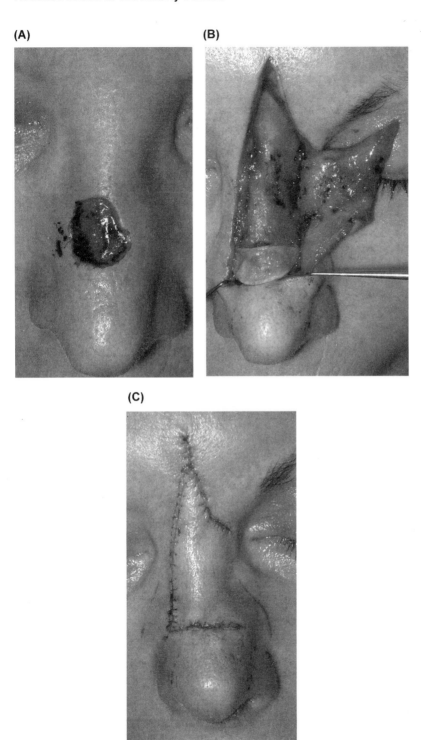

Figure 8 Reiger flap reconstruction. (**A**) A 69-year-old female after Mohs excision of a basal cell carcinoma. (**B**) Intraoperative view of laterally-based Reiger flap. Note that a cartilaginous butterfly spreader graft has been placed to prevent nasal valve collapse. (**C**) After closure of the defect.

(A)
(B)
(C)

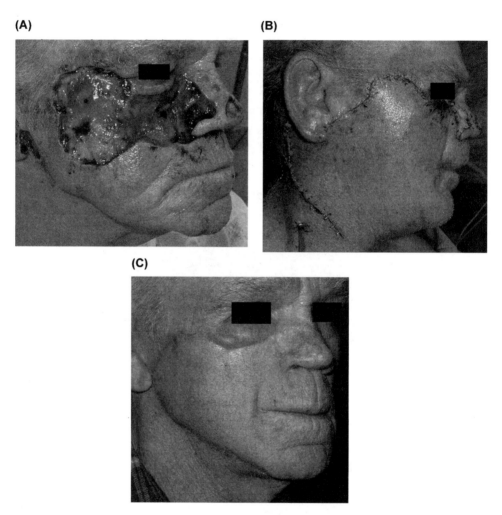

Figure 9 Cervicofacial advancement flap. (**A**) Mohs resection of the lesion from Figure 1A. (**B**) After cervicofacial advancement-rotation flap to repair the check defect, and full thickness skin grafts to the right nasal sidewall and tip. Note the lateral upward design of the incision to prevent ectropion. (**C**) The same patients four months postoperatively.

necessary to perform a bilobed flap. The disadvantage of the bilobed flap is that the circular scar often crosses aesthetic subunits, and postoperative edema can lead to pin cushioning of the scar. One must be reminded to base these flaps inferiorly to facilitate lymphatic drainage. Z-plasty, a type of interposition flap, may be used to break unsightly scars, as well as lengthen scars.

Pedicled flaps are particularly useful in certain patients as blood supply is maintained for several weeks, and then transected once the previously described stages of graft take have been completed. Paramedian forehead and melolabial flaps are examples of such flaps (Figs. 12 and 13). The superiorly based melolabial flap is excellent for alar rim defects, while the mid-forehead flap can be used to cover the skin of the entire nose down to and including the columella. In the rare case that vascular insufficiency causes distal flap loss, one should keep in mind that a contralateral flap of the same kind may be harvested, but often

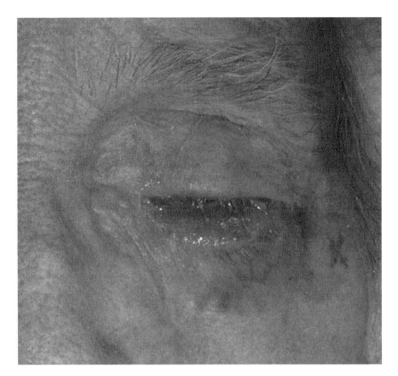

Figure 10 Cicatricial ectropion after cervicofacial advancement flap in spite of concurrent tarsal strip and lid shortening procedure.

second intention healing will be adequate. It is therefore important to design forehead flaps so that they do not involve the contralateral side.

Another useful and well-vascularized flap is the superficial temporoparietal facial flap, which is pedicled on the superficial temporal artery. This flap is vascular enough to support a skin graft, and is excellent for skull base resurfacing and auricular reconstruction.

(A)   **(B)**

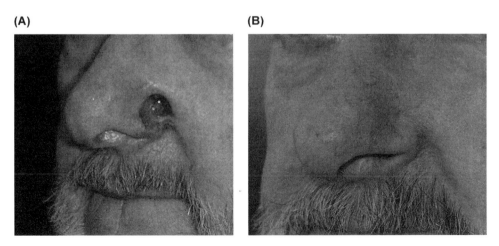

Figure 11 Rhombic flap reconstruction. (**A**) Nasal defect after Mohs resection. (**B**) Three months after rhombic flap reconstruction.

(A)   **(B)**

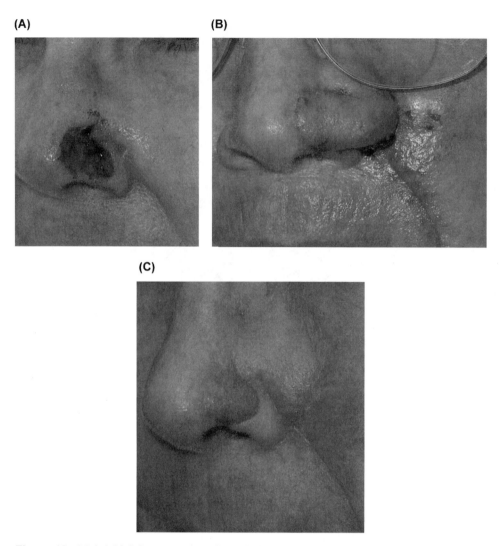

(C)

Figure 12 Melolabial flap reconstruction of alar defect. (**A**) Alar defect status post Mohs resection. (**B**) Postoperative view of melolabial flap reconstruction. (**C**) Four months after take-down of pedicled flap. Note that a bridge of skin is conserved between the check and ala to preserve the alarfacial groove.

Microvascular free flaps, covered in another chapter, are a final option of reconstruction that should be reserved only for healthy patients with large defects.

ANATOMICAL CONSIDERATIONS IN THE ELDERLY

Eyelid

Defects around the eyelid can be assessed with regard to involvement of the skin, supporting structures (tarsal plate), and the inner mucosal lining (conjunctiva). With senility, eyelids are prone to laxity of the outer lamella, causing senile ectropion. Symptoms such as excess tearing and burning of the eyes from exposure can be

(A) **(B)**

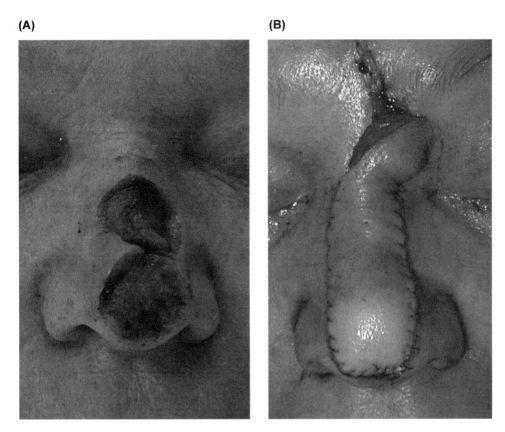

Figure 13 Paramedian forehead flap reconstruction. (A) Mohs resection of basal cell carcinoma on the nasal dorsum. (B) Paramedian forehead flap pedicled on the left supratrochlear artery. Note that the remaining skin within the dorsal nasal and tip subunits has been removed to hide the scars between subunits.

assessed using the snap test. This one finding is often overlooked when considering reconstruction of defects on or near the eyelids, and it often will require a second procedure to correct unless diagnosed properly. There should be an extremely low threshold in the elderly to perform a lid shortening procedure at the time of reconstruction.

Reconstruction of the eyelid is made easier by the facts that the eyelid skin is extremely thin, has no subcutaneous fat, and therefore is not prone to scar formation. Any defect of the lid, when closed primarily, should be closed vertically to avoid tension on the eyelid margin.

While small medial canthal defects may heal well by second intention, reconstruction of larger defects are more prone to postoperative complications, such as ectropion. Cervicofacial flaps are particularly good for anterior lamellar defects of the lower lid, but as discussed earlier, one must avoid downward pull on the lid and place incisions in the ciliary line. Especially in the elderly, any skin left under the subciliary line superior to the advancement flap will be particularly prone to unsightly edema formation.

Elderly patients, due to the redundancy of lid skin, are more likely to be adequately treated by primary closure without affecting the lid margin. Extra lid laxity also helps in the treatment of through-and-through defects of the lid, as primary closure may be performed often even when more than the usual limit of 50% of the lid is involved. Lateral cantholysis may also allow one to reduce tension for this closure as well as provide more tissue. As well, there is often an abundance of contralateral lid skin redundancy, which makes it an ideal graft for a lid defect. Upper lid skin may also be transferred to the lower lid, or if a thicker graft is needed, upper lid skin and muscle may be pedicled laterally and placed in the lower lid (often utilized for the repair of outer lamellar ectropion) (Fig. 14).

The inner lamella of the eye is best treated with free grafts from the hard palate or septum, and if the anterior lamella is involved, utilizing the cervicofacial flap for vascular support. Pedicled flaps from the adjacent lid, such as the tarsoconjunctival flap (Hughes), may be used as well for inner lamellar defects.

Forehead

Forehead reconstruction is facilitated in the elderly, as there are more prominent furrows and therefore more locations in which one can hide scars. With the anterior branch of the superficial temporal artery providing robust supply laterally and the supraorbital and supratrochlear arteries medially, the forehead has an extremely robust blood supply. Thus, defects will heal quickly by second intention (such as forehead flap donor sites unable to be closed), and flaps will not often fail. One should use the RSTLs, as well as the natural hairline and the eyebrow, to camouflage scars. Often, an O to T repair will work well for forehead lesions (Fig. 15), allowing skin to advance along the border of an aesthetic subunit or in a relaxed skin tension line. Along the hairline, a running W-plasty will help camouflage these incisions, as will beveling the incision away from the hairline so that hair may grow through the incision line.

Lesions involving the loss of eyebrow hair can be addressed using techniques that reapproximate the brow level. In this region, vertically oriented excisions may be wise, as they allow for primary closure of the brow and alignment of the remaining hair. If this is not possible and brow hair is lost, hair-bearing tissue in the form of punch grafts, strip grafts, or a pedicled flap from the temple may be used to reconstruct the eyebrow.

Temple

Lesions of the temple regions should be assessed not only for size but also, more importantly, for depth. The zygomaticotemporal and frontal branches of the facial nerve, especially above the zygoma, run superficially and are at risk during resections in this region. Patients should be asked to perform brow elevation once local anesthesia has been given time to wear off, and if the nerve has been taken, a browlift procedure should be considered.

Reconstruction of this region is more straightforward in the elderly as this region has thin and extremely mobile skin. Advancement flaps along the anterior sideburn and hairline, rhombic flaps, and bilobed flaps are excellent techniques in this region.

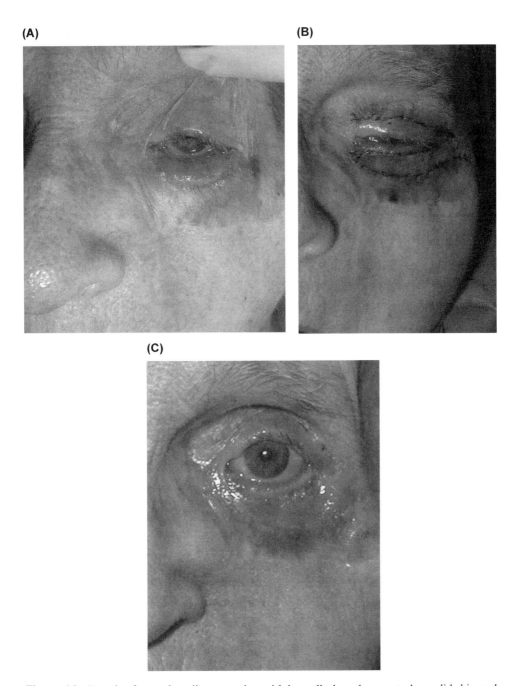

Figure 14 Repair of outer lamellar ectropion with laterally-based upper to lower lid skin and mucle transposition flap. (**A**) Severe cicatricial ectropion of the left eye three months after removal of a midface keratoacanothoma. (**B**) Intraoperative view after transposition of upper lid skin and muscle to the lower lid defect after lower lid skin muscle. (**C**) Three weeks postoperative view of the same patient.

(A)   **(B)**

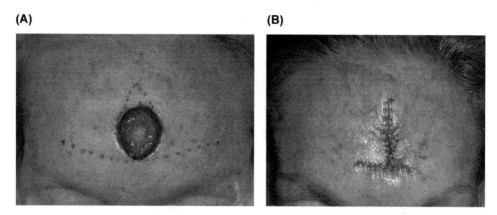

Figure 15 Reconstruction of a forehead lesion. (**A**) Mohs resection of a basal cell carcinoma. An inverted O to T closure has been marked. (**B**) After closure as planned. Note that the incisions were kept in the relaxed skin tension lines of the forehead, and they were not extended laterally to avoid injury to the supraorbital nerves.

Nasal Reconstruction

Nasal reconstruction is an extensive topic, and it is well described in the literature and in texts. The nose must be assessed using nasal aesthetic subunits to determine the extent of each lesion, and careful attention must be paid to the depth of the defect (19). I find it critical to use the concept of assessing the nose from the outside to inside and then planning reconstruction from the inside to outside. Systematic assessment will lead to an accurate diagnosis and facilitate appropriate surgical planning.

As one ages, nasal support deteriorates. A common finding in the senile patient is the ptotic nasal tip, a result of many years of gravitational force. In combination with an increase in the elasticity or supporting structures, the nose is prone to collapse. These changes may result in nasal valve collapse and nasal obstruction. Therefore, one must provide a sound structural foundation to adequately reconstruct the nose.

During any nasal work, dentures must be worn to adequately duplicate the resting nasal appearance and support. Overlooking this important step will cloud the intraoperative assessment of nasal projection and rotation. Preoperative assessment should always include nasal tip palpation to assess support. Nasal tip support can be most easily reinforced using septal cartilage or irradiated homograft cartilage as a columellar strut. Alar batten grafts or butterfly spreader grafts can reinforce lateral wall support.

Reconstructive techniques for the nose can be discussed in terms of internal lining, support, and external skin repairs. Internal lining may be obtained by septal, inferior turbinate, buccal, or epithelial turn-in grafts, and structural support can be replaced with radiated rib cartilage, calvarial bone grafting, cartilage grafts, or alloplastic materials. External skin may be replaced by skin grafts (melolabial being the best match), bilobed flaps, and rhombic flaps, as well as pedicled flaps, such as paramedian forehead flaps or melolabial flaps. These techniques will often be needed with nasal defects given the inability to close many defects primarily.

Scalp

Most scalp defects are repaired with rotational flaps, elevated in the subgaleal plane. Due to the scalp's resistance to stretch, a longer flap must be elevated (six times the diameter of the defect). Also, if it is still difficult to perform a closure, multiple incisions may be made in the galea (galeotomies) to allow more advancement.

As discussed earlier, exposed bone without periosteum presents an interesting dilemma. Without periosteum, there is no extracortical blood supply for grafts or flaps. Also, there is usually a large, deep defect that aesthetically will look abnormal if thin grafts are placed. There are two options in this scenario. The first requires that local rotation-advancement flaps be placed to fully cover the defect. The second requires that the cortical bone be drilled until bleeding begins and a split thickness skin graft be obtained and stored at 4°C. This tissue may be stored for up to 21 days. Once granulation tissue has been allowed to fill the defect, the skin graft may be placed.

Another adjunctive technique is rapid intraoperative tissue expansion (Fig. 16). In a short period of time, one may use mechanical creep to increase the amount of tissue available for reconstruction and close defects that otherwise would remain open (20). Of course, second intention healing is always an option, and this will be facilitated by exposing bleeding in the bone, as well as constant moisturization.

Face and Cheek

The elderly cheek and face rarely need grafting, as the tissues are loose enough either for primary closure or, if larger, for local flaps. The workhorse of the cheek closure is the cervicofacial advancement flap. It is important to suspend this flap superiorly either to the zygoma or lateral canthal tendon of nasal periosteum to avoid the natural downward pull of gravity and contraction. There should be no tension on the eyelid, nasal ala, or upper lip to avoid functional and cosmetic deformity. Excessive tension on the flap may result in distal flap necrosis, especially if the flap is pulled tightly over the malar eminence.

Patients with other medical comorbidities or those who have or are currently smoking are at risk to have distal flap necrosis. Flap necrosis is not only a result of tension, but also of overaggressive thinning of the flap as well as excessive cautery to control bleeding. Even with meticulous operative technique, every surgeon will eventually encounter this problem, and most often the defect will heal adequately by second intention.

Lips

Lip reconstruction is important for both function and cosmesis. It is therefore important to re-establish lip height and thickness, as well as perfectly align the vermillion border and white roll of the lip. Functional competency will be accomplished by tight reapproximation of the orbicularis muscle, and every effort must be made to salvage sensation to promote oral competence.

Defects less than one-third of the length of the lip are easily repaired primarily, whereas larger defects must be replaced by transposition flaps, such as Abbe or Estlander flaps, Gilles fan flaps, or Bernard–Burrow–Webster flaps. The karapandzic flap is particularly useful for large defects as a first-stage reconstruction of complete lip defects.

TRAUMA AND THE ELDERLY PATIENT

As a result of natural physiologic changes, elderly patients require less force to fracture facial bones. This is partly due to general bone reabsorption over time, as well as changes in the function and structure of the facial bones. Repair mechanisms are reduced in the elderly as well, and therefore both conservatism and proper technique are important to optimize one's results. Several techniques should be considered in the elderly patient while keeping in mind these physiologic changes.

A general rule in elderly patients is to apply conservatism while accomplishing functional stability. Midfacial fractures, if they are minimally displaced, are often better left untouched than aggressively reducing fractures through open approaches.

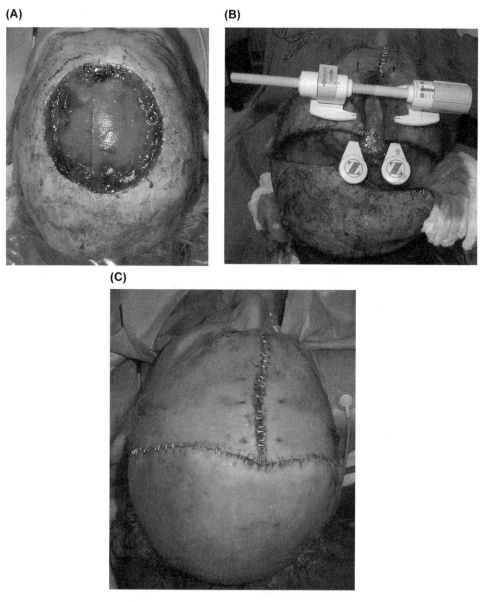

Figure 16 Intraoperative use of Sureclosure device (Zeiss, Inc.), using mechanical creep to close a large Mohs defect. (**A**) Defect prior to closure. (**B**) Sureclosure machine placed after release incisions and multiple galeotomies. (**C**) Final intraoperative closure.

Subperiosteal elevation that is often necessary in many facial fractures may compromise an already tenuous blood supply and therefore should be minimized. Although adequate occlusion should always be the goal of each repair, one should remember that occlusal perfection need not be achieved in patients with full dentures, as dentures may be remodeled after the facial fractures are allowed to heal.

If observation alone is not appropriate, one should be well equipped to utilize closed approaches to reduce fractures. There are many techniques described in the literature. A Gilles approach to elevate depressed zygomatic arch fractures is extremely effective. Zygomaticomaxillary fractures may be reduced by placing a large bone hook percutaneously under the zygomaticomaxillary buttress and pulling the fracture in the reverse direction of the force that caused the fracture. Nasal fractures may be reduced in the usual fashion, keeping in mind that elderly nasal bones are more fragile and may require extended periods of nasal splinting to set. Closed techniques are best performed as soon as swelling is reduced to visualize the defect and should be performed no later than 7–10 days after the injury, but preferably sooner.

Mandibular fractures are potentially more complicated in the elderly patient. Mandibular strength and height are maintained by the constant stress and strain applied with mastication, and with the loss of dentition, the mandible may lose over half of its height. Fractures in this population have higher rates of complications, as bony healing is slower in the elderly. Mandible repairs are more tenuous as a result of several issues. First, there is a reduced cross-sectional area of contact at the fracture repair site. Second, there is a relative decrease in the proportion of cancellous bone and marrow relative to cortical bone. This reduces the capacity for osteogenesis and accounts for a decrease in overall blood supply (21). Third, atherosclerosis and vascular disease reduce the blood supply through the inferior alveolar artery, leaving the mandible with predominantly periosteal blood supply (22). Elderly patients with poor nutritional states and reduced immune responses have a further reduction in healing capacity.

For all of these reasons, reduction of the atrophic mandible has a higher rate of nonunion. Several techniques may help improve the chances of a satisfactory result. If a closed technique is required for a favorable fracture or unilateral subcondylar fracture, interdental wires may be placed using a patient's dentures as a splint. Patients should be mobilized within 2–3 weeks to prevent ankylosis of the temporomandibular joint. If open approaches are necessary, one should minimize subperiosteal elevation to conserve blood supply. Preservation of the periosteum may be accomplished by supraperiosteal elevation. The use of 2.7-mm reconstruction plates will provide longer lasting strength to the mandible as it heals and will support greater loads over longer periods of time in the case of inadequate bony healing. Mandibular plates used for supraperiosteal plating are often designed to reduce the surface area of contact specifically to avoid disturbances in blood supply, and plates with locking screws also address this issue. Any plate placed on an atrophic mandible should be placed at the inferior aspect of the bone to avoid injury to the inferior alveolar nerve.

SUMMARY

This chapter reviews several techniques of reconstruction of various regions of the head and neck in the elderly patient. These techniques will become even more commonplace, and one should have a functional knowledge of each reconstructive option while assessing the patient's clinical status.

If a surgical course of action is taken, there is no substitute for proper surgical technique, meticulous hemostasis, and communication with the anesthesia team to reduce perioperative morbidity. Surgeons are encouraged to read the many texts dedicated to each reconstructive technique, especially the subtleties of periocular, nasal, and perioral defects.

Frequent follow-up is often indicated in this population, as complications are more frequently seen and should be identified early as you develop a relationship of trust with each patient.

Finally, chronologic age is not nearly as important as clinical age in assessing most patients, but attention paid to common problems in reconstruction in the elderly will often help us avoid these complications even in the healthy patient.

REFERENCES

1. Abrass I. Biology of aging. In: Wilson JD, Braunwald E, eds. Harrison's principles of internal medicine 12th 3d. New York, NY: McGraw-Hill Co, 1991:73–76.
2. Lapid MI, Rummans TA. Evaluation and management of geriatric depression in primary care. Proc Mayo Clin 2003; 78(11):1423–1429.
3. Hazen SE, Larsen PD, Hoot Martin JL. General anesthesia and elderly surgical patients. AORN Online 1997; 65(4):815–822.
4. Thomas DR. Age-related changes in wound healing. Drugs Aging 2001; 18:607–617.
5. Rigel DS, Friedman RJ, Kopf AW. Lifetime risk for development of skin cancer in the U.S. population: current estimate is now 1 in 5 [editorial]. J Am Acad Dermatol 1996; 35:1012–1013.
6. Karagas MR, Greenberg ER, Mott LA, et al. Occurrence of other cancers among patients with prior basal cell and squamous cell skin cancer. Cancer Epidemiol Biomarkers Prev 1998; 7:157–161.
7. Levi F, La Vecchia C, Te VC, et al. Incidence of invasive cancers following basal cell skin cancer Am J Epidemiol 1998; 147:722–726.
8. Urbach F. Ultraviolet radiation and skin cancer of humans. J Photochem Photobiol B 1997; 40:3–7.
9. Larrabee WF, Makielski K. Surgical Anatomy of the Face, Raven Press, 1992.
10. Borges AF, Alexander JE. Relaxed skin tension lines, Z-plasties on scars, and fusiform excision of lesions. Br J Plast Surg 1962; 15:242.
11. Cook TA, Parks S. Locoregional flaps for facial resurfacing. In: Myers EN, et al., eds. Advances in otolaryngology—head and neck surgery. Vol. 9. St. Louis, Mo.: Mosby, 1995:1–29.
12. Odland PB, Murakami CS. Healing by secondary intention. Oper Tech Otolaryngol Head Neck Surg 1993; 4:54–60.
13. Zitelli JA. Wound healing by secondary intention. J Am Acad Dermatol 1983; 9: 407–415.
14. Zitelli JA. Secondary intention healing: an alternative to surgical repair. Clin Dermatol 1984; 2:92–106.
15. Baillin PL, Wheeland RG. Carbon dioxide (CO_2) laser perforation of exposed cranial bone to stimulate granulation tissue. Plast Reconstr Surg 1985; 75:898–902.
16. Gibson T. Physical properties of skin. In: McCarthy J, ed. Plastic surgery. Philadelphia: WB Saunders, 1990:249.
17. Cook TA, Israel JM, Wang RD, et al. Cervical rotation flaps for midface resurfacing. Arch Otolaryngol Head Neck Surg 1991; 117:77–82.

18. Zitelli JA. The bilobed flap for nasal reconstruction. Arch Dermatol 1989; 125:957.
19. Burget GC, Menick FJ. Subunit principle in nasal reconstruction. Plast Reconstr Surg 1985; 76:239.
20. Baker SR, Swanson NA. Rapid intraoperative tissue expansion in reconstruction of the head and neck. Arch Otolaryngol Head Neck Surg 1990; 116:1431–1434.
21. Luhr H-G, Reidick T, Merten H-A. Results of treatment of fractures of the atrophic edentulous mandible by compression plating: a retrospective evaluation of 84 consecutive cases. J Oral Maxillofac Surg 1996; 54:250.
22. Pogrel MA, Dodson T, Tom W. Arteriographic assessment of patency of the inferior alveolar artery and its relevance to alveolar artery. J Oral Surg 1987; 45:767.

52
Cosmetic Surgery in the Elderly Patient

Oren Friedman
Division of Facial Plastic and Reconstructive Surgery, Department of Otolaryngology, Mayo Clinic, Rochester, Minnesota, U.S.A.

Tom D. Wang and Ted A. Cook
Department of Otolaryngology—Head and Neck Surgery, Oregon Health and Science University, Portland, Oregon, U.S.A.

INTRODUCTION

The pursuit of a permanent youthful look is an endeavor that is not unique to our time, but rather spans world history from ancient Egypt to the present. Ancient Egyptians portrayed ideal facial aesthetics in their sculptures and carvings and utilized facial makeup to enhance the appearance of the face. Greek artists, followed by artists of the Renaissance period, continued to portray aesthetic facial ideals through their works. Since these early times, the concepts of facial aesthetic ideals continue to evolve. Over the past century, surgical procedures to enhance one's external appearance have emerged from secrecy to become the fastest growing medical specialty.

The number of elderly individuals in the United States is rapidly increasing. Among all age groups, the 85-years-old and older population has the fastest growth rate. Projections from the years 1995 to 2050 indicate that the 85-plus population will increase by 401% from 3 million to 28 million in 2050 (1). The most recent U.S. census showed 35 million people over age 65, a number 12% higher than in the 1990 census (2). Between 1990 and 1994, there was an 11-fold increase in the 65 and older age group compared to a threefold increase in the population younger than 65 years. Furthermore, between 2010 and 2030, the number of people aged 65–84 will increase by 80%, while the population aged 65 and younger will increase by only 7% (1).

Advances in healthcare and hygiene, combined with an emphasis on preventative care, have allowed people to live longer and remain active through later years of life. Many individuals desire a youthful look, wanting to look as young and as well as they feel. The importance our society places on a youthful appearance may be recognized when one looks at newspapers, magazines, or television shows that popularize young beautiful individuals and spurn older, wrinkled individuals. The young, in general, view the aged as unattractive, sexually undesirable, and helpless (3). The demand for facial rejuvenation surgery will likely increase in our aging society.

Special considerations are required in addressing cosmetic surgery in the elderly, and many of these are addressed in this chapter.

THE AGING PROCESS

Aging of facial structures depends upon genetic, anatomic, chronological, and environmental factors (Fig. 1). The aging process affects the skin and underlying tissues by both intrinsic and extrinsic factors (4). Intrinsic aging refers to the effects of time, with associated hormonal and biochemical changes, on the skin. Over the course of one's lifetime, the epidermis and subcutaneous fat layers thin, and there is effacement of the dermal–epidermal junction due to a flattening of the rete ridge pattern (5). There is a progressive loss of organization of elastic fibers and collagen (elastosis) and a weakening of underlying muscles (6). These changes contribute to the wrinkling process that is characteristic of senescent skin. Extrinsic factors, such as gravity, smoking, and sun exposure, may result in keratinocytic dysplasia, coarse wrinkles, and a rough skin surface (5). Taken together, the intrinsic and extrinsic aging processes create pigmentary changes, rhytids, and texture irregularities of the skin (5,7,8).

REJUVENATION OF THE AGING FACE

While the effects of aging are normal, ubiquitous, and acceptable to many individuals, others find such changes to be problematic. Many patients desire to have their perceived age changed so that their facial appearance reflects their physical and mental state rather than their actual chronological age. Those interested in solutions for

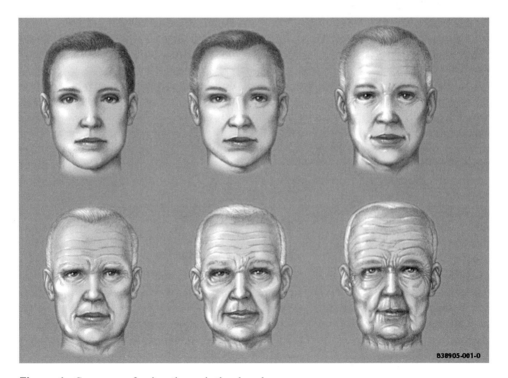

Figure 1 Sequence of aging through the decades.

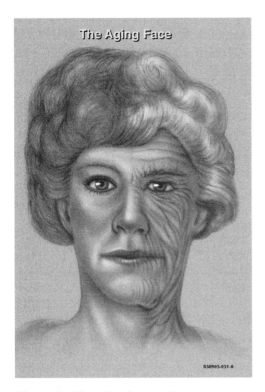

Figure 2 The aging face syndrome.

the physical stigmata of aging often start with conservative medical therapy. Sun protection and cessation of smoking are encouraged in all patients. For those with early manifestations of aging skin and excessive sun exposure, medical therapy may be effective. Retin-A (tretinoin) helps to reverse the pigment changes, fine rhytids, and roughness that are characteristic of aging facial skin (9,10). Alpha-hydroxy acids (glycolic acid, lactic acid, malic acid, citric acid, tartaric acid) may be applied to the skin in different concentrations to effect a variety of chemo-exfoliative rejuvenating changes to the skin. In addition to chemical peeling, a number of other skin resurfacing techniques are available, including laser and dermabrasion (11). Cutaneous resurfacing removes the epidermis, resulting in the growth of a fresh new epidermal layer, and injures the dermis, resulting in wound contracture and a tightening of finely wrinkled skin. In individuals with mild aging changes, primarily affecting the skin and superficial dermis, medical therapies are quite effective in maintaining a fresh and youthful appearance. As aging proceeds, changes to the facial skeleton and soft tissues predominate over the skin changes (Fig. 2). Thus, when individuals reach the fifth decade and beyond, surgical solutions to restore a youthful appearance are more often required. To create this appearance requires a fundamental knowledge of the aesthetic youthful ideals, as well as an understanding of how to achieve these goals in aging patients.

THE AGING FACE SYNDROME

Analyzing facial aesthetics can be simplified by dividing the face into thirds. The upper third of the face includes the forehead and brows; the middle third includes the midface, the eyes, and the nose; and the lower third includes the lower cheeks, jawline, and neck. For the purposes of our discussion, we will consider the eyes together with the brows and forehead because, from a practical standpoint, the periorbital area is generally rejuvenated as a single unit, including the eyes, the brows, and the forehead.

The Upper Third of the Face

Brow Aesthetics

The upper one-third of the face elongates with aging, as the hairline moves upward and the brow drifts downward (Fig. 2). Brow ptosis, lateral brow hooding, crow's feet, fine and deep rhytids in the forehead and glabella, and loss of elasticity predominate the aging upper third. The aging brow may reveal dynamic wrinkles or even wrinkles at rest. These furrows in the glabella and forehead are caused by the repeated pull on the skin by the facial mimetic muscles. Brow ptosis may be mistaken for upper eyelid skin laxity or true eyelid ptosis, and it is essential to determine the proper diagnosis before treatment is instituted.

Evaluation of the patient includes an examination in front of a mirror in both animation and repose. The patient's eyes should be closed for 10 to 20 seconds to allow for full relaxation of the forehead musculature. Upon eye opening, the true position of the brow will be noted with minimal contribution to the brow position from the upward pull of the forehead muscles. The ideal brow anatomy in the male differs from that in the female (Fig. 3). The medial brow has its medial origin at the level of a vertical line drawn to the nasal alar–facial junction. The lateral extent of the brow should reach a point on a line drawn from the nasal alar–facial junction through the lateral canthus of the eye. The medial and lateral ends should lie on

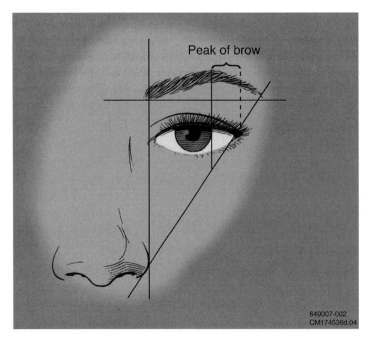

Figure 3   Ideal brow positions.

the same horizontal plane (12). The medial end should have a club-head appearance and the lateral end should gradually taper to a point. The brow should arch superiorly, at least 1 cm above the supraorbital rim in the female, with the highest point classically described as lying at the lateral limbus and more recently described as lying at the lateral canthus (Fig. 3) (13). In men, there should be less of an arch to the brow position, and more of a horizontal contour along the supraorbital ridge. The distance between the mid-pupillary line and the inferior brow border should be approximately 2.5 cm. The distance from the superior border of the brow to the anterior hairline should be 5 cm (14,15). The distance between the two medial heads of the eyebrows should be the same as the distance between the alar–facial junctions on either side of the nose.

Eyelid Aesthetics

Several reproducible features have been noted in the analysis of beautiful eyes and eyelids (Fig. 4). The palpebral fissure should be almond-shaped and symmetric between the two sides. The highest point of the upper eyelid is at the medial limbus, and the lowest point of the lower eyelid is at the lateral limbus. Sharp canthal angles should exist, especially at the lateral canthus. The lateral canthus should lie 2–4 mm superior to the medial canthus. The horizontal dimension of the palpebral fissure is 25–30 mm, while its vertical dimension is approximately 10 mm (16,17). Vertical palpebral asymmetry may indicate the presence of true ptosis of the eyelid, which would necessitate ptosis repair. The upper eyelid orbicularis muscle should be smooth and flat, and the upper eyelid crease should be crisp. The upper lid crease should lie between 8 and 12 mm from the lid margin in the Caucasian patient. A more inferior position of the upper lid crease gives a heavy and tired appearance to the eye. Excessive lid folds, tissue prolapsing over the upper eyelid crease, should be minimal to avoid the aged and tired look. The upper lid margin should cover 1–2 mm of the superior limbus, while the lower lid margin should lie at the inferior limbus or 1 mm below the inferior limbus (16,17). Note should be made of excessive skin, muscle, and orbital fat. The pinch test helps determine the degree of excess lid skin that is

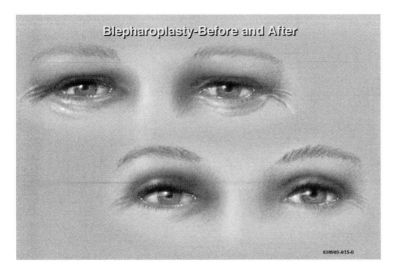

Figure 4   Eyelid aesthetics before and after blepharoplasty.

present. The snap test helps determine the degree of lower lid laxity and is useful in preoperative planning (Fig. 5) (16,18,19). Additionally, a ptotic lacrimal gland must be recognized for potential correction at surgery. Excessive lateral skin hooding may require skin excision beyond the lateral orbital rim, and prolonged wound healing would be expected in this area of greater skin thickness, a point which must be discussed with the patient before surgery (18,19).

The lower eyelid should closely appose the globe without drooping of the lid away from the globe (ectropion), or in toward the globe (entropion). Excessive lower eyelid laxity should be recognized and treated with a lid shortening/tightening procedure. Exophthalmos and enophthalmos should be recognized, as neither is favorable, and each may represent an underlying disorder. Visual acuity should be evaluated, as should the presence of Bell's phenomenon. Absence of Bell's phenomenon places the patient at increased risk for the development of postoperative corneal abrasions, should temporary or permanent lagophthalmos exist following surgery. If the patient shows signs of a dry eye, the Schirmer test should be performed, and caution should be used in deciding on surgical intervention (19,20).

Brow ptosis, glabellar rhytids, excess upper eyelid skin, pseudoherniation of orbital fat, and orbicularis muscle hypertrophy may cause an individual to unintentionally convey external expressions of boredom, fatigue, anger, and sadness, despite the fact that these expressions are not consistent with their true feelings (Fig. 2) (18–20). Not only are these age-related changes of cosmetic importance, they are frequently associated with visual field defects that may be unrecognized by the patient. As the aging brow becomes more ptotic, it descends below the supraorbital rim, and pushes additional skin over the upper eyelid, worsening the cosmetic appearance of the eyelids and aggravating the functional deficits in the superior and peripheral visual fields. Visual field changes in the elderly patient who has multiple other sensory deficits may be extremely debilitating.

Surgical correction of these functional losses, rather than cosmetic enhancement, frequently gives the patient and surgeon the greatest degree of satisfaction

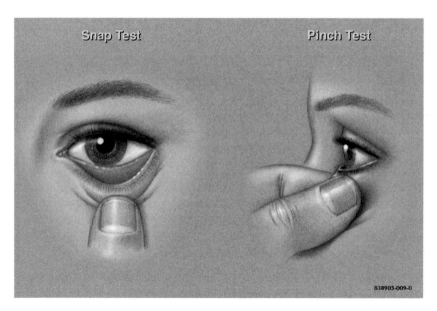

Figure 5 Snap test and pinch test.

in the postoperative period. Baggy lower eyelids are the result of weakening of the orbital septum and orbicularis oculi muscle, pseudoherniation of orbital fat, and redundant skin (3,20).

Treatment of the Upper Third—Brow Lift and Blepharoplasty

The appropriate candidates have the stigmata of an aging upper face, but they also are healthy enough to withstand surgical intervention and anesthesia. The procedures may be performed under general anesthesia or local anesthesia with sedation. Upper eyelid blepharoplasty alone may not adequately correct the patient's problem and may even worsen the degree of brow ptosis by fixing the brow in an inferior position once scar contracture has occurred (13). Therefore, attention to the repositioning of the inferiorly displaced brow is often necessary and should be achieved before performing the blepharoplasty (21).

There are several techniques for raising the brows, reducing the glabellar rhytids, and addressing the eyelid changes of aging. Traditional techniques, such as the coronal, pretrichial, mid-forehead, and direct browlifting operations, are used less frequently today as a result of the development of the endoscopic brow-lift technique (Fig. 6) (22). The endoscopic technique requires several small incisions, which are hidden behind the hairline, as compared with the high forehead techniques, which require large incisions that are often prone to visible scarring (Fig. 7). Disadvantages of the endoscopic technique include risks to the frontal branch of the facial nerve and to the sensory branches of the forehead. Advantages include a reduced rate of

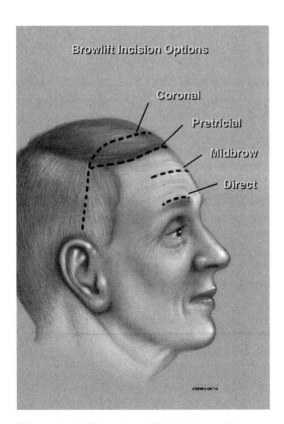

Figure 6 Different browlift incision options.

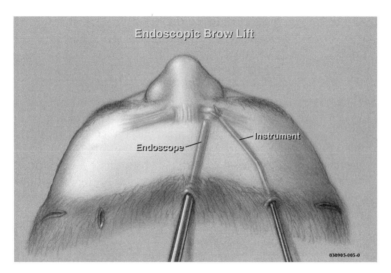

Figure 7 Endoscopic brow incision.

alopecia and postoperative scalp paresthesias and a diminished postoperative healing time (14). Surgical length does not differ between the endoscopic and open techniques, once the technique is learned and its execution becomes fluid. For these reasons, the endoscopic technique should play a prominent role in addressing the upper third of the face in the elderly patient population. In particular, elderly women with hairlines that have not receded to a great extent are ideal candidates for endoscopic browlifting techniques (Figs. 8 and 9). In contrast, males with deep forehead rhytids and receding hairlines are not always better served with the endoscopic techniques. In such patients, the mid-forehead browlift may be preferred (15). The advantages of the mid-forehead browlift include its speed, ease, low morbidity, no change in sensation superior to the incision, no distortion of the hairline or of the vascular supply to the hair follicles, and high predictability. Only a moderate amount of undermining is required, resulting in a low risk to neural structures and a lower risk of hematoma formation when compared with longer flap techniques (14). Most importantly, in the elderly patient with a functional deficit of visual field changes, the mid-forehead browlift allows precise control over brow position with a good deal of permanence. The primary disadvantage of the mid-forehead operation is in the postoperative scar. However, when performed upon the appropriate patient with care and respect for the soft tissue, the mature scar is often not noticeable. When compared with the endoscopic technique, the mid-forehead operation is more easily performed under local anesthesia and is preferred in the older individual. These patients may have multiple medical problems and both functional and cosmetic concerns relating to the upper third of the face.

In the properly selected patient, blepharoplasty can safely be performed in the elderly population. Great care is required in the preoperative assessment of the eyes and eyelids to recognize some common findings, which may be associated with potential pitfalls. Blepharochalasis, or dermatochalasis, refers to the excess lid skin that occurs as a result of loss of skin elasticity. A large amount of excess upper lid skin may cause patients to have interference in their line of sight. In such cases, blepharoplasty may restore full field of vision with the removal of excess lid skin, muscle, and fat. Blepharoptosis of the upper lid, on the other hand, must be recognized

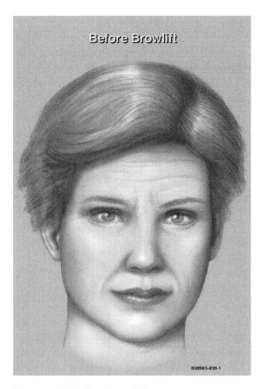

Figure 8 Before browlift.

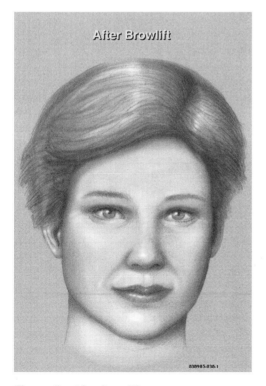

Figure 9 After browlift.

preoperatively to help avoid major complications (23). True eyelid ptosis most commonly occurs as a result of levator aponeurosis dehiscence, and it manifests as ptosis, a high or absent upper lid crease, and a thin eyelid through which the pupil may be visualized. Correcting the ptotic lid by reattaching the dehiscent levator aponeurosis to the tarsus will help to correct the patient's visual field defect and cosmetic irregularity, whereas simply performing a blepharoplasty in this situation results in potential worsening of the cosmetic and functional deficits (23). Entropion, inversion of the eyelid margin and cilia, may cause excessive tearing, burning, and irritation of the cornea, and it may be the result of eyelid skin pushing the cilia of the lid margin against the globe. Surgical repair may restore proper lid positioning to improve patient comfort and reduce the risk of lost vision due to chronic corneal irritation (24). Ectropion of the lower eyelid is the abnormal eversion of the eyelid margin and cilia away from the globe, which may cause tearing due to a malpositioned puncta and conjunctival irritation. Ectropion may occur primarily, or it may be a complication of eyelid surgery, especially common in the elderly patient (25). Failure to recognize preoperative lower lid laxity will invariably result in lower lid ectropion following blepharoplasty. If there is even the suggestion of excess lower lid laxity, a lower lid shortening or tightening procedure should be included as part of the blepharoplasty to avoid postoperative ectropion. It is essential to recognize pre operative lid laxity, ptosis, ectropion, entropion, dry eyes, and medications that cause dry eyes and increased bleeding risks before eyelid surgery in the elderly. Once a careful plan has been devised, surgery may proceed.

If performed in conjunction with a browlift, the blepharoplasty incision markings are placed after the browlift is complete and all incisions have been closed. Marking the eyelids is the single most important step in blepharoplasty, and as such, great care must be taken to insure precision (Fig. 10). There are a variety of techniques available to address both the upper and lower eyelids, each with its own merits and pitfalls. For the lower eyelid, transcutaneous and transconjunctival procedures have been described in detail elsewhere, and each has its place in the management of the elderly patient's eyelids, depending upon the goals of surgery (20). The transconjunctival

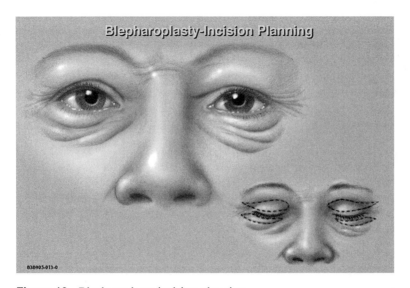

Figure 10 Blepharoplasty incision planning.

blepharoplasty (Fig. 11) has recently become increasingly popular due to the hidden incision, the maintenance of the orbicularis support structure for the lower eyelid, and a reduced rate of postoperative ectropion. Patients with pseudoherniation of fat and little need for skin excision are good candidates for this procedure. In addition, patients who heal with hypertrophic scars and patients who will not accept an external incision are good candidates. The presence of a mild to moderate amount of excess skin in the lower eyelid does not preclude the transconjunctival approach, as a pinch excision of skin and lid resurfacing techniques may be used to address the lower lid skin changes (20). The subciliary approach is most useful for those patients with a large amount of excess skin, which requires resection. It may also be used when the patient would benefit from a midface lift (26).

The Nose and the Middle Third of the Face

Age-related changes in the middle third of the face are primarily reflected by changes to the nose. In general, nasal skin, bone, muscle, and cartilage become thin and weak. The support structures that once maintained the aesthetics and function of the individual's nose may become inadequate. As the skin and subcutaneous tissues thin, the cartilaginous and bony support structures, which were once well concealed by the overlying soft tissue envelope, may become skeletonized and visible (Fig. 12) (27,28). The fibrous attachments at the scroll region slowly splay apart, resulting in the separation of the lower lateral cartilages from the upper lateral cartilages. The interdomal ligaments may weaken and stretch, resulting in a boxy nasal tip. There are also changes in the morphology of the aging face that result in distortions of the balance between the nose and other facial segments. Maxillary height is reduced and alveolar bone resorption occurs, leading to alterations in the tip relative to the remainder of the face (27). Nasal tip ptosis, dorsal irregularities, lengthening of the nose, decreasing nasolabial angle, narrowing of the nasal valve, and obstructive nasal breathing are frequent findings in the elderly patient (27–29). As the number of healthy and active elderly patients

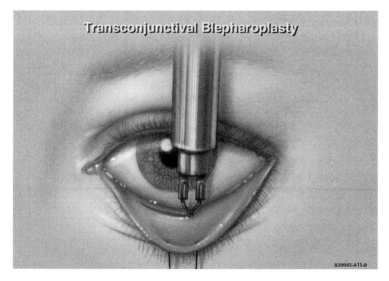

Figure 11   Transconjunctival blepharoplasty.

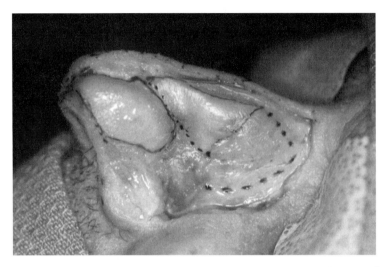

Figure 12 The upper and lower lateral cartilages and nasal bone outlined.

increases, so does the demand for functional nasal surgery. Patients may become mouth breathers and snorers, problems they did not experience in younger years. Physical activity may be limited by the individual's inability to breathe through the nose. Surgery to correct nasal aesthetics and function in the elderly patient requires care in diagnosing and treating the acquired nasal deformities.

Rhinoplasty is a challenging procedure when performed on a patient of any age. The changes associated with aging introduce new variables to the procedure and make it an even more complex challenge with greater potential risk for failure. Correcting the senescent structural changes that occur in the nose is an integral element in the rejuvenation of the entire face. While reviewing rhinoplasty techniques is beyond the scope of this chapter, certain important considerations are unique in the elderly patient's nose. The surgical management of the aging nose should involve the most conservative techniques that are least disruptive of the nasal support mechanisms. Additionally, structural support grafts may be necessary to provide strength to the weakened nose of the elderly patient.

Ptosis of the nasal tip, one of the most prevalent and distinctive findings in the patient with advancing age, is problematic for both functional and cosmetic reasons (Fig. 13). Tip ptosis, which is primarily caused by the intrinsic weakening of the lower lateral cartilages, must be recognized preoperatively to avoid postoperative complications. The drooping tip relative to the normally positioned nasal dorsum may give the illusion of a dorsal hump and dorsal septal prominence, when in fact none exists (29). In such patients, the inappropriate resection of the presumed cartilaginous dorsal excess rather than correcting the ptotic tip produces both aesthetic and functional deformities. In the elderly patient, the addition of cartilaginous support is often needed during primary rhinoplasty to correct tip ptosis, rather than resecting tissue from the dorsum. Columellar strut grafts, tip grafts, and a variety of suture techniques are available to increase tip support, projection, and rotation and thereby reverse the apparent dorsal irregularities by recreating a youthful tip position. This allows for the maintenance of a strong nasal profile by augmenting tip support rather than disrupting the structural integrity of the nose.

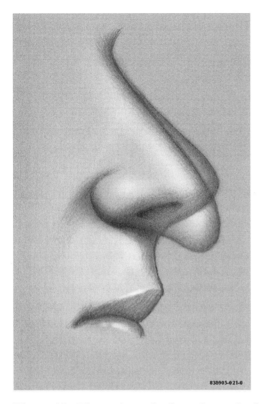

Figure 13 Tip ptosis results from the weakening of tip support mechanisms with aging.

Nasal valve obstruction is common in the elderly, and its recognition is extremely important to improve quality of life (Fig. 14). Limitations in physical activity and the development of snoring are frequent complaints among the elderly that may occasionally be attributed to nasal valve obstruction. Weakening of the upper lateral

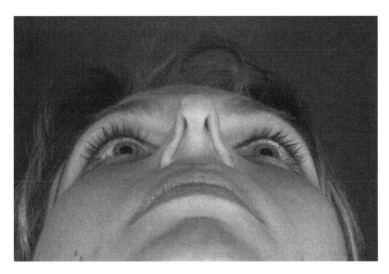

Figure 14 Nasal valve collapse.

cartilages and their support mechanisms (scroll region, lateral fibrous attachments to maxilla, sesamoid cartilages, mucosa, septal cartilage attachments) may cause collapse of the internal nasal valve and subsequent nasal obstruction. The internal nasal valve may be collapsed at rest or as a result of gentle nasal inspiration. If it is collapsed at rest, spreader grafts or nasal valve flaring stitches (30,31) may be used to widen the angle between the nasal septum and the upper lateral cartilages. If the collapse is present only with nasal inspiration, strengthening the cartilaginous support with batten grafts or with conchal cartilage butterfly grafts is the preferred treatment (32). External nasal valve collapse, due to a weakened lower lateral cartilage and subsequent collapse of the nasal vestibule, may also cause nasal obstruction in the elderly. Placement of an alar batten graft to strengthen the weakest point (the site with the greatest collapse on clinical examination) or replacing the lower lateral cartilages with conchal cartilage grafts will correct this problem.

Thinned nasal bones may be extremely fragile in the elderly patient. Therefore, every possible effort is made to maintain as much of the soft tissue support of the nasal bones. Periosteal elevation off the nasal bones is limited to the narrow area where bone alterations are required, and the attachment of the upper lateral cartilage to the nasal bones is always preserved. If osteotomies are required, they should be achieved with very sharp and small osteotomes to help minimize the amount of bone comminution and surrounding soft tissue injury. All dorsal irregularities must be smoothed to perfection, because the thinned skin of the elderly patient has little tolerance for imperfections. If there is a question of possible contour irregularities, placement of a dorsal onlay camouflaging implant (morselized septal cartilage, temporalis fascia, conchal cartilage, alloderm, vicryl mesh, Gore-tex) may help to hide the irregularity.

Midface

An important youthful attribute of the human face is the soft tissue distribution and the fullness it creates in the upper midface relative to the flatter lower midface. In youth, the orbicularis oculi muscle maintains a sling around the orbital rim, but with the loss of orbicularis tone associated with aging, descent of the orbicularis and malar soft tissue complex prevails and represents a characteristic finding in the aging middle third of the face (Fig. 15). The orbicularis oculi muscle extends beyond the eyelids to lie over the malar eminence. The convex prominences of the midface descend from their youthful location overlying the zygoma inferomedially to deepen the nasolabial crease, thereby exposing the inferior and lateral orbital rims to a greater degree. A hollowness develops in the area of transition between the lower eyelid and the cheek, and a tear trough deformity develops medially with deepening of the nasojugal fold. Overall, the midface convexity that gives the face its characteristic youthful appearance becomes flattened with increasing age (33).

Treatment of the Middle Third—Midface Lift

Midface suspension may be performed by extension of endoscopic forehead lifting procedures, by extension of standard rhytidectomy procedures, or through a subciliary approach to a lower eyelid blepharoplasty. Regardless of technique, the goals are to restore fullness to the infraorbital rim and upper cheek and to reduce the depth of the nasolabial fold (34).

Endoscopic Midface Lift.   The lateral temporal incision used for the endoscopic browlift approach may be used for endoscopic access to the midface (Fig. 16). The skin

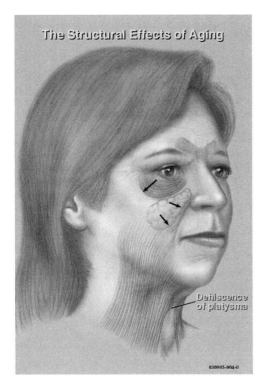

Figure 15 Midface descent associated with aging.

incision is carried down to the superficial layer of deep temporal fascia, leaving the temporoparietal fascia attached to the skin and subcutaneous tissue. Beyond the temporal line, subperiosteal dissection exposes the zygomaticofrontal suture line. Subperiosteal dissection continues inferiorly along the lateral orbital rim and inferior orbital rim to

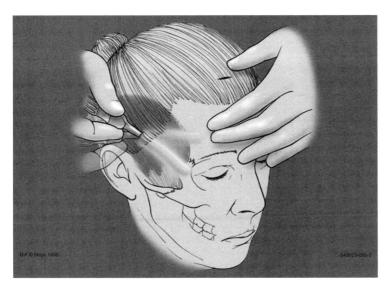

Figure 16 Lateral temporal incision made for browlift allows access for endoscopic midface elevation.

the malar eminence, maxillary face, and eventually the pyriform aperture to allow the greatest degree of mobility to the midface structures. A heavy absorbable suture then secures the periosteum of the midface to the superficial temporal fascia (34,35). A similar technique may be used by extending the standard facelift approach with a gingivo-buccal incision that allows subperiosteal elevation along the face of the maxilla to the inferior orbital rim. Subsequently, imbrication of the deep and superficial layers of the malar region allow for rejuvenation of the midface (33). The deep plane rhytidectomy may also be used to elevate the midface and flatten the nasolabial fold (36).

 Subciliary Approach. The subciliary approach to the midface lift is a simple extension of the subciliary blepharoplasty technique. When access has been obtained, the arcus marginalis is released at the inferior orbital rim. Subperiosteal dissection of the midface structures is then achieved beyond the infraorbital foramen, to the pyriform aperture and nasal bones. Once adequate elevation is achieved, some surgeons release the periosteum at the inferior-most point of subperiosteal dissection, while others leave the inferior periosteum intact. Either way, suture fixation of the midface periosteum to the orbital periosteum suspends the malar tissue. Among the elderly, a significant excess of lower lid skin is frequently noted, which requires a subciliary approach with resection of excess lower lid skin and orbicularis. Thus, the subciliary approach, which is also the most direct approach to the midface, is an excellent technique for midface rejuvenation in the elderly patient (Fig. 10) (37).

The Lower Third of the Face

Changes that accompany aging in the lower third of the face and neck are primarily cosmetic and rarely result in any functional abnormalities. With increasing skin laxity, resorption of mandibular and maxillary height, and thinning of subcutaneous fat, there is an excess of skin and soft tissue in the lower third of the face (Fig. 17). Chin ptosis and jowl formation replace the fine mandibular lines of youth. Platysmal banding, loss of the cervicomental angle, and excessive submental fullness develop in the neck. Upper lip lengthening and droopiness replace the more youthful short upper lip fullness. Ear lobe elongation is another prominent finding among the elderly. Each of these stigmata of aging may be addressed with a variety of different techniques and some are described below. Soft tissue repositioning of the face can temporarily counteract the sagging and redundant cheek skin, the loss of cervico-mental and mandibular definition, and the platysmal laxity.

Chin Ptosis

Premental fat ptosis, decreased mandibular height and projection, excess submental fullness, and prominence of the submental crease are common findings in advancing age, and may create a "witch chin" appearance. A number of techniques are available to correct this deformity, and each technique may be customized to correct deformities of varying degrees (38). If there is excessive ptosis of fibrofatty tissue and inadequate chin projection and height, a chin implant may be combined with submentoplasty in which the ptotic fatty tissue is removed. Such a technique restores the preresorption mandibular appearance and removes the ptotic premental fat (39). Other techniques aim at restoring the ptotic fat to its previous location with suture techniques either transorally or transcutaneously through the submental crease (40). Finally, by simply addressing the submental fullness with fat removal and platysma plication, a better balance in the chin may be attained.

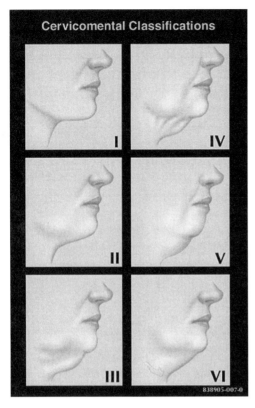

Figure 17 Cervicomental aging classification scheme.

Platysmal Banding and Obtuse Cervicomental Angle

Dehiscence and excess laxity of the platysma in the anterior neck may create two vertical bands that extend from the submentum to the clavicle, which are often visible on the anterior neck and are frequently cosmetically unappealing. This dehiscence allows for the subplatysmal soft tissue and fat to descend into the submandibular and submental region, creating fullness in the submentum and lower midline neck (turkey-gobbler) (38). The youthful and aesthetic acuteness of the cervicomental angle may be lost due to these factors. Recreation of an acute cervicomental angle and obliteration of the platysmal bands will give the elderly patient with the "turkey-gobbler" a fresh, more youthful appearance. This may be achieved through a standard facelift/necklift operation in which the platysma banding is addressed (Fig. 18). At times, particularly in the elderly male patient, the turkey-gobbler neck may be the individual's only cosmetic complaint. In such situations, a necklift procedure in which skin is directly excised with a Z plasty, T-Z plasty, W plasty, or another technique is performed (38,41). A transverse incision through the platysma at the level of the superior border of the thyroid cartilage (or hyoid bone) to better define the transition angle between the neck and the chin has also been advocated.

Jowl Formation

Fat and soft tissue descent along the mandibular body line obscures the fine bony definition of the mandible and is a central stigma of the aging face. The elderly

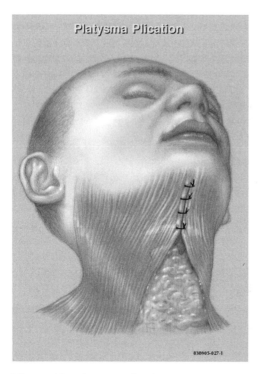

Figure 18   Platysma plication corrects platysmal banding.

patient will often complain of "bulldog-looking" cheeks due to the fullness of the jowls just lateral to the oral cavity. Jowling may be corrected with a standard facelift and necklift procedure. Descriptions of various rhytidectomy techniques is beyond the scope of this chapter, but they have been covered in detail in other sources (42–44). Suffice it to say that the goal of each of these procedures is to create a more youthful and angulated contour along the jaw line in an attempt to provide a youthful and fresh facial appearance.

Elongated Earlobe

An elongated earlobe is very common among the elderly, especially among women who have worn heavy earrings throughout their lives (Fig. 19). As the skin laxity increases, the earlobe descends and may be particularly troublesome to the older individual with great skin excess. A number of techniques are available, and each may be applied in isolation or as part of a facelift. Two full thickness triangles may be excised from the earlobe with a resultant T-shaped closure in order to reduce the size of the earlobe (45).

Upper Lip Lengthening

The upper lip elongates with advancing age. The red lip becomes thinner as the white lip increases in height. A variety of techniques are available to correct these common findings in the aging face, including surgical shortening of the white lip with simultaneous eversion of the red lip as well as a variety of augmentation techniques, such as collagen and expanded polytetrafluoroetheylene (ePTFE) implantation. The lip lift involves the excision of a segment of skin under the nostrils and elevating the skin

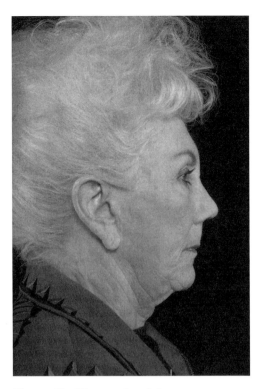

Figure 19 Elongated earlobe.

by closing it in its new position (46). Alternatively, a supravermilion lip skin excision is useful in elevating the upper lip, although the visible scar which obliterates the white roll is a major limitation of this procedure (47).

CONCLUSION

The demand for facial plastic surgery has increased dramatically in recent years as people from all socioeconomic levels and age groups have become interested in facial rejuvenation. As our population ages, the demands for aesthetic surgery in the elderly will continue to rise. Not only is it essential that the surgeon has a sound understanding of the facial plastic surgical techniques, one must also recognize that treating individuals in the later years of life requires specific considerations. With a respect for the elderly cosmetic patient's specific needs and anatomy, safe and effective surgery may be performed on these individuals in the twilight of their lives.

REFERENCES

1. American Association of Homes and Services for the Aging. (www2.AAHSA.org.).
2. www.census.gov.
3. Koblenzer CS. Psychologic aspects of aging and the skin. Clin Dermatol 1996; 14(2): 171–177.

4. Lapiere CM. The aging dermis: the main cause for the appearance of "old" skin. Br J Dermatol 1990; 122(suppl 35):5–11.

5. Bolgnia JL. Dermatologic and cosmetic concerns of the older woman. Clin Geriatr Med 1993; 9(1):209–229.

6. Montagna W, Carlisle K. Structural changes in aging skin. Br J Dermatol 1990; 122(suppl 35):61–70.

7. Gilchrest BA. Skin and photoaging: an overview. J Am Acad Dermatol 1989; 21:610.

8. Ellis CN. Management of aging skin. In: Cummings, et al., ed. Otolaryngology Head and Neck Surgery. 3rd ed. Chap. 31. St Louis: Mosby, 1998:629–639.

9. Kligman AM. Topical retinoic acid for photoaging: conceptions and misperceptions. Cutis 1996; 57:142–144.

10. Olsen EA, Katz HI, Levin A, et al. Tretinoin emollient cream: a new therapy for photo damaged skin. J Am Acad Dermatol 1992; 26:215–224.

11. Fulton JE Jr. Dermabrasion, chemabrasion, and laser abrasion: historical perspectives, modern dermabrasion techniques, and future trends. Dermatol Surg 1996; 22:619–628.

12. Ellis DAF, Masri H. The effect of facial animation on the aging upper half of the face. Arch Otolaryngol Head Neck Surg 1989; 15:710–713.

13. Miller PJ, Wang TD, Cook TA. Rejuvenation of the aging forehead and brow. Facial Plast Surg 1996; 12(2):147–155.

14. Howard BK, Leach J. Aesthetic Surgery of the Upper Third of the Face. A Self Instructional Package. Washington, D.C.: American Academy of Otolaryngology Head and Neck Surgery Foundation, Inc.

15. Cook TA, Brownrigg PJ, Wang TD, Quatela VC. The versatile midforehead browlift. Arch Otol Head Neck Surg 1989; 115:163.

16. Bergin DJ. Anatomy of the eyelids, lacrimal system, and orbit. In: McCord CD, Tanenbaum M, Nunery W, eds. Oculoplastic Surgery. 3rd ed. Chap. 2. New York: Raven Press, 1995:51–84.

17. Kikkawa DO, Lemke BN. Orbit and eyelid anatomy. In: Ophthalmic Plastic Surgery: Prevention and Management of Complications. New York: Raven Press, 1994.

18. Pastorek NJ. Upper lid blepharoplasty. In: Facial Plastic and Reconstructive Surgery. 2nd ed. Chap. 17. New York: Thieme, 2002:185–195.

19. Moses JL. Blepharoplasty: cosmetic and functional. In: McCord CD, Tantenbaum M, Nunery W, eds. Oculoplastic Surgery. 3rd ed. Chap. 11. New York: Raven Press, 1995:285–318.

20. Rankin BS, Arden RC, Crumley AL. Lower eyelid blepharoplasty. In: Facial Plastic and Reconstructive Surgery. 2nd ed. Chap. 18. New York: Thieme, 2002:196–207.

21. Koch RJ, Troell RJ, Goode RL. Contemporary management of the aging brow and forehead. Laryngoscope 1997; 107:710.

22. Ramirez OM. Endoscopically assisted biplanar forehead lift. Plast Reconstr Surg 1995; 96:323–333.

23. Millay DJ, Larrabee WF. Ptosis and blepharoplasty surgery. Arch Otolaryngol Head Neck Surg 1989; 115:198–201.

24. Martin RT, Nunery WR, Tanenbaum M. Entropion, trichiasis, and distichiasis. In: McCord CD, Tanenbaum M, Nunery W, eds. Oculopastic Surgery. 3rd ed. Chap. 8. New York: Raven Press, 1995:221–248.

25. Wesley RE. Ectropion repair. In: McCord CD, Tanenbaum M, Nunery W, eds. Oculopastic Surgery. 3rd ed. Chap. 9. New York: Raven Press, 1995:249–262.

26. Fedok FG, Perkins SW. Transconjunctival blepharoplasty. Facial Plast Surg 1996; 12(2):185–195.

27. Toriumi DM. Surgical correction of the aging nose. Facial Plast Surg 1996; 12(2):205–214.

28. Guyuron B. The aging nose. Dermatol Clin 1997; 15(4):659–664.

29. Rohrich RJ, Hollier LH. Rhinoplasty with advancing age: characteristics and management. Otolaryngol Clin North Am 1999; 2(4):755–773.

30. Park SS. The flaring suture to augment the repair of the dysfunctional nasal valve. Plast Reconstr Surg 1998; 101:1120–1122.

31. Sheen JH. Spreader graft: a method of reconstructing the roof of the middle nasal vault following rhinoplasty. Plast Reconstr Surg 1984; 73:230–239.

32. Clark JM, Cook TA. The 'butterfly' graft in functional secondary rhinoplasty. Laryngoscope 2002; 112:1917–1925.

33. Little JW. Three-dimensional rejuvenation of the midface: volumetric resculpture by malar imbrication. Plast Reconstr Surg 2000; 105(1):267–285.

34. Quatela VC, Graham D, Sabini P. Rejuvenation of the brow and midface. In: Facial Plastic and Peconstructive Surgery. 2nd ed. Chap. 16. New York: Thieme, 2002:171–184.

35. Byrd HS. The extended browlift. Clin Plast Surg 1997; 24:233.

36. Little JW, Hamra ST. The deep plane rhytidectomy. Plast Reconstr Surg 1990; 86:53.

37. Gunter JP, Hackney FL. A simplified transblepharoplasty subperiosteal cheek lift. Plast Reconstr Surg 1999; 103(7):2029–2041.

38. Dayan SH, Bagal A, Tardy ME. Targeted solutions in submentoplasty. Facial Plast Surg 2001; 17(2):141–149.

39. Gonzalez-Ulloa M. Ptosis of the chin: the witches' chin. Plast Reconstr Surg 1972; 50(1):54–57.

40. Torre JI, Martin SA, Alhakeem MS, et al. A minimally invasive approach for correction of chin ptosis. Plast Reconstr Surg 2004; 113(1):404–409.

41. Miller T, Orringer JS. Excision of neck redundancy with single Z plasty closure. Plast Reconstr Surg 1996; 97(1):219–221.

42. Hamra ST. Composite rhytidectomy. Plast Reconstr Surg 1992; 90:1–13.

43. Wang TD. Rhytidectomy for treatment of the aging face. Mayo Clin Proc 1989; 64: 780–790.

44. Alsarraf R, To WC, Johnson CM. The deep plane facelift. Facial Plast Surg 2003; 19(1):95–105.

45. McCollough EG, Hom DB. Correction of the enlarged earlobe: auricular lobuloplasty— an adjunctive facelift procedure. Laryngoscope 1989; 99:1193–1194.

46. Austin HW. The lip lift. Plast Reconstr Surg 1986; 77(6):990–994.

47. Aiache AE. Rejuvenation of the perioral area. Dermatol Clin 1997; 15(4):665–672.

53
Delirium and Dementia in the Elderly

Serge Gauthier
McGill Center for Studies in Aging, McGill University, Montreal, Quebec, Canada

In this chapter, the primary emphasis is on increasing the ability of otolaryngologists to detect acute (delirium) or long-term (dementia) cognitive impairment in their older patients. Suggestions for diagnosis and management will be offered, along with information on current hypotheses and future treatment strategies for the main causes of dementia, which include Alzheimer's disease (AD), vascular dementia (VaD), and dementia with Lewy bodies (DLB).

DELIRIUM

Delirium is a new confusional state with fluctuations and is most often caused by reaction to drugs with anticholinergic side effects such as antiemetics, antivertigo commonly used in ear, nose, and throat (ENT) practice, or because of an infectious etiology. It is usually acute but may be gradual. It can be associated with agitation but can also be of the quiet or apathetic type. Delirium is more likely to occur in patients previously diagnosed with AD. It is very common in elderly hospital patients (10–16%) and in emergency rooms (up to 10%). The key clinical features are outlined in Table 1.

Delirium requires early recognition because it carries a high mortality rate and may prolong hospital stay. It is a potentially reversible medical condition explained by a global cerebral dysfunction. The major hypothesis in terms of pathophysiology

Table 1 Clinical Features of Delirium Based on DSM-IV-TR™

Disturbances in consciousness (i.e., reduced clarity of awareness of the environment) with reduced ability to focus, sustain or shift attention
Change in cognition (memory, orientation, language) or perceptual disturbance
Short period of time (hours to days) with fluctuations during the day
Caused by a general medical condition, taking or withdrawing a specific substance (alcohol; street drugs, over-the counter, or prescribed drugs), or a combination of these factors

Source: American Psychiatric Association: Diagnostic and Statistical Manual of Mental Disorders, 4ᵗʰ ed. Text Rev. Washington, D.C.: American Psychiatric Association, 2000.

Table 2 Elements of the Confusion Assessment Method for Diagnosing Delirium

Acute onset
Inattention
Disorganized thinking
Altered level of consciousness
Disorientation
Memory impairment
Perceptual disturbances
Psychomotor agitation
Psychomotor retardation
Altered sleep–wake cycle

Source: From Ref. 1.

is a defect in neurotransmission, particularly involving the cholinergic system, sensitive to receptor blockade by many drugs, hypoxia, and deficiencies of glucose, thiamine, or niacin. Excessive activity of serotonin, dopamine, and gamma-amino-butyric acid may also play a role. These transmitters may be altered directly by drugs or indirectly through cytokines released by tissue injury and inflammatory responses.

The clinical approach to delirium is to look for it in persons at risk (older, known to have systemic illnesses or dementia) with acute and fluctuating changes in alertness. The Confusion Assessment Method (CAM) is a standardized five-minute check list that can be used by nurses or physicians (Table 2).

As a complement to the clinical assessment, an electroencephalogram (EEG) may add evidence for a global brain dysfunction rather than a primary psychiatric diagnosis by demonstrating an excess of slow activity; furthermore, it will rule out rare but possible epileptic activity.

The treatment of delirium can be preventive and symptomatic (Tables 3 and 4).

DEMENTIA

Dementia is a long-term condition with cognitive impairment representing a decline from the previous level of functioning and interference with social or occupational life. The most common causes of dementia in the elderly are AD, VaD, a combination of the two (mixed AD/VaD), and DLB. These disorders are usually gradual and progressive, although with VaD or mixed AD/VaD there may be acute worsening leading to the so-called "staircase pattern" of decline from stroke to stroke. All these disorders can be associated with depression. The key clinical features are outlined in Table 5.

Table 3 Prevention of Delirium

Avoid medications with anticholinergic side effects
Favor local anesthesia over general anesthesia
If fasting is required prior to a surgical procedure, maintain CI in patients already on such drugs until evening prior to surgery, and restart as soon as possible
Get preoperative assessment using the CAM in persons at risk and monitor for changes

Abbreviations: CI, cholinesterase inhibitors; CAM, confusion assessment method.
Source: From Ref. 2.

Table 4 Symptomatic Treatment of Delirium

Identify cause(s) with emphasis on drugs
Reduce overstimulation
Closely monitor vital signs, fluid intake/output, oxygenation
Provide familiar cues or aids (clock, calendar, photographs)
Provide sensory aids (glasses, hearing aid)
Avoid physical restraints if at all possible
Low doses of neuroleptics such as haloperidol may be used. If a parenteral route is needed (0.25–0.5 mg), cardiac monitoring is required
Low doses of benzodiazepines, such as lorazepam, oxazepam, or temazepam, may be helpful
If the delirium persists over days, case reports suggest possible beneficial effects from CI, such as donepezil and rivastigmine (not standard practice)

Abbreviation: CI, cholinesterase inhibitors.
Source: From Ref. 2.

The diagnosis of dementia tends to be made earlier than in the past as people seek reassurance that their memory complaints are not the first manifestations of AD. The typical patient with AD will be brought to the physician's office by the family, with a 1–2-year history of memory decline for recent events ("she remembers everything from the past but asks all the time when is the next appointment to see you"), hesitation with words ("she gave up her crossword puzzles"), reduced ability to find directions ("he needs a navigator to find his way to his sister's house"), reduced interest or ability to plan previously well-learned activities ("she cannot knit or cook a meal the way she used to"). The patients often deny that there is anything wrong with them. Less often, during a periodic medical examination, the physician will get positive answers when inquiring whether there has been a loss of memory in the past year, and if this has an impact on that individual's daily life. Other modes of presentation are depression and apathy ("she is very quiet and cries all the time"), false beliefs ("when he does not find his keys he thinks that people are stealing things in his house"), a long postoperative delirium ("she was confused for five days

Table 5 Key Features of the Most Common Dementias

AD	Multiple cognitive deficits with early and predominant short-term memory impairment, a gradual progression though functional losses and behavioral and psychological symptoms of dementia, with late Parkinson features
VaD	Multiple cognitive deficits with frequent impairment of executive functions, focal neurological signs and symptoms, stroke and/or white matter changes on brain imaging
DLB	Multiple cognitive deficits with early impairment of short-term memory, visual hallucinations and fluctuations, progressing to Parkinsonism

Abbreviations: AD, Alzheimer's disease; VaD, vascular dementia; DLB, dementia with lewy bodies.
Source: From Refs. 3–5.

Table 6   Diagnostic Criteria for the Amnestic Type of MCI

Memory complaint preferably corroborated by an informant
Impaired memory relative to age and education
Preserved general cognitive function
Intact activities of daily living
Not demented clinically

Abbreviation: MCI, mild cognitive impairment.
Source: From Ref. 6.

after her hip surgery, and is getting more and more forgetful since"), or a small stroke ("he had numbness on his face and right arm, and since then is getting more forgetful"). It is readily apparent that the art of making the diagnosis lies in obtaining and documenting a careful history from patients and reliable informants. This includes recognizing the pattern of cognitive symptoms, their potential impact on daily life, and their psychological impact. The diagnosis may be difficult early in the course of AD because of coexisting depression, which should be treated prior to re-evaluation.

A relatively recently recognized condition in the field of dementia is the prodromal state of mild cognitive impairment (MCI), in which the individual is not normal cognitively but not yet demented. The most widely used criteria for "amnestic" (primarily memory) MCI are listed in Table 6.

It is likely that AD and the other dementias have a noncognitive prodrome, such as mood changes, anxiety, and apathy. Unfortunately, none of these symptoms are specific enough for diagnosis before the dementia is clinically manifested, and

Table 7   Comprehensive Management of AD, VaD, DLB

In prodromal stage (amnestic MCI)
    Treat concomitant disorders (depression, hypothyroidism)
    Treat vascular risk factors (systolic hypertension, atrial fibrillation, hypercholesterolemia)
In mild stages (MMSE 18–26)
    Make accurate diagnosis
    Provide patient and caregiver education
    Recommend writing of advance power of attorney
    Recommend thinking about advance directives
    Recommend a trial of symptomatic drugs, such as CI
    Monitor driving abilities
In moderate stages (MMSE 10–17)
    Monitor for the emergence of BPSD and treat accordingly
    Recommend a trial of memantine, which can used alone or with a CI
    Plan for loss of autonomy with local community resources
    Refer to day programs
    Monitor health and well-being of caregiver
In severe stages
    Facilitate transition from home to institutional care
    Discuss cessation of symptomatic drugs, such as CI and memantine
    Make end of life decisions respecting advance directives

Abbreviations: AD, Alzheimer's disease; VaD, vascular dementia; DLB, dementia with lewy bodies; MCI, mild cognitive impairment; MMSE, mini mental state examination; CI, cholinesterase inhibitors; BPSD, behavioral and psychological symptoms of dementia.

Table 8 Suggested Use of CI

Donepezil	5 mg QD for 1 mo, then 10 mg, preferably early AM
Rivastigmine	1.5 mg BID for 1 mo, then monthly increase to 3.0, 4.5, and 6.0 mg BID as tolerated
Galantamine	4 mg BID for 1 mo, then monthly increase to 8 and 12 mg BID as tolerated

Abbreviation: CI, cholinesterase inhibitors.

neither are the current laboratory tests, including genetic markers, electroencephalogram, brain imaging, and spinal fluid examinations.

The pathophysiology of AD, VaD, and DLB is obviously diverse, but these disorders share a central cholinergic dysfunction that allows symptomatic treatment with a common class of drugs, the cholinesterase inhibitors (CI). These drugs are now part of the global management of these disorders though the different severity stages defined using the Mini Mental State Examination (MMSE) (Table 7). It should be specified that CI have not yet been formerly approved for use in VaD by regulatory authorities, although their efficacy and safety has been established in randomized clinical trials. Similarly, the use of CI has not yet been formerly approved for use in DLB. Memantine is a different class of drug acting on the N-methyl-D-aspartate glutamate receptors, currently approved in most countries for use in moderate to severe AD. There have been positive results in VaD using memantine, and we do not know yet for DLB.

The symptomatic treatment of AD, and to a certain extent VaD and DLB, is currently based on the hypothesis that many of the cognitive, functional, and behavioral symptoms result from a reduction in brain acetylcholine activity secondary to the loss of cholinergic neurons in the nucleus basalis of Maynert and/or their projections to the hippocampus, medial temporal region, and neocortex. The suggested doses and titrations for the three available CI are listed in Table 8.

It is possible that the CI will delay or attenuate some of the behavioral psychological symptoms of dementia (BPSD), but some symptoms, such as aggressivity and delusions, will require low doses of atypical neuroleptics (Table 9) for some time during the course of these dementias. It should be mentioned that a very significant neuroleptic hypersentivity has been described for patients with DLB, using any of the neuroleptics; quetiapine may be the safest one to use if necessary.

There is hope that disease modification may be achieved through new drug based on research in human populations using epidemiology, genetics, postmortem brain studies, and animal models. Current targets for AD treatment in patients with dementia or prevention in people at risk are amyloid fibrils deposition, inflammation, and cholesterol transport. For VaD, mixed AD/VaD, and even AD, control of systolic hypertension has been established as a population-based preventive strategy.

Table 9 Suggested Use of Atypical Neuroleptics

Risperidone	0.5–1 mg QD or BID
Olanzepine	5–10 mg QD
Quetiapine	12.5–50 mg HS or BID

REFERENCES

1. Inouye SK, van Dyck CH, Alessi CA, et al. Clarifying confusion: the confusion assessment method. Ann Intern Med 1990; 113:941–948.
2. Rabinowitz T, Murphy KM, Nagle KJ, et al. Delirium: pathophysiology, recognition, prevention and treatment. Expert Rev Neurotherap 2003; 3:343–355.
3. Scarpini E, Scheltens P, Feldman H. Treatment of Alzheimer's disease: current status and new perspectives. Lancet Neurol 2003; 2:539–547.
4. O'Brien JT, Erkinjunnti T, Reisberg B, et al. Vascular cognitive impairment. Lancet Neurol 2003; 2:89–98.
5. McKeith I, Mintzer J, Aarsland D, et al. Dementia with Lewy bodies. Lancet Neurol 2004; 3:19–28.
6. Petersen RC. Mild cognitive impairment as a diagnostic entity. J Int Med 2004; 256: 183–194.

54

Sensory Impairment and Deprivation in the Elderly

Allen R. Huang

Geriatric Medicine, McGill University Health Centre, Royal Victoria Hospital, Montreal, Quebec, Canada

Nothing can cure the soul but the senses, just as nothing can cure the senses but the soul.

—Oscar Wilde, *The Picture of Dorian Gray*

Mrs. S. is an 84-year-old woman who was recently admitted to the ear, nose, and throat (ENT) service for resection of a large benign right parotid tumor. She underwent uneventful surgery and immediate post-op care. On the second post-operative day the nurse calls you urgently, informing you frantically that Mrs. S. is acutely agitated, shouting for the group of men in her room chasing squirrels to leave. Mrs. S. had also got up to leave her room, tripped on a bedside table which she did not see, and had fallen. Luckily the fall did not cause any apparent injury, and she is now tied to a high-backed chair.

One of the challenges in managing health care in the elderly is the *atypical* presentation of illness. An initial reaction to the above scenario could be to request an urgent referral to psychiatry and medicine with the presumed conditions of acute psychiatric hallucinosis and delirium. However, with the knowledge and tools needed to assess the hospitalized elderly patient, clarity of diagnosis and improved management can result in satisfactory outcomes and functional recovery. Irvine (1) has described six basic principles of geriatric medicine (Table 1) that can help the health practitioner understand how to better manage the care of the elderly. These principles highlight the observation that the clinical presentation in the elderly is not necessarily caused by the first obvious diagnosis. This chapter describes how sensory impairment and deprivation can affect the presentation of health problems in the elderly and how one can assess and manage these problems.

Losses are inherent with the elderly. Physiologic changes in tissues and organs lead to functional impairments in systems. However, just because there is an age-associated decline in function does not necessarily mean that there is an accompanying clinical problem. As individuals age, they become physiologically more heterogeneous. Much of the data upon which the principles of adult medicine are based were gathered

Table 1 Six Basic Principles of Geriatric Medicine

Multiple diseases commonly coexist
The spectrum of illness is relatively unique
Illness may present in unusual ways
The ageing process plays a relatively minor clinical role
Health problems are frequently under-reported
Goals of health care become more function-based

from individuals between 18 and 65 years. The physiologic and functional reserves of those individuals are large enough to make them appear homogenous. Progressive improvements in basic hygiene, nutrition, preventative health services, and modern medical interventions have resulted in the appearance of more elderly patients presenting to consultation and surgery. In the late 1970s, Claude Oster (2) suggested that sensory deprivation could be harmful to human homeostasis. The absence of afferent inputs (i.e., sight, smell, taste, hearing, touch) to the brain removes the stressor effect, which drives the human circadian rhythm (as evidenced by experimental sensory deprivation in young adult volunteers). Prolonged bed rest is well known to have deleterious effects on bone, muscle, and cardiorespiratory function. Because of the diminished physiologic reserves of elderly patients, they may develop a deconditioning syndrome when they are put to bed for even short periods. This syndrome is similar to that of astronauts returning from space flight and weightlessness.

Sensory deprivation, like many other common problems in the elderly, is typically not spontaneously reported. Concealing their impairments allows elderly patients to ostensibly maintain their dignity and avoid embarrassment. The notions that decline is inescapable and interventions are neither effective nor efficacious are part of the mythology of aging. Unfortunately, health workers and even patients and families still support these incorrect assumptions. This nihilism needs to be overcome to enable the provision of the best care for our elderly surgical patients. Despite the potential magnitude of the problem of overwhelming numbers of frail elderly occupying acute care resources, all is not hopeless or futile. Most of the elderly are in good health and lead productive lives. Even the frail nonagenarian can be managed successfully given an understanding of geriatric issues and the use of a multiprofessional health care team (e.g., nurses, physiotherapist, occupational therapist, dietitian, pharmacist, social worker, and, as needed, recreation therapist and speech-language therapist).

VISUAL IMPAIRMENT

Men and women are visual animals. The visual system has evolved to help humans succeed in their hunter-predator functions. Binocular vision provides excellent depth perception. Color discrimination and high-resolution vision (retinal cone cells) aid in the distinction of good versus bad (foods). Low light peripheral vision (retinal rod cells) enhances the detection of movement to increase both success at hunting and avoiding predators. About 15% of the brain is dedicated to the visual cortex, which supports the importance of the visual system. It is estimated that 4% to 7% of the elderly aged 71–75 years, 16% of those over 80 years, and up to 39% of those over

Table 2 Diseases of the Eye That Can Lead to Visual Impairment

Area affected	Disease entities
Cornea	Infections and scarring, sicca syndrome, refraction (presbyopia)
Lens	Cataracts[a]
Anterior chamber	Glaucoma[a]
Retina	Macular degeneration (wet and dry)[a]
	Diabetic retinopathy
	Hypertensive retinopathy
Optic nerves and visual cortex	Ischemia and stroke syndromes

[a]Most common causes of visual impairment in elderly.

90 years have visual impairment. Visual impairment is defined as persistent vision problems (vision worse than 20/40) despite wearing the best glasses. Frequently, the impairment is severe enough to interfere with reading, driving, and watching television. Table 2 lists some typical diseases that affect the visual system and can result in impairment. Visual impairment can present in different ways. Health workers can falsely assume the presence of underlying cognitive impairment because of poor performance by an elderly patient on wayfinding and written comprehension skills secondary to low vision. Sometimes, the presentation resembles an acute psychosis. One of the most striking presentations of visual impairment is the Charles Bonnet syndrome (CBS). This entity was named after the Swiss philosopher who first described it in 1760. CBS is characterized by the presence of complex, vivid visual hallucinations in the absence of substance abuse, sleep disorders, dementia, or psychiatric or epileptic illness (3). The problem in identifying this syndrome in the elderly is that other causes of visual hallucinations, including delirium and dementia (more often in the Lewy body type), can also occur. The use of neuroleptics in the management of CBS is similar to the other treatments of visual hallucinations but the prognosis and outcomes are better. The hallmark of CBS is that patients are in a clear conscious state.

AUDITORY IMPAIRMENT

Approximately 9% of the elderly have hearing impairment. However, this estimate is likely low because of under-reporting. Causes of hearing loss in the elderly have been discussed in other chapters. The functional results are communication deficits, which can be mislabeled as confusion or even dementia. Indirect effects of hearing impairment include social isolation, embarrassment (which can lead to depression), and further social and family withdrawal.

SMELL AND TASTE DISTURBANCES

Impaired sense of smell (age-related decrease in olfactory thresholds) can lead to an accompanying loss of taste. These combined impairments can result in a decrease in food intake, leading to undernutrition and failure to thrive syndrome. Some medications (e.g., metronidazole) can impart a metallic taste while others (e.g., drugs with anticholinergic side effects) can produce or worsen xerostomia, which can worsen patient compliance with medications.

TACTILE IMPAIRMENT

Age-related changes in the peripheral nervous system result in slower nerve conduction velocities. The concomitant presence of diseases (e.g., diabetes mellitus) causing peripheral neuropathies further leads to touch-sense impairments. Falls and gait disorders may be the major presenting syndrome of these impairments. Gait and mobility problems are important factors in loss of autonomy and dependency.

> Mrs. S. had been to see you in your office several weeks ago as a referral from a family practitioner who was worried about her right neck swelling. She was accompanied by her niece. Her physician had sent a detailed medical history which included: Type 2 diabetes mellitus, chronic congestive heart failure, and bilateral macular degeneration with low vision. Her habits included: half-pack-a-day cigarette smoking and drinking at least one glass of wine daily. You had found her physical health to be intact. She was still active in her local group choir and was worried about whether any proposed surgery would have an effect on her hearing or singing. You explained the operative procedure and process to her and allayed her concerns. At the end of the visit Mrs. S. handed all the written information to her niece and said that she would trust her niece's judgment when you had asked her whether she had any further questions. As can be seen from the above descriptions of sensory impairments, it can be a struggle for older patients to continually conceal their problems. When elderly individuals are confronted by a health care institution, with its bland walls, unfamiliar layouts, unfamiliar faces, disruptive schedules, noise, and distractions, it is a wonder that they all do not decompensate. Aside from the loss of autonomy caused by these functional impairments, there can also be a loss of pleasurable activities, such as enjoyment of the visual arts, music, and speech. Sight and hearing impairment can compromise safety because of the absence of warning signals from the sights and sounds of approaching automobile traffic outside, equipment traffic within a hospital, or other alert or alarm signals. Acute confusion accompanied by physical or verbal agitation is perhaps the most common presentation that indicates to the health worker that something is wrong.

ASSESSMENT

A focused history and physical examination can eilicit the time course of the observed agitated behavior, clarify the patient's previous baseline functioning, and screen for obvious sensory impairment (4) that can be contributing to the current problem. Basic lab tests can identify any disturbances in physiologic function or medical disease control. Special diagnostic tests and referral to other specialists can further clarify the extent to which sensory impairment is involved in the elderly patient's problems. Table 3 summarizes the approach to assessing elderly patients with sensory impairment who present with an acute confusional state.

> The assessment of Mrs. S. revealed that her physiologic measures were normal, including her blood pressure when standing, oxygen saturation, electrolytes, glucose, and complete blood count (CBC). Her vision was 20/100 bilaterally using a wall sight chart. When asked about her visual hallucinations Mrs. S. calmly and clearly states that she had been troubled with "visions involving a group of men" for the past six months, but had been afraid to mention them for fear of being labeled "crazy."

Table 3 Assessing the Agitated Elderly Patient with Sensory Impairment

History	An acute onset of problems (less than 1 week) suggests delirium
	Delirium can be hyperactive (with agitated behavior) or hypoactive (stupor and coma)
	Presence of similar behavior dating back 6 months or more suggests an underlying dementia
Physical exam	Orthostatic blood pressure measurements
	Visual acuity screening using Snellen sight card
	(Pinprick sensation, position sense—in the case of falls)
Basic labs	Oxygen saturation by percutaneous measurement
	Complete blood counts
	Electrolytes, glucose, calcium
	Appropriate bacterial cultures
Special tests	Visual fields
	Fundoscopy
	Tonometry for intraocular pressures
	Audiogram
	Electromyography and nerve conduction studies
	Folstein mini-mental status examination, confusion assessment method tool (see Chapter 53, "Delirium and Dementia in the Elderly")
Referrals	Ophthalmology
	Neurology
	Psychiatry
	Geriatric medicine
	(Physiotherapy—in the case of falls)

MANAGEMENT AND INTERVENTIONS

Agitated behavior and delirium represent just the tip of the "illness iceberg." Below the surface are several layers where processes can affect functional capacity and influence the upper layers. The base of this iceberg represents the patient's physiologic reserves. As previously mentioned, this reserve is highly individualized in the elderly. The middle layers represent the patient's medical diseases and medications. These layers are where the multiple illnesses and polypharmacy so commonly found in the elderly are considered. Sensory impairment affects the interface between the person and the outside world. The iceberg model can provide a framework on which potential interventions can be organized and generate a comprehensive management scheme. Table 4 lists the layers of the illness iceberg along with potential interventions. Once sensory impairment and deprivation has been identified, several low-tech, high-touch interventions can be initiated to alleviate symptoms and anxiety. As interventions affect the respective layers in the illness iceberg and stability is achieved, the patient's coping mechanisms should re-equilibrate and the agitation resolve. Specific interventions to manage sensory impaired patients are listed in Table 5. Transfer to an alternative level of care environment with an appropriately adapted physical setup and compassionate skilled nursing is sometimes required, especially if the elderly patient's recovery is delayed. For example, balancing control of pulmonary edema secondary to heart failure and resultant hypovolemia and hypotension may take several days. Altered pharmacokinetics and pharmacodynamics in the elderly result in a prolongation of up to 48-hours observation before the full effects of medication changes are seen.

Table 4 Layers of the Illness Iceberg from Base to Tip and Potential Interventions

Layer description	Interventions
Physiologic reserves (base of iceberg)	Optimize oxygen saturation and oxygen carrying capacity (e.g., hemoglobin, cardiac output)
	Ensure adequate blood pressure, especially when standing (review hydration status, medications with hypotensive effects)
Medical conditions	Optimize disease control (e.g., heart failure, diabetes, tachyarrhythmias, COPD)
	Assistance from internal medicine or geriatric medicine consultants can be helpful
Medications	Careful review for drug–drug interactions, drug–disease interactions, drugs generally contraindicated in the elderly
	Decrease dose or avoid drugs with anticholinergic effects
	Involvement of a pharmacist is recommended
Sensory impairment	Implement environmental and behavioral modification strategies
Agitated behavior and delirium (tip of iceberg)	Implement nonpharmacologic and short-term pharmacologic strategies (see Chapter 53, "Delirium and Dementia in the Elderly")

Abbreviation: COPD, chronic obstructive pulmonary disease.

That afternoon the nurses changed her bulky head and neck dressings for a less restrictive one. Multiple sensory deprivations were suspected in contributing to the patient's agitated behaviour. Charles Bonnet syndrome was the working diagnosis for the visual hallucinations, and 2.5 mg olanzapine in the afternoon with a repeat dose in the evening was prescribed. The niece was called and asked to come in to sit with her and supervise. A small lamp was left on by the bedside during the night. A physiotherapist assessed the patient and determined that there were no mobility problems involved in the previous fall and no walking aid was required. The pharmacist reviewed the medication list and suggested a substitution of

Table 5 Interventions to Help Manage Specific Sensory Impairements in the Elderly

Impairment	Intervention
Vision	High contrast environment with horizontal edges to create multiple horizons
	Provide good, even lighting
	Reduce glare (use of low-luster floor wax)
	Provide adequate floor lighting
	Provide night lighting
	Atypical neuroleptics may be needed for cases of Charles Bonnet syndrome resistant to behavioral interventions (e.g., olanzapine 2.5–10.0 mg or risperidone 0.5–3.0 mg in divided doses)
Hearing	Use of auditory aids
	Face patients when speaking to them
Smell and taste	Decrease or avoid medications with anticholinergic or gustatory side effects
	Provide sugar-free candies to encourage salivary flow
	Offer spice supplements or salt substitutes to improve oral food intake
Touch sense	Wearing of firm supportive footwear with leather soles
	Have physiotherapist assess patient for walking aids (e.g., cane, walker)

hydromorphone (Dilaudid®) for meperidine (Demerol®). An attendant trained in the care of the elderly was hired for the evening and night.

Caution should always be used if physical restraints are being considered in the management of agitated behavior. The safety and efficacy of such devices is questionable. No physical device can replace the caring supervision of a skilled patient attendant. Although these resources may be expensive, their use is necessary for only a short time and avoids potential morbidity and mortality from physical restraint complications.

CONCLUSIONS

Sensory impairments and deprivation place elderly patients at risk for decompensation, especially in the hospital environment (5,6). Awareness of these conditions coupled with simple interventions can go a long way to providing the optimal management of the hospitalized elderly patient and accelerating a discharge process that is durable and satisfying. Empowered with the knowledge of managing these problems, the clinician can, with a low-tech, high-touch caring approach intervene to alter outcome, accelerate recovery, and subsequently return to best function and quality of life.

> Over the next two days Mrs. S. steadily improved. Her visual hallucinations became less distressing and the olanzapine was discontinued. With the increased lighting, soothing presence of her niece, and the hired attendant, she regained her "senses." She was discharged home shortly afterwards and completed her recovery quickly. She was back to her usual active lifestyle at her follow-up visit several weeks later.

REFERENCES

1. Irvine PW. Patterns of disease: the challenge of multiple illnesses. In: Cassel CK, Riesenberg DE, Sorenson LB, Walsh JR, eds. Geriatric Medicine. 2nd ed. New York: Springer-Verlag, 1990.

   Standard reference that describes the six principles of geriatric medicine: (i) multiple diseases commonly coexist; (ii) the spectrum of illness is relatively unique; (iii) illness may present in unusual ways; (iv) the ageing process plays a relatively minor clinical role; (v) health problems are frequently under-reported; and (vi) goals of health care become more function based. These principles help health workers understand why caring for the sick elderly can be a challenge. These principles also lay the foundation that the use of a multiprofessional health care team can improve the care of the elderly patient.

2. Oster C. Sensory deprivation and homeostasis. J Am Geriatr Soc 1979; 27(8):364–367.

   The primary thesis of this reference is the role of sensory inputs in the maintenance of stress in Hans Selye's general adaptation syndrome. These inputs are the triggers for normal hypothalamic–pituitary–adrenal axis function, which are necessary for homeostasis. In the situation of sensory deprivation, the entire axis activity is decreased, leading to a decrease in biogenic amine release, which has been associated with clinical depression.

3. Teunisse RJ, Cruysberg JRM, Verbeek A, Zitman FG. The Charles Bonnet syndrome: a large prospective study in The Netherlands. Br J Psychiatry 1995; 166:254–257.

This reference describes a study defining the prevalence of CBS in The Netherlands. It is important to note that the incidence of CBS is 11% to 15% in patients 65–97 years, regardless of the etiology of visual impairment. This is a surprisingly high incidence but relates to the general principle of underreporting of problems by the elderly.

4. Lachs MS, Feinstein AR, Cooney LM Jr, et al. A simple procedure for general screening for functional disability in elderly patients. Ann Intern Med 1990; 112(9):699–706.

This reference outlines a set of screening maneuvers useful in identifying important disabilities in the elderly. The tests focusing on the special senses, cognition and mobility should be applied. These tests can easily be delegated to an allied health professional to screen elderly patients during their consultation or preop visits.

5. Cranin AN, Sher J. Sensory deprivation. Oral Surg Oral Med Oral Pathol 1979; 47(5): 416–417.

This reference presents a refreshing and timeless case report of how post-op sensory deprivation can manifest and how easily it can be managed.

6. Creditor MC. Hazards of hospitalization of the elderly. Ann Int Med 1993; 118:219–223.

This reference describes the cascade to dependency that can happen to hospitalized elderly patients. Iatrogenic illness is an important cause of morbidity and mortality and has the potential to occur more frequently in elderly patients because of the principles outlined in the first reference. A few simple interventions such as using low beds for all elderly patients, keeping the bedrails down and encouraging early and frequent mobilization can limit the cascade. Again the multiprofessional health care team is an important ally.

55
Social Isolation

Vanessa Sakadakis

Social Services Department, McGill University Health Centre,
Royal Victoria Hospital, Montreal, Quebec, Canada

INTRODUCTION

Miss Brown is a 90-year-old single woman with no family who lives alone in an apartment. She had elective right hip replacement surgery in 2003, a left hip fracture in 2000, osteoporosis with kyphosis and previous multiple compression fractures, decreased vision, and decreased hearing. She does not go outdoors for fear of falling and uses a walker in the apartment. She is able to prepare a simple meal but cannot do heavy housework or go shopping independently. She weighs 103 lb and is 5 ft tall. She has a right submandibular mass that has grown significantly in the last six months and has consulted an OTL specialist.

Miss Brown is part of the fastest growing population group in Canada. In 2000, 12.5% of the population was over 65. It is projected to reach 18.9% (approximately seven million) in 2021 [1]. In 1996, 29% of seniors lived alone, an increase of 8% since 1971 [1,2].

Miss Brown also represents one in four seniors who have a long-term disability or handicap. This proportion rises sharply with age, from 21% (65–74 years), to 28% (75–85 years), and to 45% (85+) [1]. Miss Brown's level of social support and interaction needs to be more closely examined, as the patient has no family and it is uncertain what degree of involvement she has from friends or community groups. Miss Brown also has several disabilities that have an impact on her independence. This may influence her ability to cope with potential surgery to remove the mass and follow-up treatment if the mass is malignant.

SOCIAL ISOLATION AND LONELINESS

Social isolation has been defined as the voluntary or involuntary deprivation of social contact or interaction with others [3,4]. It is an objective measure of social interaction compromising a continuum ranging from high social involvement in a variety of social networks to extreme isolation [3,5]. The level of social interaction can fluctuate during different stages of an individual's life. If isolation is voluntary, it is not perceived as a problem. If it is involuntary, deprivation may affect self-image, decrease independence, and increase institutionalization (3).

Loneliness can result from perceived social isolation. It is a subjective expression of dissatisfaction with a low number of social contacts often accompanied by negative feelings about being alone. An individual can have a wide number of social contacts but can still feel subjectively lonely if the quality of the contacts is perceived to be low. Social contacts can reinforce and increase dependence on them, thus further isolating the individual from others, or they can reinforce addictive behaviors, such as alcoholism, in order for the individual to maintain some social contact.

Loneliness and social isolation is of concern to clinicians given that suicide, depression, and cognitive dysfunction are outcomes frequently associated with prolonged periods of loneliness (6). These can be reactional and transitory in response to major life events, such as retirement or bereavement.

Chappell and Badger (7) write that the quantity (size of the network and number of relationships) and the quality of social support (emotional or perceived support) appear to be linked to health; however, findings are inconsistent. It is not clear in studies whether isolation results from decreased contact with other people due to ill health or if decreased contact and the possibility of loneliness precede ill health (5). Social isolation is felt to be a risk factor for disease, for functional incapacity in general, and for disability and handicap as a result of that incapacity (8). Research is at a very early stage with inconclusive results.

Increasing attention has been placed on the biopsychosocial model examining the mechanisms linking psychological symptoms, social contributors, biological characteristics, behavioral choices, and physiological disease processes. Depression, anxiety, and social isolation influence behavior such as exercise, diet, and healthy lifestyle. A potent psychosocial risk factor that has been identified for cardiovascular disease is social isolation, such as living alone, lacking instrumental support, and/or being unable to share personal expectations with a confidant (9).

Individuals with low perceived isolation were more likely to actively cope with or solve problems and to seek instrumental and emotional support from others, whereas individuals with high perceived social isolation were more likely to behaviorally disengage or withdraw from the stressor. Negative health consequences of social isolation are particularly strong among those in need of societal support, those over 65, the poor, and minorities (10). Health care providers need to be more in tune with the types or quality of relationships maintained by their patients and whether they are satisfying (11). Social relationships also play an important role in an older person's maintenance of mental health and physical well-being by acting as buffers for stressful life events (12).

SOCIAL ISOLATION AND ELDERLY PEOPLE

Major causes of death in older adults are chronic diseases such as myocardial infarction, stroke, cancer, and diabetes. The risk factors for these diseases are usually smoking, obesity, high blood pressure, and sedentary lifestyles. One of the strongest and least understood factors for morbidity and mortality is social isolation (10).

Aging involves a constriction in roles and numerous losses (partners, family, friends, home, work) that may result in physical or social isolation. An elderly person's natural support network becomes more depleted due to illness and death (9). Changing family structures, family mobility, and the person's functional capacity may also contribute to increased social isolation (4).

When social isolation is identified as a condition of older individuals, the phenomenon is generally accepted as the continuation of a lifelong pattern rather than a development of later life (8). Loneliness is part of a negative stereotype of old age, but the problem affects only one in 10 people (13). Loneliness is not an inevitable accompaniment to old age; however, it can become a severe problem when correlated with a number of physical and psychological problems (14). The health effects of social isolation may be especially important among the aged since they commonly experience a disruption in their personal relationships by death or illness or may be removed from their social networks when they move into a nursing home.

Perceived social connectedness or support is more strongly associated with lower levels of autonomic activity, better immunosurveillance, and lower basal levels of stress hormones than is objective social connectedness (10). Negative health consequences of social isolation are particularly strong among the elderly. Socially isolated adults are characterized by increases in feelings of anxiety, depression, social stigma, hostility, and fear of negative evaluation; by increases in alcohol consumption, hospital visits, and suicide; by decreases in feelings of optimism, happiness, and life satisfaction; and decreases in nutrition and immunity (11,12,14,15). Individuals perceiving themselves to be frail and dependent may isolate themselves to disguise their loss of autonomy (8). Studies conducted by de Leeuw (16) and Katz (17) into the impact of social support in facilitating adjustment to head and neck cancer found that social support correlated with positive adjustment.

The proportions of elderly men and women describing themselves as socially isolated or lonely are equal, especially for those with fewer than three people in their support network (9). Hall and Havens (5) summarized that the odds of being socially isolated were 1.7 times greater for women than men, 1.3 times greater among those who were older with poor self-rated health, and 1.1 times greater for those with more chronic illness. An accumulation of these effects would mean that a woman over 80 and in poor health would be almost $5\frac{1}{2}$ times more likely to be socially isolated than men younger than 80 and in better health. For single individuals, increased age was associated with greater medical usage and increased estimated total health care costs, while a low perceived social environment was related to a greater number of doctor visits (12).

State-of-the-art measurement of social supports has not yet reached the point where there can be differentiation of the stage of disease at which lack of social support has the greatest impact (8). Lack of social support correlates with the incidence of chronic illness and disability with age. Social support was found to be particularly important when bedside nurturing, financial assistance, and links to bureaucratic organization are necessary. Individuals with few supports were more likely to be institutionalized when illness struck and also exhibited the poorest mental health and increased hospital and physician use. Elderly people with no source of support have been shown to have protracted recovery and hospital stays (18,19). Individuals with head and neck cancer who reported comparatively higher levels of social support also reported higher levels of well-being (17).

ASSESSMENT AND INTERVENTION

The assessment of social isolation and intervention to minimize social isolation involves training health care professionals to identify those at high risk and to teach them to manipulate the environment so as to acquire the needed social support. There are five major risk factors described below that are addressed by numerous scales measuring social isolation. These can help the health care practitioners identify what concerns can be managed by the system as well as establish links to "next-step" decisions, such as consultation to other health care professionals within the hospital, or to outpatient and community resources and planning for possible interventions (4,5,11,20,21).

1. *Physical*: mobility, history of falls, eyesight, hearing, ability to perform activities of daily living (ADL—dressing, eating, and bathing) and instrumental activities of daily living (IADL—shopping, cleaning, using the telephone, taking medication), and weight loss.
2. *Social*: living situation, involvement of family or friends, bereavement, restrictive caregiving responsibilities, and loss of home, work, volunteer, or recreational activities.
3. *Environmental*: poor housing, lack of accessible transportation, lack of local services or awareness of available community health care resources such as homecare and Meals on Wheels, or the prohibitive cost of some programs or services.
4. *Psychological*: cognitive status, motivation, problem solving ability, feeling unsafe to leave the house due to vulnerability, embarrassment regarding limitations, subjective feelings of loneliness or alienation, and self-report of depressive symptoms.
5. *Financial*: adequate finances to pay for help needed and to participate in social activities.

Although many studies have examined effective interventions for social isolation, most focus on anecdotal evidence or on individual behavioral change. Outcome studies have focused on a small number of intervention types, primarily long-term group work. There is a lack of published evidence to demonstrate the effectiveness of one-to-one intervention (4).

Prevention against social isolation involves education and training in coping mechanisms to teach a person to use social resources to maintain health. The use of peers should be capitalized because of their ability to relate to the needs and concerns of others with whom they share a similar life event (9). Isolation can be reduced by participation in meals on wheels, daily friendly visits, increasing leisure activities, and participation in day center programs (3). Isolation caused by declining health may be alleviated by a move to assisted housing or relieved temporarily by repeat contacts with the appropriate health care providers (5).

Referring back to Miss Brown, it would appear from the information we have to date that she is at high risk of being socially isolated. If the submandibular mass is to be removed surgically, we would need to determine how the support system of the patient might have an influence on health outcome, length of stay in the hospital, and her ability to keep follow-up appointments. The following risk factors would need to be assessed:

1. *Physical*: Is the patient experiencing decreased mobility, deterioration in eyesight, or decreased hearing? Is the patient having difficulty with ADL and IADL?
2. *Social*: What is the patient's living situation? Does the patient receive help from community organizations? What type and how often?
3. *Environmental*: What are the available community resources? Is the patient aware of them and prepared to use them? Does the patient have access to adequate transportation to come to the hospital and keep the appointments?

4. *Psychological*: Is the patient able to problem solve effectively? Are there any cognitive problems? Does the patient express any fears? Is the patient embarrassed by her own limitations?
5. *Financial*: Is the patient able to pay for extra services or for additional medication if needed?

When interviewed, Miss Brown explained that she walks with a walker indoors but always has a volunteer from a local community group accompany her to appointments. Although Miss Brown has access to adapted transport, it is very awkward to arrange, so she prefers to take taxis. She is able to transfer into the car independently. She has decreased vision but wears glasses. Her hearing is poor, and although she had been fitted for a hearing aid, she could not adjust to it and will not wear it. She has a telephone with volume control that she can adjust, but even with that it is sometimes difficult to communicate. She often has to ask the community social worker to help in making appointments and to do the banking on the telephone. Miss Brown states that she receives help from the same community volunteer organization for shopping and Meals on Wheels twice a week. She receives help for bathing weekly and has a private cleaning woman every two weeks. Miss Brown does not describe any financial difficulties. She learned about, and was referred to, available resources during the hip fracture in 2000, and she does not seem to have any problems asking for additional help if needed. She does not appear to have any cognitive impairment. Although Miss Brown does not seem to have any close friends or relatives, she receives regular visits from volunteers and a community social worker. She does not perceive herself as being isolated or lonely. Social isolation in this case does not appear to be a problem, and barring any complications, there does not appear to be any concern about her ability to undergo surgery and be discharged from the hospital. Had there been any cognitive impairment present and had she expressed any difficulty accepting or asking for help, or had no knowledge of available community resources, consultation and further intervention by other health care professionals would have been indicated.

CONCLUSION

Despite the fact that there is very little empirical evidence that links social isolation to ill health, it is believed to be a risk factor for disability and handicap. Physical status, age, social situation, availability and accessibility of community resources, financial situation, cognitive status, and ability to problem solve contribute to people's ability to take an active role in managing their health. Deficits in any of these areas may result in increased isolation, either voluntary or involuntary. This has an impact on the person's ability to follow up on medical concerns and prescribed treatment plans. Screening for social isolation can help health care professionals identify problems, thus allowing them to intervene directly or consult with other health care professionals to ensure that the appropriate available resources are organized to help the person cope better and decrease social isolation.

REFERENCES

1. Division of Aging and Seniors. Who are Canada's Seniors. (Accessed December 6, 2003, at http://www.hc-sc.gc.ca/seniors-aines/pubs/fed_paper/fedreport1_01_e.htm. http://www.hc-sc.gc.ca/seniors-aines/pubs/factoids/2001/toc_e.htm.).

2. Report Card by the National Advisory Council on Aging 2001. (Accessed 6 December, 2003 at http://www.hc-sc.gc.ca/seniors-aines/naca/report_card/pdf/report_e.pdf.).

3. McPherson BD. Aging as a social process. Toronto: Butterworth and Co. Ltd., 1983.

4. Cattan M, White M. Developing evidence based health promotion for older people: a systematic review and survey of health promotion interventions targeting social isolation and loneliness among older people. (Accessed September 19, 2003, at http://www.rhpeo.org/ijhp-articles/1998/13/.)

5. Hall M, Havens B. Social isolation and social loneliness. Mental Health and Aging. Ottawa, ON.: National Advisory Council on Aging, October 2002.

6. Fry PS, Debats DL. Self-efficacy beliefs as predictors of loneliness and psychological distress in older adults. Int J Aging Hum Dev 2002; 55(3):233–269.

7. Chappell NL, Badger M. Social isolation and well-being. J Gerontol Soc Sci 1989; 44(5):S169–S176.

8. Berg RL, Cassells JS. The Second Fifty Years: Promoting Health and Preventing Disability. Washington, D.C.: National Academy Press, 1992.

9. Stuart-Shor EM, Buselli EF, Carroll DL, Forman DE. Are psychosocial factors associated with the pathogenesis and consequences of cardiovascular disease in the elderly? J Cardiovasc Nurs 2003; 18(3):169–183.

10. Cacioppo JT, Hawkley LC. Social isolation and health, with an emphasis on underlying mechanisms. Perspect Biol Med 2003; 46(3):S39–S47.

11. Fioto B. Social isolation: important construct in community health. Geriatr Nurs 2002; 23(1):53–55.

12. Bosworth HB, Schaie KW. The relationship of social environment, social networks, and health outcomes in The Seattle Longitudinal Study: two analytical approaches. J Gerontol Ser B Psychol Sci Soc Sci 1997; 52B(5):P197–P205.

13. Forbes A. Caring for older people: loneliness. BMJ 1996; 313(10):352–354.

14. Donaldson JM, Watson R. Loneliness in elderly people: an important area for nursing research. J Adv Nurs 1996; 24:952–959.

15. Cacioppo JT, Hawkley LC, Crawford LE, et al. Loneliness and health: potential mechanisms. Psychosom Med 2002; 64:407–417.

16. de Leeuw JRJ, de Graeff A, Ros WJG, Hordijk GJ, Blijham GH, Winnubst JAM. Negative and positive influences of social support on depression in patients with head and neck cancer: a prospective study. Psychooncology 2000; 9:20–28.

17. Katz MR, Irish J, Devins GM, Rodin GM, Gullane PJ. Psychosocial adjustment in head and neck cancer: the impact of disfigurement, gender and social support. Head Neck 2003;25(2):103–112.

18. Ryan MC. The relationship between loneliness, social support and decline in cognitive function in the hospitalized elderly. J Gerontol Nurs 1998:19–27.

19. Mullins LC, Smith R, Colquitt R, Mushel M. An examination of the effects of self-rated and objective indicators of health condition and economic condition on the loneliness of older persons. J Appl Gerontol 1996; 15(1):23–37.

20. Phillips-Harris C. Case management: high-intensity care for frail patients with complex needs. Geriatrics 1998; 53(2):62–68.

21. Wodarski JS, Rapp-Paglicci LA, Dulmus CN, Jongma AE. The social work and human services treatment planner. New York: John Wiley and Sons, Inc., 2001.

ANNOTATED BIBLIOGRAPHY

Berg RL, Cassells JS. The Second Fifty Years: Promoting Health and Preventing Disability. Washington, D.C.: National Academy Press, 1992.

The authors define the problem, estimation of the cost of social isolation, prevention, and research issues.

Fioto B. Social isolation: important construct in community health. Geriatr Nurs 2002; 23(1):53–55.

The author provides a very good summary of the multidimensional aspect of social isolation: how it is defined, measured, and identified.

Katz MR, Irish J, Devins GM, Rodin GM, Gullane PJ. Psychosocial adjustment in head and neck cancer: the impact of disfigurement, gender and social support. Head Neck 2003; 25(2):103–112.

The authors examine the impact of social support in adjustment to head and neck cancer using numerous scales including the Medical Outcome Study Social Support Survey to measure social support.

56
Substance Misuse in the Elderly

David W. Oslin
*Department of Psychiatry, University of Pennsylvania, and Philadelphia
VA Medical Center, Philadelphia, Pennsylvania, U.S.A.*

INTRODUCTION

The use and abuse of alcohol, medications, illicit drugs, and nicotine are a significant public health concern for the growing population of elderly adults. Alcohol and drug dependence are two of the leading causes of disability worldwide; however, use and abuse of substances is often not appreciated as relevant to the care of older adults. The public health impact of substance abuse will also increase over the next several decades, as the population of elderly adults increases and the prevalence of late life addiction increases because of cohort changes. The current cohort of 30- to 50-year-old adults represents a group that was raised during the 1950s and 1960s and, as such, participated in the increased use of and addiction to heroin, cocaine, tobacco, and alcohol. Both the continued use of these substances and a history of substance abuse or dependence will likely have physical and mental health consequences for this cohort as it ages.

The elderly also represent a group of adults who are particularly vulnerable to the effects of these substances, and as such, there is a need to conceptualize the risk of use in patients who are not dependent on these substances, as well as those who are dependent. Typically, substance use problems are thought to occur only in those persons who use substances in high quantities and at regular intervals. Among the elderly, however, negative health consequences have been demonstrated at consumption levels thought of as light to moderate and in patients without a diagnosis of dependence. Thus, there is a critical need to identify and provide appropriate treatment for those older adults suffering from the effects of these substances.

GENERAL DESCRIPTION OF THE CLINICAL PROBLEM

Establishing valid criteria for defining which older adults would benefit from reducing or eliminating their substance use is a critical step. The National Institute on Alcohol Abuse and Alcoholism (NIAAA) and the Center for Substance Abuse Prevention (CSAP) recommend that persons aged 65 and older consume no more than one standard drink/day or seven standard drinks/week. In addition, older adults should consume no more than four standard drinks on any drinking day. Furthermore, in the

625

context of certain medical problems or while taking certain medications, abstinence is recommended. These recommendations are consistent with research on the relationship between heavy consumption and alcohol-related problems within this age group and consistent with the current evidence for a beneficial health effect of low risk drinking. For nicotine and illicit drugs, the accepted level of use warranting intervention is any use. The recommendation of abstinence is particularly pertinent for certain people, such as patients who are diagnosed with medical problems like cancer that are exacerbated by use of nicotine or illicit drugs.

Alcohol consumption or substance use above recommended limits is considered *at-risk use*, while *dependence* refers to a medical disorder characterized by loss of control, preoccupation, continued use despite adverse consequences, and physiological symptoms such as tolerance and withdrawal. Both at-risk use and dependence are appropriate targets for interventions to reduce use. At-risk use is also a term that may not be associated with the negative stereotypes that "dependence" does and therefore may be a useful term for discussing substance use with patients. In addition to these categories of problematic behavior, individuals may also consume alcohol at levels of low risk or be considered abstainers. It is worth noting that a previous history of at-risk use or dependence can increase the risks for developing other health problems in later life and complicate the treatment of other disorders.

MAGNITUDE OF THE PROBLEM

Drug Use

Little is known about the epidemiology of substance use disorders in the elderly other than alcoholism. Lifetime prevalence rates of drug abuse and dependence has been estimated to be 0.12% for elderly men and 0.06% for elderly women, respectively. In contrast, a more recent study of an elder-specific drug program in a veteran population found that one-quarter of patients had either a primary drug problem or a concurrent drug and alcohol problem. This more recent study may be a reflection of the growing number of elderly raised during a time of expanded drug experimentation.

Medication Misuse

Perhaps a unique problem with the elderly is the misuse or inappropriate use of prescription and over-the-counter medications. This problem includes the misuse of substances such as sedatives, hypnotics, narcotic and non-narcotic analgesics, diet aids, decongestants, and a wide variety of other over-the-counter medications. Community surveys have found that 60% of the elderly are taking an analgesic, 22% are taking a central nervous system medication, and 11% are taking a benzodiazepine. Many of these medications have the potential for inducing tolerance, withdrawal syndromes, and harmful medical consequences, such as cognitive changes, renal disease, and hepatic disease.

Alcohol Use

The prevalence of alcohol dependence among community-dwelling elderly has been estimated in two recent studies. While the prevalence of alcohol use is common (54.9% reported alcohol use in the last year), the prevalence of current alcohol dependence or problems is only 2–4%. Prevalence estimates of at-risk or problem drinking using community surveys have ranged from 1% to 15%. There is consistent evidence throughout these studies indicating that men drink more and have a greater prevalence of at-risk use or dependence than women. These studies are less clear on differences between ethnic groups, although in certain ethnic elderly minorities, such as elderly Asian populations, drinking is very uncommon. Among clinical populations, estimates of alcohol problems are substantially higher because problem drinkers of all ages are more likely to be present in health care settings. For instance, among elderly primary care patients, 10–15% of the patients screened positive for at-risk or problem drinking.

Smoking

Despite reports of significant declines in overall prevalence rates, a great number of older adults remain active smokers. Although smoking rates decrease with age (primarily due to differential mortality), one out of every five smokers is aged 50 or older. Approximately 15.2% of community-dwelling individuals aged 65–74 and 8.4% of those aged 75 and older are current smokers. Rates among African-American men are significantly higher (22.1% between the ages of 65 and 74 and 12% aged 75 or older).

WHY IS SUBSTANCE ABUSE PARTICULARLY IMPORTANT IN THE GERIATRIC POPULATION?

Beneficial Effects of Alcohol Consumption

Moderate alcohol consumption among otherwise healthy older adults has been promoted as having significant beneficial effects, especially with regard to cardiovascular disease, dementia, and mortality. The findings from the cardiovascular literature have led to a host of articles in the popular press espousing the benefits of alcohol use and have also led some people to recommend initiating alcohol consumption in persons who formerly did not drink. Alcohol in moderate amounts may also improve self-esteem or promote relaxation. While there are benefits of moderate drinking, the practice of recommending drinking to people who currently do not drink is not advocated. There is no evidence to support a therapeutic effect of alcohol for heart disease or any other condition in persons who previously did not drink.

Excess Physical Disability in Older Adults

Substance abuse has clear and profound effects on the health and well-being of the elderly in all spheres of their life. Older persons are prone to the toxic effects of substances on many different organ systems. The social and economic impact on the elderly is also tremendous. Substance abuse has effects on self-esteem, coping skills, and interpersonal relationships, which may be compounded by losses that are common in the late stages of life. The elderly are particularly prone to these toxic effects because of both the physiologic changes associated with aging and the changes associated with other illnesses common in late life.

At-risk and problem drinking have been demonstrated to impair driving-related skills and can lead to other problems, such as falls, depression, memory problems, liver disease, cardiovascular disease, cognitive changes, and sleep problems. Of particular importance to providers caring for the elderly are the potential harmful interactions between alcohol and both prescribed and over-the-counter medications, especially psychoactive medications such as benzodiazepines, barbiturates, and antidepressants. Alcohol use is one of the leading risk factors for developing adverse drug reactions and is known to interfere with the metabolism of many medications, such as digoxin and warfarin.

Older adults who consume more than an average of four drinks per day or whose drinking has led to a diagnosis of alcohol dependence are at the greatest risk for excessive physical disability and physical illness related to the drinking. The most common problems associated with alcohol dependence are alcoholic liver disease, chronic obstructive pulmonary disease (COPD), peptic ulcer disease, and psoriasis. Moreover, unexplained multisystem disease should alert the clinician to probe more closely for alcohol use. With smoking, the risks are much clearer, leading to increased rates of pulmonary disease, especially cancer. Cancer risk from both alcohol and smoking in particular are worth noting. Increased risk is observed for cancers of the oral cavity, pharynx, larynx, esophagus, and lung. Moreover, there is a synergistic effect of consuming both alcohol and tobacco such that the risk of oropharyngeal cancer increases by more than 35-fold among those who consume two or more packs of cigarettes and more than four alcoholic drinks/day. Alcohol and tobacco are also strongly negatively associated with survival rates among those who continue to use while being treated for cancer. Alcohol and, to some extent, tobacco have not consistently been associated with the development of other cancers involving the stomach, colon and rectum, liver, breast, pancreas, prostate, and ovary. Medications such as benzodiazepines are also associated with excess physical disability with increased rates of falls and driving-related impairment.

COMMON PRESENTATIONS IN THE GERIATRIC POPULATION

While it is true that substance dependence has been accepted by the medical community as imparting significant disability and warrants treatment, many older adults are not recognized as having problems related to their substance use. This lack of recognition is partly because the diagnostic criteria are often difficult to interpret and not applied in a consistent manner for older adults. For instance, many elders drink at home by themselves; thus, they are less likely to be arrested, get into arguments, or have difficulties in employment. Moreover, because many of the diseases caused or affected by substance misuse (e.g., hypertension, stroke, cancer, and pulmonary disease) are common disorders in later life, physicians may overlook the effects of substance use on certain health conditions.

Confusion about who would benefit from an intervention not only affects physician behavior in terms of offering treatment but also affects patients' behavior with regards to seeking or accepting treatment. The stereotypical older patients in need of addiction treatment are the ones who have drunk heavily all of their life, have failing health related to the alcohol, and have no social network. In contrast, the relatively healthy 70-year-olds who are drinking moderately but have some mild cognitive loss or are struggling with blood pressure control do not think that they are in need of help with their drinking and rarely ask for assistance. This diagnostic confusion is highlighted in the following case example.

> Mr. Smith is a 73 year-old man who was seen by his primary care practitioner (PCP) for a routine exam. He reports suffering from some ill-described upper abdominal discomfort and chronic cough, but otherwise he has no complaints.

Upon asking about general health habits, the PCP learns that Mr. Smith does not smoke but does drink each day at dinner and bedtime. The PCP asks him if he has problems with his drinking, which seems to upset him, but he responds negatively. His PCP makes a comment to be watchful of his drinking but does not pursue this further. He attributes the abdominal pain to gastritis and prescribes a new medication.

Six months later, at the urging of his family, the patient undergoes a mental health evaluation. The family is concerned about his ability to live alone and wants him to move into an assisted-living situation. His evaluation reveals that he is quite functional with daily activities and has no signs of dementia, although he is somewhat slowed and rarely travels outside of the house. Upon questioning him about his alcohol use, it is determined that he routinely drinks one standard drink for dinner and two standard drinks of sherry before bed. This has been his pattern of drinking for 15 years since becoming a widower. In discussing the risks of this level of use and his current medications, the patient realizes the need to cut down on his alcohol use. After several months on drinking less than one drink per day, the upper abdominal discomfort subsides, he is sleeping better, and he feels more energetic (symptoms that he had previously attributed to old age).

PHYSICAL EXAM AND LAB TESTING

The bedside exam remains the clinician's most valuable tool for identifying substance use problems. However, screening instruments help increase the sensitivity and efficiency of diagnosing various disorders. Several screening instruments have been developed for identifying alcohol use disorders, including self-administered questionnaires and laboratory studies. Self-administered questionnaires provide the busy physician with a rapid, sensitive, and low-cost method of screening for alcohol problems. Two questionnaires—the SMAST-G (Short Michigan Alcohol Screening Test: Geriatric Version) and the CAGE[a]—have been developed with these principles in mind. Both of these instruments have high sensitivity and specificity for identifying alcohol use disorders in young and middle-age subjects. The SMAST-G (Table 1) has been found to be 95% sensitive and 78% specific for identifying older persons with alcohol problems.

Biologic markers of substance use can be useful in managing patients with known alcohol use disorders, but they have proven less valuable when detecting for illness. These markers include gamma-glutamyl transferase (GGT), which has a low sensitivity and a moderate specificity for diagnosing an alcohol use disorder; mean corpuscular volume, which has a low sensitivity, but a high specificity; high density lipoprotein (HDL), which shows a linear increase with alcohol use; and carbohydrate-deficient transferring (CDT), which has a low sensitivity and low specificity. Urine drug screens are an effective method for screening or identifying illicit drug use and prescription drug use.

---

[a] C—Have you ever tried to cut down on your drinking? A—Have you gotten annoyed at someone telling you about your drinking? G—Do you feel guilty about your drinking? E—Have you ever had an eye-opener?

Table 1   Short Michigan Alcohol Screening Test: Geriatric Version (SMAST-G)

In the past year	Yes	No
1. When talking with others, do you ever underestimate how much you actually drink?	(1)	(0)
2. After a few drinks, have you sometimes not eaten or been able to skip a meal because you didn't feel hungry?	(1)	(0)
3. Does having a few drinks help decrease your shakiness or tremors?	(1)	(0)
4. Does alcohol sometimes make it hard for you to remember parts of the day or night?	(1)	(0)
5. Do you usually take a drink to relax or calm your nerves?	(1)	(0)
6. Do you drink to take your mind off your problems?	(1)	(0)
7. Have you ever increased your drinking after experiencing a loss in your life?	(1)	(0)
8. Has a doctor or nurse ever said they were worried or concerned about your drinking?	(1)	(0)
9. Have you ever made rules to manage your drinking?	(1)	(0)
10. When you feel lonely, does having a drink help?[1]	(1)	(0)
Total SMAST-G score (0–10)		

A total score of 3 or more "yes" responses is indicative of an alcohol problem.
Source: The University of Michigan Alcohol Research Center, The Regents of the University of Michigan, 1991.

TREATMENT OPTIONS

Detoxification and Stabilization

Alcohol withdrawal symptoms commonly occur in patients who stop drinking or markedly cut down their drinking after regular heavy use. During hospitalizations, patients may be particularly vulnerable to alcohol or benzodiazepine withdrawal if the clinical team is unaware of the use of these substances. Alcohol withdrawal can range from mild and almost unnoticeable symptoms to severe and life-threatening ones. The classical set of symptoms associated with alcohol withdrawal includes autonomic hyperactivity (increased pulse rate, increased blood pressure, and increased temperature), restlessness, disturbed sleep, anxiety, nausea, and tremor. More severe withdrawal can be manifested by auditory, visual, or tactile hallucinations, delirium, seizures, and coma. Other substances of abuse, such as benzodiazepines and opioids, have distinct withdrawal symptoms that are also potentially life threatening. Elderly patients have been shown to have a longer duration of withdrawal symptoms, and withdrawal has the potential for complicating other medical and psychiatric illnesses. However, there is no evidence to suggest that older patients are more prone to alcohol withdrawal or need longer treatment for withdrawal symptoms. In almost all instances, patients with signs or symptoms of withdrawal should be referred for emergent care in either an emergency room or detoxification center.

Monitoring Medication Misuse

Physicians and pharmacists should monitor prescription and over-the-counter medication use carefully, avoiding dangerous combinations with a high potential for side effects and ineffective or unnecessary medications. A practical approach to monitoring psychoactive medication use would be to re-evaluate use every three to six months. Only patients with a documented response to the treatment should continue on maintenance treatment. Patients without a response or with a partial response should be re-evaluated to consider the appropriate diagnosis and further care. This consideration is also a point in which a consultation with a specialty geriatric mental health provider could be advantageous.

Brief Interventions

Low intensity, brief interventions or brief therapies have been suggested as cost-effective and practical techniques that can be used as an initial approach to nicotine use and at-risk and problem drinking in various clinical settings. Brief intervention studies have been conducted in a wide range of health care settings, ranging from hospitals and primary health care locations to mental health clinics. Strategies have ranged from relatively unstructured counseling and feedback to more formal structured therapy and have relied heavily on concepts and techniques from the behavioral self-control literature. To date, there have been two randomized brief alcohol intervention trials with older adults. These trials have demonstrated that older adults can be engaged in treatment and that brief interventions can lead to a substantial reduction in drinking. Brief interventions can be implemented within primary and specialty medical care practices and are useful for reducing substance use. However, they can also motivate patients to engage in more formal addiction treatment (Fig. 1).

Outpatient Management

Relatively little formal research has been conducted on the comparative efficacy of various approaches to addiction treatment in older adults. In contrast to popular beliefs, older adults are quite amenable to treatment, especially in programs that offer age appropriate care with providers who are knowledgeable about aging issues. Several naturalistic studies suggest that older adults who do engage in treatment have outcomes that are as good or substantially better than younger adults. The traditional addiction clinic is focused on supportive group psychotherapy and encourages regular attendance at self-help group meetings, such as Alcoholics Anonymous (AA), Alcoholics Victorious, Rational Recovery, or Narcotics Anonymous. For older adults, peer-specific group activities are considered superior to mixed-age group activities. Outpatient rehabilitation, in addition to focusing on active addiction issues, usually needs to address issues of time management. Abstinence reduces the time spent in maintaining the substance use disorder. The management of this time, which is often the greater part of a patient's day, is critical to the prognosis of treatment. Use of resources such as day programs and senior centers can be beneficial, especially in cognitively impaired patients. Social services, such as financial support, are often needed to stabilize the patient in early recovery. Supervised living arrangements, such as halfway houses, group homes, nursing homes, and residing with relatives, should also be considered.

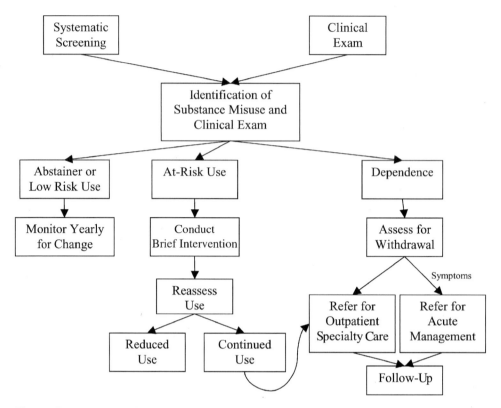

Figure 1 Treatment algorithm.

Quitting smoking is difficult at any age. It has been estimated that each year, 87% of older smokers are unsuccessful in their attempt to quit. Nicotine withdrawal symptoms, which are most severe in the first few days after cessation, often have been cited as a key factor leading to relapse. Further, many older smokers cite concerns about anticipated withdrawal symptoms as a significant barrier to cessation. Pharmacologic therapy can be beneficial for older smokers who repeatedly fail to stop smoking by other means. The majority of smokers, including older adults, prefer self-help methods for quitting. An evaluation of eight self-help trials by the National Cancer Institute (NCI) reported adult quit rates ranging from 8% to 22%.

Pharmacotherapy of Addiction

Pharmacologic treatments have not traditionally played a major role in the long-term treatment of older alcohol-dependent adults. Until recently, disulfiram was the only medication approved for the treatment of alcohol dependence, but it was seldom used in older patients because of concerns related to adverse effects. In 1995, the opioid antagonist naltrexone was approved by the Food and Drug Administration (FDA) for the treatment of alcohol dependence. The FDA approval of naltrexone was based on studies by Volpicelli et al. and O'Malley et al. demonstrating its efficacy in the treatment of middle-age patients with alcohol dependence. In both studies, naltrexone was found to be safe and effective in preventing relapse and reducing the craving for alcohol. Oslin and colleagues have extended this line of research by studying a group of older veterans aged 50–70. The results were similar to the other clinical trials, with half as many naltrexone-treated subjects relapsing to significant drinking compared to those treated with placebo. Recently, acamprosate was approved for use in the United States for the treatment of alcohol dependence. Although the exact action of acamprosate is still unknown, acamprosate is thought to reduce glutamate response. There have been no studies evaluating the efficacy or safety of acamprosate among elderly patients.

There are four forms of nicotine replacement therapy currently available: chewing gum, transdermal patches, nasal spray, and inhaler. Of these four, the transdermal patch delivers the most consistent amount of nicotine and is the easiest for older adults to use. Studies of the general population have consistently found that it is significantly more effective than placebo in providing relief from withdrawal symptoms. Orleans et al. found a 29% self-reported 6-month quit rate among low-income older adults. Although this study and clinical practice suggest that nicotine replacement is well tolerated, some authors caution that older smokers are more likely to suffer from illnesses or conditions that may prohibit its use. Coronary problems, circulatory disorders, and diabetes have been cited as possible contraindications.

Non-nicotine pharmacotherapy is available for older smokers who cannot safely use nicotine replacement therapy. Buproprion has been found to be well tolerated and to significantly reduce withdrawal symptoms. However, effectiveness for older adults has not been investigated.

SUMMARY

The misuse and abuse of substances has been problematic for humanity for centuries. Substance use disorders are associated with tremendous economic, social, psychological, and medical morbidity. Until recently, substance use disorders were an under-recognized part of aging. As the average life expectancy increases and a greater proportion of former substance users live to be over the age of 65, recognition and treatment of these problems and their consequences is increasing in importance. Fortunately, interventions are becoming available for older adults with substance use problems. These advancements can make an improved quality of life a reality for many older adults.

ACKNOWLEDGMENT

This work was supported, in part, by a grant from the National Institute of Mental Health (#) 1K08 MH01599-01 (#) P30 MH66270 and the Mental Illness Research, Education, and Clinical Center at the Philadelphia VAMC.

REFERENCES

1. Blow F. Substance abuse among older Americans. In: Center for Substance Abuse Treatment, ed. Treatment improvement protocol. Washington, D.C.: U.S. Government Printing Office, 1998.

2. Schonfeld L, et al. Cognitive-behavioral treatment of older veterans with substance abuse problems. J Geriatr Psychiatry Neurol 2000:124–129.
3. Lasslia HC, et al. Use of prescription medications in an elderly rural population: the MoVIES project. Ann Pharmacother 1996; 30:589–595.
4. Black BS, Rabins PV, McGuire MH. Alcohol use disorder is a risk factor for mortality among older public housing residents. Int Psychogeriatr 1998; 10:309–327.
5. Fleming MF, et al. Brief physician advice for alcohol problems in older adults: a randomized community-based trial. J Fam Pract 1999; 48(5):378–384.
6. Oslin DW, Pettinati H, Volpicelli JR. Alcoholism treatment adherence: older age predicts better adherence and drinking outcomes. Am J Geriatr Psychiatry 2002; 10(6):740–747.

57
Elder Abuse

Mark J. Yaffe

*Department of Family Medicine, St. Mary's Hospital Center, McGill University,
Montreal, Quebec, Canada*

INTRODUCTION

Elder abuse is an event that results in potentially devastating health and social consequences for older adults. These include poor quality of life, psychological distress, loss of property or sense of security, and overall increased morbidity and mortality (1). Yet it was not until the late 1970s that it began to receive formal attention, modeled after the literature on child abuse and domestic/marital violence (2). Detection may occur late or not at all due to lack of awareness of the problem or nonspecific and/or complex presentation. The causes of mistreatment are often multifactorial.

Primary care or consultant physicians seeing seniors for both intermittent and ongoing care are ideally positioned to recognize or suspect abuse and to initiate consultation from social service agencies. In situations involving elder abuse, doctors may be the only contact the older person has apart from the caregiver, who in fact may be the perpetrator of mistreatment. In addition, doctors may be the first professionals in contact with an abused older person following victimization, whether in the office setting or in the emergency room (3–5). Some authors have suggested routine screening for elder abuse as part of periodic health examinations, while the American Medical Association (AMA) has recommended screening of seniors if physical signs of possible abuse are present (6–8).

DEFINITION

Elder abuse represents single or multiple acts of commission or omission inflicted on an elderly person (defined as aged 60 or 65 and older, depending on the jurisdiction) by a person in a position of trust. The hurtful act is generally considered to be one that is intentional, willful, or nonaccidental (9). Nonetheless, in some cases the "intent to harm" may be difficult to demonstrate since the abuse may occur through ignorance. Elder abuse is considered to be distinct from domestic violence and from criminal violence (e.g., as an attack on a senior on the street by a stranger). The abuse is typically categorized as physical, psychological, emotional, verbal, financial, sexual, or neglectful (self-neglect is usually not considered part of an elder abuse definition).

Individual differences in judgment on the severity or implication of an act may ultimately influence the perception of that act as abusive (10). Also, the specific context or situation in which elder abuse occurs or is suspected and the background of the person observing a potential problem may determine whether it is flagged or not. Elder abuse may be identified by a number of professionals, including physicians, lawyers, notaries, social workers, law enforcement officers, nurses, psychologists, bank employees, and clergy, or it may be witnessed by members of the public. Each group brings unique perceptions and value judgments about elder abuse. Also, the specific wording that goes into definitions of elder abuse may vary according to political jurisdiction. In the United States, for example, each state has unique, but generally comparable, legal definitions for terms such as abuse, neglect, exploitation, and mistreatment, as well as for who might be an endangered, dependent, or vulnerable adult (9).

MANIFESTATIONS

Physical Abuse

Physical abuse is an injury or harm that causes pain, suffering, impairment, or disease (8). It may be characterized by hitting with hands or objects, burning, pushing, or slapping, as well as mechanical confinement or chemical restraint through unjustified medication (11).

Simple observation may reveal some of the following useful diagnostic information (12). Circumferential scars on wrists or legs can suggest use of physical or mechanical restraints. Finger- or knuckle-shaped bruises, especially on unusual accident sites such as the face, neck, chest wall, abdomen, and buttocks, may imply intentional trauma. Parallel lines on the soles and palms (sites not normally associated with accidental trauma) may be suggestive of a stick injury. Abrasions, lacerations, tears, or scars, especially on the forearms and legs of elderly (with decreased skin thickness and elasticity), force a distinction between abuse and benign trauma. Decubitus ulcers, bedsores, or pressure sores on the sacrum, hips, or heels may suggest a lack of care, and depth of such lesions may correlate with duration of neglect.

Seniors are naturally prone to fractures because of thinner, less dense bones resulting from one or more factors, which include poor nutrition, vitamin D deficiency, alcoholism, age-associated sex hormone changes, osteoporosis, steroids, Paget's disease of bone, prolonged bed rest, limb paralysis, and reduced weight bearing activity. Hip, wrist, and vertebral fractures are amongst the most common injury sites in the elderly. Fractures seen elsewhere, such as a long bone spiral fractures (suggestive of a traumatic rotational etiology), should raise the possibility of elder abuse.

Psychological, Emotional, and Verbal Abuse

Abuse that is psychological, emotional, or verbal involves the infliction of anguish, pain, or distress through verbal or nonverbal acts. This includes verbal aggression or threats, yelling, swearing, harassment, humiliation, intimidation, or abandonment (13). Since this often occurs out of public view, the presence of new psychiatric symptoms, depressed affect or speech content, social withdrawal, or agoraphobia may suggest underlying abuse (14).

Sexual Abuse

Manifestations of sexual abuse include inappropriate and indecent exposure, undesired touching that does not have a specific medical or caregiver treatment intent, and rape (10). Physical signs include bruising or edema of the vulva or similar findings on the palate from forced oral sex (12).

Neglect

The failure of mandated people to provide goods or services necessary to allow a dependent person to function or to avoid harm represents neglect (8). This includes the refusal or failure of a caregiver to provide necessary food, clothing, medicine, shelter, supervision, or medical care (13). Examples are poor or absent dental/oral care, failure to give range of movement exercises, people left in wet garments, poor wound care, irregular bathing (manifested by dirt in skin creases and insect bites from fleas, scabies, mosquitoes), inadequately staffed transfers, delays in toileting, poor hydration, not responding to calls, and confinement to rooms with too much or too little lighting (12,15). Unexplained weight loss (reflective of inadequate caloric intake, unrecognized decreased sense of smell or taste, medications that dry the oral cavity, or the presence of a swallowing dysfunction) may also portend abuse (8). Unexpected hypotension, confusion, or somnolence may be reflective of inadequate fluid intake. Medications not monitored for impact or side effects or given at prescribed times would also constitute neglect (12). Burns constitute physical abuse whether they are directly inflicted or they arise as a result of others' negligence (e.g., caregiver neglect) (12).

Financial Abuse

Compared to other forms of abuse, financial abuse is less easy to define, and rates of false positives for identification may be higher (16). It may be suspected when money is unavailable to pay for previously available treatment, care, housing, or medication and by deterioration in appearance or clothing (17). Abuse includes use of money or property without permission, forging signatures, misuse of credit cards or power of attorney, and the forceful signing of documents (e.g., deeds, wills, insurance policies) (18). Financial abuse often occurs in the hands of family members, as distinct from consumer fraud initiated by strangers who are not in positions of trust (19,20).

EPIDEMIOLOGY

Reliable incidence and prevalence data are absent for a number of reasons. First, gradients of severity of harm make labeling difficult. For example, should a single episode of poor care be categorized in the same fashion as chronic mistreatment? Or, since elderly bruising can be due to innocent bumping of a limb, the effects of anticoagulation, or abusive behavior, how can the etiology be clearly identified?

Second, some elder abuse studies have examined incidence, while others have looked at prevalence. Data collecting strategies and definitions of elder abuse have differed as a function of social settings: seniors in institutions (long-term or chronic care) versus community-based situations (home with or without help, assisted living complexes, nursing homes). Few population-based studies have been reported (21). Reliable reporting of abuse has further been hampered by the reluctance of some victims to report and the sometimes poor cognitive functioning of the elderly, which may skew thought content and recall. Perpetrators may themselves be sources of information and deliberately hide possible clues of abuse.

Published estimates of elder abuse report prevalence estimates ranging from 1% to 10%, with two of the most methodologically rigorous surveys reporting 3.2% and 4%, respectively (22–25). These statistics are almost certainly conservative since under-recognition may occur in as many as 80% of cases, and reporting may occur in only anywhere from 1 in 6 to 1 in 15 cases (3,26,27). Common perpetrators are spouses, children, other relatives, acquaintances, paid caregivers, and other persons in positions of trust. Neglect appears more frequently than emotional and psychological abuse, which in turn are more common than financial abuse (16,28). Women are victimized more often than men; for example, older white females are the most frequent victims of financial abuse (29). Such observations may be skewed, however, because of the gender disparity in the elderly population (30). Similar kinds of statistical bias may be seen in the finding that elder abuse in North America is reported more often in the home setting; indeed, 80% of all such seniors are living at home (31–33).

RISK FACTORS

Risk factors associated with elder abuse should help raise the index of suspicion and focus attention on potential victims. However, differences in working definitions of abuse, sampling techniques, data collection strategies, age groups studied, and low utilization of control groups as well as few prospective studies have collectively limited the usefulness of research in this area (34). For example, while some studies have linked female sex, frailty, cognitive impairment, and increased age to an increased incidence or prevalence of elder abuse, other reports have failed to do so or have demonstrated an opposite association (35).

The "geriatric syndrome" is the recognition that a single underlying pathophysiological process (e.g., falls, incontinence, or functional decline) has multiple possible interacting etiologies and that components of such syndromes may hide or copy possible markers of elder abuse (11). This "geriatric syndrome" concept further limits the attempt to establish clear risk factors for abuse. Such complex interfaces might be seen in the example of elder abuse associated with those who are sufficiently ill as to be dependent. Dementia (seen in 5% to 10% of those 65 and older, or in 30% to 39% of those 85 and over) would be such a condition (36,37). Yet within a cohort study of those 75 and over, 70% rated their health as good to excellent (38). However, such a generally independent group could still fall prey to victimization, neglect, and financial abuse.

Despite the limitations of clearly identifying risk factors, support exists for clinician/physician use of them in clinical assessments. Table 1 summarizes the strength of association of suspected risk factors with elder abuse (35).

MORTALITY CONSEQUENCES OF ELDER ABUSE

Beyond extensive physical and psychological morbidity, there is also a direct relationship between elder abuse and mortality that goes beyond that which might be directly attributable to specific acts of abuse. A 13-year prospective cohort study of

Table 1 Association of Possible Risk Factors and Elder Abuse

Weak association	Moderate association	Strong association
Social isolation (CR)	Females (CR)	Poor physical health/frailty (CR)
Dementia (CR)	Blacks (CR)	Childhood violence (CG)
Mental illness (CG)	Passive/dependent (CR)	Stress (CG)
Hostility (CG)	CG dependent on CR	CR dependency on CG
Drugs/alcoholism (CG)	CG related to CR	Institutional care (CG)

CR and CG live together
Abbreviations: CR, care receiver; CG, caregiver.

2812 community-dwelling older adults showed statistically significant differences for survival between nonabused (40%) versus abused (9%) elderly, but when potential confounding factors (demographic characteristics, chronic diseases, functional status, cognitive status, social networks, and depression) were adjusted for, deaths were found not to be directly attributable to injuries caused by the abuse (1). Rather it was postulated that the outcomes could be the effects of severe stress experienced by the abuse victims over time, or that elder abuse could be an extreme form of negative social support (an entity linked causally in other contexts to morbidity and mortality).

PHYSICIAN DETECTION

The morbidity and mortality findings suggest an important role for physicians in the identification and referral of possible victims of elder abuse to social service agencies. Doctor involvement, however, appears to be unfortunately low. In the United States, 18% of reports to adult protective services for suspected elder abuse came from all health care professionals, with only 2% coming from physicians (1,5). Social workers, followed by nurses, were the key professionals in detecting elder abuse (20), with physicians ranking no higher than 10th amongst health care professionals reporting elder abuse (35).

Low detection/reporting rates by doctors have been attributed to: (i) lack of awareness of the problem and knowledge about how to identify it (35,39); (ii) absence of a clear working definition (3); (iii) lack of protocols for detecting and intervening (39,40); (iv) ethical issues (e.g., confidentiality) (41); (v) complexity of the geriatric syndrome and physicians attitudes that tend to dismiss worrisome abnormalities as part of normal aging (11,42); and (vi) victim reluctance to report abuse (due to denial, shame, fear of retaliation or placement) (39,40). For financial abuse the latter may be especially true (43,44). Health professionals may be more likely to report physical than financial abuse due to concerns that the latter is beyond their scope or competence or because of fear of offending or insulting suspected victims (5,11,17,32).

Office visit time constraints represent another serious concern since an optimal assessment might include many of the following (3,4): (i) direct visual observations (appears poorly cared for, or fearful of caregiver); (ii) detailed medical history (injuries, emergency room visits, "doctor-hopping,"); (iii) social history (family dysfunction or violence); (iv) comprehensive, head-to-toe medical examination; (v) laboratory tests; (vi) cognitive evaluation; (vii) separate interviews for patient and caregiver; and (viii) home visit (4,32,45).

ELDER ABUSE SCREENING

Such comprehensive elder abuse assessments are beyond the practical scope of most physicians. However, screening for abuse may be more realistic, and an array of classification inventories and screening instruments exist [SHCIEA, O APSIR, PIAEAN (protocol for the identification and assessment of elder abuse and neglect), SPIANE (screening for identification of abuse and neglect of the elderly), EADI (elder abuse detection indicators), HALF (health attitudes towards aging, living arrangements, and finances), and BASE (brief abuse screen for the elderly)] (46–52). A critique of these tools shows that they have limited use since they differ in focus, definition of abuse, format, structure, and type of data generated, plus for the most part psychometric properties have not been reported (53). When some of the latter properties are identified, construct and content validity are only moderate or have not been addressed. Reliability has been tested only for the BASE (52), and sensitivity and specificity of the measures to detect abuse are lacking overall, resulting in lack of confidence for either detecting or ruling out abuse.

Existing validated instruments [BASE, HSEAST (Hwalek Sengstock elder abuse screening test), CASE (caregiver abuse screen), and IOA (indicators of abuse)] are of limited use for the majority of doctors because of excessive length or questions that do not fit an office encounter with a doctor, require a home visit, or are based on interviews with the caregiver (a possible source of abuse) and not the care receiver (52,54–56).

While elder abuse and domestic violence are generally perceived as discrete and different entities, the literature on screening for the latter may have parallels for the former. The AMA has recommended routine screening for abuse of all female patients in primary care settings (57), while other groups favor screening only in suspicious cases (58). A British systematic review of programs screening women for domestic violence found little justification for them, while the Canadian Task Force on Preventive Health Care observed that "while there is insufficient evidence to recommend for or against universal screening for violence clinicians need to be alert to signs and symptoms of potential abuse" (59,60).

Physician-researchers are calling for brief, practical screening tools for doctor use that may overcome existing problems (3,27). Models exist in the four-question CAGE [C = desire to cut down the number of drinks; A = anger at someone who tells you to stop or cut down the drinking; G = guilt over drinking; E=desire for a morning "eye opener" drink (if two are positive, one has a drinking problem)] screen for alcoholism, the five-question Family APGAR (a measure of the health of family functioning) tool for family dysfunction, and two-question inquires for depression (61–64). In this vein, Canadian researchers have developed and are attempting to validate a five-question Elder Abuse Suspicion Index (EASI) for physician office use (65). The "value-added" of using such screening tools is that while they may initially generate negative findings, their use connotes to patients that the doctor is familiar with the topic and is prepared to discuss it should the patient try to initiate it at a later date.

OUTCOMES FROM DETECTION

Most physicians lack expertise to confirm suspected elder abuse or the wherewithal for follow-up and intervention. Some countries have mandatory reporting laws for elder abuse to facilitate the process. In the United States this is regulated by state law, with some states having voluntary reporting, while others have mandatory signaling (which may be a requirement for all or only specified occupations). In some states, a privileged professional confidential relationship may eliminate the obligation to report (33,66). Depending on the jurisdiction, referrals are usually made to adult protective services (APS), family services, or social services; the minimum age for which they are reportable also varies (age 60 or 65). Variability in the level of training to respond, the speed of response, and the nature of protocols used is also noted between and within communities.

It would appear that few systems of mandatory reporting, prevention techniques, or intervention strategies have been submitted for formal evaluation (59,60,67). While controlled trials are absent, in one Canadian descriptive study, 80% of 473 intervention strategies (relating to 83 cases of confirmed elder abuse) were reported successful or partially successful, while in another study of 208 cases there was success in stopping (31%) or diminishing (29%) the abuse in 60% of the cases (68,69).

SUMMARY

Elder abuse carries significant morbidity and mortality. It may be suspected or identified by an informed physician through one or more patient encounters. Some reports have raised questions about the value of screening; however, such pronouncements may be premature in that the measures to detect elder abuse, document its incidence and prevalence, and evaluate effectiveness of interventions are in their relative infancy. Physicians therefore are encouraged to be attentive to this important medical and social problem in their patients.

ACKNOWLEDGMENTS

Appreciation is gratefully expressed to Christina Wolfson, Maxine Lithwick, Sylvia Straka, and Elizabeth Podnieks. As members of the Elder Abuse Suspicion Index (EASI) research team, they have contributed important ideas on elder abuse from their respective disciplines of epidemiology, social work, and nursing. The research of this group is funded by a grant from the Institute of Aging of the Canadian Institutes of Health Research.

REFERENCES

1. Lachs MS, Williams C, O'Brien S, Pillemer K, Charlson M. The mortality of elder mistreatment. J Am Med Assoc 1998; 280(5):428–432.
2. Committee on National Statistics and Law, Division of Behavioral and Social Sciences and Education. In: Bonnie RJ, Wallace RB, eds. Elder Mistreatment: Abuse, Neglect, and Exploitation in an Aging America. National Research Council Panel to Review Risk and Prevalence of Elder Abuse and Neglect. Washington, D.C.: National Academies Press, 2003:14–17.
3. Allison EJ, Ellis PC, Wilson SE. Elder abuse and neglect: the emergency medicine perspective. Eur J Emerg Med 1998; 5(3):355–363.
4. Aravanis SC, Adelman RD, Breckman R, et al. Diagnostic and treatment guidelines on elder abuse and neglect. Arch Fam Med 1993; 2(4):371–388.

5. Rosenblatt DE, Cho KH, Durance PW. Reporting mistreatment of older adults: the role of physicians. J Am Geriatr Soc 1996; 44:65–70.

6. Fulmer T, Birkenhauer D. Elder mistreatment assessment as part of everyday practice. J Gerontol Nurs 1992; 18:42–45.

7. Mouton CP, Espino DV. Health screening in older women. Am Fam Phys 1999; 59: 1835–1842.

8. American Medical Association. Diagnostic and treatment guidelines on elder abuse and neglect. 1996; AA25:96–937:4M: 12/96.

9. Hamp LF. Analysis of elder abuse and neglect definitions under state law. In: Bonnie RJ, Wallace RB, eds. Elder Mistreatment: Abuse, Neglect, and Exploitation in an Aging America. National Research Council Panel to Review Risk and Prevalence of Elder Abuse and Neglect. Committee on National Statistics and Law, Division of Behavioral and Social Sciences and Education. Washington, D.C.: National Academies Press, 2003:181–237.

10. Committee on National Statistics and Law, Division of Behavioral and Social Sciences and Education. In: Bonnie RJ, Wallace RB, eds. Elder Mistreatment: Abuse, Neglect, and Exploitation in an Aging America. National Research Council Panel to Review Risk and Prevalence of Elder Abuse and Neglect. Washington, D.C.: National Academies Press, 2003:35–38.

11. Lachs MS, Pillemer K. Abuse and neglect of elderly persons. N Engl J Med 1995; 333:437.

12. Dyer CB, Connelly M-T, McFeeley P. The clinical and medical forensics of elder abuse and neglect. In: Bonnie RJ, Wallace RB, eds. Elder Mistreatment: Abuse, Neglect, and Exploitation in an Aging America. National Research Council Panel to Review Risk and Prevalence of Elder Abuse and Neglect. Committee on National Statistics and Law, Division of Behavioral and Social Sciences and Education. Washington, D.C.: National Academies Press, 2003:339–381.

13. Clarke ME, Pierson W. Management of elder abuse in the emergency department. Emerg Med Clin North Am 1999; 17:631–644.

14. Committee on National Statistics and Law, Division of Behavioral and Social Sciences and Education. In: Bonnie RJ, Wallace RB, eds. Elder Mistreatment: Abuse, Neglect, and Exploitation in an Aging America. National Research Council Panel to Review Risk and Prevalence of Elder Abuse and Neglect. Washington, D.C.: National Academies Press, 2003:54.

15. Hawes C, Blevins D, Shanley L. Preventing abuse and neglect in nursing homes: the role of the nurse aide registries. Report to the Centers for Medicare and Medicaid Services (formerly HCFA) from the School of Rural Public Health, Texas A&M University System Health Science Center School of Rural Public Health, 2001.

16. National Center on Elder Abuse. The National Elder Abuse Incidence Study: Final Report. Washington, D.C.: National Aging Information Center, 1998.

17. Tueth MJ. Exposing financial exploitation of impaired elderly persons. Am J Geriatr Psychiatry 2000; 8:104–111.

18. Hafemeister TL. Financial abuse of the elderly in domestic settings. In: Bonnie RJ, Wallace RB, eds. Elder Mistreatment: Abuse, Neglect, and Exploitation in an Aging America. National Research Council Panel to Review Risk and Prevalence of Elder Abuse and Neglect. Committee on National Statistics and Law, Division of Behavioral and Social Sciences and Education. Washington, D.C.: National Academies Press, 2003:388–389.

19. National Center on Elder Abuse. Elder abuse: Questions and Answers. Washington, D.C.: National Center on Elder Abuse, 1996.

20. Hafemeister TL. Financial abuse of the elderly in domestic settings. In: Bonnie RJ, Wallace RB, eds. Elder Mistreatment: Abuse, Neglect, and Exploitation in an Aging America. National Research Council Panel to Review Risk and Prevalence of Elder Abuse and Neglect. Committee on National Statistics and Law, Division of Behavioral

and Social Sciences and Education. Washington, D.C.: National Academies Press, 2003:385.

21. Branch LG. The epidemiology of elder abuse and neglect. Panel on elder abuse and neglect, Committee on National Statistics. Durham, NC: Duke University School of Medicine, October 1, 2001.

22. Kozak JF, Elmslie T, Verdon J. Epidemiological perspectives on the abuse and neglect of seniors: a review of the national and international research literature. In: MacLean MJ, ed. Abuse and Neglect of Older Canadians: Strategies for Change. Toronto: Thompson Educational Publishing, 1995:129–142.

23. Patterson C, Podnieks E, Gass DA. Helping your patient deal with elder abuse. Canad J Geriatr 1992; 8(7):37–42.

24. Pillemer K, Finkelhor D. The prevalence of elder abuse: a random survey. The Gerontol 1988; 28(1):51–57.

25. Podnieks E, Pillemer KA, Nicholson JP, Shillington T, Frizzel A. National survey on abuse of the elderly in Canada. Toronto: Ryerson Polytechnical Institute, 1990.

26. Jones JS. Elder abuse and neglect: responding to a national problem. Ann Emerg Med 1994; 23(4):845–848.

27. Bird PE, Harrington DT, Barillo DJ, McSweeney A, Shirani KZ, Goodwin CW. Elder abuse: a call to action. J Burn Care Rehabil 1998; 19(6):522–527.

28. National Center for Elder Abuse. Summaries of the statistical data on elder abuse in domestic settings: an exploratory study of state statistics for FY 93 and FY 94, 2000. (Available at http://www.aoa.gov/abuse/report/Cexecsum.html.)

29. National Clearinghouse on Family Violence. Health Canada (NCFV). Financial abuse of older adults, 2001. (Available at http://www.hc-sc.gc/hppb/family violence/html/financialaben.html.).

30. Committee on National Statistics and Law, Division of Behavioral and Social Sciences and Education. In: Bonnie RJ, Wallace RB, eds. Elder Mistreatment: Abuse, Neglect, and Exploitation in an Aging America. National Research Council Panel to Review Risk and Prevalence of Elder Abuse and Neglect. Washington D.C.: National Academies Press, 2003:60.

31. Kosberg JI, Nahmiash D. Characteristics of victims and perpetrators and milieus of abuse and neglect. In: Baumhover LA, Beall SC, eds. Abuse, Neglect and Exploitation of Older Persons: Strategies for Assessment and Intervention. Baltimore: Health Professions Press, 1996.

32. Marshall CE, Benton D, Brazier JM. Elder abuse: using clinical tools to identify clues of mistreatment. Geriatrics 2000; 55:42–53.

33. Moskowitz S. Saving granny from the wolf: elder abuse and neglect—the legal framework. Connecticut Law Rev 1998; 31:77–201.

34. Committee on National Statistics and Law, Division of Behavioral and Social Sciences and Education. In: Bonnie RJ, Wallace RB, eds. Elder Mistreatment: Abuse, Neglect, and Exploitation in an Aging America. National Research Council Panel to Review Risk and Prevalence of Elder Abuse and Neglect. Washington D.C.: National Academies Press, 2003:88–103.

35. Lachs MS, Fulmer T. Recognizing elder abuse and neglect. Clin Geriatr Med 1993; 9(3):665–681.

36. Rice DP, Fillit HM, Max W, Kropman DS, Lloyd JR, Duttagupta S. Prevalence, costs, and treatment of Alzheimer's disease and related dementias: a managed care perspective. Am J Managed Care 2001; 7:809–818.

37. Henderson S. Epidemiology of dementia. Ann Med Interne (Paris) 1998; 149:181–186.

38. Eberhardt MS, Ingram DD, Makuc DM, et al. Urban and rural health chartbook. Hyattsville, Md.: National Center for Health Statistics.

39. Fulmer T, McMahon DJ, Baer-Hines M, Forget B. Abuse, neglect, abandonment, violence, and exploitation: an analysis of all elderly patients seen in one emergency department during a six-month period. J Emerg Nurs 1992; 18(6):505–510.

40. Clarke ME, Pierson W. Management of elder abuse in the emergency department. Emergency Medical Clinics of North America 1999; 17(3):631–644.

41. Blakely B, Dolon R, May D. Improving the responses of physicians to elder abuse and neglect: contributions of a model program. J Gerontol Soc Work 1993; 19(3/4):35–47.

42. Lachs MS. Preaching to the unconverted: educating physicians about elder abuse. J Elder Abuse Neglect 1995; 7(4):1–12.

43. Podnieks E. National survey on abuse of the elderly in Canada. J Elder Abuse Neglect 1992; 4:5–58.

44. Dessin CL. Financial abuse of the elderly. Idaho Law Rev 2000; 36:203–226.

45. Paris BE, Meier DE, Goldstein T, Weiss M, Fein ED. Elder abuse and neglect: how to recognize warning signs and intervene. Geriatrics 1995; 50(4):47–51.

46. Sengstock MC, Hwalek M. A review and analysis of measures for the identification of elder abuse. J Gerontol Soc Work 1987; 10(3/4):21–37.

47. Pennsylvania Department of Aging. Older adult protective services investigation report. Pittsburgh, PA.: Pennsylvania Department of Aging, 1988.

48. Tomita S. Detection and treatment of elder abuse and neglect: a protocol for health care professionals. Phys Occup Ther Geriatr 1982; 2:37–51.

49. Higginson G. Political considerations for changing medical screening programs. J Am Med Assoc 1999; 282(15):1472–1474.

50. Bloom J, Ansell P, Bloom M. Detecting elder abuse: a guide for physicians. Geriatrics 1989; 44(6):40–44.

51. Ferguson D, Beck C. H.A.L.F.—a tool to assess elder abuse within the family. Geriatr Nurs 1983:301–304.

52. Reis M, Nahmiash D, Shrier R. A brief abuse screen for the elderly (BASE): its validity and use. Paper presented at the 22nd Annual Scientific and Educational Meeting of the Canadian Association on Gerontology, Montreal, Canada, October 1993.

53. Kosma A, Stones MJ. Issues in the measurement of elder abuse. In: MacLean MJ, ed. Abuse and Neglect of Older Canadians: Strategies for Change. Toronto: Thompson Educational Publishing, 1995:117–128.

54. Hwalek MA, Sengstock MC. Assessing the probability of abuse of the elderly: towards the development of a clinical screening instrument. J Appl Gerontol 1986; 5:153–173.

55. Reis M, Nahmiash D. Validation of the caregiver abuse screen (CASE). Canad J Aging 1995; 14(suppl 2):45–60.

56. Reis M, Nahmiash D. Validation of the indicators of abuse (IOA) screen. Gerontologist 1998; 38(4):471–480.

57. American Medical Association, Council on Scientific Affairs. Violence against women: relevance for medical practitioners. JAMA 1992; 267:3184–3189.

58. Ferris LE, Nurani A, Silver L, for the Family Violence Prevention Unit HC. A handbook dealing with woman abuse and the Canadian criminal justice system: guidelines for physicians. Ottawa: Minister of Public Works and Government Services Canada, 1999; Cat. H72–21/164–1998E.

59. Ramsay J, Richardson J, Carter YH, Davidson LL, Feder G. Should health professionals screen for domestic violence? Systematic review. BMJ 2002; 325:314–324.

60. Wathen CN, MacMillan HL. Canadian Task Force on preventive health care. Recommendation statement on violence against women. Can Med Assoc J 2003; 169:582–584.

61. Savitsky J. Early diagnosis and screening. In: Barnes H, Aronson MD, Delbanco T, eds. Alcoholism: A Guide for the Primary Care Physician. New York: Springer-Verlag, 1987: 47–58.

62. Smilkstein G, Ashworth C, Montano D. Validity and reliability of the Family APGAR as a test for family function. J Fam Pract 1982; 15:303–311.

63. Arroll B, Khin N, Kerse N. Screening for depression in primary care with two verbally asked questions: cross sectional study. BMJ 2003; 327:1144–1146.

64. Kroenke K, Spitzer RL, Williams JBW. The Patient Health Questionnaire—2: validity of a two-item depression screener. Med Care 2003; 41:1284–1292.

65. Yaffe MJ, Lithwick M, Wolfson C, Straka S, Jasserand F. Physician screening for elder abuse. Unpublished plenary presentation at Fifth Annual Meeting of the Minds Conference: elder abuse and domestic violence. Clearwater, FL.: University of South Florida Harrell Centre for Domestic Violence, July 15–18, 2001.

66. Roby JL, Sullivan R. Adult protection services laws: a comparison of state statutes from definition to case closure. J Elder Abuse Neglect 2000; 12:17–51.

67. Committee on National Statistics and Law, Division of Behavioral and Social Sciences and Education. In: Bonnie RJ, Wallace RB, eds. Elder Mistreatment: Abuse, Neglect, and Exploitation in an Aging America. National Research Council Panel to Review Risk and Prevalence of Elder Abuse and Neglect. Washington D.C.: National Academies Press, 2003:121.

68. Nahmiash D, Reis M. Most successful intervention strategies for abused older adults. J Elder Abuse Neglect 2000; 12(3/4):53–70.

69. Lithwick M, Beaulieu M, Gravel S, Straka SM. The mistreatment of older adults: perpetrator–victim relationships and interventions. J Elder Abuse Neglect 1999; 11(4): 95–112.

58
Anxiety and Depression in Older Patients

Jeffrey P. Staab
*Departments of Psychiatry and Otorhinolaryngology—Head and Neck Surgery,
The Balance Center, University of Pennsylvania Health System,
Philadelphia, Pennsylvania, U.S.A.*

INTRODUCTION

The last two decades have witnessed increasing attention to the psychological aspects of otorhinolaryngologic diseases. Anxiety and depression have been recognized as frequent concomitants of conditions affecting the ears, nose, and throat, exacerbating morbidity, driving up medical costs, and reducing quality of life for patients. Diagnostic techniques have improved, moving the field beyond the dichotomous thinking that previously divided patients between otorhinolaryngologic and "psychogenic" conditions. An increasingly sophisticated medical-psychiatric approach to differential diagnosis is emerging, which recognizes that psychiatric disorders may be a primary cause of ear, nose, and throat symptoms, but focuses greater attention on the more common situation in which otorhinolaryngologic and psychiatric illnesses coexist.

Very few studies have investigated psychiatric disorders in geriatric patients with otorhinolaryngologic conditions. As a result, older individuals with diseases of the ears, nose, and throat may not benefit from recent advances in geriatric psychiatry. Refinements in psychiatric diagnosis have made it possible to recognize previously overlooked anxiety and depressive disorders in the elderly. Advances in treatment have brought safer and more effective psychiatric interventions to the geriatric population. This chapter will attempt to close the gap between otorhinolaryngology and psychiatry for older patients. It will review the presentation, differential diagnosis, and treatment of anxiety and depression in individuals with otologic, rhinologic, and laryngologic conditions and head and neck cancer. Whenever possible, it will focus on studies that included patients older than age 65. Where data on the elderly are scarce, information will be extrapolated from investigations of younger cohorts in otorhinolaryngology and psychiatry, recognizing the limitations of this approach.

OVERVIEW OF ANXIETY AND DEPRESSION IN THE ELDERLY

Anxiety and depression are common in patients older than age 65, but two important differences exist between older and younger patients with these disorders. First, older patients with anxiety and depression are much more likely to have coexisting medical problems. Medical morbidity, not advancing age, determines the prevalence of anxiety and depression in the elderly. Interestingly, the rate of depression is lower in healthy, community dwelling elders (5%) than in younger adults (8%), but as medical morbidity increases, so does the prevalence of depression. Clinically significant depressive symptoms occur in about 9% of older primary care outpatients and 25% of nursing home residents (1). The otorhinolaryngologist caring for older patients is most likely to encounter anxiety and depression in conjunction with medical or surgical problems. Primary psychiatric causes of ear, nose, and throat symptoms are relatively uncommon in the elderly.

The second difference between older and younger adults is the manner in which they manifest anxiety and depression. Older adults are less likely to report the psychological symptoms of anxiety or depression. More commonly, they will present with somatic symptoms or functional impairment. These somatic presentations confound diagnostic evaluations by mimicking or exacerbating symptoms of coexisting medical conditions. Patients with anxiety and depression also have a poorer response to medical and surgical interventions than their nonanxious, nondepressed counterparts with similar medical problems (1). This may prompt the otorhinolaryngologist to pursue more aggressive medical or surgical therapies than are needed for patients' physical illnesses, increasing the risk of adverse medical outcomes and worsening patients' quality of life. For example, a woman with generalized anxiety may report chronic, nonspecific dizziness that severely limits the woman's physical activities, despite successful treatment for benign paroxysmal positional vertigo. A man with depression and head and neck cancer may complain of throat pain and loss of appetite, even though the man's cancer treatment is progressing well. The desire to help such patients is great, but interventions must be targeted effectively at the cause of the ongoing morbidity. Fortunately, simple techniques have been developed to detect anxiety and depression in nonpsychiatric settings (1). These methods can be employed in otorhinolaryngologic practice to identify patients who may benefit from psychiatric treatment in addition to their otorhinolaryngologic interventions.

MANIFESTATIONS OF ANXIETY AND DEPRESSION IN OTORHINOLARYNGOLOGIC PRACTICE

Anxiety Disorders

Anxiety disorders are related to physical symptoms of the ears, nose, or throat in three ways. Anxiety may be the primary cause of such symptoms, develop secondary to otorhinolaryngologic disease, or coexist with otorhinolaryngologic illnesses (2). Panic disorder is far and away the most common psychiatric cause of symptoms suggesting otorhinolaryngologic illness. Panic attacks commonly cause dizziness, lightheadedness, or choking sensations. However, de novo panic disorder is unusual in the elderly. Therefore, the otorhinolaryngologist caring for older patients will encounter pathological anxiety almost exclusively as a secondary complication of ear, nose, and throat diseases or as a comorbid condition that predated the onset of otorhinolaryngologic illness.

Three types of pathological anxiety are important in otorhinolaryngologic practice: (i) conditioned hypersensitivity, (ii) phobic behaviors, and (iii) generalized anxiety (2). Patients with illnesses of the ears, nose, or throat may become highly sensitized to internal physical symptoms (e.g., pharyngeal sensations in patients with dysphagia) and to relevant external stimuli (e.g., visual motion cues in patients with imbalance). Hypersensitivity is thought to arise from classical conditioning, in which new or unexplained physical sensations are linked (i.e., conditioned) to instinctive anxiety responses. Dizziness, tinnitus, and dysphagia are potent triggers of this phenomenon. Patients may experience physical symptoms that mimic otorhinolaryngologic illnesses for months or even years. In younger adults, the inciting events are often transient, leaving patients with persistent hypersensitivity symptoms after the triggering illnesses have resolved (e.g., maxillary fullness that lingers after adequate control of sinusitis). In older individuals, the precipitating events are more likely to be chronic physical diseases, creating situations in which conditioned hypersensitivity exacerbates the functional disability of the underlying medical problems (e.g., excessive caution when walking after a stroke). Patients with conditioned hypersensitivity may not appear overtly anxious, and queries about anxiety often elicit negative responses. Instead, hypersensitivity should be suspected in patients who are excessively vigilant about their physical symptoms or have persistent symptoms despite adequate medical or surgical interventions.

Phobic behaviors include avoidance of situations that patients associate with their physical symptoms (phobic avoidance) and trepidation when facing these circumstances (anticipatory anxiety). Examples include patients with mild dysphagia who avoid solid foods because of a fear of choking and dizzy patients who become anxious in advance of highway driving. Phobic behaviors may be confined to specific situations or generalize to many areas of patients' lives. Phobic behaviors may dominate the clinical picture, causing more disability than the comorbid physical illnesses. Phobic symptoms are easily overlooked in the elderly. Patients, families, and physicians frequently accept frailty and poor physical functioning in the face of medical diseases. Prudent adaptations to physical limitations are not phobic behaviors, but excessive changes may be symptoms of phobic avoidance (e.g., a patient with mild peripheral neuropathy who refuses to walk unaided). Phobic behaviors may be accompanied by panic attacks, but this is almost always a secondary development in the elderly. Therefore, older patients with new onset panic attacks should be evaluated for medical precipitants. Central and peripheral vestibular deficits are the most common otorhinolaryngologic triggers of panic attacks.

Generalized anxiety is a condition in which patients worry excessively about many different topics. Its prevalence in community dwelling elderly is about 2%. Patients with generalized anxiety are lifelong worrywarts. In otorhinolaryngologic settings, they seek excessive reassurance about their diagnoses, treatment, and prognosis. They are pessimists who focus on catastrophic possibilities, frequently asking "What if ... " questions. In the elderly, generalized anxiety often coexists with major depression (1).

Depression

Unlike anxiety disorders, depression does not cause symptoms that mimic otorhinolaryngologic diseases, but it may complicate their clinical course (2). Patients with major depression report higher levels of physical symptoms than nondepressed individuals with similar medical problems, and they are less likely to comply with treatment recommendations. Depression also has far ranging physiological effects, such as alterations in hypothalamic–pituitary–adrenal axis function, autonomic activity, platelet adherence, glucose metabolism, and cytokine activation. Research in coronary artery disease, diabetes, cancer, and HIV infection suggest that depression-related physiological changes may adversely affect the biological course of those medical conditions (3). It is not known if depression has similar effects on otorhinolaryngologic diseases.

Risk factors for depression are similar in older and younger adults, including female gender, low socioeconomic status, social isolation, and a previous history of depression. Older individuals bear additional burdens, such as caregiving of debilitated loved ones, loss of companions, and their own failing health. Sleep, appetite, stamina, and cognitive capabilities decline with age. As a result, many people expect depression to be a normal part of aging. Older individuals experience periods of dysphoria as do younger adults, but it is not normal to be impaired by depressive symptoms at any age (1).

Elderly individuals suffering from depression may appear sad and admit that their mood is low. However, they are more likely to experience anhedonia, a loss of pleasure in activities, that causes them to forego their usual pastimes. Changes in sleep and appetite are cardinal features of depression in both young and old, but their assessment is often confounded by medical problems in the elderly. Otorhinolaryngologic conditions, such as obstructive sleep apnea and dysphagia, may cause profound alterations in sleep and appetite, whether patients are depressed or not. Older patients may contemplate death, but rarely consider suicide in the absence of depression. Therefore, anhedonia, social withdrawal, sleep or appetite changes that have no medical cause, functional impairment out of proportion to medical illness, poor treatment adherence, and suicidal thoughts all suggest the presence of clinically significant depression in the elderly.

ASSOCIATION OF ANXIETY AND DEPRESSION WITH OTORHINOLARYNGOLOGIC ILLNESSES

Otology and Neurotology

Hearing Loss

The relationships among hearing loss, anxiety, and depression are complex. One small study found that 45 prelingually deaf patients who used sign language reported a high quality of life, but the study suggested that they may be prone to depression (4). Fifteen patients reported depressive symptoms on the Geriatric Depression Scale, a rate that was significantly higher than a normal hearing cohort. Among patients who acquired hearing loss late in life, one large study ($N = 1332$) found a strong correlation ($r = 0.85$) between hearing loss and depression (5). Another ($N = 624$) found that hearing loss and other physical impairments contributed to disability, whereas depression had an independent effect on handicap (6). One small investigation ($N = 40$) found no link between hearing loss and depression among well-to-do elders (7). Interestingly, three investigations (e.g., Ref. 5) demonstrated significant reductions in depression among older patients with hearing loss after they were fitted with hearing aids.

Tinnitus

Research on the psychiatric correlates of tinnitus is inconsistent, and available studies have not focused on geriatric patients. An investigation of 100 adults with tinnitus found normal psychological profiles on the Minnesota Multiphasic Personality

Inventory, whereas another study of 82 patients using a standardized clinical examination found that 62% had a depressive illness and 45% an anxiety disorder (8,9).

Dizziness and Imbalance

Older individuals frequently present to primary care clinicians and otorhinolaryngologists with complaints of dizziness and imbalance. Four diagnostic subtypes of dizziness in the elderly have been proposed (vertigo, disequilibrium, pre-syncopal lightheadedness, and other dizziness) based on research into the cardinal features of patients' histories (10). The other dizziness subtype includes patients who are frequently diagnosed with "psychogenic dizziness," a nonspecific term suggesting that patients' symptoms are caused by psychiatric disorders. However, a careful analysis of the longitudinal patterns of illness in 132 adults with medically unexplained dizziness found that two-thirds of patients had medical problems that triggered both dizziness and conditioned hypersensitivity to motion cues. Hypersensitivity sustained their symptoms, with or without phobic behaviors and generalized anxiety (2). Figure 1 is an extension of that study, showing the distribution of psychiatric diagnoses by age in patients whose dizziness could not be explained fully by active neurotologic illnesses. Among patients with panic disorder and phobias, 50% had primary anxiety disorders (e.g., dizziness caused solely by anxiety), whereas the other 50% had secondary anxiety disorders complicating neurotologic conditions. Patients with generalized anxiety and depression always had coexisting medical problems. These results indicate that it is unusual for elderly patients to have primary psychiatric causes of dizziness.

On the other hand, it is quite common for anxiety and depression to complicate neurotologic illnesses in the elderly. For example, 28 patients older than age 60 with benign paroxysmal positional vertigo rated themselves significantly below population norms on the 36-item Standard Form (SF-36) health questionnaire, a patient self-report of physical and psychological symptoms and quality of life that is

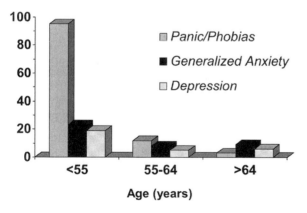

Psychiatric Diagnoses in 180 Patients with Chronic Subjective Dizziness

Figure 1 The type of psychiatric disorders found in patients with chronic subjective dizziness varies with age. In younger adults, panic disorder and specific phobias of dizziness-related situations predominate. In older individuals, generalized anxiety disorder and major depression are more common.

commonly used in medical settings. After treatment with particle repositioning maneuvers, 23 (82%) had no vertigo on exam. Their mean SF-36 physical and mental health scores returned to normal (11).

Rhinology

Two reasonably large studies have investigated psychiatric symptoms in adults with sinus disease, though neither focused on the elderly. In a prospective observational study (12), 95 patients with chronic sinusitis completed physical examinations, had computed tomography scans of the sinuses, and answered standardized questionnaires about sinus symptoms, mental and physical health status, and psychiatric distress at baseline and again at 1, 3, 6, and 12 months after sinus surgery. Individuals with clinically significant anxiety or depression reported more sinus symptoms and a lower quality of life at baseline and throughout their surgical management. However, they had a similar degree of improvement with surgery as patients without psychiatric distress. A study of 109 adults with chronic sinusitis showed that level of depressive symptoms and patients' perceptions of their ability to manage their illness accounted for 26% of quality of life scores, after controlling for the severity of sinus disease (13). Though these investigations did not specifically address the geriatric population, their findings that depression, anxiety, and sense of control affect symptom burden and quality of life throughout treatment are consistent with data from older patients with other medical problems.

Laryngology

Voice Disorders

Psychosomatic interpretations of voice dysfunction have existed for decades. Since the 1980s, however, systematic research has provided a more detailed understanding of the relationships between biological and psychological causes of voice disorders. Spasmodic dysphonia is no longer considered to have a psychological cause, and modern investigations have yielded inconsistent results about the rates of anxiety and depression in patients with this condition (14,15). Nevertheless, botulinum toxin treatment appears to reduce psychological distress, as it improves voice quality in patients with spasmodic dysphonia (15). Individuals with vocal cord paralysis may suffer significant rates of anxiety and depression. One study, which included older patients, found a moderate positive correlation between the level of psychological distress and physical voice impairment (14).

In contrast to the secondary nature of psychological factors in spasmodic dysphonia and vocal cord paralysis, personality traits have a primary role in functional dysphonia. In two studies, one with subjects up to age 84, patients with functional dysphonia had high levels of interpersonal sensitivity, anxiety, and obsessiveness (14,16). This suggests that functional dysphonia is a condition that affects self-conscious individuals who are highly reactive to interactions with others. Figure 2 shows that the relative rate of biological and psychological voice disorders varies with age. Geriatric patients are more likely to have a biological basis to their voice disorders, but this does not spare them from psychological comorbidity.

One study systematically measured the efficacy of six weeks of voice therapy on physical and psychological variables in 204 patients from age 17 to 87 with hoarseness lasting at least two months. Self-perceived and blinded observer ratings of voice quality improved, but anxiety and depressive scores did not change (17).

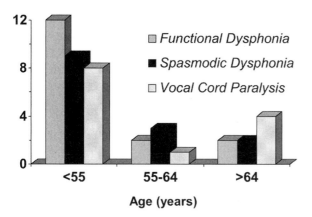

Diagnostic Categories for 43 Patients with Voice Symptoms

- ▨ Functional Dysphonia
- ■ Spasmodic Dysphonia
- ☐ Vocal Cord Paralysis

Age (years)

Figure 2 The diagnostic categories of persistent voice disorders vary with age. In younger adults, functional and spasmodic dysphonias are most likely, whereas vocal cord paralysis was found more often in patients older than 65 years of age.

Sleep Apnea

Several studies have found higher rates of depression and poorer quality of life in patients with obstructive sleep apnea than in the general population. Patients with sleep apnea also have deficits in executive function (e.g., decision-making) and other cognitive tasks. In the largest community-based study, 18,980 individuals from 15 to 100 years of age in five European counties were surveyed by telephone. Eighteen percent of patients with probable sleep apnea, based on their answers to the telephone questionnaire, had major depression, and 18% of patients with major depression had probable sleep apnea (18). Both illnesses have an adverse effect on sleep architecture, and their interactions are now being investigated in sleep laboratories. Several investigations have demonstrated improvement in both apnea and depression with continuous positive airway pressure treatment. A recent study demonstrated significant improvements in depression, anxiety symptoms, and anxious personality traits in 51 patients after one and three months of continuous positive airway pressure (19). Surgical treatment with extended uvulopalatal flap procedures produced a moderate degree of improvement in depressive symptoms in 84 Taiwanese patients. Curiously, improvements in psychological symptoms did not correlate with changes in sleep indices or daytime sleepiness after surgery (20).

HEAD AND NECK SURGERY

Studies of patients with squamous cell carcinoma of the head and neck (SCCHN) provide a consistent picture of the psychiatric symptoms associated with this condition. In the early stages of diagnostic evaluation and treatment, nearly one-half of patients suffer through periods of anxiety (33%) or depression (15–21%). Treatment interventions, both surgery and radiation therapy, exacerbate psychological distress and worsen quality of life during the first 3–6 months after diagnosis (21,22). This holds true for older and younger adults with cancers located in the oral cavity, pharynx, or larynx (22). Women, patients with more advanced cancers, and those who receive combined treatments are more likely to suffer deterioration in psychological status and quality of life (21). As is the case with other medical conditions, moderate levels of anxiety and depression may interfere with treatment adherence and self-care (e.g., medication compliance, adequate dietary intake). However, a three-year prospective study of patients with SCCHN who were treated with surgery and/or radiation therapy showed a reduction in depressive symptoms and improvement in quality of life by one year after diagnosis (21). At three years, patients' principal complaints were about expected physical consequences of their disease and its treatment (e.g., dry mouth, loss of taste). Explanations about these physical sensations and their unlikely association with cancer recurrence were helpful. Therefore, patients recently diagnosed with SCCHN need support, education, and reassurance during the early stages of therapy. From a psychological standpoint, resilience is the expected outcome, but some patients will have a level of anxiety or depression that interferes with daily functioning, treatment adherence, and self-care. These patients may require psychiatric intervention, but there are few specific studies to guide psychiatric treatment.

DIAGNOSIS AND TREATMENT OF ANXIETY AND DEPRESSION IN OTORHINOLARYNGOLOGIC PRACTICE

The most important tool for detecting anxiety and depression in otorhinolaryngologic practice is a high index of suspicion. The most important therapeutic intervention is a willingness to address psychological factors as part of a comprehensive treatment plan for otorhinolaryngologic disease. Figure 3 is a time-efficient algorithm for identifying clinically significant anxiety and/or depression in older patients referred for evaluations of ear, nose, and throat symptoms. It requires little, if any, alteration in otorhinolaryngologic procedures and is based on research on effective methods for identification of psychiatric illnesses in primary care and specialty medical settings (1).

History and Physical Examination

The clinical history and physical examination are paramount in detecting anxiety and depression. Do they reveal *active* otorhinolaryngologic disease? This question is important because conditioned hypersensitivity can cause persistent ear, nose, or throat symptoms long after the illnesses that triggered it have resolved. A common example is the patient who reports a past history of position-related vertigo typical of benign paroxysmal positional vertigo, but has only chronic nonspecific dizziness with a negative Dix-Hallpike test at the time of consultation. In cases such as this, screening for anxiety and depression is warranted. If the only evidence of physical disease is found in past history, treatment for the identified medical problem is helpful only if relapse is likely (e.g., migraine prophylaxis). Otherwise, treatment of a resolved physical illness will not bring the patient relief from current symptoms.

A more common scenario in the elderly is the situation in which the clinical history and physical examination detect an otorhinolaryngologic condition, but they cannot explain the full extent of the patients' symptoms or impairment in function. This strongly suggests the presence of comorbid otorhinolaryngologic and psychiatric disorders. In this scenario, treating the otorhinolaryngologic illness and screening for anxiety and depression will produce the best clinical outcomes.

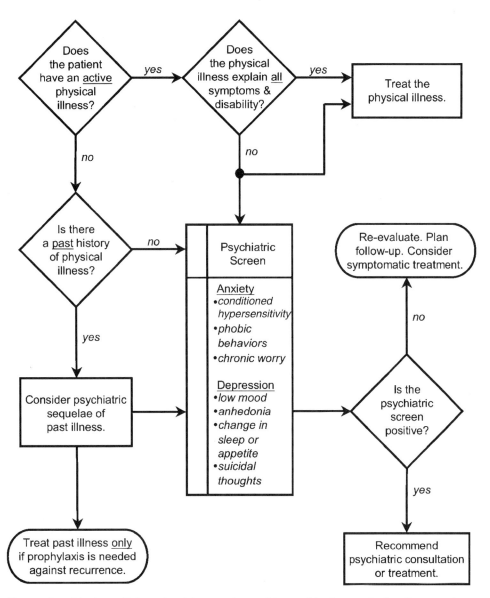

Figure 3 This time-efficient algorithm can be used in otorhinolaryngologic office practice to identify patients who may need psychiatric evaluation and treatment. The signs and symptoms listed in the "Psychiatric Screen" panel are described in the text.

Psychiatric Screen

A reasonable screen for anxiety disorders involves three questions:

1. Do the patient's physical symptoms mimic past otorhinolaryngologic disease, or is the patient overly vigilant about present physical deficits (conditioned hypersensitivity)?
2. Does the patient avoid situations associated with his or her symptoms or anticipate these circumstances with excessive anxiety (phobic behaviors)?
3. Is the patient a worrywart (generalized anxiety)?

For depression, only two screening questions are needed (1):

1. Has the patient felt depressed, sad, or blue for most of the last two weeks?
2. Has the patient lost pleasure in the usual activities?

The second question may be more sensitive for depression in the elderly. A positive result to either of the depression questions can be followed by queries about sleep and appetite to increase the specificity of detecting major depression rather than lesser reactions to transient life events. A simple question about suicide may reduce the chance that a dangerous situation is missed. Examples include, "Have you thought that life is not worth living?" or "Have you thought about hurting yourself?" A positive or equivocal result would warrant urgent psychiatric consultation.

Differential Diagnosis

Dementia and delirium are much more common in older patients than in younger adults. Complaints of memory loss or periods of confusion suggest these cognitive disorders. Conversion disorder, hypochondriasis, and malingering are part of the differential diagnosis of medically unexplained physical symptoms. These disorders are uncommon in the elderly. Conversion disorder manifests with unusual (aphysiological) motor or sensory deficits that have no physical cause. The hallmark of hypochondriasis is a strong preoccupation with being ill, usually with a catastrophic disease, not just hypervigilance about physical symptoms as in conditioned hypersensitivity. Malingering is quite rare in the elderly, but should be considered whenever compensation for injury is a prominent concern of the patient.

Testing

Research in primary care settings suggests that the screening questions above may be just as sensitive, though not as specific, as formal psychiatric instruments for detecting depression in nonpsychiatric settings (1). Evidence supporting the anxiety screen is emerging. Therefore, the otorhinolaryngologist who follows the algorithm of Figure 3 can be confident in making a psychiatric referral or recommending psychiatric intervention, as indicated.

Several psychiatric questionnaires are available to supplement the diagnostic algorithm of Figure 3 (1). All are short self-reports that can be completed by patients in the waiting room prior to consultation. The Patient Health Questionnaire is a three-page survey that screens for five psychiatric illnesses commonly encountered in primary care settings (depression, anxiety, alcohol abuse, psychosomatic illnesses, and eating disorders). It can be used in its entirety, or any of its five parts can be used independently. The anxiety and depression modules were recently tested in 268 adults presenting to an otorhinolaryngology clinic for evaluation of dizziness (23). Ninety-seven patients had follow-up psychiatric examinations that demonstrated excellent validity of the two Patient Health Questionnaire modules for detecting anxiety and depression in this patient population. The Geriatric Depression Scale is a 15-item questionnaire that was designed specifically for older patients whose medical illnesses may confound other assessment scales (1)

Extensive laboratory testing is not needed for diagnosing anxiety or depression (1). A thyroid stimulating hormone level is the only test that should be considered routinely. Other laboratory tests may be ordered as indicated by history or examination findings.

TREATMENT OPTIONS

Though the field of geriatric psychiatry has advanced considerable in the last 2 decades, there are very few examples of its application to otorhinolaryngology. Therefore, the treatment options discussed below are adapted from geriatric psychiatry largely on the basis of clinical experience. They may be refined in future research.

Otorhinolaryngologic Disease-Specific Therapies

Otorhinolaryngologists treating older patients are much more likely to encounter anxiety and depressive disorders in conjunction with otorhinolaryngologic diseases than as the primary causes of the ear, nose, and throat symptoms. Therefore, it is reasonable to ask if treatment of the medical condition will improve coexisting psychiatric symptoms or if specific psychiatric interventions are required. The available data are mixed. In patients with spasmodic dysphonia and hearing loss, anxiety and depression are likely to improve with medical intervention. However, anxiety and depressive symptoms tend to be mild in these patients. Patients with SCCHN may have significant anxiety and depression as they negotiate the early stages of therapy, but most adapt to their circumstances and do not require psychiatric treatment. With other conditions, otorhinolaryngologic interventions seem not to affect psychiatric morbidity, even if they are successful in reducing physical symptoms (e.g., voice therapy for hoarseness and surgery for sleep apnea). Given the inconsistency of these findings and the natural variability among patients, it seems prudent to recommend psychiatric interventions in four situations: (i) when anxiety or depression interfere with medical diagnosis and treatment, (ii) when patients are distressed by their psychiatric symptoms, (iii) when patients are functionally impaired by their psychiatric symptoms, and (iv) when patients may be unsafe (i.e., when they may be suicidal, assaultive, or unable to care for themselves). In other circumstances, patient education and support may be all that is required during the course of otorhinolaryngologic illness.

Psychiatric Interventions

Pharmacotherapy

Selective serotonin reuptake inhibitors have become first-line agents for treating anxiety and depressive disorders in both younger and older patients. Six of these medications [fluoxetine (Prozac®, Prozac Weekly®, Sarafem®), sertraline (Zoloft®), paroxetine (Paxil®, Paxil CR®), fluvoxamine (Luvox®), citalopram (Celexa®), and escitalopram (Lexapro®)] are available in the United States. Other antidepressants available in the United States include venlafaxine (Effexor®, Effexor XR®), duloxetine (Cymbalta®), bupropion (Wellbutrin®, Wellbutrin SR®, Wellburtrin XL®), mirtazapine (Remeron®, Remeron Sol-Tabs®), and generic nefazodone, as well as the older tricyclic antidepressants and monoamine oxidase inhibitors. Additional antidepressants are available in other countries. Nefazodone has been withdrawn from the market in many countries other than the United States in the face of case reports of fulmitant hepatic failure. All antidepressants except sertraline, escitalopram, venlafaxine, and duloxetine are available as generic preparations.

Elderly patients are likely to be taking multiple medications and have several concurrent medical problems. Therefore, the major consideration in choosing an antidepressant is to minimize potential drug–drug and drug–disease interactions (3). In this regard, citalopram, escitalopram, low to moderate dose sertraline, venlafaxine, duloxetine, bupropion, and mirtazapine have minimal effects on cytochrome P450 isoenzymes in the liver. As a result, they are not likely to cause significant drug–drug interactions. Of these agents, venlafaxine and duloxetine may cause dry mouth, which could be problematic in patients undergoing treatment for SCCHN. Mirtazapine is most likely to promote weight gain, which may be desirable in patients with cancer-related anorexia. Regardless of the antidepressant chosen, geriatric patients should be prescribed one-half of the usual adult starting dose, with gradual titration upward as tolerated.

Benzodiazepines are effective anxiolytics and vestibular suppressants, but they can be problematic in the elderly, who are more susceptible to cognitive impairment and falls when taking these medications. Therefore, prescriptions are best limited to the lowest effective dose for the shortest necessary duration in situations where benzodiazepines are indicated. Antipsychotic medications do not have a primary role in the treatment of anxiety or depressive disorders but may be used as adjunctive agents.

Systematic investigations of antidepressant efficacy for patients with anxiety, depression, and otorhinolaryngologic disease are just beginning to emerge. One published case series of selective serotonin reuptake inhibitors for patients with chronic dizziness and anxiety or depression included patients older than age 65 (24). Two-thirds of patients had a significant reduction in physical and psychiatric symptoms, but treatment response was not analyzed by age.

Psychotherapies

Psychotherapy may play an important role in the treatment of elderly patients with psychiatric symptoms. For mild to moderate anxiety or depression, psychotherapy is as effective as anxiolytic or antidepressant medications, and many patients prefer this treatment modality. For patients with cancer, many psychosocial intervention programs have been developed. Psychotherapies have not been studied systematically in elderly otorhinolaryngology patients, though a few pilot studies have been published recently (25).

CONCLUSION

Anxiety and depressive disorders can be expected in elderly patients with a variety of conditions affecting the ears, nose, and throat. Almost always, these psychiatric disorders coexist with otorhinolaryngologic diseases. Primary psychiatric causes of ears, nose, and throat symptoms are unusual in the elderly. Anxiety and depression increase symptom burden, confound otorhinolaryngologic diagnosis, reduce treatment adherence, and adversely affect therapeutic outcomes. Recognition of anxiety and depression requires a high index of suspicion but little time beyond the usual otorhinolaryngologic consultation. A streamlined algorithm is available to assist the otorhinolaryngologist in detecting anxiety and depression and determining when psychiatric consultation would be beneficial. Recent advances in geriatric psychiatry have produced a wealth of treatment interventions for older patients with anxiety and depressive disorders, but these have not been studied systematically in the geriatric population with otorhinolaryngologic diseases.

REFERENCES

1. Staab JP, Datto, CJ, Weinrieb RM, Gariti P, Rynn M, Evans DL. Detection and diagnosis of psychiatric disorders in primary medical care settings. Med Clin North Am 2001; 85:579–596.
2. Staab JP, Ruckenstein MJ. Which comes first? Psychogenic dizziness versus otogenic anxiety. Laryngoscope 2003; 113:1714–1718.
3. Evans DL, Staab JP, Petitto JM, et al. Depression in the medical setting: biopsychological interactions and treatment considerations. J Clin Psychiatry 1999; 60(suppl 4):40–55.
4. Kempen GI, Verbrugge LM, Merrill SS, Ormel J. The impact of multiple impairments on disability in community-dwelling older people. Age Ageing 1998; 27:595–604.
5. Cacciatore F, Napoli C, Abete P, Marciano E, Triassi M, Rengo F. Quality of life determinants and hearing function in an elderly population: Osservatorio Geriatrico Campano Study Group. Gerontology 1999; 45:323–328.
6. de Jonge P, Ormel J, Slaets JP, et al. Depressive symptoms in elderly patients predict poor adjustment after somatic events. Am J Geriatr Psychiatry 2004; 12:57–64.
7. Sloan MM, Dancer J. Should identification audiometry include a screening for depression among residents of upper socioeconomic retirement centers? Percept Mot Skills 2001; 92(3 Pt 2):1251–1254.
8. Collet L, Moussu MF, Disant F, Ahami T, Morgon A. Minnesota Multiphasic Personality Inventory in tinnitus disorders. Audiology 1990; 29:101–106.
9. Zoger S, Svedlund J, Holgers KM. Psychiatric disorders in tinnitus patients without severe hearing impairment: 24 month follow-up of patients at an audiological clinic. Audiology 2001; 40:133–140.
10. Salles N, Kressig RW, Michel JP. Management of chronic dizziness in elderly people. Z Gerontol Geriatr 2003; 36:10–15.
11. Gamiz MJ, Lopez-Escamez JA. Health-related quality of life in patients over sixty years old with benign paroxysmal positional vertigo. Gerontology 2004; 50:82–86.
12. Davis GE, Yueh B, Walker E, Katon W, Koepsell TD, Weymuller EA. Psychiatric distress amplifies symptoms after surgery for chronic rhinosinusitis. Otolaryngol Head Neck Surg 2005; 132:189–196.
13. Chen H, Katz PP, Eisner MD, Yelin EH, Blanc PD. Health-related quality of life in adult rhinitis: the role of perceived control of disease. J Allergy Clin Immunol 2004; 114: 845–850.
14. Mirza N, Ruiz C, Baum ED, Staab JP. The prevalence of major psychiatric pathologies in patients with voice disorders. Ear Nose Throat J 2003; 82:808–814.
15. Liu CY, Yu JM, Wang NM, et al. Emotional symptoms are secondary to the voice disorder in patients with spasmodic dysphonia. Gen Hosp Psychiatry 1998; 20:255–259.
16. Lauriello M, Cozza K, Rossi A, Di Rienzo L, Coen Tirelli G. Psychological profile of dysfunctional dysphonia. Acta Otorhinolaryngol Ital 2003; 23:467–473.
17. MacKenzie K, Millar A, Wilson JA, Sellars C, Deary IJ. Is voice therapy an effective treatment for dysphonia? A randomised controlled trial. BMJ 2001; 323:658–661.
18. Ohayon MM. The effects of breathing-related sleep disorders on mood disturbances in the general population. J Clin Psychiatry 2003; 64:1195–1200.
19. Sanchez AI, Buela-Casal G, Bermudez MP, Casas-Maldonado F. The effects of continuous positive air pressure treatment on anxiety and depression levels in apnea patients. Psychiatry Clin Neurosci 2001; 55:641–646.
20. Li HY, Huang YS, Chen NH, Fang TJ, Liu CY, Wang PC. Mood improvement after surgery for obstructive sleep apnea. Laryngoscope 2004; 114:1098–1102.
21. de Graeff A, de Leeuw JR, Ros WJ, Hordijk GJ, Blijham GH, Winnubst JA. Long-term quality of life of patients with head and neck cancer. Laryngoscope 2000; 110:98–106.
22. Derks W, De Leeuw JR, Hordijk GJ, Winnubst JA. Elderly patients with head and neck cancer: short-term effects of surgical treatment on quality of life. Clin Otolaryngol 2003; 28:399–405.

23. Persoons P, Luyckx K, Desloovere C, Vandenberghe J, Fischler B. Anxiety and mood disorders in otorhinolaryngology outpatients presenting with dizziness: validation of the self-administered PRIME-MD Patient Health Questionnaire and epidemiology. Gen Hosp Psychiatry 2003; 25:316–323.
24. Staab JP, Ruckenstein MJ, Solomon D, Shepard NT. Serotonin reuptake inhibitors for dizziness with psychiatric symptoms. Arch Otolaryngol Head Neck Surg 2002; 128: 554–560.
25. Johansson M, Akerlund D, Larsen HC, Andersson G. Randomized controlled trial of vestibular rehabilitation combined with cognitive-behavioral therapy for dizziness in older people. Otolaryngol Head Neck Surg 2001; 125:151–156.

ANNOTATED BIBLIOGRAPHY

Davis GE, Yueh B, Walker E, Katon W, Koepsell TD, Weymuller EA. Psychiatric distress amplifies symptoms after surgery for chronic rhinosinusitis. Otolaryngol Head Neck Surg 2005; 132:189–196.

This prospective study investigated the adverse effects of depression on surgical management of chronic sinusitis, including links between severity of depression and burden of physical symptoms before and after surgery.

de Graeff A, de Leeuw JR, Ros WJ, Hordijk GJ, Blijham GH, Winnubst JA. Long-term quality of life of patients with head and neck cancer. Laryngoscope 2000; 110:98–106.

This prospective study details the clinical course of anxiety and depression in patients with squamous cell cancer of the head and neck, beginning with high levels of psychiatric symptoms encountered early in the course of treatment and following patients through the gradual emergence of resilience.

Mirza N, Ruiz C, Baum ED, Staab JP. The prevalence of major psychiatric pathologies in patients with voice disorders. Ear Nose Throat J 2003; 82:808–814.

This small study is one of the only investigations to compare and contrast psychiatric symptoms and personality features found in patients with spasmodic dysphonia, functional dysphonia, and vocal cord paralysis.

Staab JP, Datto CJ, Weinrieb RM, Gariti P, Rynn M, Evans DL. Detection and diagnosis of psychiatric disorders in primary medical care settings. Med Clin North Am 2001; 85:579–596.

This paper presents a comprehensive review of research on the detection of psychiatric disorders in nonpsychiatric settings. It includes a section that deals specifically with the problems of psychiatric diagnosis in elderly patients.

Staab JP, Ruckenstein MJ. Which comes first? Psychogenic dizziness versus otogenic anxiety. Laryngoscope 2003; 113:1714–1718.

This paper extends previous psychosomatic theories of dizziness to describe three ways in which anxiety and dizziness relates to one another: (i) anxiety may be a primary psychiatric cause of dizziness, (ii) anxiety may be a secondary complication of neurotologic illness, and (iii) anxiety may pre-date dizziness, but interact with an incident neurotologic illness to magnify symptoms and disability. Older patients are included in the study cohort.

59
Coordination of Care

Steven C. Zweig
Department of Family and Community Medicine, University of Missouri–Columbia School of Medicine, Columbia, Missouri, U.S.A.

CARE COORDINATION

The goal of care coordination is to enhance the quality of health care, improve health outcomes, prevent unnecessary hospitalizations, and reduce preventable expenditures. Care coordination programs should serve chronically ill people who are at risk for adverse outcomes by three primary strategies: first, identifying those medical, functional, and psychosocial needs that increase the risk of adverse health events; second, addressing those needs through education in self-care, optimization of medical treatment, and integration of care (including across settings and providers); and third, monitoring patients for progress and early signs of problems (1).

Not surprisingly, care coordination fits the complex needs of frail elderly people, although there are also common examples of disease-specific programs fitted to persons of varying age groups. Two types of care coordination programs address these needs: case management and disease management. Case management emphasizes the care of high-risk patients to minimize adverse medical events and poor health outcomes. Patient education and care coordination are highly individualized, with relatively less reliance on disease specific guidelines and protocols and more attention to arranging referrals and community resources and engaging family caregivers. Disease management programs use a standardized patient education curriculum, relying on disease specific guidelines and protocols with less emphasis on care coordination, as patients tend to not be as frail. The locus of care coordination may be at the level of the practice, hospital, or insurer. Its motivations include improving quality of care, enhancing function, and reducing costs.

In their comprehensive examination of 29 programs, Chen and coworkers found that programs went through a three-step process with each patient reflecting the strategies described above: assess and plan, implement and deliver, and reassess and adjust. Each step had a number of important tasks (Table 1).

The nurse partner model is an example of the *case management* form of care coordination. Based on one developed at the Carle Clinic, this program identifies and coordinates the care of frail elderly patients with complex comorbidities who are members of a family medicine practice at the University of Missouri—Columbia. An advanced practice nurse works with over 200 elderly patients in collaboration

Table 1 Steps and Tasks of Care Coordination

Assess and plan
  Uncover all important problems
  Address all important problems and goals
  Draw from a comprehensive arsenal of proven interventions
  Produce a clear, practical plan of care with specific goals
Implement and deliver
  Build ongoing relationships with the primary care physicians and other providers
  Build ongoing relationships with patient and families
  Provide excellent patient education
  Make certain that planned interventions get done
Reassess and adjust
  Perform periodic reassessments
  Be accessible. Patients must have an easy way to reach a care coordinator
  Nurture the relationships with primary care physicians and providers
  Nurture the relationships with patient and family
  Make prompt adjustments to the plan of care as needed

Source: From Ref. 1.

with faculty and resident physicians. Compared with similar patients on another team of the same practice, patients in the care coordination group were less likely to be hospitalized or visit the emergency room. The patients in the care coordination group experienced a relative decrease in hospitalization of 12%, compared with a 27% increase in the control group. Similarly, emergency department visits dropped by 17% in the care coordination group versus an increase of 44% in the control group (2).

This model of care coordination resides in the primary care practice, including patient interactions in the office, by telephone, and during home visits. Activities in the office include: needs assessment, medication review at each visit, and patient education. Telephone coordination includes follow-up after office visits or hospital discharge, facilitation of discharge plans with the hospital team, arrangement of consultations and diagnostic tests, and contact with providers whenever the patient touches another part of the health care system. Home visits include assessment of patient safety, medication adherence, and functional assessment. Direct and immediate contact with the nurse partner is available to patients and their family members/caregivers. The system's electronic medical record enables the nurse partner to know immediately when patients interact with another part of the system. Care coordination depends on daily close collaboration with physician colleagues. The nurse partner communicates with physicians at all times and adds patients to clinic schedules as needed. An example of case management is described as follows:

> Mrs. R. was an 81-year-old retired dean with interstitial lung disease who entered the practice after a hospitalization for influenza and pneumonia. She was cared for by a family physician/geriatrician with periodic consultation from pulmonary specialists. She developed delirium during her stay that was slow to resolve after discharge, requiring close phone follow-up and nurse visits. Fortunately, Mrs. R. lived with her daughter, but her daughter frequently traveled out of state. Mrs. R. used oxygen continuously and needed help with many of her activities of daily living. Over the next year, the nurse partner established a trusting relationship with the patient and her daughter, arranged needed outpatient services and equipment, and acted as liaison between consulting physicians and other outpatient

services, ensuring that all had accurate and up to date information in order to make appropriate medical decisions. Mrs. R. began to attend an exercise class for cardiopulmonary strengthening, which helped decrease her oxygen requirement and increased her exercise tolerance from 6 to 45 minutes. Her condition stabilized and she needed less help and less frequent medical visits.

In other arrangements, the health plan employs case managers to work with physicians in different practices. Integrating the physician, patient, and case manager in this arrangement is much more difficult due to lack of proximity and different organizational allegiances (3). Methods that facilitate closer communication include assigning one case manager to a physician or group and developing modes of communication with which the physician and case manager are comfortable (e.g., phone, fax, electronic mail).

There are also many examples of *disease management* programs in the United States. They may target patients with diabetes, asthma, congestive heart failure, depression, and other chronic diseases (4). In the primary care-based model, physicians work with specialized teams in treating patients with specific chronic diseases. Group Health's electronic medical record enables primary care physicians to view longitudinal information on their diabetic patients, such as when they were last seen, glycohemoglobin levels, dates for eye examinations and microalbumin checks, and medication lists. The system notifies patients and providers when more follow-up is indicated. An endocrinologist and nurse are available to help coach the primary care physicians in making the best of a brief office visit, and group visits are created for patient education (5). In the carve-out model, contracts are made with disease management companies, separate from primary care. Some of these programs are run by pharmaceutical companies with interest areas in specific chronic diseases. For example, a program may help identify patients with diabetes and target those who are poorly controlled using communications by phone or mail to encourage self-monitoring and to provide patient education materials.

Other models of care coordination have focused on specific high-risk periods for patients, such as following discharge from the hospital. This model has been tested in patients with congestive heart failure and in older patients with complex care needs, and it has been shown to reduce readmission rates, length of subsequent hospitalization, and costs (6–10). Elements include close collaboration with care providers in various settings of care, a follow-up phone call to the patient and/or care setting within 48 hours of hospital discharge, and immediate access to the care coordinator by a direct phone number. Roles of the transitional case manager include: facilitating interdisciplinary collaboration between the sending and receiving care teams; serving as a single contact person who can address patient/family questions or concerns before, during, and immediately after a transfer; reviewing medications for potential errors after discharge; following up with the patient to make sure that the patient has received durable medical equipment and appointments with the receiving providers; empowering the patient and caregiver to participate more in their care by providing patient education; and educating the patient and caregiver about the plan of care.

The otolaryngologist may play a series of important roles in the care coordination of elderly patients. The otolaryngologist may serve as the primary provider in a patient with a complex head and neck cancer that may have other comorbidities contributing to frailty. The otolaryngologist may also serve as a consultant to a primary care provider coordinating the care of a complex elderly patient with dizziness or hearing loss, as well as work collaboratively with care coordinators in helping patients transition from hospital to community-based care.

THE FUTURE OF CARE COORDINATION

One of the challenges of all such programs is aligning costs and reimbursement. For example, insurers are interested in programs that reduce morbidity and hospitalization because they are at risk for the costs of those outcomes. Outside of staff model HMOs or risk bearing provider-based programs, providers may not benefit financially from care coordination programs. Care coordination takes time and money, which may improve care but may not save money for the sponsoring program, at least in the short run. Traditional forms of Medicare or Medicaid have not provided reimbursement for care coordination or disease management outside the fee for service model for physician payment.

There are exceptions. The Program for All-Inclusive Care of the Elderly (PACE) provides a financial platform and incentive for groups to provide comprehensive care coordination of the frail elderly who are dually eligible for both the Medicaid and Medicare programs (11). At a rate of 2.39 times the usual average adjusted per capita cost (AAPC) for Medicare and a state-negotiated Medicaid rate, PACE programs provide comprehensive care (including hospital care) for community-living frail elders who have functional needs similar to nursing home residents. This requires intensive team-based management across settings of care, including the use of adult day health centers, transportation systems, and home-based care, with the goal of keeping patients functional and out of hospitals and nursing homes. PACE programs have typically operated in urban areas, with each program caring for about 200–400 people.

The Centers for Medicare and Medicaid services has developed a Capitated Disease Management Demonstration to test models aimed at beneficiaries who have one or more chronic conditions that are related to high costs to the Medicare program, such as stroke, congestive heart failure, or diabetes. This program provides an adjusted payment for services based on full capitation with the goal of improving quality of services and reducing costs (12). More of such programs may be created in the future.

Ultimately, even fee for service models may financially benefit from effective care coordination. If length of stay can be reduced by safely transitioning patients to community settings, hospitals can save money based on Medicare's DRG system of inpatient reimbursement. Also, if unreimbursed readmissions can be avoided, quality of care is improved and the hospital saves money. Finally, if physicians can deliver more effective billable services by extending their care with a care coordination program, then they can help support the program financially while improving the quality of care for their patients.

REFERENCES

1. Chen A, Brown R, Archibald N, Aliotta S, Fox PD. Best practices in coordinated care. Princeton, NJ: Mathematica Policy Research, Inc., 2000.
2. Rastkar R, Zweig S, Delzell JE, Davis K. Nurse care coordination of ambulatory frail elderly in an academic setting. Case Manager 2002; 13(1):59–61.

3. The HMO Workgroup on Care Management. Essential components of geriatric care provided through health maintenance organizations. J Am Geriatr Soc 1998; 46(3): 303–308.

4. Bodenheimer T. Disease management—promises and pitfalls. N Engl J Med 1999; 340(15):1202–1205.

5. McCulloch DK, Price MJ, Hindmarsh M, Wagner EH. A population-based approach to diabetes management in the post-DCCT era. Diabetes Care 1994; 17:765–769.

6. Parry C, Coleman EA, Smith JD, et al. The care transitions intervention: a patient-centered approach to ensuring effective transfers between sites of geriatric care. Home Health Care Serv Q 2003; 22:1–17.

7. Naylor MD, Brooten D, Campbell R, et al. Comprehensive discharge planning and home follow-up of hospitalized elders: a randomized controlled trial. JAMA 1999; 281:613–620.

8. Rich MW, Beckham V, Wittenburg C, et al. A multidisciplinary intervention to prevent the readmission of elderly patients with congestive heart failure. N Engl J Med 1995; 333:1190–1195.

9. Stewart S, Pearson S, Horowitz JD. Effects of a home-based intervention among patients with congestive heart failure discharged from acute hospital care. Arch Intern Med 1998; 158:1067–1072.

10. Coleman EA, Fox PD. One patient, many places: managing health care transitions, part II: practitioner skills and patient and caregiver participation. Ann Long-Term Care 2004; 12(10):34–39.

11. National PACE Association. A PACE profile 1996: an integrated model of medical and long-term care services. National PACE Association, Washington, DC, April 1996.

12. Centers for Medicare and Medicaid Services. Capitated Disease Management Demonstration. (Accessed January 5, 2005 at http://www.cms.hhs.gov/healthplans/research/cdm.asp?)

60

Polypharmacy in Older Adults

Emily R. Hajjar
Philadelphia College of Pharmacy, University of the Sciences in Philadelphia, Philadelphia, Pennsylvania, U.S.A.

Joseph T. Hanlon
Department of Medicine (Geriatrics), University of Pittsburgh, Pittsburgh, Pennsylvania, U.S.A.

INTRODUCTION

Prescribing medications for older persons is a complex task because they often require multiple medications for multiple chronic conditions. The goal of this chapter is to provide information to otolaryngologists regarding the definitions, epidemiology, and consequences of polypharmacy. We will end with a discussion on principles of geriatric pharmacotherapy. The focus of this book chapter will be on older persons in outpatient settings, as 95% of elders reside in the community.

POLYPHARMACY DEFINITIONS AND EPIDEMIOLOGY

Polypharmacy is commonly defined in one of two ways. The first definition is the concomitant use of multiple drugs, simply classified by medication count (1). Elderly patients often have multiple comorbidities requiring multiple medications. This definition is controversial because it does not take appropriateness into account. Community-based surveys reveal that elders take a daily average of two to three prescription medications (2–4). It is also important to carefully consider the use of nonprescription medications (over-the-counter agents and dietary supplements) in older adults. In a study of rural community dwelling elders, it was found that 87% took at least one and almost 50% took two to four over-the-counter medications (5). Kaufman et al. (6) reported data on dietary supplements from a national survey and found that 47% to 59% of older patients took a vitamin or mineral, and 11% to 14% took herbal supplements. Kaufman et al. (6) also found that 12% of those greater than 65 years old take 10 or more prescription or nonprescription medications combined. There are new data suggesting that polypharmacy is increasing among the elderly, especially in the oldest old (7).

The second definition of polypharmacy is the administration of more medications than are clinically indicated, representing excessive or unnecessary drug use (8). This definition necessitates clinical review of medications to determine polypharmacy. Few studies have evaluated this definition of polypharmacy (unnecessary drug use). A study by Lipton et al. (9) found that 59% patients in an ambulatory setting were taking medications that were prescribed without indication or were determined to be suboptimal. In another outpatient study by Schmader et al. (10), 55% of patients were taking drugs without an indication, 32.7% were taking ineffective drugs, and 16.8% were taking drugs with therapeutic duplication. Schmader et al. (11) also evaluated unnecessary drug use, defined by the Medication Appropriateness Index criteria, and demonstrated no indication, ineffectiveness, and duplication in nearly 400 of elderly outpatients. They found that the daily average number of unnecessary drugs was 0.65 per person.

Most Common Drugs

When evaluating polypharmacy, it is important to consider the types of prescription and nonprescription medications being consumed. Kaufman et al. (6) reported that the most common prescription medications used among noninstitutionalized people were estrogen products, levothyroxine, hydrochlorothiazide, atorvastatin, and lisinopril. In a study of more than 30,000 Medicare patients in Massachusetts, Gurwitz et al. (12) found that cardiovascular agents, antibiotics, diuretics, opioids, and antihyperlipidemics were the most frequently used classes of prescription medications. Regarding nonprescription agents, Kaufman et al. (6) found that acetaminophen, ibuprofen, aspirin, pseudoephedrine, diphenhydramine, multivitamins, vitamin E and C, ginseng, ginko biloba extract, and allium sativum (garlic) were the most common ones used. Stoehr et al. (5) also found that analgesics, vitamins, minerals, antacids, and laxatives were commonly used nonprescription agents among the elderly.

Predictors

Various risk factors for polypharmacy, defined by medication count, have been identified. Risk factors can be separated into three categories: demographic, health status, and access to health care characteristics. Demographic characteristics associated with polypharmacy include increased age, white race, and education (4,13,14). Health status characteristics associated with polypharmacy include poorer health, depression, and certain types of health care problems (e.g., hypertension, respiratory diseases) (2,13–15). Access to health care characteristic predictors of polypharmacy include number of health care visits and having supplemental insurance (14,15). Future studies are needed to evaluate predictors for unnecessary drug use in the elderly.

CONSEQUENCES OF POLYPHARMACY

Polypharmacy has many negative consequences in the elderly. The risk of adverse drug reactions (ADRs), drug interactions, and patient nonadherence may increase with increased number of drugs. Moreover, risk of negative health outcomes in older persons (e.g., geriatric syndromes, functional decline) is increased with use of multiple medications. The following provides additional information about these specific consequences associated with polypharmacy.

ADRs

An ADR, defined by the World Health Organization, is a reaction that is noxious and unintended and occurs at dosages normally used in humans for prophylaxis, diagnosis, or therapy (16). ADRs have been reported to occur in between 5% and 35% of outpatients and account for as many as 12% of hospital admissions in older patients (12,17–20). The risk of ADRs is strongly associated with multiple comorbidities, use of specific types of drugs, and increasing number of drugs taken (1,20).

Drug Interactions

Use of multiple prescription drugs is a strong risk factor for inappropriate prescribing (10,21). One concern is the increased risk of drug interactions. Drug–drug interactions can be defined as the effect that the administration of one medication has on another drug (22). The main types of drug–drug interactions can be classified into two categories: pharmacokinetic interactions and pharmacodynamic interactions. Other possible drug interactions include drug–disease interactions.

Pharmacokinetic Drug–Drug Interactions

Pharmacokinetic interactions pertain to those interactions wherein one drug affects the absorption, distribution, metabolism, and excretion of another drug. For example, absorption of medications (e.g., tetracycline and quinolone antibiotics) may be altered by the presence of multivalent cations (e.g., antacids, sucralfate, iron, calcium supplements). Drug distribution interactions are mainly related to plasma protein binding (22–24). Drug distribution interactions involving the displacement of drugs from protein binding sites are rarely clinically significant. Drug–drug interactions most likely to be clinically significant are those that involve alterations in the hepatic metabolism of narrow therapeutic range drugs (e.g., warfarin). Common medications that can inhibit drug metabolism include ciprofloxacin, erythromycin, and cimetidine. Inhibiting drug metabolism may result in higher drug levels and enhanced side effects. Induction of hepatic metabolism will result in reduced drug efficacy due to lower drug levels. Examples of medications that can induce drug metabolism include rifampin and carbamazepine. Clinically significant interactions can also been seen with the inhibition of renal clearance of one drug by another drug (22–24). Many of these drug interactions involve competitive inhibition of tubular secretion of anionic (e.g., penicillin, cephalosporins) or cationic drugs (e.g., trimethoprim).

Pharmacodynamic Drug–Drug Interactions

Pharmacodynamic interactions occur when administration of one drug alters the response of another drug and produces enhanced or adverse effects. For example, concomitant administration of multiple central nervous system medications (e.g., benzodiazepines and opioid analgesics) can result in delirium, falls, and other problems (23,25).

Drug–Disease Interactions

Medications used to treat one disease state can have deleterious effects on other diseases (26,27). Elderly patients are more prone to drug–disease interactions because they are more likely to be taking multiple medications for multiple comorbid conditions. They are also likely to suffer greater consequences, as they have alterations in homeostatic mechanisms and diminished physiological reserve (23). For example, use of nonsteroidal anti-inflammatory drugs (e.g., ibuprofen, naproxen) can exacerbate peptic ulcer disease. Another example is that drugs that are highly anticholinergic (e.g., diphenhydramine, meclizine) may worsen pre-existing constipation, cognitive impairment, or xerostomia (26–29). Opioids may also cause hip fractures in those with a history of falls and worsen pre-existing confusion (26–30).

Medication Adherence

Polypharmacy creates complex medication regimens that make nonadherence a common problem in the elderly, with prevalence rates averaging 50% (31–33). However, overall, elderly patients are adherent with about 75% of their individual medications (31,32). When compared to younger patients taking the same number of drugs, the elderly have similar adherence rates to the younger patients (34).

Other Health Outcomes

Polypharmacy is also associated with geriatric syndromes, decline in functional status, and increased health care costs. The geriatric syndromes whose risk increases with use of multiple drugs include cognitive impairment and delirium, falls and hip fractures, and urinary incontinence (35,36). Increased number of prescription medications in community-dwelling women were also associated with greater decline in physical and instrumental activities of daily living (37). Finally, the use of multiple unnecessary drugs increases drug costs.

PRINCIPLES OF GERIATRIC PHARMACOTHERAPY

Multiple medications are a potentially modifiable risk factor. The following reviews some principles to improve polypharmacy and reduce its negative consequences (38).

The first priority in prescribing is to complete a thorough medication history. Asking the patient to bring in all prescription and nonprescription medications to each office visit will aid in this. The provider must then decide whether new drug therapy is necessary. Many medical problems in the elderly do not require a pharmacological solution, or the risks associated with drug therapy outweigh potential benefits. Once a drug is determined to be necessary, providers need to consider the drug's pharmacokinetics and side effect profile and the patient's renal and hepatic function for proper dosing. Most often, starting doses in the elderly are reduced, and many medications must be given in extended intervals to prevent toxicity from occurring. Providers should also become experts in prescribing a few drugs to manage common problems in the elderly. Other comorbid conditions and medications also need to be taken into account to avoid drug–disease or drug–drug interactions. Screening for drug–drug and drug–disease interactions before prescribing will help to reduce adverse outcomes. There are a number of software packages available (e.g., ePocrates®, Micromedex®) to aid clinicians in assessing drug–drug and drug–disease interactions (39,40). Limiting the prescribing of "prn" drugs and considering medications that can be dosed once or twice daily will help to enhance adherence. Educating both patients and their families verbally and in writing about their medications can improve adherence. Considering generic options, utilizing compliance aids (e.g., pill boxes, medication calendars), and encouraging family support can help to improve medication adherence (41–43). Establishment of clear and reasonable therapeutic endpoints and periodic review of medications are also important.

SUMMARY

Polypharmacy is a common phenomenon in older persons. Multiple drug use can increase the risk of negative patient health outcomes. Otolaryngologists need to be aware of these issues when dealing with older patients and adhere to the principles of geriatric pharmacotherapy when prescribing.

REFERENCES

1. Stewart RB. Polypharmacy in the elderly: A fait accompli? DICP 1990; 24:321–323.
2. Stewart RB, Cooper JW. Polypharmacy in the aged: practical solutions. Drugs Aging 1994; 4:449–461.
3. Nolan L, O'Malley K. Prescribing for the elderly: Part II. Prescribing patterns: differences due to age. J Am Geriatr Soc 1988; 36:245–254.
4. Hanlon JT, Fillenbaum GG, Burchett B, et al. Drug-use patterns among black and nonblack community dwelling elderly. Ann Pharmacother 1992; 26:679–685.
5. Stoehr GP, Ganguli M, Seaberg EC, Echement DA, Belle S. Over-the-counter medication use in an older rural community: the MoVIES project. J Am Geriatr Soc 1997; 45: 158–165.
6. Kaufman DW, Kelly JP, Rosenberg L, Anderson TE, Mitchell AA. Recent patterns of medication use in the ambulatory adult population of the United States: the Slone survey. JAMA 2002; 287:337–344.
7. Linjakumpu T, Hartikainen S, Klaukka T, Veijola J. Use of medications and polypharmacy are increasing among the elderly. J Clin Epidemiol 2002; 55:809–817.
8. Montamat SC, Cusack B. Overcoming problems with polypharmacy and drug misuse on the elderly. Clin Geriatr Med 1992; 8:143–158.
9. Lipton HL, Bero LA, Bird JA, McPhee SJ. The impact of clinical pharmacists' consultations on physicians' geriatric drug prescribing. A randomized controlled trial. Med Care 1992; 30:646–658.
10. Schmader K, Hanlon JT, Weinberger M, et al. Appropriateness of medication prescribing in ambulatory patients. J Am Geriatr Soc 1994; 42:1241–1247.
11. Schmader KE, Hanlon JT, Pieper CF, et al. Effectiveness of geriatric evaluation and management on adverse drug reactions and suboptimal prescribing in the frail elderly. Am J Med 2004; 116:394–401.
12. Gurwitz JH, Field TS, Harrold LR, et al. Incidence and preventability of adverse drug events among older persons in the ambulatory setting. JAMA 2003; 289:1107–1116.
13. Chrischilles EA, Foley DJ, Wallace RB, et al. Use of medications by persons 65 and over: data from the established populations for epidemiologic studies of the elderly. J Gerontol 1992; 47:M137–M144.
14. Fillenbaum GG, Horner RD, Hanlon JT, Landerman LR, Dawson DV, Cohen HJ. Factors predicting change in the prescription and nonprescription drug use in a community-residing black and white elderly population. J Clin Epidemiol 1996; 49:587–593.
15. Espino DV, Lichtenstein MJ, Hazuda HP, et al. Correlates of prescription and over-the-counter medication usage among older Mexican Americans: the Hispanic EPESE study. J Am Geriatr Soc 1998; 46:1228–1234.
16. Venulet J, Ham MT. Methods for monitoring and documenting adverse drug reactions. J Clin Pharmacol 1996; 34:112–129.

17. Hanlon JT, Schmader KE, Gray S. Adverse drug reactions. In: Delafuente JC, Stewart RB, eds. Therapeutics in the elderly. 3rd ed. Cincinnati: Harvey Whitney Books, 2000:289–314.
18. Gray SL, Mahoney JE, Blough DK. Adverse drug events in elderly patients receiving home health services following hospital discharge. Ann Pharmacother 1999; 33: 1147–1153.
19. Grymonpre RE, Mitenko PA, Sitar DS, Aoki FY, Montgomery PR. Drug-associated hospital admissions in older medical patients. J Am Geriatr Soc 1988; 36:1092–1098.
20. Nolan L, O'Malley K. Prescribing for the elderly. Part I: Sensitivity of the elderly to adverse drug reactions. J Am Geriatr Soc 1988; 36:142–149.
21. Hanlon JT, Artz MB, Pieper CF, et al. Inappropriate medication use among frail elderly inpatients. Ann Pharmacother 2004; 38:9–14.
22. Seymour RM, Routledge PA. Important drug–drug interactions in the elderly. Drugs Aging 1998; 12:485–494.
23. Guay DRP, Artz MB, Hanlon JT, Schmader KE. The pharmacology of aging. In: Tallis RC, Fillit HM, eds. Brocklehurst's Textbook of Geriatric Medicine and Gerontology. 6th ed. London. U.K.: Churchill Livingstone, 2003:155–161.
24. Hansten PD, Horn JR. Drug interactions analysis and management. Facts and comparisons. St. Louis, Mo., 2002.
25. Weiner D, Hanlon JT, Studenski S. CNS drug related falls liability in community dwelling elderly. Gerontology 1998; 44:217–221.
26. Fick DM, Cooper JW, Wade WE, Waller JL, Maclean R, Beers MH. Updating the Beers criteria for potentially inappropriate medication use in older adults. Arch Intern Med 2003; 163:2716–2724.
27. McLeod PJ, Huang AR, Tamblyn RM, Gayton DC. Defining inappropriate practices in prescribing for elderly people: a national consensus panel. CMAJ 1997; 156:385–391.
28. Tune LE. Anticholinergic effects of medication in elderly patients. J Clin Psychiatry 2001; 62(S 21):11–14.
29. Lewis IK, Hanlon JT, Hobbins MJ, Beck JD. Use of medications with potential oral adverse drug reactions in community-dwelling elderly. Spec Care Dent 1993; 14:171–176.
30. Shorr RI, Griffin MR, Daugherty JR, Ray WA. Opioid analgesics and the risk of hip fractures in the elderly: codeine and propoxyphene. J Gerontol 1992; 47:M111–M115.
31. Ryan AA. Medication compliance and older people: a review of the literature. Int J Nurs Stud 1999; 36:153–162.
32. Lipton HL, Bird JA. The impact of clinical pharmacists' consultations on geriatric patients' compliance and medical care use: a randomized controlled trial. Gerontologist 1994; 34:307–315.
33. Benner JS, Glynn RJ, Mogun H, Neumann PJ, Weinstein MC, Avorn J. Long term persistence in the use of statin therapy in elderly patients. JAMA 2002; 288:455–461.
34. German PS, Klein LE, McPhee SJ, Smith CR. Knowledge of and compliance with drug regimens in the elderly. J Am Geriatr Soc 1982; 30:568–571.
35. Larson EB, Kukall WA, Buchner D, Reifler BV. Adverse drug reactions associated with global cognitive impairment in elderly persons. Ann Intern Med 1987; 107:169–173.
36. Hogan DB. Revisiting the O complex: urinary incontinence, delirium, and polypharmacy in elderly patients. Can Med Assoc J 1997; 157:1071–1077.
37. Magaziner J, Cadigan DA, Fedder DO, Hebel JR. Medication use and functional decline among community dwelling older women. J Aging Health 1989; 1:470–484.
38. Hanlon JT, Lindblad CI, Maher R, Schmader KE. Geriatric pharmacotherapy. In: Tallis R, Fillit H, eds. Brocklehurst's textbook of geriatric medicine. 6th ed. London, U.K.: Churchill Livingstone, 2003:1289–1296.
39. Micromedex. (Accessed December 12, 2003 at: http://www.micromedex.com/.)
40. ePocrates. (Accessed December 12, 2003 at: http://www.epocrates.com/index.do.)

41. Murray MD, Darnell J, Weinberger M, Martz BL. Factors contributing to medication noncompliance in elderly public housing tenants. Drug Intell Clin Pharm 1986; 20:146–152.
42. Murray MD, Birt JA, Manatunga AK, Darnell JC. Medication compliance in elderly outpatients using twice-daily dosing and unit-of-use packaging. Ann Pharmacother 1993; 27:616–621.
43. Cramer JA. Enhancing patient compliance in the elderly: role of packaging aids and monitoring. Drugs Aging 1998; 12:7–15.

61

Preoperative Evaluation

Christopher D. Newell
Department of Anesthesia and Perioperative Medicine, Oregon Health and Science University, Portland, Oregon, U.S.A.

INTRODUCTION

The preoperative care of patients is crucial in optimizing perioperative outcomes. Evaluation of patients by history, physical examination, and review of medical records is the first step in this process. This information can be used to determine if further diagnostic tests are needed and to adjust medical therapy. An important part of the preoperative evaluation is assessing the patients' surgical and anesthetic risks, as this is critical in decision making regarding which procedure, if any, is best for the patient. Geriatric patients coming for surgery are a heterogeneous group, but a number of important generalizations can be made. As patients age, the incidence of concomitant illness increases (individuals older than 65 have on average 3.5 medical diseases) as functional reserves decrease (1). This chapter covers important preoperative considerations by organ system, guidelines for ordering diagnostic tests, and risk stratification.

CARDIOVASCULAR SYSTEM

Special attention must be paid here; cardiovascular complications are serious and concerns about cardiovascular disease are one of the most common causes of delays and cancellations of surgery. Aging causes structural changes to the heart: conducting tissue degeneration, calcification of valves, and ventricular hypertrophy (2). Peripheral vascular resistance and blood pressure increase because of arterial stiffening. Maximum obtainable heart rate, oxygen consumption, and ejection fraction all progressively decline with age. All of these changes put the elderly patient at risk for complications such as congestive heart failure (CHF), myocardial ischemia, and arrhythmias.

Despite all this, advanced age is a minor clinical predictor of increased perioperative cardiovascular risk. The major clinical predictors are recent myocardial infarction (<1 month), unstable angina, decompensated CHF, significant arrhythmias, and severe valvular disease (3). Exercise tolerance has been found to be an important determinant of perioperative risk. Poor exercise tolerance (could not walk four blocks and climb two flights of stairs) has been shown to independently predict complications with an odds ratio of 1.94 (4). In this study, the chance of a serious

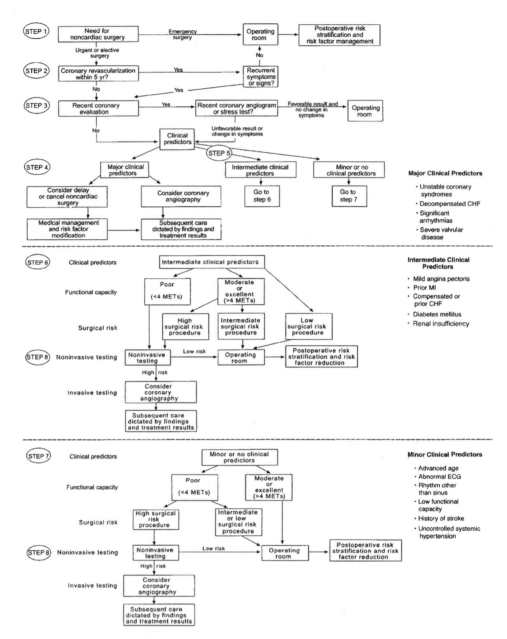

Figure 1 Stepwise approach to preoperative cardiac assessment. Steps are discussed in text. *Subsequent care may include cancellation or delay of surgery, coronary revascularization followed by noncardiac surgery, or intensified care. *Source*: From Ref. 3.

adverse event was inversely related to the number of blocks that could be walked. Indeed, functional capacity is a key element of the guidelines recently published by the American College of Cardiology/American Heart Association (ACC/ AHA) Task Force on Perioperative Evaluation of Cardiac Patients Undergoing Noncardiac Surgery (Fig. 1) (3). The majority of ear, nose, and throat (ENT) procedures would fall into intermediate or low surgical risk categories. Using this algorithm, most ENT patients without major clinical predictors who had adequate exercise tolerance could proceed to surgery without further workup. Park (5) pointed out in a review of these guidelines that the use of beta-blockers has not been taken into consideration. A number of studies have shown that beta-blockers can reduce the perioperative risk of cardiovascular complications, yet they remain underutilized (6–8).

Hypertension is a frequently encountered problem in the preoperative evaluation, and much debate remains about how high is too high. Poorly treated or untreated hypertension leads to intravascular volume contraction, labile blood pressure intraoperatively, and concerns that this will increase complications. Patients with evidence of end-organ changes (renal insufficiency of left ventricular hypertrophy) or pressures greater than 180/110 should have surgery delayed for further treatment (9).

PULMONARY SYSTEM

Aging causes structural changes in the lungs, leading to decreased lung elasticity, chest wall compliance, and mucociliary clearance. Physiologic changes include decreased respiratory drive, increased dead space, and increased ventilation to perfusion mismatching (2). The alveolar-to-arterial gradient for oxygen widens by approximately 4 mmHg per decade of life (10). Elderly patients are at increased risk perioperatively for apnea, hypoxemia, hypercarbia, aspiration, and pneumonia.

A careful assessment of the patients' current pulmonary function and any preexisting pulmonary diseases, such as asthma, chronic obstructive pulmonary disease, or sleep apnea, will dictate preoperative therapy. Patients with underlying respiratory infections should be treated with antibiotics, and surgery should be delayed. Some patients may benefit from the perioperative use of bronchodilators and/or steroids (11). Smoking cessation for 24 hours will decrease methemoglobin and carboxyhemoglobin levels and increase oxygenation, but it also leads to decreased mucociliary clearance (9). Studies suggest that smoking cessation for greater than six weeks is required to improve perioperative risks (12).

ENDOCRINE SYSTEM

The incidence of diabetes increases with age, and the development of end-organ damage is a function of the duration of the disease. Management of the diabetic patient in the perioperative period is worthy of its own chapter. These patients are at increased risk of silent myocardial ischemia, hypoglycemia, hyperglycemia, and have greater hemodynamic lability secondary to autonomic dysfunction (9). There has been a trend in recent years to more tightly control blood glucose management perioperatively. There are various protocols described elsewhere to achieve this, all of which are dependent on the type of diabetes and the patient's current medications.

Age has a variable role in diseases of the thyroid, parathyroid, and adrenal and pituitary glands, much of which may be related to an increase of specific diseases over a lifetime (2). Evaluation should cover the history of the patient's endocrine disease and the type and adequacy of the patient's current therapy.

RENAL SYSTEM

Glomerular filtration rate and creatinine clearance decrease with age as renal function declines. This puts the elderly patient at increased risk for postoperative renal failure (2). Maintaining adequate renal perfusion is essential, but these same patients may not tolerate fluid challenges because of cardiac disease. Patients with chronic renal failure are at increased risk of CHF, hyperkalemia, platelet dysfunction, and anemia. Those patients who require hemodialysis should have their surgical procedures scheduled shortly after dialysis, even though this may leave them hypovolemic. Dealing with this hypovolemia perioperatively is much simpler than having a volume-overloaded patient who is anuric.

NERVOUS SYSTEM

Neurologic function declines with age, affecting memory, coordination, sensory functions, intellectual activity, and autonomic responses (2). For many of these reasons, elderly patients are at increased risk of postoperative delirium (13). Those patients with a history of stroke are also at increased risk of a perioperative stroke. Similar to a history of recent myocardial infarction, recent cerebral ischemia may be a relative contraindication to surgery. Evaluation should include baseline neurologic deficits in order to compare any changes postoperatively (9).

NUTRITION

Nutritional depletion is a frequent problem in elderly patients and can lead to problems with wound healing, infection, and recovery from surgery (14). Preoperative evaluation should include an assessment of nutritional status to help guide plans for perioperative nutritional supplementation. Patients with compromised nutritional status ($>10\%$ weight loss and serum albumin $<2.5\,\mathrm{g/dL}$) should be considered for 7–10 days of nutritional repletion (preferably enteral) prior to surgery (15).

PREOPERATIVE TESTING

The purpose of preoperative laboratory testing is to guide clinical decision making, thereby optimizing patient outcome. No test is 100% sensitive and specific, and the test must be interpreted in the context of the clinical situation. Bayes' theorem implies that a test is most useful in a population with a moderate probability of disease (16). A positive test in a population with a very low prevalence of disease is likely a false positive, whereas a negative test in a population with a very high prevalence of disease is likely a false negative. It must also be remembered that "normal" reference ranges are based on 95% confidence intervals, such that 5% of normal individuals will fall into the "abnormal" range (9). If you order enough laboratory tests, almost everyone will have an abnormal value. Normal reference ranges are also based on younger patients and may increase the incidence of abnormal results in the geriatric population.

The use of routine preoperative laboratory tests has been discouraged because of concerns about cost and risk versus benefit (17). Routine preoperative laboratory tests are estimated to cost over $30 billion each year in the United States. Several studies have looked at the value of such tests; 60–70% of these tests were not specifically indicated, and only 0.2% might influence perioperative management (18,19). The benefit of routine tests is obviously low, and they are not without risk (20).

Different types of risks have been suggested: invasive tests to follow up on false positive results have associated morbidity and mortality (e.g., coronary angiography complications), medical therapy for abnormal test results is also not without risk (e.g., adverse reaction to potassium replacement), and there are medical–legal risks associated with ignoring abnormal results or not following up on tests that were ordered preoperatively. Instead of routine testing, it is recommended to only order those tests that, given the clinical situation, have a reasonable chance of yielding meaningful results. One should always anticipate test results and have a plan in mind to deal with these results. If a positive or negative test result will have no impact on clinical management, then do not bother ordering the test. The current guidelines for Oregon Health and Science University Pre-Admission Testing Clinic are shown in Table 1. Previous test results from less than six months of the planned procedure are acceptable if the patient's medical condition and treatment have been stable.

Electrocardiogram

Age is frequently used as an indication for electrocardiogram (ECG), but it is difficult to reach a consensus on what age, if any, is most appropriate. Abnormal preoperative ECGs are common in elderly patients, but a recent study found that this was not associated with an increased risk of postoperative cardiac complications (21). Clinical indications for preoperative ECG include known or suspected cardio circulatory disease, respiratory disease, and risk factors for coronary artery disease (22).

Chest Radiograph

Chest radiographs and pulmonary function tests rarely reveal information that would change management in patients without risk factors (11). The most useful information can be gained by history and physical examination. Routine preoperative chest radiographs are not indicated and generally are not covered by medical insurance. Indications include new or changing lung disease and those patients at high risk for pulmonary complications (23).

Hemoglobin

Even in healthy patients, the measurement of hemoglobin preoperatively is reasonable for those procedures with risk of significant blood loss. Patients who are likely to be anemic (hematologic disorder, chemotherapy, renal disease, etc.) and those patients who because of systemic disease will not tolerate anemia should also be tested (9,23). The lowest acceptable hemoglobin preoperatively will be dependent on the patient and the planned procedure. In patients without systemic disease, hemoglobin of 7 g/dL is usually acceptable. Preoperative transfusion should be considered for those patients with coronary artery disease and hemoglobin of less than 10 g/dL (24).

Coagulation Tests

Several different tests are available to assess coagulation function, including prothrombin time, international normalized ratio, partial prothrombin time, platelet count, and bleeding time. Each test has its own advantages and disadvantages and measures different aspects of the coagulation system. Routine testing is not

Table 1 OHSU Preoperative Testing Guidelines

	Hgb/Hct	PT/PTT	Plt	Elect	BUN/Creat	Glucose	SGOT/SPGT	EKG	CXR	hCG	T/S T/C
Age >64	X							X			
Procedure with expected/ possible blood loss	X										X
Cardiovascular disease	X				X			X			
Pulmonary disease	X							X	±		
Hepatic disease	X	X	X				X				
Renal disease	X			X	X						
Bleeding disorder	X	X	X								
Diabetes				X	X	X		±			
Possible pregnancy										X	
Use of diuretics				X	X						
Digoxin				X	X			X			
Steroids				X		X					
Anticoagulants	X	X		X	X						
CNS disease				X	X	X		X			

Tests done within six months prior to surgery may be used in patients whose medical conditions have remained stable during that period, including no changes in relevant medications.

The physician's own judgment is needed regarding patients with diseases not listed in the table.

Symbols: ±, perhaps obtain; X, obtain.

Abbreviations: HGB, hemoglobin; PT, prothrombin time; PTT, partial thromboplastin time; PLT, platelet count; Elect, electrolytes (i.e., sodium, potassium, chloride, carbon dioxide, and proteins); Creat/BUN, creatinine and blood urea nitrogen; SGOT/SGPT, serum glutamic-oxaloacetic transminase and alkaline phosphatase; CXR, chest X ray; ECG, electrocardiogram; hCG, human choriogonadotropin; T/S, T/C, blood typing and screening for unexpected antibodies or type and crossmatch; CNS, central nervous system; OHSU, Oregon Health and Science University.

Source: Modified from Roizen MF. Preoperative evaluation. In: Miller RD, ed. Anesthesia. 5th ed. Chapter 23. Section 3. New York: Churchill Livingston, 2000.

recommended as coagulation tests are only indicated in patients with known or suspected bleeding disorders, hepatic disease, or on anticoagulant medication (23,25).

Serum Chemistries

Serum chemistries are most often ordered as panels and can include electrolytes,
glucose, renal function tests, and liver function tests. Indications include renal
disease, hepatitis, cirrhosis, diabetes, significant cardiovascular disease, and patients
on diuretics, digoxin, or steroids (9).

RISK STRATIFICATION

In determining surgical risk, one must take into account not only the risk of the procedure (and some procedures are clearly riskier than others) but also the risks of
delaying or forgoing the operation. The urgency of the situation must also be considered; emergent surgery has a much higher complication rate than elective surgery
(2). The surgical mortality rate increases with age. In a study comparing surgical
mortality for various operations in older versus younger patients, those patients
<60, 60–69, 70–79, and ≥80 undergoing radical neck dissection had mortality rates
of 0.0%, 2.8%, 5.9%, and 13.6%, respectively (26).

Cardiac complications are frequently life threatening and are the leading
cause of postoperative deaths (9). A variety of indices have been proposed to stratify the risk of cardiac complications. One of the most widely used has been the
Goldman Cardiac Risk Index, which uses a point system to place patients in
one of four risk classes (I–IV) (27). The latest update of the Goldman Cardiac
Risk Index uses six predictors of complications: high-risk type of surgery, history
of ischemic heart disease, history of congestive heart failure, history of cerebrovascular disease, preoperative treatment with insulin, and preoperative serum
creatinine >2 mg/dL. Patients with 0, 1, 2, or ≥3 of these factors had major cardiac complication rates of 0.4–0.5%, 0.9–1.3%, 4–7%, and 9–11%, respectively (28).
The ACC/AHA guidelines are similar but divide patients into three risk groups.
Major clinical predictors are unstable coronary syndromes, decompensated
CHF, significant arrhythmias, or severe valvular disease. Intermediate clinical
predictors are mild angina, prior myocardial infarction (MI), compensated or prior
CHF, diabetes mellitus, or renal insufficiency. Minor clinical predictors include
advanced age, abnormal ECG, rhythm other than sinus, low functional capacity, his-
tory of stroke, or uncontrolled systemic hypertension (3).

Pulmonary complications are the most common form of postoperative morbidity
(29). Age alone is not an independent risk factor for postoperative pulmonary complications, but elderly patients more frequently have cardiopulmonary disease. Chronic lung
disease is the most important predictor of postoperative pulmonary complications (11).
The severity of disease will make a difference in risk. Pulmonary function tests can help
assess the presence and severity of lung disease, but they are generally no more sensitive
or specific than history and physical examination (30). Arterial blood gas measurement
may be useful in identifying those patients with hypercapnia or hypoxia. Patients with
hypercapnia ($PaCO_2$ >45 mmHg) have a higher incidence of postoperative pulmonary
complications, and patients with chronic obstructive pulmonary disease (COPD)
and hypercapnia have a decreased life expectancy (31,32). Arterial hypoxemia
(PaO_2 <50 mmHg) is also associated with increased risks.

CONCLUSION

A thorough history and physical examination preoperatively can be used to identify concomitant disease. Obtaining indicated tests and consultations will add to this information and can then be used to adjust medical therapy as needed, assess surgical risk, and decide on the most appropriate surgical procedure. The goals of preoperative evaluation should be to optimize the patient's condition, avoid unnecessary testing, minimize delays and cancellations of surgery, and minimize perioperative complications.

REFERENCES

1. Muravchick S. Geroanesthesia. Principles for management of the elderly patient. St. Louis: Mosby-Year Book, 1997.
2. McLeskey CH, ed. Geriatric anesthesiology. Baltimore: Williams & Wilkins, 1997.
3. Eagle K, Berger P, Calkins H, et al. ACC/AHA Guideline update for perioperative cardiovascular evaluation for noncardiac surgery—executive summary. Circulation 2002; 105:1257.
4. Reilly DF, McNeely MJ, Doerner D et al. Self-reported exercise tolerance and the risk of serious perioperative complications. Arch Intern Med 1999; 159:2185.
5. Park KW. Preoperative cardiology consultation. Anesthesiology 2003; 98:754.
6. Mangano DT, Layug EI, Wallace A, Tateo I. Multicenter Study of Perioperative Ischemia Research Group. Effect of atenolol on mortality and cardiovascular morbidity after noncardiac surgery. N Engl J Med 1996; 335:1713.
7. Wallace A, Layug B, Tateo I, et al. Prophylatic atenolol reduces postoperative myocardial ischemia. Anesthesiology 1998; 88:7.
8. Poldermans D, Boersma E, Bax JJ, et al. Echocardiographic Cardiac Risk Evaluation Applying Stress Echocardiography Study Group. The effect of bisoprolol on perioperative mortality and myocardial infarction in high-risk patients undergoing vascular surgery. N Engl J Med 1999; 341:1789.
9. Barash PG, Cullen BF, Stoelting RK, ed. Clinical anesthesia (4/e). Philadelphia: Williams & Wilkins, 2001.
10. Sorbini CA, Grassi V, Solinas E, et al. Arterial oxygen tension in relation to age in healthy human subjects. Respiration 1968; 25:3.
11. Doyle RL. Assessing and modifying the risk of postoperative pulmonary complications. Chest 1999; 115:77S.
12. Warner MA, Offord KP, Warner ME, et al. Role of preoperative cessation of smoking and other factors in postoperative pulmonary complications: a blinded prospective study of coronary artery bypass patients. Mayo Clin Proc 1989; 64:609.
13. Marcantonio ER, Goldman L, Mangione CM, et al. A clinical prediction rule for delirium after elective noncardiac surgery. JAMA 1994; 271:134.
14. Corish CA. Preoperative nutritional assessment in the elderly. J Nutr Health Aging 2001; 5:49.
15. McClave SA, Snider HL, Spain DA. Preoperative issues in clinical nutrition. Chest 1999; 115:64S.
16. Shuman P. Bayes' theorem: a review. Cardiol Clin 1984; 2:319.
17. Smetana GW, Macpherson DS. The case against routine preoperative laboratory testing. Med Clin North Am 2003; 87:7.
18. Roizen M. Preoperative patient evaluation. Can J Anaesth 1989; 36:S13.
19. Johnson RK, Mortimer AJ. Routine preoperative blood testing: is it necessary? Anaesthesia 2002; 57:914.

20. Marcello PW, Roberts PL. "Routine" preoperative studies. Which studies in which patients? Surg Clin North Am 1996; 76:11.
21. Liu LL, Dzankic S, Leung JM. Preoperative electrocardiogram abnormalities do not predict postoperative cardiac complications in geriatric surgical patients. J Am Geriatr Soc 2002; 50:1186.
22. Pasternak LR, Arens JF, Caplan RA, et al. Practice advisory for preanesthesia evaluation. Anesthesiology 2002; 96:485.
23. Fischer SP. Cost-effective preoperative evaluation and testing. Chest 1999; 115:96S.
24. Consensus Conference. Perioperative red cell transfusion. JAMA 1988; 260(18): 2700–2703.
25. Ng KF, Lai KW, Tsang SF. Value of preoperative coagulation tests: reappraisal of major noncardiac surgery. World J Surg 2002; 26:515.
26. Ziffren SE, Hartford CE. Comparative mortality for various surgical operations in older versus younger age groups. J Am Geriatr Soc 1972; 20:485.
27. Goldman L, Caldera DL, Nussbaum SR, et al. Multifactorial index of cardiac risk in noncardiac surgical procedures. N Engl J Med 1977; 297:845.
28. Lee TH, Marcantonio ER, Mangione CM, et al. Derivation and prospective validation of a simple index for prediction of cardiac risk of major noncardiac surgery. Circulation 1999; 100:1043.
29. Ferguson MK. Preoperative assessment of pulmonary risk. Chest 1999; 115:58S.
30. Zibrak JD, O'Donnell CR, Marton K. Indications for pulmonary function testing. Ann Intern Med 1990; 112:763.
31. Milledge JS, Nunn JF. Criteria of fitness for anesthesia in patients with chronic obstructive lung disease. BMJ 1975; 3:670.
32. Hodgkin J. Prognosis in chronic obstructive pulmonary disease. Clin Chest Med 1990; 3:555.

62

Anesthesia for Otorhinolaryngologic Surgery in the Elderly

Myrdalis Díaz-Ramírez
Department of Anesthesiology and Perioperative Medicine, Oregon Health and Science University, Portland, Oregon, U.S.A.

INTRODUCTION

Advances in medicine and anesthesiology over the last century have made it more feasible to consider operative intervention in elderly patients for a wide range of disease processes. One-third of all surgical procedures in the United States are performed on patients who are 65 years old or older, with a proportionate number of these performed by otolaryngologists (1). Surgery for extirpation of head and neck cancer is common in the elderly since aging patients have a higher rate of malignancy. Overall, more than one-half of all cancer patients are older than 65 years of age at the time of diagnosis. As this population increases, ever larger numbers of elderly patients will present with diseases that require surgical management. As the number of healthy elderly patients increases, so will the number seeking operative management of diseases affecting their quality of life. Finally, coincident with these increases will be the number of patients presenting with significant comorbid conditions, which will affect both treatment plans and decision making.

The general state of health, as determined by the American Society of Anesthesiologists (ASA) status, is a better predictor of outcomes and complications than chronological age itself (Table 1) (2–4). Two-thirds of patients older than 80 who are undergoing head and neck surgery have coexisting major medical conditions, with ASA classification 3 or 4 in over 40% of these patients (5).

A thorough history and physical examination facilitates the classification of patients and the selection of the optimal anesthetic plan. Discussion between the surgeon and patient's primary physician is often necessary to clarify specific issues. A history of congenital or acquired disease of the airway and coexisting diseases or conditions may determine anesthetic choice. Physiological changes occurring naturally in this population may be as important as comorbidities in directing modification of the anesthetic plan. Physical examination should include a detailed exam of the upper airway, and radiological studies need to be reviewed in detail.

Discussion between the surgeon and the anesthesiologist is pivotal in preparation for the anesthetic since access to the airway will often be shared. Issues of access,

Table 1   Standard ASA Patient Classification

ASA 1—a normal healthy patient

ASA 2—a patient with a mild systemic disease, for example, well controlled asthmatic, hypertensive, or diabetic patient

ASA 3—a patient with a severe disease that limits activity but is not incapacitating, for example, uncontrolled hypertension

ASA 4—a patient with an incapacitating systemic disease that is a constant threat to life, for example, active congestive heart failure

ASA 5—a moribund patient not expected to survive 24 hours with or without operation, for example, post-trauma patient with dilated and fixed pupils

The letter *E* can be used to specify emergency surgical procedure. It is added to any level on the classification.

Abbreviation: ASA, American Society of Anesthesiologists

tracheal displacement, patient positioning, sequence of surgical events, and use of specific medications (muscle relaxants, nitrous oxide) need to be addressed preoperatively. Checklists and other "memory tricks" are useful to facilitate this discussion, and are particularly valuable in the absence of a long history of cooperation.

PHYSIOLOGIC CHANGES IN THE ELDERLY AND COMMON COMORBIDITIES

Cardiovascular System

The prevalence of cardiovascular disease is as high as 50–65% in the elderly (6,7). It is often asymptomatic, increasing the risk for potential unidentified serious comorbidities. Elderly patients demonstrate diminished elasticity of blood vessels with a higher predisposition to atherosclerosis and reduced cardiac and arterial compliance. Ventricular hypertrophy and calcification of cardiac valves will be more common. They will also have a relatively depressed autonomic nervous system with diminished beta-adrenergic responsiveness. This leads to decreased maximal cardiac output and heart rate, as well as decreased response to adrenergic agents. Over 20% of head and neck patients have been reported to have cardiac disease, and nearly 14% will have a history of myocardial infarction (2,8). Given the prevalence of cardiac comorbidities in this age group, it is important that an adequate preoperative evaluation and patient stabilization be performed. The American College of Cardiology/ American Heart Association Task Force on Practice Guidelines developed the 1996 guidelines on perioperative cardiovascular evaluation for noncardiac surgery (9). This task force identified a series of clinical predictors of increased perioperative cardiovascular risk (Table 2). Although age was identified as a minor factor, the group defined head and neck surgery as intermediate cardiac risk. The detailed algorithm for preoperative evaluation developed is shown in Figure 1. Cardiovascular stabilization should be achieved preoperatively for any elective procedure.

Respiratory System

Pulmonary disease that may not be clinically evident prior to surgery may become significant during and following anesthesia. Pulmonary elasticity, alveolar surface area, and forced expiratory volume in 1 second (FEV_1) are diminished in the elderly.

Table 2 Clinical Predictors of Increased Perioperative Cardiovascular Risk (Myocardial Infarction, Heart Failure, Death)

Major

Unstable coronary syndromes
- Acute or recent MI[a] with evidence of important ischemic risk by clinical symptoms or noninvasive study
- Unstable or severe[b] angina (Canadian Class III or IV)[c]

Decompensated heart failure

Significant arrhythmias
- High-grade atrioventricular block
- Symptomatic ventricular arrhythmias in the presence of underlying heart disease
- Supraventricular arrhythmias with uncontrolled ventricular rate

Severe valvular disease

Intermediate

Mild angina pectoris (Canadian Class I or II)

Previous MI by history or pathological Q waves

Compensated or prior heart failure

Diabetes mellitus (particularly insulin-dependent)

Renal insufficiency

Minor

Advanced age

Abnormal ECG (left ventricular hypertrophy, left bundle-branch block, ST-T abnormalities)

Rhythm other than sinus (e.g., atrial fibrillation)

Low functional capacity (e.g., inability to climb one flight of stairs with a bag of groceries)

History of stroke

Uncontrolled systemic hypertension

---

[a]The American College of Cardiology National Database Library defines recent MI as greater than 7 days, but less than, or equal to 1 month (30 days); acute MI is within 7 days.
[b]May include "stable" angina in patients who are unusually sedentary.
[c]Campeau L. Grading of angina pectoris. Circulation. 1976; 54:522–523.
Abbreviations: ECG, electrocardiogram; MI, myocardial infarction.
Source: From the ACC/AHA Guideline Update for Perioperative Cardiovascular Evaluation for Noncardiac Surgery. A Report of the American College of Cardiology/American Heart Association Task Force on Practice Guidelines (Committee to Update the 1996 Guidelines on Perioperative Cardiovascular Evaluation for Noncardiac Surgery).

There is increased thoracic stiffness, residual volume, and alveolar and anatomic dead space (10). These changes result in decreased vital capacity and increased effort and work of breathing. Gas exchange will be impaired due to ventilation–perfusion mismatch. Arterial oxygenation decreases as we age; hence, supplemental oxygen is employed routinely in the perioperative period. Pulmonary comorbidities may require further workup and stabilization prior to surgery. These include chronic heavy smoking, chronic obstructive pulmonary disease (COPD), obstructive sleep apnea, and respiratory tract infections. Cigarette smoking and pack-years smoked have been identified as among the most important factors in the development of postoperative pulmonary complications. McCulloch et al. (11) noted that 15% of head and neck patients in their series developed pulmonary postoperative complications, including pneumonia, adult respiratory distress syndrome, and inability to wean off the ventilator. Functional status has been identified as an important predictor of these postoperative complications.

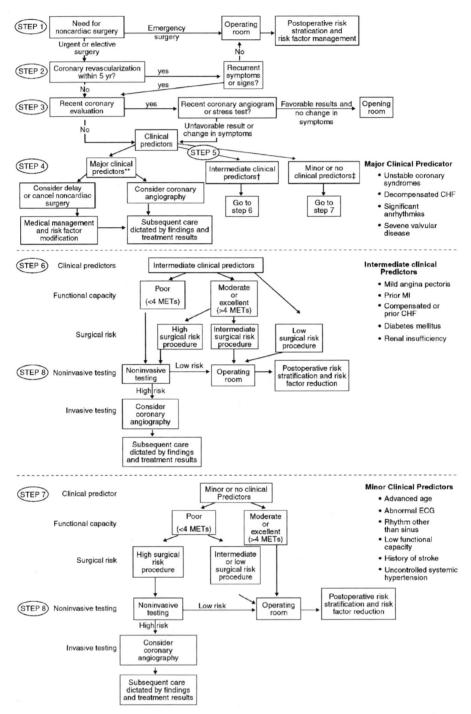

Figure 1 Stepwise approach to preoperative cardiac assessment. *Source*: From the ACC/AHA Guideline Update for Perioperative Cardiovascular Evaluation for Noncardiac Surgery. A Report of the American College of Cardiology/American Heart Association Task Force on Practice Guidelines (Committee to Update the 1996 Guidelines on Perioperative Cardiovascular Evaluation for Noncardiac Surgery).

Central and Peripheral Nervous System

Progressive loss of neurons, diminished central neurotransmitter activity, and deafferentation contribute to an increased sensitivity to administered anesthetic agents; hence, anesthetic requirements diminish in the elderly (12). The decrease in neuronal density that occurs with age is accompanied by a reduction in cerebral blood flow and cerebral oxygen consumption. Aging also results in decreased neural plasticity and impaired autonomic homeostasis. On the other hand, response to blood pressure, CO_2, O_2, and cerebral autoregulation is unchanged when compared with younger patients. A decline in serotonin receptors, acetylcholine, acetylcholine receptors, and dopamine in several regions of the brain occurs. Sleep is usually affected with a decrease in slow-wave, or delta, sleep, which is the most restoring and deepest level of sleep. Memory and reasoning performance are decreased with advancing age. Conditions like cerebral arteriosclerosis, Alzheimer's disease, and Parkinson's disease are more common with aging. These diseases, along with polypharmacy and drug interactions, alcohol–sedative–hypnotic withdrawal, endocrine and metabolic problems, depression, pre-existing dementia, anxiety, perioperative hypoxia, hypocarbia, and sepsis can contribute to postoperative delirium (13). Assessment of mental status, medications, and pre-existing motor or sensory deficits is important in the prevention or diagnosis of postoperative central nervous system (CNS) and peripheral nervous system complications.

Thermoregulation

Thermoregulation is impaired in the elderly, especially in those older than 80 years of age, due to an impaired ability to vasoconstrict and shiver (14). The threshold for heat conservation is at a lower temperature than the younger population, so heat loss to the environment will also be greater. In addition older patients have an impaired ability to produce and maintain heat, so their ability to tolerate cold declines. The risk of hypothermia enhances drug effects on the thermoregulatory response. These effects are even greater in the presence of the delayed drug metabolism that accompanies normal aging.

Intraoperative hypothermia also increases the risk of wound infection and delayed healing, prolongs bleeding due to alteration of platelets and the coagulation cascade, reduces drugs clearance, and increases the risk of myocardial infarction. Maintenance of normothermia before, during, and after the procedure is critical and is achieved by a variety of techniques, including warming of inhaled gases, fluids, and room and the use of convection and direct heating blankets.

Renal System

Decreased drug clearance and difficulty tolerating salt or water loads are a result of decreased renal vascularity, perfusion, and loss of renal tissue mass (1). Approximately 30% of the renal mass is lost by the eighth decade, and up to half of the glomeruli may be absent or nonfunctional by that age. Total renal blood flow decreases 10% per decade in adults. Aging results in reduced response to antidiuretic hormone and reduced maximal absorption rate for glucose. There is an increased risk of renal ischemia. Acute renal failure is associated with more than one-fifth of perioperative deaths among elderly surgical patients. Intraoperative monitoring of fluid and electrolyte balance is required to prevent acute renal failure. Medications that are excreted through the kidneys will demonstrate prolonged clearance, with signs of prolonged effects or toxicity at doses that would be normal in a young healthy patient.

Hepatic System

Liver mass decreases with aging, and hepatic blood flow decreases in proportion to the decrease in tissue mass. The pharmacokinetics of hepatically metabolized drugs will be altered in the elderly. Hepatic drug metabolism is primarily mediated by the cytochrome P (450) system, which progressively declines after the fifth decade (15). Drug elimination will also be diminished due to the changes in hepatic blood flow. Many commonly used anesthetics, like opioids, barbiturates, benzodiazepines, propofol, and etomidate, and most nondepolarizing relaxants are affected.

A history of alcoholism will be present in up to 35% of the patients undergoing otolaryngologic surgery. These patients may demonstrate a paradoxical response to administered agents. In the chronic alcoholic, the minimum alveolar concentration (MAC) of anesthetic gases must be *increased* due to hepatic enzyme induction and more rapid metabolism. However, in the setting of *acute* alcohol consumption, a *decrease* in required anesthetic gas concentration is to be expected. Chronic alcohol use is often associated with nutritional depletion. Malnutrition with reduced hepatic function can decrease drug metabolism. Reduced levels of serum albumin accompany malnutrition and are associated with an increased rate of major postoperative complications. The nutritional status of the patient should be addressed and treated aggressively in the preoperative period prior to elective surgery.

Hematopoietic System

Aging seems to have minimal influence on available red blood cell mass, white blood cell count, the number or function of platelets, or coagulation, despite resorption of bone marrow (6). Loss of myeloid function will, however, lead to diminished immune competence and loss of hematopoietic reserve, manifested by reduced ability to respond to anemia. Involution of thymic tissue does not seem to be associated with a significant impact on the neuroendocrine response to stress.

Musculoskeletal System

Skeletal muscle and other lean tissue components are lost during aging, simultaneously with increases in the lipid fraction (16). This contributes to prolonged drug effects, reduced metabolism, and heat production, as well as a diminished resting cardiac output. This population will also demonstrate an increased incidence of multiple types of arthritis, such as rheumatoid, psoriatic, degenerative, and ankylosing spondylitis. The presence of any of these can interfere with anesthetic management, especially airway management due to decreased cervical spine range of motion or mouth opening.

Head and Neck

Loss of vision and hearing can result in perioperative difficulties, particularly in communication with patients (17). Elderly patients undergoing surgical procedures will typically be instructed to leave their glasses and hearing aids with relatives for safe keeping. Despite this fact, no difficulties with communication were noted in the preoperative evaluation, yet the same patient may present a significant problem in the OR holding area! Visual acuity is diminished and blindness will be increased. Presbyopia and lens opacification contribute to increased sensitivity to glare and decreased accommodation.

Presbycusis is the most common auditory dysfunction of the elderly. When severe, it will impair communication and can lead to social and emotional disturbances. Physiological changes result in decreased high-frequency acuity, making it difficult to discriminate words from background noise, such as in the operating room prior to induction. Appropriate accommodations, such as reduction of background noise, speaking face to face, and speaking loudly, can reduce the risk of poor communication.

PREOPERATIVE EVALUATION AND TREATMENT

During the preoperative evaluation of an elderly patient, a thorough medical history, physical exam, necessary laboratory testing, and imaging studies will be performed and reviewed, as in the case for surgery in younger patients (6). In the event of an emergency procedure, sufficient time to obtain all the desired information may not be available. Decisions must be made based on multiple assumptions, utilizing available personal information and expected aging changes.

Medical History

A review of care, medications taken, and allergies is key in the history of a patient scheduled for surgery. A history of problems with previous anesthetics is obtained, both for the patient as well as the immediate family. The patient's level of function and comorbidities are reviewed as well as the use of any assistive devices or existing implants. The initial interview dictates the rest of the examination.

Physical Examination

A basic examination would include determination of arterial blood pressure, auscultation of lungs and heart, and examination of pulses. Assessment of the patient's general heath, neurological function, extremities, and skin is obtained as well.

A thorough evaluation of the airway is always of main importance in the preanesthetic evaluation. Its importance increases even more when surgery of this part of the body is contemplated. The basic evaluation of the airway has been described as having 11 main components, listed in Table 3 (18). Suboptimal findings that predict a difficult airway include a Mallampati score greater than 2, a highly arched or very narrow palate, a noncompliant mandibular space, a short or thick neck, less than three fingerbreadths on thyromental distance, decreased cervical range of motion, or less then 3 cm of interincision distance. The presence of a congenital syndrome (craniofacial dysostoses), a beard, facial scars, facial injuries, facial dressings, absence of teeth, obesity, acromegaly, and gastric reflux can also indicate a potential problem with airway management.

Preoperative Testing

An extensive literature addressing the requirements for preoperative testing exists, and controversy and local practice variation persist. A task force of the American

Table 3 Practice Guidelines for Sedation and Analgesia by Non-anesthesiologists

- Pre-procedure evaluation with history, physical examination, and appropriate laboratory testing required
- Pre-operative patient optimization performed
- Full discussion of procedure, alternatives, risks, and questions by the patient answered
- Follow pre-procedure fasting ASA guidelines
- Follow monitoring as per ASA recommendations
- Personnel:
  - Individual, other than the practitioner performing the procedure, present to monitor the patient throughout the procedure
    - Trained in basic and advanced life support
    - Knowledgeable in pharmacology of sedatives and analgesics
    - Able to assist in minor interruptible tasks only if patient is stable
- Intravenous equipment, pharmacologic antagonists, and basic resuscitative medications
  - Oxygen and defibriliator immediately available
  - Agents chosen should include analgesics and sedatives, mostly administered intravenously
  - Agents chosen should be carefully titrated to effect
  - Reversal agents should be available
- Emergency Equipment
  - Suction, appropriately sized airway equipment, means of positive-pressure ventilation
- Post-Anesthesia Care Unit
  - Observation area available
  - Patients to be discharged once stable and no risk of cardiopulmonary depression
- Complex cases to be done under the care of an anesthesiologist

Source: A report by the American Society of Anesthesiologists Task Force on Sedation and Analgesia by Non-Anesthesiologists. Anesthesiology 1996; 84:459–71.

Society of Anesthesiologists has made recommendations for routine preoperative evaluation in order to standardize practices (19). A summary of these recommendations follows.

Electrocardiogram—It is agreed that an electrocardiogram may be indicated for patients with known cardiovascular risk factors or for patients with risk factors identified in the course of a preanesthesia evaluation. However, no consensus was obtained as to the minimal age at which a routine ECG should be obtained prior to surgery. It is understood, though, that the elderly population is at increased risk for cardiovascular disease; hence, an ECG is considered to be routine.

Chest roentgenogram (CXR) and other pulmonary evaluation—The routine requirement for a CXR should be based on a history of smoking, recent upper respiratory infection, unstable chronic obstructive pulmonary disease, and cardiac disease. Additional pulmonary testing should be based on the type and invasiveness of the surgical procedure, interval from previous evaluation, and the presence of symptomatic asthma, COPD, or scoliosis with restrictive function. Most centers set a minimum cut-off age for the obtaining of a CXR; hence, one is obtained routinely in the elderly preoperative patient.

Hemoglobin or hematocrit—Either extreme of age is an indication for routine determination. Other factors will be type and invasiveness of procedure, presence of liver disease, a history of anemia, bleeding, and other hematologic disorders.

Coagulation function—Studies have demonstrated that a history is reliable in the identification of patients who are at increased risk of bleeding. The routine obtaining of a coagulation profile is therefore not recommended. Patients with a history of bleeding disorders, renal or liver dysfunction, exposure to medications that affect coagulation, or in whom significant blood loss is anticipated should undergo preoperative determinations.

Serum chemistries—The recommendations are to base preoperative determinations on likely perioperative therapies, endocrine disorders, risk of renal and liver dysfunction, and use of certain medications or alternative therapies. Nonetheless, preoperative values are known to vary at the extremes of age.

Urinalysis—It is only indicated with the suspicion of urinary tract infection or specific urologic procedures.

An in-depth preoperative evaluation is routinely obtained for patients undergoing head and neck surgery. The evaluation may include anatomical and function studies such as computed tomography (CT) scans, magnetic resonance imaging, high-resolution magnetic resonance imaging, functional magnetic resonance (fMR) imaging, single photon emission computed tomography (SPECT), and positron emission tomography. The anesthesiologist may need to review the available studies and discuss the plan for airway access and maintenance with the surgeon. Anatomical and functional derangements identified can significantly impact on airway strategies in anesthetic planning.

Premedication

The need for specific premedication will be primarily determined by the pre-existing comorbidities and level of anxiety regarding the procedure. The optimal treatment for anxiety is a full discussion with the patient, including appropriate details about the procedure, alternatives, and risks and answering any specific questions the patient might have. A short-acting benzodiazepine, such as midazolam, can be administered in titrated doses as a specific pharmacological treatment for anxiety. The risks and benefits of these medications should be considered individually in any specific case to avoid prolonged postoperative sedation due to the delayed metabolism associated with aging. Antiemetic prophylaxis, antireflux prophylaxis, B-blockers for chronic hypertensive patients, beta agonists for patients with COPD, and anti-inflammatories for post-operative pain control should also be considered in selected patients.

INTRAOPERATIVE CARE

Positioning

The patient's head will typically be positioned away from the anesthesiologist's reach during head and neck surgery. Special attention to positioning is made *before* final draping is performed. The eyes are protected to prevent possible trauma, either from physiologic, chemical, or mechanical damage (20). The head is positioned to avoid extremes of torsion, flexion, or extension in order to diminish the likelihood of injuries to the cerebral circulation system and spine. The arms must be padded and positioned at less than 90° to reduce the risk of brachial plexus injury. Pressure points are carefully padded. The intravenous access and monitors are placed in a position accessible to the anesthesiologist. The responsibility for positioning is shared, and both the surgeon and anesthesiologist must ensure that any pressure points are adequately protected. Access to the airway should be considered during positioning, particularly since both surgeon and anesthesiologist may share in this responsibility as well.

Monitoring

Intraoperative monitoring should include standard ASA monitors. This implies the presence of an anesthesia machine, fully checked, with a ventilator. It also includes pulse oximeter, stethoscope, alarm system, and monitors for inspired oxygen, end-tidal carbon dioxide, respiratory rate, heart rate, blood pressure, motor blockade, and temperature. The need for further invasive monitoring will depend on type of procedure and coexisting disease. For example, one may consider the use of spirometer, arterial blood gas tension, central venous pressure, and arterial blood pressure measurement in a patient with moderate pulmonary disease. The use of specific intraoperative monitoring for head and neck surgery may require different equipment that will impact the anesthetic plans. Evoked facial nerve monitoring may be necessary to help preserve facial nerve integrity during surgery in the mastoid/temporal bone area (21). Intermediate or long-acting muscle relaxants must not be used in these patients. Communication between surgeon and anesthesiologist is necessary.

Anesthetic Drugs

Pharmacokinetic and pharmacodynamic changes in the elderly are multifactorial. Reduction in lean body mass and cardiac output, decrease in metabolism and excretion of metabolites, and loss of brain neurons contribute to these changes (22). These changes affect some of the most common anesthetic drugs like hypnotics, volatile anesthetics, and opioid analgesics when used in elderly patients. Several studies have shown that the dosage of hypnotics required to achieve a loss of consciousness and slowing of the EEG is reduced in the elderly (23–25). Martin noted diminished drug requirement with increasing age with *all* the commonly administered anesthetic medications. Age affected the amount of drug required for anesthesia in patients older than 40–45 years of age (26).

Inhaled Anesthetics

Age seems to have minimal effect on the *pharmacokinetic* behavior of volatile inhalational anesthetics. Reductions in concentrations required are due to age-related alterations in *pharmacodynamics*. MAC is the alveolar partial pressure of gas at which 50% of humans will not move in response to a surgical skin incision. A decrease in MAC with increasing age has been observed for all the volatile drugs (27).

Of particular importance is the use of nitrous oxide in the trauma patient and the patient undergoing ear surgery. Nitrous enters a closed space more rapidly than nitrogen can leave. This can lead to increased pressure in an enclosed space. Therefore, in order to decrease the risk of expansion of a pneumothorax or pneumoencephalus or a middle ear pressure increase, nitrous is best avoided in trauma patients. Negative pressures in the middle ear can develop after discontinuation of high concentrations of nitrous oxide in the presence of a malfunctioning Eustachian tube. The sudden decrease in pressure could lead to serous otitis media or disruption of a middle ear reconstruction. This is problematic at concentrations greater than 50% (28). Nitrous typically is either avoided completely or turned off 15 minutes before closure of the middle ear. In head and neck surgery, inhaled anesthetics are favored because they cause bronchodilation, diminish the airway reflexes, allow the use of high concentrations of oxygen, and may help in decreasing blood loss by inducing moderate hypotension.

Opioids

Opioids also have greater effect in the elderly because of changes in *both* pharmacokinetics and pharmacodynamics (29,30). High initial plasma levels are present because of decreased volumes of distribution. The prolonged effects of morphine are due to diminished hepatic blood flow, among other factors. Reduced dose requirements of fentanyl are seen with the CNS changes that occur with aging. Opioid increments during titration, however, are not significantly different than other age groups (31,32). The approximate equianalgesic doses for intravenous fentanyl, hydromorphone, and morphine are 200 μg, 2 mg, and 10 mg, respectively. Their half-lives are 1.5–6 hours for fentanyl, 2–3 hours for hydromorphone, and 3–7 hours for morphine. Both hydromorphone and morphine are metabolized by glucoronidation, while fentanyl undergoes oxidation. All of them can produce rigidity with high doses; this is especially seen with fentanyl. Fentanyl is highly lipophilic, and high or repeated doses can result in drug accumulation. Morphine can release histamine and it also has active metabolites, which can accumulate, especially in renal insufficiency. Even though meperidine has been popular in the past, its use has markedly diminished due to the production of active metabolites, which can result in neuroexcitation and subsequent seizure activity. Its current use is, for the most part, limited to postoperative shivering treatment at a dose of 12.5–25 mg intravenously. The mechanism of action for this particular use is unknown. The latest synthetic opioid is remifentanil, metabolized by plasma esterases. It does not have any active metabolite, and its half-life is only 3–5 minutes due to redistribution and ester hydrolysis (20). It is an excellent choice for cases in which the prolonged effects of opioids are to be avoided. It does not provide any postoperative analgesia, so appropriate adjustment in analgesia will be necessary. The use of opioids during head and neck surgery should be minimized in an attempt to achieve an adequate balance between analgesia and side effects, especially since opioid use increases the risk of postoperative nausea and vomiting.

Induction Agents and Sedatives

Essentially all commonly-used induction agents require a dose reduction in the elderly. The age-related dose reductions of etomidate, thiopental sodium, and propofol in the elderly appear to be due to changes in pharmacokinetics. Thiopental, for example, has a prolonged effect due to CNS changes in the elderly. The rapid onset and prolonged half-life of propofol is due to its high lipid solubility (20). The induction dose of barbiturates for a 70-year-old adult is approximately 30% less than that required for individuals 40–50 years younger. Changes in pharmacodynamics seem to be the reason for the reduced requirements for midazolam. The usual onset of action for midazolam in a young and healthy patient is 2–5 minutes, with a half-life of 3–11 hours. It does have an active metabolite, which will be accumulated, especially in the patient with renal dysfunction. All of these medications must be titrated to effect in the elderly population in order to avoid prolonged undesired effects.

Muscle Relaxants

Muscle relaxants are classified as either depolarizing or nondepolarizing. The depolarizing agents (i.e., succinylcholine) imitate the action of acetylcholine at the neuromuscular junction. They bind and activate the nicotinic cholinergic receptors, leading to depolarization of the end plate and the adjacent muscle membrane. Succinylcholine is metabolized by pseudocholinesterases, which are diminished in the elderly male, resulting in dose reductions in that population. Other adverse effects include severe hyperkalemia, transient increase in intracranial and intraocular pressures, myalgias, cardiac arrythmias, malignant hyperthermia, and prolonged paralysis in patients with atypical pseudocholinesterase (20). If there are no contraindications, its use is preferred by many surgeons in cases that require neuromuscular monitoring due to its short duration.

The nondepolarizers (i.e., pancuronium) compete with acetylcholine at the neuromuscular junction. They are classified by relative length of action. A short-acting nondepolarizer is mivacurium, with 1.5–2 minutes to intubation. Among the intermediate acting are atracurium, cisatrascurium, rocuronium, and vecuronium. Their average recovery time is 10–15 minutes. Rocuronium and vecuronium are primarily excreted by the liver. In the long-acting classification are pancuronium, pipecuronium, d-tubocurarine, and doxacurium. Their average recovery time is above 25 minutes. The length of procedure and comorbidities of the patient will affect the choice of muscle relaxants.

Local Anesthetics

Local anesthetics (LAs) are classified into esters and amides. Procaine, cocaine, chloroprocaine, and tetracaine are esters. A major degradation product for these is *para*-amino benzoic acid, which may cause allergic reactions. Lidocaine, mepivacaine, bupivacaine, etidocaine, ropivacaine, and levo-bupivacaine are amides. LAs block sodium channels and impair the propagation of the action potential. Lipid solubility increases the potency. Duration of the block is increased in LAs with high protein binding and increased dose. The onset is determined by the characteristics of the LA and the tissue pH. Systemic effects and toxicity are determined by specific drug choice as well as dose. For example, a dose of 6–8 mg/kg of lidocaine will result in a peak plasma concentration of 3–5 μg/mL. A dose of 1.5–2 mg/kg of bupivacaine results in serum levels of 0.5–1 μg/kg. Lidocaine toxicity can be manifested at 7–10 μg/mL and bupivacaine toxity at 1.5–2 μg/mL.

Cocaine is often used in head and neck surgery since it provides local anesthesia and vasoconstriction (33). Cocaine blocks the reuptake of dopamine and norepinephrine, producing accumulation of these at the nerve synapses. Increased accumulation can lead to CNS and cardiovascular toxicities, which could be pronounced in the debilitated or predisposed patient. Patients with cholinesterase deficiencies will be at a higher risk for sudden death, as cocaine is metabolized by plasma and liver cholinesterases. The maximum recommended dose in a *young healthy* adult is 1.5 mg/kg, but its use should be avoided or the dose decreased in the elderly, especially if halothane or epinephrine is being used as well.

Addition of epinephrine provides vasoconstriction, increased duration of action, faster onset, and lower systemic toxicity due to reduced absorption. An adequate and safe dose of epinephrine is 0.1 mg (10 mL of 1:100,000 concentration). This may be repeated after 20 minutes. The injector needs to remember that tissues of the head are very vascularized and absorption of epinephrine will be increased, particularly with inadvertent intravascular injection. This can lead to severe cardiovascular complications or death. Addition of bicarbonate to the local anesthetics decreases pain with injection but will precipitate ropivacaine or bupivacaine.

Regional Anesthesia of the Head and Neck

Regional anesthesia is occasionally utilized for head and neck procedures. Pertinent anatomy must to be delineated and the injections done under sterile conditions. The patients monitored as per standard ASA guidelines and emergency airway management equipment should be readily available. As with any procedure, there are contraindications and potential complications of which the surgeon and anesthesiologist must be aware.

Cervical Plexus Block

A cervical plexus block is useful for anterior neck surgery (34,35). This block provides anesthesia of the sensory and motor fibers of the neck and posterior scalp. The superficial branches supply the skin of the back of the head, side of the neck, and anterior and lateral area of the shoulder. A *superficial cervical plexus* block is performed by injecting 10 mL of local anesthetic subcutaneously along the posterior border of the sternocleidomastoid muscle to block the greater auricular and transverse cervical nerves. A *deep cervical block* is performed by injecting deeply along the transverse processes and carries significantly greater risk. Inadvertent phrenic nerve block is the most common complication, but subarachnoid or epidural injection, vertebral artery injection, recurrent laryngeal nerve block, and cervical sympathetic block are also possible. Due to the risk of phrenic and recurrent laryngeal nerve blocks, this procedure should not be performed bilaterally or in patients with respiratory compromise. Other regional blocks include the trigeminal and occipital nerve blocks (34–36). These blocks are usually employed for chronic pain rather than for surgery.

Airway Anesthesia

Regional anesthesia of the airway is usually performed to facilitate awake instrumentation or intubation of the airway (37). Premedication with an anticholinergic such as robinol is often employed. Topical anesthesia of the mucosal membranes is achieved with 4% lidocaine, care being taken to avoid overdoseage. A superior laryngeal nerve block can be performed with 2–3 mL of local anesthetic injected via a 25-gauge needle directed just inferior to the greater cornu of the hyoid bone and superior to the thyroid cartilage. The trachea can be anesthetized by injecting topical anesthetic directly through the cricothyroid membrane.

Intubation

Preparation for the anesthetic includes a complete evaluation of the airway, which includes an estimate of the likelihood for potential difficult airway, need for orotracheal or nasotracheal approach, device to be used and size, and the need for an awake or asleep procedure. The ASA has developed a difficult airway algorithm, which serves as a guideline in case of difficult airway, either recognized or unrecognized preoperatively (Fig. 2) (18). An awake tracheostomy might be indicated in patients with upper airway trauma, infection, or tumor.

    Potential complications of intubation can include nasal mucosal injuries as a result of nasotracheal intubation, sinusitis, dental trauma, temporomandibular joint dislocation, mucosal injuries (nasal or laryngotracheal), arytenoid dislocation, vocal cord paralysis, granulations or granulomas of larynx, and laryngotracheal stenosis.

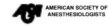

AMERICAN SOCIETY OF
ANESTHESIOLOGISTS

DIFFICULT AIRWAY ALGORITHM

1. Assess the likelihood and clinical impact of basic management problems:
   A. Difficult Ventilation
   B. Difficult Intubation
   C. Difficulty with Patient Cooperation or Consent
   D. Difficult Tracheostomy

2. Actively pursue opportunities to deliver supplemental oxygen throughout the process of difficult airway management

3. Consider the relative merits and feasibility of basic management choices:

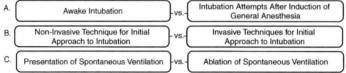

4. Develop primary and alternative strategies:

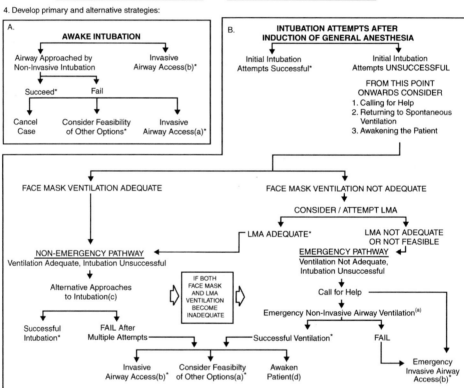

*Confirm ventilation, tracheal intubation or LMA placement with exhaled co₂

a. Other options include [but are not limited to]: surgery utilizing face mask or LMA anesthesia, local amesthesia infiltration or regional nerve blockade. Pursuit of those options usually implies that mask ventilation will not be problematic. Therefore, these options may be of limited value if this step in the algorithm has been reached via the Emergency Pathway.

b. Invasive airway access includes surgical or percutaneous tracheostomy or crioothyrotomy.

c. Alternative non-invasive approaches to difficult intubation include (but are not limited to): use of different laryngoscope blades, LMA as an intubation conduit (with or without fiberoptic guidance), fiberoptic intubation, intubating stylet or tube changer, tight wand, retrograde intubation, and blind oral or nasal intubation.

d. Consider re-preparation of the patient for awake intubation or cancelling surgery.

e. Options for emergency non-invasive airway ventilation include (but are not limited to):rigid bronchoscope, nasophageal-tracheal comtube ventilation, or transtracheal jet ventilation.

Figure 2 Difficult airway algorithm american society of anesthesiologists. *Source*: From Ref. 18.

Extubation

Extubation is considered a part of the continuum of the anesthetic management. The risks and benefits of an asleep versus an awake extubation must be considered. Factors contributing to the decision are the patient's ability to maintain an adequate oxygen tension, ventilation and breathing pattern, level of consciousness, adequacy of muscle relaxation reversal, and ability to protect the airway. The throat and stomach are suctioned, and there should be a plan for emergency reintubation, if needed. Extubation is performed after an adequate evaluation and careful planning has been done.

POSTOPERATIVE COMPLICATIONS

Nausea and vomiting are common complications after head and neck surgery. It is often helpful to initiate treatment with preoperative antiemetics like ondansetron, dolasetron, and metoclopramide even before the surgery has started. Limiting the amount of opioids, inhaled anesthetics (including nitrous), and the use of muscle relaxants and reversal therapy will reduce postoperative nausea and vomiting. Total intravenous anesthetic with propofol (which has been associated with antiemetic properties) can be utilized as well.

SPECIFIC CASES

A number of specific types of cases require modifications of anesthetic technique to avoid complications. These include ear surgery, laser surgery, nasal surgery, surgery for epistaxis, laryngoscopy, and bronchoscopy (38–40). Anesthetic considerations for these procedures performed in the elderly population are the same as those in the younger population, so they are not addressed further in this text.

Anesthesia for Thyroid and Parathyroid Surgery

Anesthetic management of patients undergoing thyroid and parathyroid surgery can be challenging in a number of ways. Elderly patients may demonstrate different physiologic responses to hypo- or hyperthyroidism than those of younger patients. A significant percentage of elderly patients who undergo thyroidectomy do so to treat obstructive airway symptoms; hence, the airway is of concern and must be considered (41). Thyroid storm after surgical manipulation presents an unusual but difficult management problem. It usually occurs 6–19 hours after surgery but can begin intraoperatively during surgery of an acutely hyperthyroid patient. Elective surgery can be performed in the presence of mild to moderate hypothyroidism; however, only emergency surgery should be done on a severely hypothyroid patient due to the risk of myxedema coma.

Disorders of the parathyroid glands can result in either hyper- or hypocalcemia, with physiologic changes affecting multiple systems. Hypercalcemia that cannot be corrected before the surgery should be normalized intraoperatively with normal saline and furosemide. The effect of serum calcium levels on muscle relaxants is unpredictable. Muscle relaxants are carefully titrated with the use of a muscle stimulator. These patients may be osteopenic as well, so careful positioning is necessary to prevent fractures.

Postoperative complications can include hypocalcemia, recurrent laryngeal nerve paralysis, bleeding with hematoma obstructing the airway, thyroid storm, and laryngospasm (41). Hypocalcemia can occur in 1–40% of the patients undergoing total thyroidectomy due to removal of the parathyroid glands (42). Postoperative determination of calcium and phosphate is required in these patients.

Oncological Surgery

The elderly patient undergoing head and neck oncological surgery will present multiple challenges for the anesthesiologist (43). Alcoholism can be present in as much as a third of the patients, with up to a fourth of the patients abusing alcohol at the time of surgery (2,8). Patients with difficulty eating due to the tumor might be malnourished and dehydrated (44). Electrolytes should be checked and any derangement corrected preoperatively. Other frequent comorbidities are pulmonary and cardiovascular diseases, such as chronic obstructive pulmonary disease and coronary artery disease (45). The risk for excessive blood loss is increased. Patients who have previously undergone radiation have unique problems. Their mucosa is friable and specifically susceptible to bleeding. They may present with airway edema that is undetected until intubation is performed. The cervical range of motion and mouth opening might be limited as well.

Besides the tumor itself and comorbidities, the surgical approach will also be a major determinant of the technique used to secure the airway. An elective tracheotomy may be required before induction of general anesthesia. Patient position and equipment setup will be very important, especially in large multi-team procedures such as skull base surgery or procedures that require free-flap reconstruction. Multiple surgical specialties may be involved simultaneously in the care of the patient. The surgical and donor sites will be exposed, thus decreasing vascular and monitoring access as well as increasing the area exposed to heat and fluid loss.

Specific postoperative complications can include loss of multiple cranial nerves, such as after excision of paragangliomas (46). Patients might have hypothyroidism after non-thyroid cancer head and neck surgery, and hypoparathyroidism after thyroid cancer surgery (47). Patients need to be monitored postoperatively for difficulty compensating for any lost cranial nerve and for signs of hypothyroidism and hypoparathyroidism.

Infection of the Upper Airway

Ludwig's angina has become much less frequent with the development of antibiotics but is still encountered, even in the elderly patient (41). Airway obstruction can occur suddenly due to swelling of the floor of the mouth and tongue. Patients with neck infections may also have trismus, supraglottic edema, and nuchal rigidity. Additional comorbidities and complications may include aspiration and mediastinal, lung, or systemic infection. Upper airway obstruction can occur in the presence of laryngeal and soft tissue edema. Emergent intubation may be required. Tracheotomy under local anesthesia is considered safer than general anesthesia in the case of the patient with stridor at rest.

Supraglottitis or epiglottitis has been identified in adults and is clinically distinct from children (41). Classic symptoms encountered in children, such as fever, hoarseness, and drooling, may not be as marked, leading to delays in diagnosis. Peritonsillar abscesses occasionally present in the elderly and can predispose a patient to airway obstruction and trismus (48). Any plan for management of the airway needs to take into account the possibility of abscess perforation and trismus (48).

When the temporomandibular joint motion is limited, access to the airway might be a problem, even requiring awake intubation (49). Nasotracheal intubation is the method of choice for surgery of the temporomandibular joint or patients with severe trismus.

Office-Based Head and Neck Surgery

Multiple head and neck procedures have been performed safely in an outpatient setting for many years. These include procedures performed in both the younger population and the elderly (50–52). The decision to do a procedure in this setting is dependent on multiple factors, not only the specific procedure proposed.

Office-based anesthesia carries unique risks and mandates that identical standards to those used in a regular operating room be in effect. Selected patients should be ASA 1 or 2, eliminating many elderly patients. Patients with a recognized potential for difficult airway should not undergo anesthesia in this environment. Guidelines for preoperative care are unchanged. All the surgical and anesthetic equipment, including emergency cardio respiratory equipment, must be available. Local anesthesia with mild to moderate sedation is employed most commonly. Procedures that are minimally invasive but still require general anesthesia are done with an anesthesiologist in a specially prepared procedure room. The American Society of Anesthesiologists, the American Association of Nurse Anesthetists, and the Joint Commission on Accreditation of Healthcare Organizations have recommended guidelines that help to regulate office-based surgery.

CONCLUSION

Anesthesia for the geriatric patient is a growing field. Both the surgeon and the anesthesiologist will face new challenges, as advances in medicine and surgery will enable surgical treatment of ever more complex patients in this growing population. A substantial knowledge of the physiologic changes in the elderly and pharmacology is essential. Tailoring of the anesthetic is always individual, taking into account the different comorbidities and type of surgery. Communication between surgeon and anesthesiologist is of extreme importance for a smooth flow in the operating room.

REFERENCES

1. Beliveau MM. Perioperative care for the elderly. Med Clin North Am 2003; 87(1): 273–289.
2. McGuirt WF, Davis III SP. Demographic portrayal and outcome analysis of head and neck cancer surgery in the elderly. Arch Otolaryngol Head Neck Surg 1995; 121:150–154.
3. Robinson DS. Head and neck considerations in the elderly patient. Surg Clin North Am 1994; 74:431–439.
4. Pelczar BT, Weed HG, Schuller DE, et al. Identifying high-risk patients before head and neck oncologic surgery. Arch Otolaryngol Head Neck Surg 1993; 119:861–864.
5. Jan MY, Strong EW, Saltzman EI, et al. Head and neck cancer in the elderly. Head Neck Surg 1983; 5:376–382.

6. American Society of Anesthesiologists. Syllabus on geriatric anesthesia. ASA, 2003.
7. Muravchick S. Anesthesia for the elderly. In: Miller, ed. Anesthesia. 5th ed. New York: Churchill Livingstone, 2000:2140–2165.
8. Arriaya M, Johnson JT, Kanel KT. Medical complications in total laryngectomy: incidence and risk factors. Ann Otol Rhinol Laryngol 1990; 99:611–615.
9. Eagle KA, Berger PB, Calkins H, et al. ACC/AHA guideline update for perioperative cardiovascular evaluation for noncardiac surgery update. A report of the American College of Cardiology/American Heart Association Task Force on Practice Guidelines (Committee to Update the 1996 Guidelines on Perioperative Cardiovascular Evaluation for Noncardiac Surgery), 2002.
10. Zeleznik J. Normative aging of the respiratory system. Clin Geriatr Med 2003; 19(1): 1–18.
11. McCulloch TM, Jensen NF, Girod DA, et al. Risk factors for pulmonary complications in the postoperative head and neck surgery patient. Head Neck 1997; 372–377.
12. Muravchick S. Anesthesia for the elderly. In: Miller, ed. Anesthesia. New York: Churchill Livingstone, 2000:2144–2146.
13. Chung F. Postoperative mental dysfunction. In: McLeskey CH, ed. Geriatric anesthesiology. Williams & Wilkins, 1997:487–495.
14. De Witte J. Perioperative shivering: physiology and pharmacology. Anesthesiology 2002; 96(2):467–484.
15. Anantharaju A. Aging liver. A review. Gerontology 2002; 48(6):343–353.
16. Naguib M. Advances in neurobiology of the neuromuscular junction: implications for the anesthesiologist. Anesthesiology 2002; 96(1):202–231.
17. Goodwin WJ, Balkany T, Casiano RR. Special considerations in managing geriatric patients. In: Cummings, ed. Otolaryngology: Head and Neck Surgery. Mosby-Year Book, 1998:315–320.
18. American Society of Anesthesiologists Task Force on Management of the Difficult Airway. Practice guidelines for management of the difficult airway: an updated report by the American Society of Anesthesiologists Task Force on Management of the Difficult Airway. Anesthesiology 2003; 98(5):1269–1277.
19. American Society of Anesthesiologists Task Force on Preanesthesia Evaluation. Anesthesiology 2002; 96(2):485–496.
20. McRae K. Anesthesia for airway surgery. Anesthesiol Clin North Am 2001; 19(3): 497–541, vi.
21. Khan A, Pearlman RC, Bianchi DA, et al. Experience with two types of electromyography monitoring electrodes during thyroid surgery. Am J Otolaryngol 1997; 18:99.
22. Jones AG, Hunter JM. Anaesthesia in the elderly. Special considerations. Drugs Aging 1996; 9:319–331.
23. Avram MJ, Krejcie TC, Henthorn TK. The relationship of age to the pharmacokinetics of early drug distribution the concurrent disposition of thiopental and indocyanine green. Anesthesiology 1990; 72:403–411.
24. Avram MJ, Sanghvi R, Henthorn TK, et al. Determinants of thiopental induction dose requirements. Anesth Analg 1993; 76:10–17.
25. Kirkpatrick T, Cockshott ID, Douglas EJ, Nimmo WS. Pharmacokinetics of propofol (Diprivan) in elderly patients. Br J Anaesth 1988; 60:146–150.
26. Martin G. A study of anesthetic drug utilization in different age groups. J Clin Anesth 2003; 15(3):194–200.
27. Mapleson WW. Effect of age on MAC in humans meta-analysis. Br J Anaesth 1996; 76:179–185.
28. Chinn K, Brown OE, Manning SC, et al. Middle ear pressure variation: effect of nitrous oxide. Laryngoscope 1997; 107:357.
29. Owen JA, Sitar DS, Berger L, Brownell L, Duke PC, Mitenko PA. Age-related morphine kinetics. Clin Pharmacol Ther 1983; 34:364–368.

30. Scott JC, Stanski DR. Decreased fentanyl and alfentanil dose requirements with age. A simultaneous pharmacokinetic and pharmacodynamic evaluation. J Pharmacol Exp Ther 1987; 240:159–166.

31. Rooke GA. Anesthesiology and geriatric medicine: mutual needs and opportunities. Anesthesiology 2002; 96(1):2–4.

32. Aubrun F, Monsel S, Langeron O, Coriat P, Riou B. Postoperative titration of intravenous morphine in the elderly patient. Anesthesiology 2002; 96:17–23.

33. Ahlstrom KK. Local anesthetics for facial plastic procedures. Otolaryngol Clin North Am 2002; 35(1):29–53, v–vi.

34. Wedel DJ. Nerve Blocks. In: Miller, ed. Anesthesia. New York: Churchill Livingstone, 2000:1538–1543.

35. Rosenberg M, Phero JC. Regional anesthesia and invasive techniques to manage head and neck pain. Otolaryngol Clin North Am Dec 2003; 36(6):1201–1219.

36. Ward JB. Greater occipital nerve block. Semin Neurol 2003; 23(1):59–62.

37. Simmons ST. Airway regional anesthesia for awake fiberoptic intubation. Reg Anesth Pain Med 2002; 27(2):180–192.

38. Sosis MB, Braverman B, Caldarelli DD. Evaluation of a new laser resistant fabric and copper foil wrapped endotracheal tube. Laryngoscope 1996; 106:842.

39. Donlon JV. Anesthesia for ear surgery. In: Albert PW, Ruben RJ, eds. Otologic medicine and Surgery. New York: Churchill Livingstone, 1988:995.

40. Weeks DB. Use of jet venturi ventilation during microsurgery of the glottis and subglottis. Anesth Rev 1985; 12:32.

41. Bansal A, Miskoff J, Lis RJ. Otolaryngologic critical care. Crit Care Clin 2003; 19(1): 55–72.

42. Bhattacharyya N, Fried MP. Assessment of the morbidity and complications of total thyroidectomy. Arch Otolaryngol Head Neck Surg 2002; 128:389–392.

43. Garantziotis S. Critical care of the head and neck patient. Crit Care Clin 2003; 19(1): 73–90.

44. Bachmann P, Marti-Massoud C, Blanc-Vincent MP, et al. Standards, options and recommendations: nutritional support in palliative or terminal care of adult patients with progressive cancer. Bull Cancer 2001; 88:985–1006.

45. Daugherty TM. Anesthesia management for head and neck surgery. J Clin Anesth 1994; 6:74.

46. Sniezek JC. Paraganglioma surgery: complications and treatment. Otolaryngol Clin North Am 2001; 34(5):993–1006, vii.

47. Sinard RJ, Tobin EJ, Mazzaferri EL, et al. Hypothyroidism after treatment for nonthyroid head and neck cancer. Arch Otolaryngol Head Neck Surg 2000; 126:652–657.

48. Doyle DJ. Upper airway diseases and airway management: a synopsis. Anesthesiol Clin North Am 2002; 20(4):767–787, vi.

49. Stackhouse RA. Fiberoptic airway management. Anesthesiol Clin North Am 2002; 20(4):933–951.

50. Tonin HA. Office surgery in otolaryngology. Otolaryngology 1978; 86(2):176–180.

51. Krouse HJ. Innovations in office-based surgery. Head Neck Nurs 1998; 16(3):20–26.

52. Koch ME. Office-based anesthesia: an overview. Anesthesiol Clin North Am 2003; 21(2):417–443.

63

Postoperative Care for the Geriatric Patient

Robert L. Cross Jr. and Richard Hanson
Department of Anesthesiology and Perioperative Medicine, Oregon Health and Science University, Portland, Oregon, U.S.A.

INTRODUCTION

Ear, nose, and throat (ENT) surgery has been implicated as an important preoperative predictor of prolonged discharge from the postanesthesia care unit (PACU). Additionally, the majority of morbidity and mortality of surgery occurs in the postoperative setting. Declines in health and cognitive function associated with aging further increase the risk in elderly patients undergoing a surgical procedure. For these reasons, many adverse outcomes can be avoided with proper care and foresight in the management of the postoperative elderly patient. To adequately delineate concerns in the first postoperative week, a systems-based review follows, highlighting key components in the management of the elderly ENT patient.

CARDIOVASCULAR SYSTEM

Reduced vascular capacitance, stiffened ventricles, and higher prevalence of coronary artery disease (CAD), arrhythmias, and congestive heart failure (CHF) all make hemodynamic stability in the elderly more difficult to achieve and result in an increasing incidence of postoperative morbidity and mortality. Mangano estimated the prevalence of CAD in patients over the age of 80 exceeds 80%, while another study by Kannel suggests the prevalence of CHF approaches 10%.

As with the prevention of many other causes of postoperative morbidity and mortality, a large part of the cardiac management lies in effective screening and optimization of the patient in the preoperative period. In the initial postoperative period, the goal is to decrease the strain on the aging heart by controlling heart rate and blood pressure. Perioperative β-adrenergic blockade has been shown to reduce analgesic requirements, speed recovery from anesthesia, and improve hemodynamic stability. Concern for hypotension with the administration of beta-blockers is mostly unfounded, with the reduction of mean arterial blood pressure (MAP) less than 10%. Adequate pain management will have the greatest impact on further control of heart rate and blood pressure in the immediate postoperative time course. Additionally, adequate oxygenation must be maintained as hypoxia can also lead to a demand increase in cardiac output, supplying itself with blood of low oxygen content leading to an increased likelihood of cardiac ischemia.

Head and neck surgery is generally considered a high-risk surgery from a cardiovascular standpoint, with a risk of perioperative death or myocardial infarction that may exceed 4%. The majority of myocardial infarctions occur in the first 48 hours of the postoperative period. Approximately 45% of the mortality in the first 30 days following surgery has a cardiac cause. For these reasons, cardiac protection is paramount in the postoperative period. As mentioned above, heart rate control through the use of β-blockers and appropriate pain management is the cornerstone of postoperative cardiac protection. Opiates, in addition to their pain management properties, have been shown to provide ischemic preconditioning, which may result in further cardiac protection. A case-control study by Poldermans et al. reported an 80% reduction in cardiac mortality in patients treated with HMG Co-A reductase inhibitors in the perioperative period, suggesting there may be a role for these medications in the perioperative period as well.

PULMONARY SYSTEM

Issues involving airway obstruction are the most common life-threatening problems in the postoperative ENT patient. Laryngospasm is one of the most severe sources of airway obstruction; it occurs immediately post-extubation and results in complete airway obstruction. Initial treatment involves application of positive pressure ventilation with 100% FiO$_2$ by mask accompanied by jaw lift. Ultimately, a 0.15–0.3 mg/kg IV dose of succinylcholine may need to be administered to break the laryngospasm. A further complication of laryngospasm is negative pressure pulmonary edema, which results from inspiratory attempts on a closed glottis. Hypoxia is the most common presenting sign, occurring up to 80 minutes after the episode of laryngospasm. Treatment is supportive, with supplemental oxygen and close monitoring. Once laryngospasm occurs, these patients often require positive pressure bag-mask ventilation to regain an open airway. In severe cases, endotracheal intubation with mechanical ventilation may be required to maintain adequate oxygenation.

Partial airway obstruction usually presents as stridor. Inspiratory stridor suggests a supraglottic or glottic obstruction. Supraglottic obstruction is commonly due to relaxation of the posterior pharyngeal structures in a sedated postoperative patient or edema as a direct result of surgery in the area. In either case, initial treatment includes jaw lift while providing supplemental oxygenation. An oral– or nasal–pharyngeal airway may need to be inserted to help maintain patency of the airway. Ultimately, endotracheal intubation may be required. This can be a challenging task in the face of an edematous post-procedure airway. Edema of the vocal cords, injury to the recurrent laryngeal nerve, and cricoarytenoid joint arthritis are all reasons for partial glottic obstruction. Humidified oxygen and continuous positive airway pressure (CPAP) are the mainstays of treatment.

Expiratory or combined inspiratory and expiratory stridor points toward a subglottic source of obstruction. Subglottic obstruction will not resolve with the treatments outlined above. If the trachea does not appear compromised by external sources (i.e., hematoma, edema), tracheal stenosis or foreign body aspiration must be considered. Definitive diagnosis of either of these causes requires bronchoscopy.

If edema or hematoma formation is the cause of obstruction, surgeons must be notified and the airway needs to be secured. During intubation, the goal should be to maintain spontaneous respirations during induction as this will result in retained muscular tone of the pharynx, optimizing intubating conditions. Ultimately, awake intubation may need to be performed. If airway patency is lost, emergent reduction of the hematoma must occur with either endotracheal intubation or emergent crycothyrotomy.

Patients taken intubated to the intensive care unit (ICU) due to airway edema will need to be assessed for an adequate airway patency prior to extubation. A plan for extubation must be well thought out, including provisions for reintubation should it be necessary. Prior to extubation, a trial of breathing can include deflation of the endotracheal cuff to assess space around the endotracheal tube while the lumen of the tube is occluded. Detection of air movement around the tube with a stethoscope placed over the trachea at a peak pressure of 20 cm H_2O or less suggests that there will not be airway closure with extubation. A more quantitative assessment of airway leak (edema) can also be achieved by determining the difference between expiratory and inspiratory tidal volume with the endotracheal tube cuff inflated and deflated at a constant set tidal volume of 10–12 mL/kg. Using this technique, patients with a cuff leak of less than 12% of inspiratory volume are at increased risk of demonstrating post-extubation stridor. In questionable cases, the patient may be extubated with a jet-ventilating stylet inserted through the endotracheal tube. After removal of the endo-tracheal tube, spontaneous ventilation can be assessed with the stylet in place. Adequate ventilation and oxygenation can be maintained via jet ventilation if required, and the stylet can be used to reintubate the patient via Seldinger technique, as it remains in the tracheal lumen.

Changes in function make pulmonary morbidity a large concern in the post-operative elderly patient. The stiffening of the thorax, coupled with reduced musculature results in diminished compliance. Forced expiratory volume in one second (FEV_1) is reduced. Inspiratory and expiratory reserve function decline with age. Response to hypoxia, cough, and ciliary function are all reduced as well. Despite all of these things, no guidelines have been developed to address these concerns in the postoperative setting. Ultimately, adequate oxygenation and ventilation must be maintained with measures to help prevent aspiration in the postoperative period. This requires a balance between neurologic responsiveness and the inevitable sedation that accompanies adequate pain control.

Postoperative atelectasis and pneumonia account for significant morbidity and mortality. It has been reported that almost 25% of deaths in the first six days following surgery are related to pulmonary complications. Atelectasis has been shown to be present within five minutes of induction of general anesthesia and may persist for up to 48 hours postoperatively. Pneumonia is the third most common postoperative infection and occurs in up to 40% of patients. There is likely a continuum between atelectasis formation and the development of postoperative pneumonia; therefore, maneuvers to eliminate atelectasis likely lead to a reduction in postoperative complications and pneumonia. Many treatments have been used to improve pulmonary function in the postoperative period including incentive spirometry CPAP, positive end expiratory pressure (PEEP) if mechanically ventilated, deep breathing exercises, and chest physiotherapy. Although all these techniques appear effective, the only proven technique to reduce postoperative pulmonary complications is incentive spirometry. Prophylactic postoperative antibiotic therapy has not been shown to reduce the incidence of pneumonia.

Deep vein thrombosis (DVT), which may lead to a pulmonary embolism (PE), can have grave consequences in the postoperative patient. The American College of Chest Physicians (ACCP) state the incidence of calf DVT is 20% to 40%, proximal DVT is 4% to 48%, clinically significant PE is 2% to 4%, and fatality due to PE is 0.4% to 1% in the untreated, high-risk patient (any patient greater than 60 years of age). Graduated compression stockings (GCSs) can reduce the risk of DVT by approximately 50%. The use of low-density unfractionated heparin (LDUH) 5000 U bid or low-molecular weight heparin (LMWH) 3400 U once daily can reduce the risk by 60% to 70%. GCSs have been shown to further reduce the risk of DVT when coupled with heparin therapy by an additional 75% compared to heparin therapy alone. The ACCP recommends the above LDUH or LMWH alone for all patients greater than 60 years of age. If theses patients have further risk factors (previous DVT, hypercoagulable state, malignancy, etc.) the recommendation is to combine LDUH or LMWH with GCS. If the patient is at a high risk of bleeding, the very least is GCS therapy. Most patients should be treated until they are ambulatory.

GASTROINTESTINAL SYSTEM

Postoperative nausea and vomiting (PONV) is a significant reason for delay in discharge from the PACU as well as unanticipated inpatient admission. Overall incidence of PONV approaches 30%, with ENT procedures accounting for an increased risk. One must also consider the emetic properties of blood that may be swallowed during the surgical procedure. Apfel et al. devised a PONV risk assessment score consisting of four predictors: female gender, history of PONV or motion sickness, nonsmoker, and use of postoperative narcotics. The incidence of PONV following general anesthesia, given these risk factors, can be found in Table 1.

Treatment of PONV needs to be multimodal in its approach. Antiemetic medications include the $5HT_3$ antagonists, droperidol (dopamine antagonist), promethazine, and dexamethasone. All four modalities have been proven efficacious individually and further beneficial when used in combination. Ondansetron in combination with droperidol reduced the incidence of PONV by 90%. Droperidol, however, currently carries an FDA "black box" warning for prolonged QT syndrome and cardiac arrhythmias. For this reason, it should be considered a second-line medication. The use of droperidol requires a preoperative 12 lead electrocardiogram (EKG) and continuous cardiac monitoring for two hours following administration. Metoclopromide, although not shown to significantly reduce PONV, may hold a place in the perioperative regimen of ENT surgery, as it increases gastric emptying, which could decrease stomach transit time for swallowed blood.

Table 1   PONV Risk Assessment

Risk factors	Incidence of PONV (%)
1	20
2	39
3	61
4	79

Risk factors: Female gender, history of PONV or motion sickness, nonsmoker, the use of postoperative narcotics.
Abbreviation: PONV, postoperative nausea and vomiting

Another concern in the postoperative time course is reduced gut motility and constipation as a result of inactivity and narcotic pain medications. Any patient placed on opioids should be started on a bowel regimen at the same time.

In the ambulatory setting, it has been standard practice to require patients to take oral fluids prior to discharge. Several studies have investigated this practice and the results are mixed; however, there is no clear benefit shown in requiring patients to drink fluids prior to discharge. As a result, current Practice Guidelines for Postanesthetic Care recommends that drinking fluids not be included in discharge criteria and only used on an individual case basis.

The nutritional status of elderly patients is more likely to be impaired when compared to the young. This, coupled with the pain, sedation, and nausea that may be present after a surgical procedure, places them at increased risk for malnutrition in the postoperative setting. It is therefore important to initiate nutritional support as soon as possible. Bastow et al. found that enteral supplements were beneficial and reduced postoperative complications in elderly hip fracture patients. Any patients deemed at risk may warrant a nutrition consult in the postoperative setting. Although nutrition is paramount to a smooth recovery, parental supplementation has been associated with increased complications when administered to adequately nourished patients and therefore should only be used in patients with marked nutritional deficits.

RENAL SYSTEM

The reduction of renal blood flow, loss of parenchyma, and increasing sclerosis of nephrons all lead to reduced glomerular filtration rate in elderly patients, placing them at increased risk for postoperative renal impairment. These changes reduce the aging kidneys' effectiveness in maintaining electrolyte and pH balance and make them less able to withstand and compensate for the sometimes large volume and blood pressure shifts that can be associated with a surgical procedure. Hypervolemia in the elderly patient may be beneficial to the kidney, but can result in CHF in a patient with impaired cardiac function. Postoperative care of the elderly patient requires diligent management to maintain a euvolemic state while monitoring electrolytes for trends that may suggest increased renal impairment.

Until recently, it has been a standard requirement that a patient void prior to discharge home from the PACU in ambulatory patients. Recent studies suggest that even patients at high risk for urinary retention (a history of urinary retention or intraoperative catheterization) need not be required to void prior to discharge. Current practice guidelines for postanesthetic care do not require voiding as a routine discharge criterion.

ENDOCRINE SYSTEM

Diabetes mellitus has an increasing prevalence in the elderly patient. Blood sugars will likely be more labile in the perioperative setting owing to increased catacholamines, no or minimal enteral intake, and influence of various medications (example: corticosteroids). Hypoglycemia at best may result in altered mental status and at worst permanent cognitive delay, coma, or death. Recently, hyperglycemia has been implicated in prolonged wound healing, inhibition of the immune system, and increased risk of infection. Glycemic control needs to be actively monitored and controlled in any patient showing signs of lability. The most consistent approach is use of an insulin drip in the intraoperative and immediate postoperative setting. Most institutions have a standard insulin drip protocol that may be used. A modest goal would be to maintain blood sugars in the range of 100–150.

Hypoparathyroidism can occur following surgery involving the thyroid. This results in postoperative hypocalcemia in up to 30% of patients. For this reason, calcium and phosphate levels should be monitored in all patients with surgery involving the thyroid, parathyroid, and immediately surrounding structures. Calcium should be supplemented when appropriate. Usually this is a self-limited condition, with only a small number of patients progressing to chronic hypoparathyroidism.

Head and neck cancer surgery can result in postoperative hypothyroidism. Sixty-one percent of patients undergoing total laryngectomy, thyroid lobectomy, and radiation therapy developed hypothyroidism in one study. The time course is such that there will likely be no clinical indicators in the immediate postoperative period.

NEUROLOGIC SYSTEM

Delirium is a common postoperative sequelae in the elderly patient and has been shown to increase time to recovery, length of hospital stay, and hospital costs. The leading predictor of postoperative delirium is preoperative cognitive impairment. Other factors associated with postoperative delirium include older age, poor physical function, high-risk surgery, undertreated pain, infection, and metabolic derangements. Pain is an area that can readily be impacted when treated properly in the postoperative setting. In reviewing the results of several studies, Liu et al. concluded that the quality, as opposed to the type of pain management, has much more to do with the incidence of delirium.

Two common postoperative medications implicated in the incidence of postoperative delirium were benzodiazepines and meperidine. These two should therefore be avoided in the elderly surgical patient if at all possible.

Stroke is a known perioperative complication that may result in devastating morbidity and mortality. The incidence of stroke associated with non-head and neck surgery is between 0.08% and 0.2%, whereas the incidence in major head and neck surgery has been reported to be as high as 4.8%. As postoperative stroke can be ischemic or hemorrhagic, there is no definitive prophylaxis for its prevention. However, appropriate management of risk factors may help reduce the incidence of postoperative stroke. These risk factors include uncontrolled hypertension, hypotension, hyper- or hypo-coagulable states, arrhythmias, and intravascular plaques.

Postoperative pain is the one of the most common reasons for delay in discharge from the PACU and an important overall concern in the postsurgical time course. Optimal treatment of postoperative pain should be multimodal in its approach and start well before the end of the case and in many instances prior to its inception. Generous use of local anesthetics by field block infiltration or specific nerve block should be used when possible to prevent postoperative pain. Once significant pain has been observed (i.e., greater than a visual pain score of 4 or less or back to baseline pain score, if baseline is greater than 4), treatment should also include both pharmacologic and nonpharmacologic methods.

The first step in pain management needs to be an effective method of assessment. There are several methods available, but all have limitations in an elderly

Table 2 FPS Designed for and Standardized in a Senior Population

0 = No pain
1 = Tolerable (but does not prevent any activities)
2 = Tolerable (and does prevent some activities)
3 = Intolerable (but can use telephone, watch TV, or read)
4 = Intolerable (and cannot use telephone, watch TV, or read)
5 = Intolerable (and unable to verbally communicate because of pain)

Functional pain scale incorporates three levels of assessment. First, pain is rated as "tolerable" or "intolerable." If pain is reported as intolerable, this should be considered an urgent matter and further evaluation and intervention rendered immediately with frequent follow-up to assure improvement into the "tolerable" range as rapidly as possible. Second is a functional component. Some patients are likely to rank pain at the highest level, especially if apprehension over receiving adequate pain medication exists. With the FPS, the problem of having a patient who always report pain at the highest level "5," even when there is clear improvement, is obviated. Because of the functional component associated with verbal communication, this instrument adjusts the score based on the fact that a person can verbally respond about pain. This functional portion of the scale provides a more objective component to the assessment and makes the instrument more sensitive to changes in pain level. Finally, the 0–5 scale presents a means of rapidly comparing to prior pain level responses (responsiveness). Ideally, all patients should reach at a 0–2 level, preferably 0–1.
Abbreviation: FPS, functional pain scale
Source: Gloth FM. Principles of perioperative pain management in older adults. Clin Geriatr Med 2001; 17(3):553–573.

population that has an increased prevalence of hearing and/or visual disturbance, cognitive delay, and limited education. A simplified scale proposed by Gloth for specific use in the elderly includes a basic self-assessment of tolerable versus intolerable pain, combined with a functional assessment by patient and caregiver to reach a pain score of 0–5 (Table 2).

Nonpharmacologic modalities of treatment are often overlooked but can be an effective adjunct to traditional medicinal interventions. Application of cold compresses can inhibit the release of tissue breakdown byproducts. Warm compresses stimulate the release of endogenous opiates. Relaxation or diversion techniques can help to redirect focus from pain and help to allay anxiety.

Pharmacologic pain management remains the standard postoperative treatment of ENT cases. A combination of opiate and non-opiate analgesics should be used whenever possible to optimally control pain in the postoperative setting. Of the nonopioid analgesics, acetaminophen is the most commonly used. It works well in the elderly population and has fewer gastrointestinal side effects than non-steroidal anti-inflammatory drugs (NSAIDs). Caution must be used, however, as acetaminophen is found in combination with many other medications, and it is easy to exceed the maximum daily dosage of 4 g. NSAIDs have been proven to work well in conjunction with opioids. Naproxen premedication at least 30 minutes prior to laparoscopic surgery resulted in lower postoperative pain scores, fewer opiates, and earlier discharge from the PACU. Postoperative bleeding, gastrointestinal side effects, hypertension, and renal impairment are all concerns with conventional NSAID administration and cannot limit their use in the elderly. Newer cyclooxygenase-2 inhibitors have greatly lessened the risk of gastrointestinal (GI) bleeding and have proven safe to use with warfarin. However, rofecoxib (Vioxx®™) was voluntarily removed from the market in September of 2004 after a trial showed a significant increase in the risk of myocardial infarction associated with its use. Until further scrutiny of the Cox-2 class of drugs occurs, alternative NSAIDS may be necessary.

The mainstay of postoperative analgesia continues to be opioids. In the hospital setting, patient-controlled analgesia (PCA) devices have proven very effective at maintaining a baseline level of analgesia by using a basal rate of administration while providing the flexibility to self-medicate a predetermined dose prior to activity or during times of increased pain. To attain a proper basal rate, it might be prudent to initially program the pump without a basal rate and assess usage over 24 hours. A basal rate can then be calculated equal to 1/2 the total used and averaged over the entire time period. Usage of a patient-controlled analgesia assumes a level of competency to be able to follow directions and self-administer medications when appropriate. As cognitive impairment is of concern in the elderly, dosing of pain medications may become the responsibility of their immediate care provider. Again, it is best to use sustained release opioids whenever possible. This results in fewer peaks and troughs and ultimately a reduced total dose of medication. Specific requests for analgesic medication from a nurse [pro re nata (PRN) medications] should be avoided whenever possible. Most opioids come in several preparations, including parenteral, tablet, liquid, and suppository, providing innumerable options for dosing.

Meperidine should not be considered for chronic analgesia in the elderly. Its metabolite, normeperidine, can accumulate, resulting in an increased risk of falls, increased sedation, and a reduction in the seizure threshold. It has proven effective in small doses (12.5–25 mg times one dose) to alleviate shivering that is often encountered after emergence from general anesthesia.

Several side effects are associated with opioid administration. Decreased bowel motility and ultimately constipation can be expected. A proper bowel regimen should be instituted, which includes adequate hydration, high fiber diet, and ambulation. In addition, senna works well to increase peristalsis and gut motility. If a cathartic must be used, sorbitol works well and has minimal effects on the GI tract when taken long term. Other side effects are often self-limiting and resolve with tolerance to the medication. Side effects such as nausea and vomiting often resolve over several days and should be treated with antiemetic medications in the interim.

CONCLUSION

There are many potential opportunities for morbidity and mortality in the postoperative elderly patient. All of the organ systems are likely impaired to some degree. This requires diligent care and attention to detail, as elderly patients are less likely to tolerate extreme changes from their baseline level of function. Ultimately, the best way to avoid postoperative morbidity and mortality is to identify at-risk patients prior to surgery and optimize their medical condition before any surgical intervention is undertaken.

BIBLIOGRAPHY

Apfel CC, Laara E, Koivuranta M, et al. A simplified risk score for predicting postoperative nausea and vomiting: conclusions from cross-validations between two centers. Anesthesiology 1999; 9:693–700.

Berge KH, Lanier WL. Problems after head, neck and maxillofacial surgery. Post Anesthesia Care 1992; 282–291.

Beliveau MM, Multach M. Perioperative care for the elderly patient. Med Clin North Am 2003; 87:273–289.

Chung F, MezeiG. Factors contributing to a prolonged stay after ambulatory surgery. Anesth Analg 1999; 89:1352–1359.

Comfort VK, Code WE, Rooney ME, Yip RW. Naproxen premedication reduces postoperative tubal ligation pain. Can J Anesth 1992; 4:349–352.

Cook DJ, Rooke GA. Priorities in perioperative geriatrics. Anesth Analg 2003; 96:1823–1836.

Duncan KO, Leffell DJ. Preoperative assessment of the elderly patient. Dermatol Clin 1997; 15:583–593.

Garantziotis S, Kyrmizakis DE, Liolios AD. Critical care of the head and neck patient. Crit Care Clin 2003; 19:73–90.

Gloth FM. Pain management in the elderly: principles of perioperative pain management in older adults. Clin Geriatr Med 2001; 17:188–199.

Guigoz Y, Lauque S, Vellas BJ. Identifying the elderly a risk for malnutrition: the mini nutritional assessment. Clin Geriatr Med 2002; 18:737–757.

Halaszynski TM, Juda R, Silverman DG. Optimizing postoperative outcomes with efficient preoperative assessment and management. Crit Care Med 2004; 32:S76–S86.

Howell SJ, Sear JW. Perioperative myocardial injury: individual and population implications. Br J Anaesth 2004; 93:3–8.

Jin F, Chung F. Multimodal analgesia for postoperative pain control. J Clin Anesth 2001; 13:524–539.

John AD, Sieber FE. Age associated issues: geriatrics. Anesthiol Clin North Am 2004; 22:45–58.

Kannel WB, Belanger AF. Epidemiology of heart failure. Am Heart J 1991; 121:951–957.

Liu LL, Wiener-Kronish JP. Perioperative anesthesia issues in the elderly. Crit Care Clin 2003; 19:641–656.

Mangano DT. Perioperative cardiac morbidity. Anesthesiology 1990; 12:153–184.

McGrath B, Chung F. Postoperative recovery and discharge. Anesthiol Clin North Am 2003; 21:367–386.

Ong SK, Morton RP, et al. Pulmonary complication following major head and neck surgery with tracheostomy, a prospective, randomized, controlled trial of prophylactic antibiotics. Arch Otolaryngol Head Neck Surg 2004; 130:1084–1087.

Practice guidelines for postanesthetic care. A Report by the American Society of Anesthesiologists Task Force on Postanesthetic Care. Anesthesiology 2002; 96:742–752.

Richardson JD, Cocanour CS, Kern JA, et al. Perioperative risk assessment in elderly and high-risk patients. J Am College Surg 2004; 199:133–146.

Rosenthal RA, Kavic SM. Assessment and management of the geriatric patient. Crit Care Med 2004; 32:S92–S105.

Shyong EQ, Lucchinetti E, Tagliente, et al. Interleukin balance and early recovery from anesthesia in elderly surgical patient exposed to β-adrenergic antagonism. J Clin Anesth 2003; 15:170–178.

Stierer T, Fleisher LA. Challenging patients in an ambulatory setting. Anesthiol Clin North Am 2003; 21:243–261.

Warner DO. Preventing postoperative pulmonary complications. The role of the anesthesiologist. Anesthesiology 2000; 92:1467–1472.

64
Informed Consent

Cheryl Ellis Vaiani
Institute for the Medical Humanities, University of Texas Medical Branch, Galveston, Texas, U.S.A.

Informed consent is the process by which fully informed patients can participate in decisions about their own health care. The ethical principle underlying informed consent is respect for persons, or autonomy. Informed consent reflects both the legal and ethical right of patients to make choices about what happens to their bodies in accordance with their values and goals, and the ethical duty of the physician to enhance the patient's well-being. The older patient may present a challenge to the practice of informed consent. It may be difficult to establish effective communication with the elderly patient secondary to sensory limitations (impaired sight, hearing, speech), pain, confusion, or limitations in memory, each of which may be worsened with hospitalization. Because overcoming these communication obstacles may require time and patience, it is not uncommon for family members to assume decision-making for the elderly (or to be given that role by the health care team). It is important that the patient who is able to participate in decision-making not be bypassed for convenience or by family request. Evaluating, promoting, and protecting the decision-making capacity of the elderly patient is an important responsibility of the physician. This chapter will discuss the process and elements of informed consent and the evaluation of decisional capacity and how to proceed if the patient is determined not to be able to make medical decisions.

There is no absolute formula for obtaining informed consent for a procedure, treatment plan, or therapy. A consent form should best be considered the documentation of the *process* of informed consent, not a single event or a guarantee that the process has occurred. The process should include explanations from the physician in language the patient can understand and the opportunity for the patient to ask questions and consult with others, if necessary. Clarification of the patient's understanding is an important part of the consent process. Asking the patients to explain in their own words what they expect to happen and possible outcomes is much more indicative of their understanding than their ability to merely repeat what the physician has stated (What do you understand about the surgery that has been recommended to you?). The geriatric patient who nods or fails to question a treatment plan is sometimes thought to have given consent when, in fact, that patient has no ability to understand or evaluate alternatives. Ideally, the process of informed consent should really be one of shared decision-making, where the physician and patient work together to choose a course of treatment utilizing the physician's expertise and the patient's values and goals.

There are four major exceptions to the requirement for informed consent; generally they reflect the balancing of the patient's self-determination and best interest. The first exception deals with emergency situations. In situations when emergency treatment is required and the patient is unable to give consent (patient is unconscious, incoherent, or unable to communicate), consent can be presumed on the basis that a reasonable person would agree to the treatment. The emergency exception does not apply if it is known that the patient would refuse the treatment, e.g., the Jehovah's Witness patient who is known to refuse blood transfusions in all situations or the patient who has indicated a desire not to be resuscitated. Incapacity is the second exception to the requirement for informed consent and will be discussed in detail later in this chapter. If a patient is incapable of making medical decisions, a surrogate decision-maker can guide appropriate treatment according to the decision-maker's knowledge of the patient's wishes or best interest. Therapeutic privilege is the third exception and allows information to be withheld from the patient, but only in very circumscribed situations. If the physician believes that providing the patient information would seriously harm the patient, information could potentially be withheld or postponed until the potential harm to the patient is mitigated. Therapeutic privilege is not permission to avoid delivering bad news. Neither is therapeutic privilege permission to withhold information because the physician fears that honest and accurate information might result in the patient's refusal of treatment (1). The final exception to informed consent is when the patient chooses to waive informed consent. A patient's informed choice not to participate in decision-making or to delegate the decision-making to another person should be respected. The elderly patient may say, "Let my daughter decide." It is important that the physician explore both the reasons for and the limitations of the waiver by the patient and to insure that the patient remains committed to that choice over time (1,2). Family members sometimes seek to protect the geriatric patient from disturbing or stressful news or decision-making by assuming the patient's role in communicating with the health care team. While the family motives may be good ones, only the patient can waive their right to informed consent.

A 65-year-old man presents to you with failing eyesight. Your history and physical exam indicate the probability of rapidly progressing loss of sight culminating in blindness. You re-enter the exam room, but before you can say anything, he nervously shakes his head and says: "Boy, I sure hope I'm not going blind . . . my father was totally blind for years and it was horrible. If you tell me I'm going blind, I think I'd end it all."

Is it allowable to withhold the prognosis from this patient?

- While this could be considered a situation where the therapeutic waiver to informed consent might be appropriate, more information is needed.
- It is important to evaluate the risk of this patient's threat. Is the patient depressed? Have there been previous suicide threats/attempts? Or are the patient's words more an indication of the seriousness of this diagnosis to his way of life and expectations for the future?
- If you determine the patient's threat to be a realistic concern, how can you help the patient? Should supportive family members or friends be present? Do you recommend psychiatric evaluation and guidance and/or hospitalization?
- The seriousness of this diagnosis indicates that careful and considerate presentation of diagnosis, prognosis, and options may require planning and timing but does not justify withholding diagnosis from patient.

Informed consent includes three major components: disclosure, capacity, and voluntariness. Disclosure is the provision of relevant information, such as the nature and purpose of the decision/therapy/procedure, the relevant risks, benefits, and uncertainties, feasible alternatives, and the prognosis if treatment is not given (3). Capacity is the patient's ability to understand the relevant information and to appreciate those consequences of their decision. Voluntariness implies that the person has the ability to make a free choice absent of coercion, manipulation, or positive or negative controlling influences.

Physicians sometimes struggle with the application of informed consent in practice. Since patients cannot be expected to comprehend information at the same level as the physician, what information is important to include and what can be omitted? The guidance provided by state law usually indicates a legal standard of disclosure: professional standard (what a reasonable physician would disclose), reasonable person standard (what a reasonable patient in the same or similar situation would want to know), or particular person standard (what a reasonable person in the same particular circumstances would want to know) (2). While it is important to be cognizant of your state's law, it may not provide specific guidance in dealing with a particular patient or situation. As a general recommendation, although it is not necessary to disclose every risk, it is important to include those that are common, likely, or indicative that the potential of harm is severe. If the informed consent process is one of two-way communication and interaction, the questions and concerns of the patient can guide the physician in appropriate disclosure (3). Patients seek and expect a recommendation based on the physician's knowledge and experience, not merely a listing of available options. While some patients may appreciate and benefit from access to an article about a procedure and its statistical outcomes, it is not a substitute for disclosure of information by the physician and may confuse and be disingenuous to the patient.

Voluntariness means that a choice has been made free of coercion, manipulation, or other forms of controlling influence. Decisions are made in the context of various pressures: competing needs, familial interests, legal obligations, religious beliefs, and persuasive arguments; physicians need to be alert to situations when these influences may be interfering with the patient's free choice (3). Talking to the patient alone and allowing adequate time for discussion may serve to augment the patient's decision-making. Persuasion is central to the consent process. Physicians present a plan of care and convincing reasons why that particular choice is indicated. A patient's reluctance to agree to that plan should signal the clinician that further discussion is necessary. Persuasion may respect and enhance patient autonomy by improving the patient's understanding of the circumstances and options. Persuasion can also be negative if it involves manipulation of information in order to convince the patient.

Determining a patient's capacity to participate in decision-making is an important physician role. While capacity is generally assumed in adult patients, there are numerous occasions when capacity for decision-making is questionable or absent. Illness, medication, and altered mental status may result in an inability to participate independently in medical decision-making. Hospitalization may cause fear, confusion, or intimidation in the elderly and compound other sensory deficits associated with aging. Capacity for decision-making occurs along a continuum, and the threshold capacity is dependent on the decision to be made: the more serious the consequences of the decision, the higher the level of capacity that should be required. Decisional capacity may also change over time; an individual may be capable of medical decisions one day or even one time of day but not at another. The elderly patient may have diminished or fluctuating capacity and the physician may need to schedule communication early in the day to avoid "sundowning" or confusion that occurs at the end of the day (4). Probably the most common reason for questioning a patient's capacity is patient refusal of a treatment, procedure, or plan that the physician feels is indicated. While a patient refusal certainly raises a "red flag" and may be an appropriate indicator for an evaluation of capacity, it should not be the only one. Determination of capacity should be an essential part of the informed consent process for any decision.

Although we commonly use them interchangeably, competence and capacity have different meanings in the legal context. Competence is a legal term and considers globally whether one is capable of self-care and managing their own business affairs. Competence is determined by a judge in a court of law. If a person is judged to be incompetent, another decision-maker, a legal guardian, is generally appointed. Capacity is determined by the physician and is one's actual, present ability to understand and appreciate the nature of their condition and the consequences of their decision to consent to treatment or refuse it.

But how does a physician best evaluate a patient's capacity? There is no one definitive assessment tool for capacity. Although there are many guides and standards to evaluating capacity, it is most generally a common sense judgment that arises from a clinician's interaction with the patient. Mental status tests that assess orientation to person, place, and time are less useful than direct assessment of a patient's ability to make the particular medical decision. Simple questions such as,

- What do you understand about what is going on with your health right now?
- What treatment/diagnostic test/procedure has been proposed to you?
- What are the benefits/risks?
- What have you decided and why?

more directly assess the evaluation of capacity in the clinical setting (2,6). A psychiatric consult may contribute to the assessment, particularly if mental illness may be contributing to the incapacity. Depression in the elderly and chronically or terminally ill patient may influence capacity, and psychiatry may be helpful in identification and treatment of depression to enhance a patient's capacity. An ethics consultation may also help address the ethical dimensions of the capacity assessment.

Mrs. Whitehead is an 84-year-old patient with multiple medical problems, including end stage renal disease requiring hemodialysis, diabetes, and hypertension. She lives alone with minimal assistance (meals on wheels, transportation), but recent hospitalizations have left her less able to maintain her independence. She is hospitalized for cataract surgery and you are discussing the surgery with her at the end of a long day of surgery. After your presentation of information about the procedure, its risks and benefits, and expected outcome, you ask for Mrs. Whitehead to sign her surgical consent form. Although she picks up the pen and seems ready to sign, she says, "I am not so sure I want this surgery. I am really tired of dialysis three times a week." What should your response be?

- Patient may be expressing her concern about the effect of the surgery on her independence, or may need reassurance, or may be making a decision about further interventions. She also could be depressed or confused at the end of the day. Further questioning and discussion is clearly necessary to evaluate her capacity and her reasons for questioning the surgery.

If the patient is determined to be incapacitated for medical decision-making, clinicians must turn to a surrogate decision-maker to provide consent. Ideally, all patients would have a designated proxy appointed in a living will or power of attorney for health care. This proxy would be aware of the patient's values and preferences and would be able to make treatment decisions in the patient's stead according to their wishes. Since this is rarely the case, relatives, according to the hierarchy designated by state law, are frequently utilized as surrogate decision-makers. Family members are considered to be able to best know and represent the patient's best interests. If an incapacitated patient has not indicated a proxy and no relatives are available, individual state law sometimes designates institutional committees to assist in decision-making. For a patient who is felt to be permanently incapacitated for decision-making, particularly one without available family members, a legal guardian may be necessary.

Surrogate decision-makers are expected to make their decisions according to the wishes of the incapacitated patient and to represent the patient's best interests. If the physician suspects that other motives or issues may be influencing the surrogate's decision-making, further discussion, consultation, or even legal action may be necessary. Surrogates are required to first make decisions according to the substituted judgment standard. They are asked to make the decision that the patient would have made in the same circumstances. Unfortunately, surrogates may not always know what decision the patient would have made, or there may be disagreement among relatives about the patient's wishes. In circumstances when the patient's wishes are unknown, surrogates are asked to base decisions on what they believe is best for the patient, the best interests standard (6).

Ethically and legally, informed consent is at the heart of the relationship between the physician and the patient. It is the process of educating the patient and assessing that the patient has understood. It is dependent not on the information provided but the understanding of that information by the patient. The limited physiologic, psychologic, and social reserves of the elderly make them particularly vulnerable to disempowerment. Enhancing decision making for an elderly patient may be as simple as facing the patient, speaking slowly and distinctly, and decreasing background noise. It also may involve providing the patient adequate time to consider the issues and make a decision. Or it may require the physician to make the difficult decision that an elderly patient is incapable of independent medical decision-making and seek a surrogate for help. Shared decision-making for the geriatric patient is a goal that is worthwhile and achievable but requires time, effort, and interest on the part of the physician. Further information on informed consent can be found on the Web sites in References 7 and 8.

REFERENCES

1. Meisel A, Kuczewski M. Legal and ethical myths about informed consent. Arch Intern Med 1996; 156:2521–2526.
2. Lo B. Resolving ethical dilemmas: a guide for physicians. 2nd ed. Lippincott: Williams & Wilkins, 2000.
3. Boyle RJ. The process of informed consent. In: Fletcher JC, Lombardo PA, Marshall MF, Miller FG, eds. Introduction to Clinical Ethics. 2nd ed. Hagerstown, MD: University Publishing Group, 1997:89–105.

4. Dubler NN. Legal and ethical issues. In: The Merck Manual of Geriatrics. 3rd ed. Published by Merck Research Laboratories, Whitehouse Station, NJ, 2000:1–16.
5. Lo B. Assessing decision-making capacity. Law Med Health Care 1990; 18:193–201.
6. Boyle RJ. Determining patients capacity to share in decision making. In: Fletcher JC, Lombardo PA, Marshall MF, Miller FG, eds. Introduction to Clinical Ethics. 2nd ed. Hagerstown, MD: University Publishing Group, 1997:71–88.
7. http://eduserv.hscer.washington.edu/bioethics/topics/consent.html.
8. http://www.research.umn.edu/consent/menu_med.html.

65
Pain Management in the Elderly

David Sibell
Department of Anesthesiology and Perioperative Medicine, Oregon Health and Science University, Portland, Oregon, U.S.A.

Old age is not so bad when you consider the alternatives.

—Maurice Chevalier (1888–1972)

THE SIZE OF THE PROBLEM

"You're just going to have to learn to live with it." This is what many patients suffering from chronic pain hear from their physicians. Until the mid-20th century, the idea that chronic pain conditions could and should be treated was relatively novel. People with chronic pain conditions have been viewed as weaklings or malingerers, when, in fact, these perceptions likely represent physicians' discomfort in assessing and treating chronic pain conditions. As there are consistently more effective options for the treatment of chronic pain conditions, and as pain management is becoming required both in medical education and practice, it is now considered a fundamental patient right (1). This reflects a complete change in beliefs about a physician's obligation to treat pain. While this is a sign of both improved ability to treat pain and societal expectations, the concept of treating suffering has long been at the core of medical ethics and philosophy.

Changes in medical practice regarding pain management have been relatively slow to affect the treatment of older Americans. There are numerous barriers to the treatment of pain in the elderly, including societal, patient, and medical care team factors (Fig. 1) (2). Overcoming these and others is not only useful, but is incumbent on the treatment team involved in the care of older patients with chronic pain.

But how common is chronic pain among American elders? Almost a quarter of the U.S. population is 55 years old or older, and the most rapidly growing segment of this population is octogenarians (3). The aged population is more likely to suffer from painful medical disorders, such as osteoarthritis, painful diabetic neuropathy, postherpetic neuralgia, and cancer [the American Cancer Society states that 77% of cancer patients are 55 years of age or older (4)]. The prevalence of diabetes mellitus

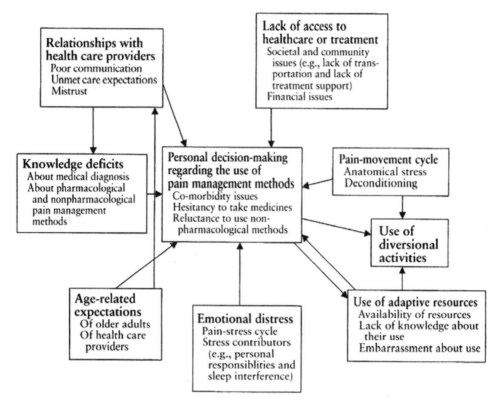

Figure 1 Barriers to treatment of chronic pain of older adults with arthritis.

is increasing over time, and its intensity increases with age, as well. The occurrence of painful diabetic neuropathy equals approximately 20–30% among diabetics. Six hundred thousand to eight hundred thousand cases of postherpetic neuralgia occur annually, and amongst PHN patients over 50 years of age, the prevalence of postherpetic neuralgia is nearly 15 times greater than in those younger than 50 (5). In addition, there is a 70% incidence of osteoarthritis in this age group, with at least another 42,000,000 elderly Americans at risk for a chronic pain condition (6). Clearly, chronic pain in elderly Americans is a problem that requires the attention of the medical community.

BASIC SCIENCE OF CHRONIC PAIN

It is beyond the scope of this chapter to review the entire physiology of pain reception, transmission, and processing. Instead, the focus is on physiological issues pertinent to geriatric patients with chronic pain. The comparison between young and old patients with chronic pain differs most greatly with respect to assessment, sensory apparatus, and pharmacological effects of pain medications. There is a vocabulary utilized in the study of pain. A small glossary can be found in Table 1.

Painful conditions are disproportionately under-assessed in elderly patients. These patients, as a group, may underreport painful conditions or have barriers to communicating their symptoms to their providers. These occur often in patients who have lost cognitive or language skills as a result of neurological injury. Another factor in age-related assessment failure is the patient's own inhibitions. Geriatric patients may

Table 1 Glossary of Pain Terminology

Term	Definition
Allodynia	Painful response to an innocuous stimulus
Dysesthesia	Abnormal, unpleasant sensation
Hyperalgesia	Exaggerated response to a normally mildly noxious stimulus
Hyperpathia	Abnormal painful reaction to a repeated stimulus, associated with an increased threshold to the initiating stimulus
Hypoesthesia/hypesthesia	Decreased sensation to a normal stimulus
Neuralgia	Pain in the distribution of a nerve or nerves
Neuropathic pain	Pain initiated or caused by a primary lesion to the nervous system
Nociceptor	Neuronal receptor sensitive to noxious stimulus
NSAID	Nonsteroidal anti-inflammatory drug

feel that their painful condition is normal for their age or fear seeking medical attention for complaints that may lead to ominous diagnoses (7). However, the most significant impairment to pain assessment in elders is inadequate evaluation by the physician (8). In order to maximize patient access to effective treatment for specific disorders, the clinician must conduct an active, targeted history and physical examination.

Many investigators have hypothesized age-related changes in pain sensation. Clinical efforts have largely outpaced understanding of these changes, however. This has led to problematic developments, such as patent ductus arteriosus surgery on neonates without anesthesia. Although this practice is no longer condoned, there are those who believe that the nervous systems of elders are also incapable of experiencing pain in a manner similar to younger cohorts. There have been no studies demonstrating a clear difference in pain sensation between young and old subjects. There may be a slight difference between the sensation of "fast pain," mediated by small, myelinated A-δ fibers, and "slow pain," mediated by c-fibers, but this does not appear to be clinically significant (9). There are differences in nociception relating to disease states, however, which may occur as complications of disease accumulate with age. This is due principally to changes in the central and peripheral nervous system.

Cerebrovascular accidents, spinal injuries, and peripheral polyneuropathies effect sensation in predictable, if problematic, ways. These can include hypesthesia to normal stimuli, as well as allodynia and hyperalgesia. While not associated with age per se, these changes are found in increasing frequency in elderly patients with neurological diseases.

By far, the most relevant differences in the treatment of elderly patients have to do with changes in pharmacology that occur with age and with diseases that occur more commonly in older patients. Protein binding is affected by age. However, this is less frequently relevant in pharmacological concerns than are changes in proportion of adipose tissue and decreases in renal and hepatic function that occur with age. Furthermore, there may be offsetting influences, such as decreased protein binding compensating for decreased receptor sensitivity to a given drug. Generally speaking, changes in protein binding are present with advancing age, but they are not of primary physiological relevance (10).

Of principal interest in geriatric pharmacology are the age-related decreases in hepatic and renal function and their effects on biotransformation. Reduction in efficiency of demethylation results in prolonged half-lives of substances that depend on this mechanism. This is especially problematic in drugs such as diazepam, whose half-life is prolonged from 24 hours in younger patients to more than 90 hours in older patients. Phase I metabolism is generally more effected than phase II so that the duration of action of drugs whose hepatic metabolism primarily involves demethylation by cytochrome P40 reductase enzymes are more prolonged than those that are primarily conjugated (11).

Decreases in renal function have the most important effect on pharmacology in elderly patients. As humans age, there is an expected progression of glomerulosclerosis and interstitial fibrosis. Tubular function also decreases. These and other factors serve to reduce glomerular filtration rate (GFR) by approximately 8 mL/min/decade after age 30. Add changes associated with hypertension and/or diabetes, exposure to toxins (including NSAID-induced nephropathy), and other disease-related effects, and GFR may be further impaired. This has significant effects on drug clearance. These changes mandate dose reductions for certain drugs, such as lorazepam (12). The worst-case scenario is meperidine. Meperidine's volume of distribution is decreased in older patients. It undergoes prolonged hepatic metabolism and has a principal metabolite, normeperidine, whose elimination half-life is inversely proportional to creatinine clearance. As the parent compound is re-dosed, normeperidine levels increase until patients become hyper-reflexic, myoclonic, or suffer generalized tonic–clonic seizures.

Finally, older people are more susceptible to drug toxicities and adverse effects. This is, in part, due to interactions secondary to polypharmacy. It is also due to primary degenerative processes leading to physiological states exacerbated by pharmaceuticals. One key example is the increased risk of constipation with opioids due to age-related decreases in colonic transit; another is increased susceptibility to NSAID-induced nephropathy due to underlying glomerulosclerosis and decreased GFR.

It is also worth mentioning that adherence to drug therapy may be hindered in older patients. Adherence to therapeutic regimens is especially low when the risk factors of dementia, use of "safety bottles," and complicated therapeutic regimens are present. Clinicians amplify adherence by paying increased attention to in-office patient education, as well as clear take-home instructions. Simple dosing regimens, including reduced frequency of dosing, improve adherence as well.

DIAGNOSIS OF PAINFUL DISORDERS IN THE ELDERLY

A common failing in pain diagnosis is the use of the pain *complaint* as a *diagnosis*. "Chronic back pain" is not a diagnosis; rather, it is a complaint. A differential diagnosis for this complaint includes such varied diagnoses as lumbar facet arthritis, myofascial dysfunction, and metastatic cancer. Therefore, a firm diagnosis starts with a good history and physical examination. Since this topic comprises a wide variety of pathological conditions, focusing on particular historical and physical examination points would be problematic. Instead, this section will focus on general concepts. Where applicable, specific findings will be discussed in the differential diagnosis section.

As with any pain history, it is important to ask the patient detailed questions about the pain complaint. There is a popular mnemonic device to assist with this: PQRST (Table 2). While these questions do not often suffice for a complete history, they are essential in forming the differential diagnosis of pain conditions. The quality of pain is particularly important, as this can help with the initial branch point in the differential diagnosis.

Table 2   PQRST Pain History Mnemonic

P: provoke	What provokes or improves the pain? What do you think causes it?
Q: quality	What type of pain sensation (e.g., sharp, dull, achy, burning, stinging)?
R: radiates	Does the pain radiate? If so, where? If not, where is it localized?
S: severity	How severe is the pain? You may use a 0–10 scale.
T: time	When did the pain start? Is it worse at any particular time of day?

Source: From Ref. 13.

Pain that is sharp and well localized is often referred to as somatic nociception. It is predominantly mediated by A-δ neuronal fibers and is typically found in conditions involving inflammatory pain (e.g., fracture, laceration, arthralgias). In contrast, achy and/or colicky, anatomically vague pain is generally visceral in etiology. This is served primarily by c-fibers (e.g., colonic distension, biliary colic, ureteral distension, pancreatitis). Pain that is lancinating, electrical, burning, and/or itchy is usually associated with a neuropathic condition (e.g., diabetic neuropathy, glossopharyngeal neuralgia). These distinctions are extremely important, as the therapy for one type of pain condition may be less effective for another. One example would be the relatively high efficacy of NSAIDs in rheumatoid arthritis in comparison to diabetic neuropathy.

The anatomic location and radiation pattern of a pain complaint are key to understanding the underlying lesion, as are the exacerbating and ameliorating features. Jaw pain may be primary, as in a mandibular fracture or temporomandibular dysfunction, or secondary, as in angina pectoris, which radiates to the jaw.

The clinician should also inquire as to prior treatments. How effective were they? Were there side effects that limited treatment with a particular medication? What dose was achieved before the treatment was abandoned? Did an interventional treatment or surgery lead to improvements or complications? Thorough knowledge of these historical points improves therapeutic efficiency by reducing duplicative efforts but allowing retrial of incomplete medical trials.

The physical examination is also critical. This involves a general health examination (the clinician that fails to examine the abdomen of a patient complaining of back pain is the one who misses the diagnosis of a metastasis of a primary abdominal tumor), as well as specific examination techniques involving pain conditions. The goal of this examination is to refine the differential diagnosis created by the chief complaint and history of present illness by including and excluding differential diagnoses. Although it is uncomfortable for the patient, the clinician must duplicate, or at least simulate, in the examination those exacerbating factors mentioned in the history. If cervical extension duplicates pain, for instance, it is important to measure the degree of cervical extension, and to specify where the pain is duplicated. This yields not only a suggestion as to the anatomical etiology of the painful condition (e.g., myofascial vs. radicular vs. arthropathic), but serves as a functional measurement that may be reassessed over time. If therapy leads to improved range of motion, this finding serves as an objective measurement of success.

There is a 40% decrease in lumbar flexion and a 76% decrease in lumbar extension associated with age (axial rotation remains constant across age groups) (14). This factors into physical examination, with respect to what is considered normal in older patients. The neurological examination is particularly important. In addition to measurement of power and reflexes, the sensory examination is particularly important. Examination with light touch reveals areas of hypesthesia and allodynia. Further careful investigation with a pin in these areas reveals hyperalgesia and hyperpathia. When taken together, these findings generate the anatomic and pathophysiologic criteria by which neuropathic pain conditions are diagnosed. If an intraoral examination is necessary for assessment of a pain complaint, examination with a cotton swab may replace the light touch examination.

DIFFERENTIAL DIAGNOSIS

Effective pain treatment begins with a thorough clinical assessment. In order to optimize the efficiency of this assessment, the clinician must have a sense of the epidemiology of painful conditions in the elderly population. There are a few key diagnoses that increase in frequency with age, and that predispose patients to chronic pain conditions.

Neuropathic Pain States

Approximately 770,000 Americans suffer symptomatic strokes annually (15). Of these, approximately 3% to 5% will have central post-stroke pain syndrome (CPSP) a neuropathic pain syndrome that occurs after stroke (16). Others will have related, non-neuropathic pain complaints, having to do with rehabilitation (e.g., shoulder pain due to transfers to and from a wheelchair, pressure ulcerations, etc.). CPSP is diagnosed by neurological examination: The patient will have typical neuropathic pain findings (e.g., allodynia, hyperalgesia, hyperpathia, and/or lancinating spontaneous pains) in the distribution of the stroke. There may be associated cognitive and/or affective changes that complicate diagnosis and therapy. These symptoms often present up to two years after the stroke.

There are several painful cranial neuropathies. These are not strictly age related, but deserve mention, given the nature of this text. One of the most problematic is glossopharyngeal neuralgia (GN). GN has multiple etiologies, including an elongated styloid process (Eagle syndrome) or tumor in the area of the lateral posterior pharynx to the middle ear. It may also be idiopathic. It is characterized by spontaneous lancinating pain in the tongue and throat, often exacerbated by deglutition. There is often a dull, achy component in between attacks. It is a principal differential diagnosis in the complaint of odynophagia. There is also a frequent association with cardiac dysrhythmias, which may be life threatening (17).

Another, more common painful cranial neuropathy is trigeminal neuralgia (TN), also known as *tic doloreux*. This is characterized by intermittent lancinating pain in the distribution of one or more of the trigeminal branches. The pain may be spontaneous or brought on by physical contact or stress. Trigeminal neuralgia may be due to compressive effects on the trigeminal ganglion within the foramen ovale. Anatomic causes include an overriding artery, aneurysm, tumor, or other structure, in which case foraminal decompression may be indicated. This therapy is frequently effective, but the long-term success rate is variously reported between 20% and 70% (18). Therefore, the therapy is considered as a long-term palliation, rather than a complete cure. Radiofrequency neurotomy offers a less invasive alternative. It is associated with lower surgical risk and a higher initial response rate, but a lower frequency of long-term pain relief. There is insufficient evidence at present to make a global recommendation regarding these two options, so this decision must be made on an individual basis (19).

If the pain is of a different character (e.g., not lancinating) or anatomic description, it is considered atypical facial pain or chronic facial pain (20). This set of complaints is typically more resistant to medical and/or interventional therapies. Typically, the therapeutic choices involve medical treatments, presuming a neuropathic underlying, and often involve nonmedication therapy such as cognitive behavioral psychological therapy as well.

Postherpetic neuralgia (PHN) occurs in adults who suffer a reactivation of the varicella-zoster virus, which remains dormant in dorsal root ganglia (DRG) or trigeminal ganglia after a childhood infection. Zoster occurs in a dermatomal or cranial nerve distribution, and destruction of the DRG by zoster infection correlates directly with severity of PHN. This disease is more common in elderly patients, who for a variety of reasons have reduced cellular immunity. The disease appears most commonly in thoracic dermatomes, but cranial nerves are second in frequency (21). While the zoster infection itself can be severely painful, it is the prolonged pain after resolution of the infection that is even more devastating. This occurs in between 3% and 30% of patients suffering a single episode of zoster infection and is more common in older patients.

Early intervention with antivirals has been shown to reduce the prevalence of PHN by approximately 50% (22). However, for those patients who are in pain, gabapentin, pregabalin, topical lidocaine patch (Lidoderm®, Endo Pharmaceuticals), and opioids may be effective. The first three of these are now FDA approved for the treatment this disorder. The role for interventional treatment in this population is not as clear, with the exception of the use of intrathecal opioids when systemic opioids are effective but not tolerated. Some have advocated the use of nerve blocks during the acute zoster outbreak as a means of reducing the prevalence of PHN, but many of these studies lack adequate controls and appear to be charting the natural history of the illness (23). However, there is evidence that early analgesia reduces some of the secondary changes associated with chronic neuropathic pain. Therefore, early treatment of zoster-related pain is important in the immediate term, and may have long-term benefits as well.

Diabetes mellitus is the most common etiology of neuropathy in the United States and Europe, with approximately one-third of diabetics developing neuropathy (24). There are many presentations of diabetic neuropathy, but the most common is as a peripheral polyneuropathy. This presents typically with stocking-like lower extremity hypesthesia and allodynia, eventually involving the upper extremities in a glove-like distribution. Adequate glycemic control is important to retard the rate of disease progression, but the neuropathy will typically advance despite this control.

Postherpetic neuropathy and diabetic neuropathy are the most frequently studied neuropathic pain syndromes, and therefore have the largest variety of proven therapies. The data from these studies, as well as that from smaller disease-specific studies, demonstrate that there is significant cross-effectiveness in the treatment of neuropathic pain states.

Primarily Musculoskeletal Pain States

Musculoskeletal pain states are the most common pain complaints registered by older patients. Some estimates are that 100% of elderly patients will complain of muscle aches and weakness during their lives. Osteoarthritis is also ubiquitous, as mentioned earlier in this chapter.

Muscular pain can be divided into two major types: primary and secondary. Primary muscular pain is further divided into localized muscular pain, generally attributed to an injury, and generalized muscular pain. Localized muscular pain is generally acute, resolving on a time course of days or, at most, weeks. Patients are more prone to acute muscular trauma if they are deactivated and deconditioned. If these conditions are apparent, activating physical therapy, defined by engagement in some form of physical conditioning, has more long-term efficacy than passive physical therapy (i.e., primarily associated with modalities such as ultrasound or muscle stimulation). Furthermore, there are far-reaching health and physical performance benefits associated with improved physical conditioning (25).

For generalized myofascial pain states, more involved programs often are necessary. While the mechanism of fibromyalgia is still unclear, the American College of Rheumatology has stipulated diagnostic characteristics. These involve the presence of generalized myofascial pain and a positive Myofascial Tender Point Survey (26). The physiology and exact treatment regimens available for fibromyalgia go beyond the scope of this chapter, but several excellent reviews are available on the subject (27). Generalized myofascial pain not conforming to the diagnosis of fibromyalgia still shares much of the treatment concepts, as does that due to fibromyalgia.

Oncological Pain States

The American Cancer Society estimates that 50% to 70% of cancer patients experience pain, but that less than half of them receive adequate treatment for it (28). Despite the fact that there has been a worldwide effort to improve the treatment for patients with cancer over the past two decades, this sobering fact persists. Approximately 17% of patients with cancer pain complain of their primary symptom in the head and/or neck (29). "Cancer pain" is a misleading term, as it encompasses many etiologies for pain. Primary tumor involvement, invasion of surrounding tissues, metastases, and results of treatments such as radiation, surgery, and/or chemotherapy may all cause pain and other unpleasant symptoms. As in the treatment of nonmalignant pain, the treatment of pain in patients with cancer should be focused on the etiology, type of pain (e.g., nociceptive vs. neuropathic), and the patient's other multidimensional factors. Therefore, while an anatomic diagnosis is essential, so is an understanding of the patient's anxiety and affect.

Patients with anxiety disorders and/or depression have higher requirements for analgesics than matched patients without these factors. This is not because these patients are somehow embellishing their symptoms; rather, there are complicated interactions between mental and emotional influences and pain. Medications alone are often insufficient in the treatment of cancer-related pain, and much of the time, this is due to the concomitant affective, cognitive, and familial influences on the patient and their diagnosis (30,31).

Therefore, the treatment of pain in patients with cancer is not fundamentally different from that for those patients with nonmalignant pain. Diagnosis, multidimensional assessment, and attention to the type of pain complaint are the most important factors. The major differences, especially in otolaryngology practice, have to do with associated challenges involving disfigurement, nutrition, and death from the disease.

TREATMENT OPTIONS

Rather than attempt to outline specific treatments for each painful disorder, it is more fitting to describe treatment strategies for categories of painful disorders, as the mechanisms of painful disorders tend to respond in kind (e.g., painful diabetic neuropathy is apt to respond to treatments that are effective for other neuropathic pain states, such as postherpetic neuralgia).

Neuropathic Pain States

Historically, the most well-validated therapies for neuropathic pain have included tricyclic antidepressants and certain anticonvulsants. It is still true that these agents have the most substantial volume of medical literature to support their use, but recently, other medical and nonmedical therapies have emerged as equally or more effective.

Tricyclic antidepressants are not technically analgesic medications, but can reduce allodynia, hyperalgesia, and spontaneous pain in neuropathic pain conditions. They all require gradual dose titration and have anticholinergic, adrenergic, and cardiac conduction side effects that can make them unsuitable for elderly patients. Therefore, their use must be carefully monitored in older patients, and it may be advisable to avoid them in patients more subject to these adverse effects. This is an off-label but generally accepted and well-validated use for this class of medications. The most commonly used tricyclic antidepressants for painful conditions are amitriptyline, nortriptyline, and desipramine. These are listed here in decreasing order of anticholinergic properties. Typically, the dose of any of these medications for elderly patients starts at 10–25 mg daily. These drugs are usually started at night with the ultimate dose goal being in the 100–150 mg/day range. Nortriptyline is generally associated with fewer adverse effects than amitriptyline, but still may be hazardous in older adults at risk for its adverse effects (32). Not all patients tolerate the higher doses, however, and the clinician must be careful in using these drugs in patients prone to xerostomia, cardiac dysrhythmias, orthostatic hypotension, urinary retention, constipation, or sedation. The beneficial effects of these drugs are typically delayed by four to six weeks after reaching the effective dose, whereas the adverse effects are generally apparent immediately.

Unfortunately, there is no convincing evidence to support the use of selective serotonin reuptake inhibitors specifically to treat pain (33). There is some early clinical evidence to support the use of some of the newer, atypical agents, but it is insufficient to merit the same level of endorsement as with tricyclic antidepressants at this time. Recently, the novel serotonin or norepinephrine reuptake inhibitor antidepressant, duloxetin, was FDA approved for the treatement of painful diabetic neuropathy. This drug, when taken at a dose of 60 mg. once daily, produces a 50% reduction in average pain over 24 hours and is generally well tolerated (34).

Not all anticonvulsants are effective in treating neuropathic pain, but three of the five drugs currently FDA approved for the treatment of neuropathic pain conditions are anticonvulsants (carbamazepine, gabapentin, and pregabalin). There is also scientific evidence supporting the use of several other anticonvulsants in a variety of neuropathic pain conditions. Carbamazepine has been used to treat trigeminal neuralgia since the 1960s. It has established efficacy in this condition, but also has significant safety concerns. It may cause hepatic injury, myelosuppression, and numerous drug–drug interactions. Although it may be used with care in elderly patients, there are generally better alternatives available.

Gabapentin is a more recent development. This antiepileptic has demonstrated efficacy in numerous randomized, controlled trials in several neuropathic pain conditions. Among the most frequently studied are painful diabetic neuropathy and postherpetic neuralgia, diseases more frequently seen in elderly populations (35).

This drug appears to bind to the "2-" protein subunit of voltage-gated calcium channels and reduce excitatory neurotransmitter release. However, it is generally well tolerated, produces no significant drug–drug interactions, and has no end-organ toxicities. The effective daily dose is generally between 1800 and 3600 mg/day, but the initial dose should be limited to 300 mg/day in elderly patients, to avoid the evanescent side effects, including sedation and ataxia. Increases of 300 mg/day are generally well tolerated. Pregabalin, an anticonvulsant similar in its mechanism to gabapentin, has proven efficacy in the treatment of both PHN and PDN and is FDA approved for the treatment of pain due to both disorders. Pregabalin is more potent than gabapentin and has linear absorption kinetics all through its typical dose range of 300–600 mg/day, in twice daily dosage (36,37).

Aside from carbamazepine and gabapentin, few of the numerous alternative anticonvulsants have a significant body of evidence to support their use. However, there is a growing body of evidence that suggests that lamotrigine, in particular, shows efficacy in a number of neuropathic pain states. It is difficult to use, however, when compared with gabapentin. The dose escalation period from 25 or 50 to 150 mg is measured in weeks, as most patients only tolerate increases of 25–50 mg/week. The principal side effect of this medication is a nonallergic rash, which, in the worst case, may proceed to Stevens–Johnson syndrome. However, it may be an effective second-line anticonvulsant (38). It is possible that ongoing studies will define the roles for the other anticonvulsant drugs for painful conditions in the near future.

Traditionally, opioids have been disparaged as ineffective in the treatment of neuropathic pain. More recent evidence, however, points to the contrary. While early negative studies reflected societal prejudices against opioid medications or poor study design, more recent work has demonstrated that opioids compare favorably with tricyclic antidepressants and anticonvulsants in reducing both pain and allodynia in neuropathic pain states (39–41). Given the safety profile of these medications alongside recent information demonstrating efficacy, opioids should most definitely be considered for analgesia in chronic neuropathic pain states. A more thorough description of appropriate opioid utilization in the elderly follows this section.

Myofascial Pain States

As mentioned above, primary myofascial pain may be localized due to an acute injury, or may be either regional or generalized in the chronic condition. In any of these cases, the greatest importance should be to restore natural posture and muscle activity where possible. Activating physical therapy is the most common treatment likely to accomplish this goal of restoration of muscle activity. This involves an exercise regimen done by the patient on a daily basis, or at least several days per week. It may be land-based or pool therapy, and it may be facilitated by physical therapy modalities at times. However, the greatest importance is on the independent home exercise plan, as this is what retrains posture and physiological range of motion.

The use of opioids and other analgesics in primary myofascial pain states is controversial. There is limited evidence both for and against their use, and the only consensus is that the physicians should use their best judgment in these cases, using the medication to facilitate physical performance and withdrawing it if its use results in deterioration. NSAIDs may be effective for *acute* myofascial injuries, but are also not generally effective in *chronic* myofascial pain. NSAIDs administration also carries a substantial risk of toxicity in chronic, high-dose use. Antidepressant treatment, on the other hand, is efficacious in chronic myofascial pain states, such as fibromyalgia.

Interventional treatment with trigger point injections (injection of local anesthetic or other agents directly into the painful muscular trigger point) may have acute benefits, such as improving adherence to a single physical therapy appointment. However, this therapy has only limited benefit in the long term (42). Botulinum toxin injections have been proven effective in some primary dystonias, as well as in spasticity; both of these conditions may result in pain. In primary myofascial pain, the quality and quantity of studies has yet to produce compelling evidence of long-term utility for this substance (43).

Nociceptive Pain States

In a condition where pain is initiated by tissue damage, the pain is generally described as sharp and well localized. While it may occur at rest, movement or pressure exacerbates it. This accounts for most pain states caused by trauma (including surgery) and/or inflammation. It is the type of pain most intellectually accessible to clinicians assessing patients, as it is a universal experience. Nociceptive pain states are most closely associated with acute pain, but there are chronic nociceptive states, as well. Nonhealing wounds, oral ulcerations, arthritis, and mechanical instability (e.g., some postoperative temporomandibular surgery patients) are some diagnoses leading to chronic nociceptive pain states. Generally speaking, treatment of the underlying cause of the painful condition ameliorates the pain. However, the definition of chronic pain is that it lasts longer than anticipated. In this case, the focus must be less on curing the underlying problem, if it is incurable, and more on symptom reduction and functional improvement.

Pharmacologically, the etiology of the pain complaint determines what the analgesic options are. Most chronic nociceptive pain responds to either NSAIDs or opioids, with appropriate pharmacological attention paid to concomitant pain-related comorbidities (e.g., neuropathies). In elderly patients, the clinician must pay special heed to the risk of NSAIDs. Classic, nonselective NSAIDs are responsible for approximately 16,500 deaths annually in the United States (44). They cause gastritis and stomach ulcerations, platelet inhibition, and renal failure, and older patients are more prone to all of these complications. Therefore, any older patient on chronic NSAID therapy should have appropriate monitoring for gastric bleeding (e.g., complete blood count, fecal occult blood assay, and/or endoscopic visualization), as well as laboratory studies to check for trends in creatinine or alternate assessments of renal function. The newer cyclooxygenase-2-specific agents (Cox-2 inhibitors) are associated with a lower potential for gastropathy and bleeding diathesis, but are equally nephrotoxic.

Acetaminophen is one of the most common over-the-counter analgesics and is combined in many prescription analgesics. It can be an effective component of therapy for numerous painful disorders, including osteoarthritis. However, it is also responsible for more overdose-related hospitalizations than any other drug (45). There is also an association between chronic acetaminophen use and end-stage renal disease (46). Therefore, while acetaminophen is indicated in patients with osteoarthritis, its total daily dose should not exceed 4 g/day, in healthy young adults, and 2 g/day in elderly patients. It should be reduced further, or omitted entirely, in patients with liver disease (47). The clinician must pay special attention during the history for acetaminophen-containing compounds, both prescription and nonprescription. Patients will often forget to mention these. Therefore, specific queries are warranted.

Opioids

Of all the analgesic medications, the most historically controversial are the opioids. Recent data also indicate that they are the safest and most effective, as a class. Furthermore, opioids are available in oral, buccal, sublingual, nebulized, transcutaneous, subcutaneous, intravenous, epidural, intrathecal, intraventricular, and rectal forms, making them the most versatile class of analgesics, by far. This is particularly important in the practice of otolaryngology, where patients may have frequent inability to take oral agents.

In 1998, the American Geriatric Society released guidelines on the treatment of chronic pain in older persons. This document stated, for the first time in such a publication, that opioids were underutilized in the geriatric population, and that they were safe and effective in this population, when used appropriately (48). These guidelines were updated in 2002 and are required reading for any clinician treating elderly patients (49). They were also restructured to include a more multidimensional approach to the assessment and treatment of chronic pain in geriatric patients.

Tramadol is not technically an opioid, but has approximately 5% μ-receptor activity. This drug can cause seizures when administered in excess doses. Its maximum dose in patients over the age of 70 is 300 mg/day, and drug dose should be less in patients with renal dysfunction. It interacts with numerous other drugs, including antidepressants and some cardiac drugs. Therefore, while appropriate for use in selected patients, this drug must be employed with care in older patients.

Methadone also merits special considerations. It is the only long-acting opioid that can be made into a liquid, or have its tablet disrupted to yield lower dose. This may be invaluable in otolaryngology patients who require enteral feeding, or who only tolerate liquids. It is also quite inexpensive. However, in larger doses, the β-elimination half-life of this drug is unpredictable and may extend dangerously in patients with impaired liver function. Therefore, it is inappropriate in some patients and should always be used with extra caution in elderly patients. Recent changes in pharmacoeconomics have caused a large-scale transition from other analgesics to methadone, sometimes with disastrous consequences, including increased mortality (50). Therefore, this is another drug with both unique benefits and hazards, and should be used with caution in older patients.

Meperidine is outdated and has no place in the treatment of chronic pain. Its primary metabolite, normeperidine, has a half-life of at least 14 hours, and is essentially infinite in anephric patients. It causes cerebral excitation and induces generalized tonic–clonic seizures in a predictable manner, given even routine use in patients with postoperative patient-controlled analgesia (51,52). There are no longer any convincing indications for the use of this substance for painful conditions. Even the indication involving a putative sphincter of Oddi spasm-sparing effect is based on studies from the 1930s in which it was felt to be equivalent in potency to morphine. At equipotent doses, there is no sparing effect.

Generally speaking, the other opioids are somewhat interchangeable. Most studies tout the effectiveness of a single opioid against a nonopioid, or an older preparation of the same drug. However, the principal concept in the use of this class of drugs in the treatment of chronic pain is the strategy involving scheduled (time-contingent) long-acting opioid doses, as opposed to symptom contingent ("prn") doses. Morphine, oxycodone, and fentanyl are available in slow-release matrices, which allow for time-contingent dosing. Methadone may also be used in this capacity, with the aforementioned caveats. Time-contingent dosing is less intrusive into patients' lives and allows for reduced adverse effects by creating more consistent blood levels than frequent short-acting doses. Patients may also be classically conditioned to desire pills by the psychological mechanisms inherent in symptom-contingent dosing. The separation in time between administration and perceived effect in the long-acting, time-contingent medications may ameliorate this effect. Therefore, it is more important to choose a strategy involving the primary use of time-contingent opioid dosing than to select any particular drug. With the exception of methadone, the opioid equivalencies are fairly well understood (Obtain permission for use of opioid table from AGS).

There is also therapeutic benefit in rotating opioids if adverse effects or tolerance becomes problematic (53). This involves the wholesale substitution of one time-contingent opioid for another. The initial step is to add the opioid equivalences of the current regimen, and calculate a 24-hour total, usually in morphine equivalence. Due to incomplete cross-tolerance, there is generally a 20% to 50% reduction in overall dose accompanying any change. It may be prudent to allow for some increased symptom-contingent dosing during the first few days of the new regimen to allow for the decrease, followed by prudent increases in the scheduled dose based on the temporary increase in symptom-contingent drug.

INTERVENTIONAL TREATMENTS

Aside from the otolaryngological approaches outlined elsewhere in this text, there are interventional therapies specific to painful conditions. While a detailed explanation of all conceivable interventional therapies is beyond the scope of this chapter, a few of these treatments may be relevant to elderly otolaryngology patients with chronic pain conditions.

While individual practitioners maintain enthusiasm for stellate ganglion block, the injection of local anesthetic in the vicinity of the cervicothoracic sympathetic ganglion, there is a paucity of supportive studies in the medical literature. Most of these are small, uncontrolled studies and do not constitute an appropriate base of evidence to recommend a discrete role for this therapy in the treatment of chronic pain. Traditionally, it has been used for diagnosis and therapy of sympathetically mediated pain of the face and upper extremity. While it may have immediate results, no long-term studies have demonstrated efficacy in populations of patients with chronic pain. Therefore, it is difficult to state an evidence-based role for it in this population.

Cervical facet arthropathy is common and a frequent cause of cervicogenic headache. Patients complaining of mechanical (movement-related) cervical pain radiating either to the occiput or trapezius may have painful facet arthropathy. The most validated confirming diagnostic regimen involves the injection of local anesthetic into the immediate vicinity of the medial branch of the primary posterior ramus of the segmental spinal nerve, which innervates the facet joint. If a series of at least two of these injections reduces the axial pain substantially, the likelihood of prolonged improvement with radiofrequency facet denervation is approximately 70% (54). In this procedure, an insulated cannula is placed in the vicinity of the medial branch, and the nerve is heated by radio frequency energy. The neurolytic process does minimal collateral damage and is effective for a median duration of 422 days (55). This process may aid greatly in the patient's ability to participate in physical therapy, thereby facilitating myofascial improvement as well.

For chronic neuropathic pain refractory to medical therapy, spinal cord stimulation (SCS) represents a validated therapy. Originally used fairly indiscriminately in its early development, this technology has more recently proven to be effective in selected patients, and to provide long-term relief for neuropathic pain, predominantly in the extremities.

The mechanism of SCS is still incompletely understood. Originally, the Gate Control theory led to the development of this technology (56). This theoretical mechanism led to a conceptual understanding of the complexity of influences that modify pain impulses in the periphery, spinal cord, and brain. The exact mechanism of SCS is still somewhat unclear but includes the following components:

- electrical stimulation of the posterior spinal cord alters patients' perception of pain and dysesthetic sensation in the affected area by antidromic stimulation of sensory nerves,
- stimulation of hypoactive inhibitory neurons,
- suppression of sympathetic activity, leading to increased perfusion (57).

The process involves the placement of catheters or plates containing electrodes into the epidural space. These are connected to an internal pulse generator/battery, which is programmable. The operator then programs the device to achieve maximum symptomatic relief.

While the principal application for SCS in the United States is for extremity neuropathic pain (e.g., spinal nerve injury, complex regional pain syndrome), in Europe, this technology is used more frequently for ischemic heart and extremity disease. It has been demonstrated effective in improving blood flow in inoperable ischemic disease and improving numerous quality-of-life indicators, as well as improving wound healing in ischemic lower extremities (58).

Although originally intended for patients with end-stage cancer-related pain, the intrathecal drug delivery system (IDDS) is also used for selected patients with pain of nonmalignant origin. In this system, a biocompatible catheter is placed into the intrathecal space via a translaminar spinal approach. It is tunneled subcutaneously and connected to a pump implanted subcutaneously in the abdominal subcutaneous tissue. The most common type of pump is programmable, so that the dose may be adjusted. There are also models available that are not adjustable, but do not have a battery that will eventually require replacement. Generally, the programmable model reduces the frequency of pump access required and may be advantageous for most patients. Any of these pumps is refilled via a transcutaneous injection of drug into the pump's refill port.

The principal advantage of this method of opioid delivery is the substantial overall dose reduction possible by conversion to the intrathecal route. Three hundred milligrams of oral morphine converts to roughly 1 mg of intrathecal morphine. This has the benefit of sparing dose-related adverse effects, notably, constipation. The decrease in toxicity, when compared with comprehensive systemic medical therapy, facilitates analgesia. Therefore, both toxicity and analgesia improve with conversion to an intrathecal drug delivery system.

While these implantation therapies may be expensive initially, there is increasing evidence that they are significantly more cost-effective over time than more traditional therapies for chronic pain conditions (59,60). This differential is likely to increase as the costs associated with prescription drugs increase. In either of these implantation therapies, patient selection is crucial. Along with a thorough medical evaluation, these patients must have good understanding of the strengths, limitations, and responsibilities associated with implanted therapeutic devices. Therefore, a psychological evaluation is considered standard of care as a component of the evaluation. This serves to further assess and educate the patient, as well as to prepare them for the therapeutic process.

GENERAL TREATMENT CONCEPTS

While much of this chapter has focused on the identification and classifications of different painful conditions and their medical management, the most effective management of chronic pain conditions involves a broader, multidisciplinary approach. The classical distinction between what is organic and what is imagined is an artifice created by centuries of focus on partial understanding of pain physiology and on curative treatments. Unfortunately, for many patients with chronic pain, the underlying condition is not amenable to complete restoration to the premorbid condition. For this reason, any treatment program should include measures to restore optimal conditioning, as well as adaptation and coping strategies. While it is the responsibility of the treating clinician to minimize the patient's symptoms, often through medication and/or interventional care, there is an equal responsibility to facilitate normalization and a return to a healthful state.

For many of these patients, only an approach incorporating assessment and plans outside of the traditional role of medicine-as-cure model will be effective. Having said that, a broad understanding of the pathophysiology of chronic pain conditions and their appropriate therapeutic options can be the key to symptom reduction and functional improvement in patients with chronic, intractable pain.

REFERENCES

1. American Pain Foundation Pain Care Bill of Rights. (c) 2001 American Pain Foundation, 201 N. Charles St. Ste 710, Baltimore, Md. 21201. (Reprinted with permission. The American Pain Foundation is an independent nonprofit organization serving people with pain through information, advocacy, and support.)
2. Davis GC, Hiemenz ML, White TL. Barriers to managing chronic pain of older adults with arthritis. J Nurs Scholarship 2002; 34(2):121–126.
3. United States Census Bureau. Census 2000. (www.census.gov.)
4. American Cancer Society Website: "Who Gets Cancer?" (www.cancer.org.)
5. Schmader KE. Epidemiology and impact on quality of life of postherpetic neuralgia and painful diabetic neuropathy. Clin J Pain 2002; 18:350–354.
6. Sowers M. Epidemiology of risk factors for osteoarthritis: systemic factors. Curr Opin Rheumatol 2001; 13:447–451.
7. Ferrell BA. Overview of aging and pain. In: Ferrell BR, Ferrell BA, eds. Pain in the Elderly. Seattle: IASP Press, 1996:6–7.
8. Cleeland CS, Gonin R, Hatfield AK, et al. Pain and its treatment in outpatients with metastatic cancer. NEJM 1994; 330(9):592–596.
9. Harkins SW, David MD, Bush FM, Kasberger. Suppression of first pain and slow temporal summation of second pain in relation to age. J Gerontol Med Sci 1996; 51A(5): M260–M265.

10. Grandison MK, Boudinot FD. Age-related changes in protein binding of drugs. Clin Pharmacokinet 2000; 38(3):271–290.
11. Beyth RJ, Shorr RI. Principles of drug therapy in older patients: rational drug prescribing. Clin Ger Med 2002; 18(3):577–592.
12. Mühlberg W, Platt D. Age-dependent changes of the kidneys: pharmacological implications. Gerontology 1999; 45:243–253.
13. Bauman T. Pain management. In: Pharmacotherapy: A Pathophysiologic Approach. 5th ed. McGraw-Hill, 2002:1103–1117.
14. Troke M, Moore AP, Maillardet FJ, Hough A, Cheek E. A new, comprehensive normative database of lumbar spine ranges of motion. Clin Rehabil 2001; 15:371–379.
15. Leary MC, Saver SL. Annual incidence of first silent stroke in the United States: a preliminary estimate. Cerebrovasc Dis 2003; 16(3):280–285.
16. Andersen G, Vestergaard K, Ingeman-Nielsen M, Jensen TJ. Incidence of central post-stroke pain. Pain 1995; 61:187–193.
17. Soh KB. The glossopharyngeal nerve, glossopharyngeal neuralgia and the Eagle's syndrome—current concepts and management. Singapore Med J 1999; 40(10):659–665.
18. Elias WJ, Burchiel KJ. Microvascular decompression. Clin J Pain 2002; 18(1):35–41.
19. Kondziolka D, Lunsford LD, Flickinger JC. Stereotactic radiosurgery for the treatment of trigeminal neuralgia. Clin J Pain 2000; 18(1):42–47.
20. Madland G, Feinmann C. Chronic facial pain: a multidisciplinary problem. J Neurol Neurosurg Psychiatry 2001; 71(6):716–719.
21. Brown GR. Herpes zoster: correlation of age, sex, distribution, neuralgia, and associated disorders. Southern Med J 1976; 69(5):576–578.
22. Dworkin RH, Boon RJ, Griffin DR, Phung D. Postherpetic neuralgia: impact of famciclovir, age, rash severity and acute pain in herpes zoster patients. J Infect Dis 1998; 178(suppl 1):76S–80S.
23. Winnie AP, Hartwell PW. Relationship between time of treatment of acute herpes zoster with sympathetic blockade and prevention of post-herpetic neuralgia: clinical support for a new theory of the mechanism by which sympathetic blockade provides therapeutic benefit. Regional Anesth 1993; 18(5):277–282.
24. Simmons Z, Feldman EL. Update on diabetic neuropathy. Curr Opin Neurol 2002; 15:595–603.
25. Seguin R, Nelson ME. The benefits of strength training for older adults. Am J Prev Med 2003; 25(3Sii):141–149.
26. Okifuji A, Turk DC, Sinclair JD, Starz TW, Marcus DA. A standardized manual tender point survey. I. Development and determination of a threshold point for the identification of positive tender points in fibromyalgia syndrome. J Rheumatol 1997; 24(2): 377–383.
27. Buskila D. Fibromyalgia, chronic fatigue syndrome, and myofascial pain syndrome. Curr Opin Rheumatol 2001; 13:117–127.
28. American Cancer Society. Cancer Facts & Figures, 2003. (http://www.cancer.org/downloads/STT/CAFF2003PWSecured.pdf.)
29. Grond S, Zech D, Diefenbach C, Radbruch L, Lehmann KA. Assessment of cancer pain: a prospective evaluation in 2266 cancer patients referred to a pain service. Pain 1996; 64(1):107–114.
30. Fernandez E, Milburn TW. Sensory and affective predictors of overall pain and emotions associated with affective pain. Clin J Pain 1994; 10(1):3–9.
31. Jamison RN, Taft K, O'Hara JP, Ferrante FM. Psychosocial and pharmacologic predictors of satisfaction with intravenous patient-controlled analgesia. Anesth Analg 1993; 77(1):121–125.
32. Watson CP, Vernich L, Chipman M, Reed K. Nortriptyline versus amitriptyline in postherpetic neuralgia: a randomized trial. Neurology 1998; 51(4):1166–1167.

33. Max MB, Lynch SA, Muir J, Shoaf SE, Smoller B, Dubner R. Effects of desipramine, amitriptyline, and fluoxetine on pain in diabetic neuropathy. NEJM 1992; 326(19): 1250–1256.

34. Goldstein DJ, Lu Y, Detke MJ, Lee TC, Iyengar S. Duloxetine vs. placebo in patients with painful diabetic neuropathy. Pain 2005; 116(1–2):109–118.

35. Backonja M, Glanzman RL. Gabapentin dosing for neuropathic pain: evidence from randomized, placebo-controlled clinical trials. Clin Therap 2003; 25(1):81–104.

36. Frampton JE, Foster RH. Pregabalin: in the treatment of postherpetic neuralgia. Drugs 2005; 65(1):111–118.

37. Frampton JE, Scott LJ. Pregabalin: in the treatment of painful diabetic peripheral neuropathy. Drugs 2004; 64(24):2813–2820.

38. Tremont-Lukats IW, Megeff C, Backonja MM. Anticonvulsants for neuropathic pain syndromes. Drugs 2000; 60(5):1029–1052.

39. Rowbotham MC, Twilling L, Davies PS, Reisner L, Taylor K, Mohr D. Oral opioid therapy for chronic peripheral and central neuropathic pain. NEJM 2003; 348(13): 1223–1232.

40. Watson CPN, Babul N. Efficacy of oxycodone in neuropathic pain: a randomized trial postherpetic neuralgia. Neurology 1998; 50(6):1837–1841.

41. Gimbel JS, Richards P, Portenoy RK. Controlled-release oxycodone for pain in diabetic neuropathy. Neurology 2003; 60:927–934.

42. Forseth KO, Gran JT. Management of fibromyalgia. Drugs 2002; 62(4):577–592.

43. Lang AM. Botulinum toxin type a therapy in chronic pain disorders. Arch Phys Med Rehabil 2003; 84(3 suppl 1):S69–S73.

44. Singh G. Recent considerations in nonsteroidal anti-inflammatory drug gastropathy. Am J Med 1998; 105(1B):31S–38S.

45. Lane JE, Belson MG, Brown K, Scheetz A. Chronic acetaminophen toxicity: a case report and review of the literature. J Emerg Med 2002; 23(3):253–256.

46. Fored CM, Ejerblad E, Lindblad P, et al. Acetaminophen, aspirin, and chronic renal failure. NEJM 2001; 345(25):1801–1808.

47. American College of Rheumatology Subcommittee on Osteoarthritis. Recommendations for the medical management of osteoarthritis of the hip and knee. Arthritis Rheumatism 2000; 43(9):1905–1915.

48. AGS Panel on Chronic Pain in Older Persons. The management of chronic pain in older persons. J Am Geriatr Soc 1998; 46:635–651.

49. American Geriatrics Society Panel on Persistent Pain in Older Persons. The management of persistent pain in older persons. J Am Geriatr Soc 2002; 50:S205–S224.

50. Oregon Department of Human Services CD summary. Methadone deaths (and distribution) on the rises, 52(14). (Web address: http://www.dhs.state.or.us/publichealth/cdsummary/2003/ohd5214.pdf.).

51. Kaiko RF, Foley KM, Grabinski PY, et al. Central nervous system excitatory effects of meperidine in cancer patients. Ann Neurol 1983; 13:180–185.

52. Simopoulos TT, Smith HS, Peeters-Asdourian C, Stevens DS. Use of meperidine in patient-controlled analgesia and the development of a normeperidine toxic reaction. Arch Surg 2002; 137(1):84–88.

53. Indelicato RA, Portenoy RK. Opioid rotation in the management of refractory cancer pain. J Clin Oncol 2002; 20(1):348–352.

54. Lord SM, Barnsley L, Wallis BJ, McDonald GJ, Bogduk N. Percutaneous radiofrequency neurotomy for chronic cervical zygapophyseal-joint pain. N Engl J Med 1996; 335(23):1721–1726.

55. McDonald GJ, Lord SM, Bogduk N. Long-term follow-up of patients treated with cervical radiofrequency neurotomy for chronic neck pain. Neurosurgery 1999; 45(1):61–67.

56. Melzak R, Wall P. Pain mechanisms: a new theory. Science 1965; 150:971–979.

57. Oakley JC, Prager JP. Spinal cord stimulation mechanisms of action. Spine 2002; 27:2574–2583.

58. Kumar K, Toth C, Nath RK, Verma AK, Burgess JJ. Improvement of limb circulation in peripheral vascular disease using epidural spinal cord stimulation: a prospective study. J Neurosurg 1997; 86(4):662–669.

59. Kemler MA, Furnee CA. Economic evaluation of spinal cord stimulation for chronic reflex sympathetic dystrophy. Neurology 2002; 59:1203–1209.

60. De Lissovoy G, Brown RE, Halpern M, Hassenbusch S, Ross E. Cost-effectiveness of long-term intrathecal morphine therapy for pain associated with failed back surgery syndrome. Clin Therap 1997; 19(1):96–112.

66

Advance Directives and Do Not Resuscitate Orders

Cheryl Ellis Vaiani
Institute for the Medical Humanities, University of Texas Medical Branch, Galveston, Texas, U.S.A.

Advance care planning is the process by which an individual considers the personal values about the end of life, discusses those values with family or others close to them and health care providers, and completes those documents that record those decisions for the future when the individual is unable to make his wishes known. While this process is important for all age groups, it is perhaps most pertinent for the geriatric population who will likely face this decision and may not have a spouse or family member to speak on their behalf. And even when family is available, studies have demonstrated that relatives are seldom better than chance in guessing a patient's choices for care. Advance directives allow a person to ensure that their preferences for treatment will be known and can be used to direct care even when that person is no longer able to make informed decisions. Knowing a patient's directions for care relieves stress, guilt, and emotional burden for relatives who are asked to make those decisions.

The Patient Self-Determination Act of 1991 requires that all patients entering federally funded hospitals and nursing homes be offered the opportunity to complete an advance directive. All states have laws governing advance directives but there is variability from state to state. In general, advance directive documents are of three types: a living will, appointment of an agent to make health care decisions, and decisions about out-of-hospital resuscitation. Advance directive documents for each state can be found in Reference 1. Documents can be downloaded and printed from that site.

The living will documents the interventions a patient would or would not want in future situations such as when the patient has been diagnosed with a terminal or irreversible illness or condition. Although most patients use such instructions to refuse life-sustaining treatments when they would merely prolong the dying process or support a vegetative state, a living will may also direct that life-sustaining treatments be provided in all situations. Living wills can usually be completed without the services of an attorney or notary and can be changed at any time. A living will becomes effective only when the appropriate conditions are met—the patient has a terminal or irreversible condition and the patient is incapable of communicating their own wishes. There are difficulties with living wills; sometimes interpretation is difficult (does no ventilator mean no ventilator even for a short-term, likely reversible condition?), many times the document is unavailable (your family should have copies, know where copies are, and it should not be stored in safe deposit box), and the complexities of health care make it impossible to anticipate every possible situation that may occur and define treatment choices (how would the patients evaluate their quality of life if dyspnea prevents them from walking across the room; make a choice about chemotherapy if the chances of success are very slim and the side effects likely disabling; decide on the use of artificial nutrition if Alzheimer's disease is progressing and the patients are no longer aware of their surroundings?).

A "medical power of attorney," "durable power of attorney for health care," or "health care agent" are terms for the document that appoints an agent or proxy authorized to make health care decisions on behalf of the incapacitated patient (the patient must be incapacitated for the agent to have authority). The proxy is expected to represent the choices of the patient, hopefully on the basis of a clear understanding of the patient's values, beliefs, and wishes. A proxy that states, "I just can't bear to lose John, I want you to do everything to keep him alive," may be expressing their own wishes instead of the patient's and should be gently reminded that a proxy's legal and ethical responsibility is to make the choice John would have made. A health care agent is particularly useful in guiding decision making in complex situations because the agent has the flexibility to respond according to a patient's wishes in a complex and rapidly changing medical environment. The third type of advance directive, the Out of Hospital Do Not Resuscitate (OOHDNR) order, may not exist in all states but is a document used primarily to guide treatment by emergency medical personnel in the out-of-hospital setting (in some states this includes emergency rooms, outpatient clinics, and nursing homes). This document and the accompanying identifying bracelet or necklace alerts emergency personnel that the patient does not wish resuscitation in the case of cardiac or respiratory arrest. Because in many situations emergency medical personnel are required to initiate resuscitation without such a document, this document ensures that the patient will not be forced to receive unwanted treatment. Utilizing this document is particularly important when a terminally ill patient is discharged from the hospital with a palliative care plan and hospice services.

The decision concerning cardiopulmonary resuscitation (CPR) is frequently required during hospitalization, when completing advance directives, and when discussing treatment choices. Unfortunately, there is frequently misunderstanding on the part of patients and sometimes health care workers about resuscitation orders. Cardiopulmonary resuscitation was developed and proved efficacious in the 1960s for a particular type of patient, the cardiac patient. Over the next 20 years, the use of CPR was extended to apply to all patients, sometimes without regard to whether it will provide benefit to the patient (2). Unlike other treatments and procedures when a patient's consent is required, CPR, in most situations, will be provided unless the patient has refused consent. From the ethical perspective, this approach errs on the side of life, but it also may mean that patients are provided a treatment that most likely will not work, and may actually cause harm.

Cardiopulmonary resuscitation in the hospital setting is successful in allowing the patient to survive to hospital discharge an average of 15% of the time. In patients with stroke, metastatic cancer, sepsis, or in nursing home residents, survival is even less likely (3). Patients frequently believe that CPR has a much higher success rate than is realistic, an impression clearly influenced by the frequently portrayed success of CPR on television (4). Even the terminology of orders not to initiate

CPR, do not resuscitate orders, may contribute to misunderstanding. It suggests that resuscitation would be successful if performed. Some hospitals have changed the words to Do Not Attempt Resuscitation (DNAR) in an effort to more accurately reflect the reality.

Informed decisions about resuscitation require that patients have an accurate understanding of their diagnosis, prognosis, the likelihood of CPR's success in their situation, and the risks involved. Ideally, the discussion is held routinely with all hospitalized patients, not just those who are judged to be a high risk for cardiac arrest. Routine use of resuscitation should be questioned in many situations: patients with terminal/irreversible illness where death is imminent and/or expected (patient with widely metastatic cancer); when resuscitation would not be expected to provide substantial improvement in the patient's ultimate outcome (patient with persistent vegetative state or catastrophic neurological injury); and when death is thought to be inevitable despite the application of resuscitative measures (ICU patient with rapidly falling blood pressure despite maximal support). Discussions about resuscitation are best aimed at the patient's goal for care in the context of the patient's present condition and future prognosis. Patients and families should be reassured that a decision not to utilize resuscitative efforts does not mean no treatment and that a plan of care that emphasizes comfort and palliation can be just as aggressive as a plan for curative treatment. The patient's decision should be routinely revisited over time and as disease progression occurs. Good communication skills are essential to introduce and conduct these conversations with patients and families, and many current end-of-care curricula including the American Medical Association (AMA) sponsored Education for Physicians in End of Life Care (EPEC) can provide tools for physicians to develop and reinforce these skills.

Although the term futility is commonly utilized in discussions about resuscitation by health professionals, there is no consistently agreed upon definition of futility. In a strict sense, when a treatment or procedure is futile, it is physiologically impossible to succeed (for example, if the patient has rigor mortis or has been decapitated in a motor vehicle accident). Many discussions of futility are instead clinical judgments based on a low likelihood of success or moral judgments that the quality of life would be so poor as to make continued existence not worthwhile, such as when a patient is in a vegetative state or unable to survive outside the intensive care unit (ICU). From an ethical perspective, quality-of-life assessments and the balancing of risks and benefits should reflect the patient's perspectives and values, not those of the health care providers.

Honoring patients' requests not to be resuscitated may also become an issue when the patient has an operative procedure. Patients with terminal illness may desire surgery for palliation, pain relief, or vascular access yet not desire resuscitation if they experience cardiac arrest. Both the American College of Surgeons (5) and American Society of Anesthesiologists (6) reject the unilateral suspension of orders not to resuscitate in surgery without a discussion with the patient, but some physicians feel that patients cannot have surgery without being resuscitated and view a DNR order as "an unreasonable demand to lower the standard of care" (7). Some provider concern may result from the tendency to extend the resuscitation order to other treatment modalities. Controlling bleeding and maintaining blood pressure are clearly intraoperative responsibilities and differ from resuscitation in the event of arrest. The situation where inability to control bleeding or hypotension by usual measures leads to arrest or the arrest is the result of a medical error is less clear cut. Discussions with the patient or surrogate about their goal for care and desires in various scenarios can help guide decision making. Such conversations allow a mutual decision that respects both the patient's and physician's autonomy. A patient who refuses resuscitation because the patient's current life is burdensome can clearly be harmed by intervening to resuscitate while in the operating room (OR). On the other hand, a patient who refuses resuscitation because the low likelihood of success and possibility of return to a prearrest state may be convinced to change their decision based on the more favorable outcomes of intraoperative arrest (8). If uncomfortable with the patient's decision about interventions, a physician can certainly choose to transfer the care of the patient to another physician, but the physician's wishes should not be imposed upon the patient.

A 62-year-old man with severe emphysema has had multiple ICU admissions over the past year. He requires oxygen to relieve shortness of breath while sitting still. He feels his life is so restricted that he would not want aggressive treatment (further ICU treatment, ventilator, or resuscitation) and has completed both living will and out-of-hospital DNR documents. The patient's eyesight is also deteriorating from macular degeneration, and he desires surgery to prevent further deterioration. You are uncomfortable with taking him to surgery with the DNR order in place.

- This is a patient who judges his current quality of life as poor and does not want life-sustaining treatment to maintain such a poor quality of life. Yet he would like surgery to make his remaining life as comfortable and self-sufficient as possible. The patient desires all necessary intraoperative support but does not want to be intubated or cardioverted; although volume expansion and blood pressure support is acceptable to the patient. If the patient were to arrest, even as a result of an iatrogenic mistake, he does not desire resuscitation.
- If the surgeon is reluctant to perform the surgery he should assist the patient in finding another surgeon. It would not be appropriate to insist that the DNR order be rescinded for surgery.

Cardiopulmonary resuscitation is not appropriate for every patient who has a cardiac or pulmonary arrest, even if that patient is in the OR. Physicians need to develop skill in communicating accurate information about the risks and benefits of resuscitation with patients and families in light of the patient's condition and prognosis and make this discussion a routine part of their plan of care.

REFERENCES

1. Http://www.partnershipforcaring.org/Advance/index.html.
2. Burns JP, Edwards J, Johnson J, Cassem NH, Truong RD. Do-not-resuscitate order after 25 years. Crit Care Med 2003; 31:1543–1549.
3. Schneider AP II, Nelson, DJ, Brown DD. In-hospital cardiopulmonary resuscitation: a 30-year review. J Am Board Fam Pract 1993; 6:91–101.
4. Diem SJ, Lantos JD, Tulsky JA. Cardiopulmonary resuscitation on television. NEJM 1996; 334:1378–1382.
5. Statement of the American College of Surgeons on Advance Directives by Patients. "Do not resuscitate" in the operating room. Am Coll Surg Bull 1994; 79(9):29. (Available at http://www.facs.org/fellows_info/statements/st-19.html.)

6. Ethical guideline for the anesthesia care of patients with do-not-resuscitate orders or other directives that limit care. Park Ridge, Il: American Society of Anesthesiologists, 1999:746–747. (Available at http://anestit.unipa.it/mirror/asa2/Standards/09.html)

7. Younger SJ, Cascorbi HF, Shuck JM. DNR in the operating room: not really a paradox. JAMA 1991; 266:2433–2434.

8. Girardi LM, Barie PS. Improved survival after intraoperative cardiac arrest in noncardiac surgical patients. Arch of Surg 1995; 130:15–18.

67

End-of-Life Issues in the Otolaryngology—Head and Neck Surgery Patient

Gerry F. Funk

Department of Otolaryngology—Head and Neck Surgery, University of Iowa College of Medicine, Iowa City, Iowa, U.S.A.

INTRODUCTION

This chapter focuses on a number of the aspects of terminal care that are pertinent to the otolaryngologist. The otolaryngologist's involvement in the terminal care of patients frequently centers on issues related to the airway and dysphagia. However, there are a number of aspects of terminal care for head and neck cancer (HNC) patients within which the otolaryngologist may contribute expertise. Several specific issues that pertain to terminal HNC patients, and that set them apart from other terminal patients, are highlighted. Conversely, a number of other issues may be generalized to the terminal care of most geriatric patients. This chapter is written with the assumption that otolaryngologists managing terminal patients will not be working in isolation and that consultation and multidisciplinary interaction with a palliative care team is available.

HNC MANAGEMENT FROM A PALLIATIVE CARE PERSPECTIVE

The curative approach to disease predominates in the daily practice of most otolaryngologists. This approach utilizes the history, symptom identification, physical examination, and diagnostic studies to identify and characterize the disease process. The underlying disease is then treated with the goal of cure (1). This is frequently the approach taken with most early-stage and many late-stage HNCs. In the early stages of disease this approach is appropriate. However, when there is little hope of cure or absolutely no hope of cure, physicians should consider the dynamic transition to a more palliative approach to the patient's management. This type of dynamic transition through the natural history of a severe disease is diagrammed in Figure 1 (2). Approaching patients with this concept opens possibilities for management appropriate to a particular patient at a particular stage of the disease that may have not otherwise been considered. At the palliative end of the spectrum, the history is used

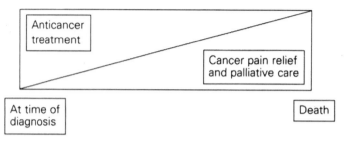

Figure 1 The proposed allocation of effort for cancer patients in developed countries. A continuum of care that promotes a shift from curative to palliative care throughout the natural history of the disease is demonstrated. *Source*: From Ref. 2.

to identify patients' goals and symptoms are treated rather than used as diagnostic indicators, diagnostic studies are ordered only if they will facilitate symptom relief, and interventions are used to relieve symptoms, not cure disease. This dynamic approach to disease runs counter to the classic teaching most of us received in medical school and residency, and it requires discipline to implement.

From a statistical standpoint, roughly 40% to 50% of HNC patients will end up being candidates for palliative care related to the HNC (3). From a practical standpoint, many advanced-stage HNC patients are in the gray area between curative intent and palliative care. Many patients are treated with interventions that are designed to optimize locoregional control and maximize quality of life. The overt intent is to cure the cancer, but the reality is that maximizing local control and quality of life in order to prevent disability and death from locoregional disease are the goals of many treatment regimens for advanced-stage disease (4). This is appropriate and indicates that management plans are being designed with a curative–palliative continuum in mind. Moving along the continuum is a shared experience between the physician, patient, and the patient's family. The physician's role is to educate the patient and family about the best potential options throughout the treatment course and communicate to the patient that support will be available regardless of which direction the patient chooses to move along the continuum at any given stage in the natural history of the disease (5). If radiotherapy or chemotherapy are selected for palliation, a specific palliative goal should be identified.

SPECIAL CONSIDERATIONS IN THE TERMINAL CARE OF HNC PATIENTS

Although HNC patients have many of the same concerns and face many of the same problems as other elderly patients with terminal cancer, there are a number of challenges that are relatively unique to the HNC patient population.

As a group, HNC patients demonstrate an overall compromise in health status (6,7). This compromise involves many areas of health as measured by general health status instruments and may be related to the prolonged alcohol and tobacco abuse often associated with HNC. This group also contains an over-representation of people in the lowest socioeconomic strata (3). The practical result is that HNC patients as a group tend to have comorbid conditions and adverse psychosocial circumstances that exert a detrimental influence on their treatment. They also have fewer resources and support systems to call on. Advanced age compounds the problem.

HNC patients, particularly those with terminal disease, frequently present with a compromised ability to speak and communicate easily. This may be the result of treatment to the larynx, pharynx, or oral cavity. Often it is due to a tracheostomy (8).

Airway obstruction is a very frightening prospect for anyone. The worst possible death many of us can imagine is to die from acute loss of the airway. Family members of terminal HNC patients are frequently worried that the patient will suffocate, and the issue of airway management must be very clearly addressed early in the palliative care of HNC patients.

One of the greatest fears many terminal patients have is the fear of dying alone and isolated. Unfortunately, many factors in the terminal phase of HNC, in particular uncontrolled disease above the clavicles, predispose these patients to isolation. This is particularly true when patients are in an acute care hospital in which the overriding treatment model is curative. Patients may have malodorous, ulcerated masses that distort the face and neck, and even the most dedicated medical and nursing teams may find it difficult to interact with the patient for more than a brief period of time (9). Communication difficulties compound the potential for isolation of these patients.

Compromised nutrition is a multifactorial problem for many HNC patients, both cured and terminal. Many patients who are able to take an oral diet struggle with decreased swallowing ability, inadequate dental rehabilitation, xerostomia, and a decreased sense of taste. The work of preparing nutritious meals that can be easily consumed is a burden. Family and community support may be lacking. Many patients with terminal, locally recurrent HNC will not be able to take anything by mouth. In this circumstance, all calories and hydration must come through tube (nasogastric or gastrostomy tube) feeding. Maintaining a functioning feeding tube and using it to maintain adequate caloric intake is a burden, and particularly so for those with terminal disease in whom nausea and vomiting are frequent problems (8,10).

The pain experienced by patients with terminal HNC that is due to local recurrence is frequently challenging to treat due to components of neuropathic and bone pain (11–13). Opioids, traditionally used to manage terminal cancer pain, are less effective against these types of pain. This situation is not unique to the HNC patient, but does highlight the need for palliative care and pain experts to be consulted.

Although in terminal HNC the brain and carotid arteries are frequently in close proximity to the recurrent cancer, the actual incidence of death due to carotid rupture or brain invasion is relatively low (14). In effect, HNC patients may live for some time with locally advanced recurrent disease, because the vital organs of the chest and abdomen are spared (15). This may create a very difficult situation for all parties involved in the protracted death of a patient from locally advanced cancer.

In this section a number of challenges, which are in some measure peculiar to the terminal management of HNC patients, have been identified. However, the terminal HNC patient in many instances does have an advantage over many other terminal cancer patients. The gastrointestinal system distal to the esophagus is usually spared. With access to this system, delivery of fluids, nutrition, and medications are not hampered. However, in many circumstances a feeding tube is required.

HISTORY AND INFORMATION GATHERING

The initial history obtained from a HNC patient entering a palliative care program is similar to any other medical history with an emphasis on current symptoms and prior treatment. It is important to identify any symptoms that are currently having a severe negative impact on the patient's life quality. The otolaryngologist will want to focus on symptoms suggesting current or impending airway compromise, swallowing or tube feeding difficulties, and prior treatment that may put the patient at risk for carotid rupture.

Specific issues that frequently need to be addressed with elderly, terminal patients include adequacy of pain management, mode of nutritional support, medication regimen, and wound care. In more debilitated patients, potential placement in a care facility and the feasibility of the patient staying at home need to be discussed. In this context, the realistic availability of family to help with patient care needs to be discussed. If the oral route for medication and nutrition is currently being used, will a feeding tube be required in the future? Many of these patients are taking a large number of medications and may be very confused about what they should be taking and when. Can the pain medication regimen be simplified? With few exceptions, all patients on opioids should be on a stimulant laxative and stool softener in order to prevent constipation.

PHYSICAL EXAMINATION

From the standpoint of the otolaryngologist, the key points of the physical examination are the status of the airway, the swallowing ability of the patient, the potential for carotid rupture, and fungating wounds that are causing symptoms. These aspects of the examination need to be viewed as they are at the time of the exam, and with an eye toward future growth of the tumor.

From a more general perspective, the global status of the patient is important in formulating a management plan. If the patient is ambulatory and has desires to travel and see family in the near future, this is likely a realistic goal. Conversely, if the patient is bedridden and extremely cachectic, this is likely not a realistic goal, and interventions to shape realistic goals for the patient are indicated.

If the patient will be traveling, and the airway is tenuous or swallowing ability severely compromised, a gastrostomy tube and a tracheostomy may be necessary to help the patient with their desired plans.

The examination should include a comprehensive examination of the head and neck including a detailed look at the larynx. Often advanced, local recurrence will result in lymphedema and potential airway compromise even if the pharynx and larynx are not directly involved with tumor. Cranial nerve deficits that may compromise swallowing should be identified. Local tumor invading in the region of the tracheostomy that may require the use of a custom-made, long tracheostomy tube should be recognized. Tumor invading the deep neck with potential vascular space invasion should be identified.

The examination should also include a general survey focusing on indicators of hydration status, nutritional status, thyroid function, focal neurologic deficits, pressure wounds, deep vein thromboses, hepatic or renal failure, and bowel obstruction. Terminally ill patients in whom death is likely to occur within weeks will exhibit severe cachexia associated with advanced cancer. The physician should recognize this general appearance. The loss of appetite and utilization of body fat stores is a natural phenomenon at this stage of dying. Enteral feeding is very unlikely to alter this progression (16).

As a general approach, the laboratory workup is minimal for most patients entering palliative care. However, the physician managing the patient should order any laboratory test that will help clarify the patient's clinical situation and facilitate symptom management. A reasonable minimum for HNC patients with terminal ill-ness would include a recent hematocrit and thyroid function tests. These are parti-cularly important if the patient is demonstrating fatigue out of proportion to the clinical situation. However, it is certainly reasonable to order a computed tomogra-phy (CT) or any other radiographic study to clarify the patient's clinical status or to potentially prophylax against an acute vascular or airway problem. In some cases, an extensive locoregional and metastatic workup may be appropriate in order to clarify the palliative status of the patient. This may include a trip to the operating room for endoscopy and biopsies.

DEVELOPING A PLAN

Within the first several visits, there are several key issues that must be clarified: (i) Is the patient comfortable with the palliative care approach, and does the patient clearly understand that symptom management, not cure of disease, is now going to be the goal of treatment? (ii) The physician in charge of the overall palliative care plan needs to be clearly identified as do the other participants in the patient's care such as the hospice personnel, social workers, and contact nurses. (iii) What are the resources available (or not available) to the patient? These should be reviewed with a social worker on the palliative care team (e.g., family members willing to help in patient care, friends willing to help with transportation, financial resources, and insurance resources). (iv) What are the patient's primary goals for their remaining life, and how can the palliative care team help the patient meet these goals?

The first aspect of the management plan is to clarify that the patient is an appropriate candidate for palliative care intervention. If potential curative options exist, these need to be clarified and presented to the patient and family. Similarly, if there are experimental protocols appropriate for the patient, these options need to be discussed. These decisions can be very difficult. For some patients, the partici-pation in an experimental protocol would raise false hope, result in discomfort, and ultimately be a large disappointment. However, for others, participation in an experimental protocol would provide a purpose and focus, allow the patient to estab-lish new relationships, and regardless of whether the intervention was oncologically useful or not, the patient would obtain palliation simply by participating. In most circumstances, the best way to address these difficult issues is to directly ask the patient what they would like to do.

In terms of approaching the patient's goals, a useful model is the concept of total pain set forth by Dame Cicely Saunders in her pioneering work as a leader in the field of palliative care. She defined the total pain of a dying individual to include physical, emotional, social, and spiritual pain (17). It is very helpful to elicit the patient's goals within each of these areas. In most circumstances, the otolaryn-gologist will be focusing on the physical goals, and other members of the palliative care team will address the other areas. For example, some of the physical goals may include pain relief that enables the patient to travel and visit family or relief of upper airway obstruction that is interfering with sleep.

In the remainder of this section, we look at the management of specific pro-blems confronting the terminal patient with HNC. A number of these problems are tied with the physical goals the patient may have identified. Many of these prob-lems are also encountered in the care of debilitated, elderly patients without HNC.

SPECIFIC MANAGEMENT ISSUES

Pain

A modest body of literature has been devoted to the management of pain associated with terminal or advanced HNC (11–13,18–21). The pain of uncontrolled HNC above the clavicles may be very severe, and of a type that does not respond well to opioid medication alone. A systematic approach to pain management employing a wide armamentarium of medications is mandatory for optimal results. A structured pharmacologic approach will often be effective in bringing cancer pain under control (22,23). It is important to bring severe pain under control as rapidly as possible because persistent pain may result in both peripheral and central nervous system physiologic changes that can make pain management very difficult (24).

The sensation of pain has a number of origins and can be classified using a variety of different schemes. Within the head and neck, pain may be of several types: (i) Somatic-nociceptive pain is due to the stimulation of nociceptors richly distributed through all tissues of the head and neck. This is pain transmitted through pain fibers, and includes mucosal, muscle, periosteal, bone, and cutaneous pain. The nociceptors are stimulated by pressure, injury, and inflammation. (ii) Nociceptive-nerve pain results from the stimulation of nociceptive nerves that run along cranial nerves or other large nerves in the head and neck (the nervi nervorum) (11). This pain is associated with tumor invasion and is distributed in the sensory territory of the parent nerve. (iii) Neuropathic pain in the head and neck is the pain that results from direct injury or irritation (e.g., tumor invasion, compression, surrounding inflammation) of a cranial nerve, cervical rootlet, or brachial plexus. This type of pain has been likened to deafferentation pain (18,24). Neuropathic pain is poorly responsive to opioid medication and is frequently treated with tricyclic antidepressants or anti-seizure medications. (iv) Bone pain is a form of somatic-nociceptive pain but deserves special attention because of its prevalence in terminal HNC patients and its resistance to treatment with opioid medications alone. The skull base and mandible are frequent sites of bone pain for HNC patients with locoregional recurrence, and these may present as some of the most difficult patients to manage (18). (v) Complex regional pain syndromes involving the sympathetic nervous system may also occur in HNC patients following treatment or as a result of local disease. These syndromes are quite rare and are frequently very difficult to treat (25). Complex regional pain syndromes mandate consultation with a pain specialist and are beyond the scope of this chapter. Patients may have one or all of these different types of pain as well as other somatic and visceral pain related to the HNC, other illnesses, or prior treatment.

A wide variety of nonsteroidal, opioid, antidepressant, anticonvulsant, anxiolytic, corticosteroid, bisphosphonate, and other medications are available for use in the management of pain in the HNC patient. The overall key to success is a systematic and structured approach that can then be individualized for each patient (23). Ongoing evaluation and modification of the pain management regimen is necessary to produce the best results and minimize unwanted side effects. The approach must allow for an escalation in both potency and dose of medication as well as the incorporation of adjunctive medications. No patient with cancer should live or die with unrelieved pain (22).

Before a pain management regimen is planned, it is crucial that the pain experienced by the patient be defined both in character and severity. A number of visual analog or rating scales are available for this purpose. A simple rating of 0 to 10 along with the patient's description of the pain is simple and effective. The character of the pain should be described. Lancinating, electric shock-type pain often suggests a neuropathic origin. A deep, boring, constant, dull pain suggests a bone origin. Pain with motion often indicates muscular or joint involvement. The sensation of heat suggests inflammation. The association of the pain with any type of stimulation, activity, or time of the day should be investigated. This information will help in tailoring the pain regimen and use of adjunctive medications. Finally, the effectiveness of the current pain management regimen should be defined in order to establish a baseline from which changes will potentially be made.

A proven approach to cancer pain management is the three-step process outlined by the World Health Organization (WHO) (2,13,12,26). The WHO three-step process first assigns a severity to the pain (Fig. 2). A useful means of determining a starting point is with a 10-point pain scale. For example, on a scale from 0 to 10: 1 to 4 = mild, 5 to 6 = moderate, 7 to 10 = severe. Medications are assigned to three steps. Step-1 medications are used to treat mild pain. This is most frequently the nonopioid, nonsteroidal, anti-inflammatory drugs (NSAIDs) and acetaminophen group of medications. For moderate pain or pain not relieved by step-1 medications, step-2 medications are instituted. These include the weaker opioids and fixed drug combination medications with these opioids such as acetaminophen-codeine. Oxycodone is considered a step-2 medication when used in a fixed-drug combination. Finally, for severe pain or pain not relieved by step-2 medications the step-3, strong opioids, are utilized (Fig. 3).

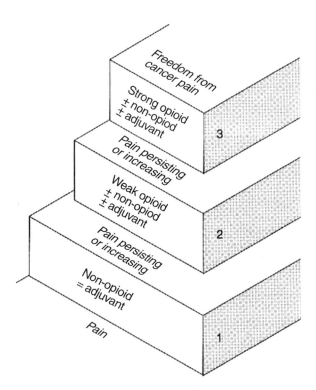

Figure 2 The WHO three-step approach to cancer pain. *Abbreviation*: WHO, World Health Organization. *Source*: From Ref. 2.

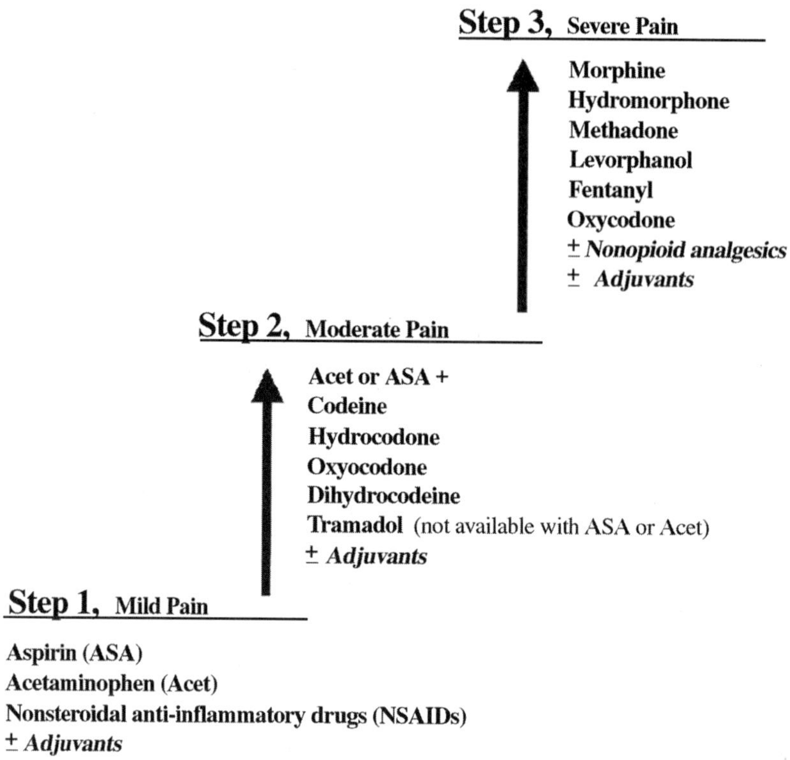

Step 3, Severe Pain

Morphine
Hydromorphone
Methadone
Levorphanol
Fentanyl
Oxycodone
± *Nonopioid analgesics*
± *Adjuvants*

Step 2, Moderate Pain

Acet or ASA +
Codeine
Hydrocodone
Oxyocodone
Dihydrocodeine
Tramadol (not available with ASA or Acet)
± *Adjuvants*

Step 1, Mild Pain

Aspirin (ASA)
Acetaminophen (Acet)
Nonsteroidal anti-inflammatory drugs (NSAIDs)
± *Adjuvants*

Figure 3 Medications used at each step in the WHO three-step approach to cancer pain. *Abbreviation*: WHO, World Health Organization. *Source*: From Ref. 16.

The WHO pain management ladder includes the use of adjunctive medications and nonopioids at each step. This is extremely important for HNC patients. It is likely that over half of the patients treated for severe pain due to terminal, locoregional HNC have some component of neuropathic pain (18). This type of pain may not respond well to opioids alone. Although there are a number of patients in whom opioids and anti-inflammatory medications will be adequate for pain relief (27), in patients who fail to respond to NSAID and opioids, the use of tricyclic antidepressants such as amitriptyline, nortriptyline, or desipramine may prove beneficial (28). The use of anticonvulsants such as carbamazepine or gabapentin should also be considered if a tricyclic antidepressant does not reduce the neuropathic pain (11,19,22,28). When neuropathic pain is due to compression of a nerve or invasion of a bony foramen containing a nerve, corticosteroids may also be of significant benefit.

Patients with uncontrolled, locoregional HNC frequently have bone invasion, most frequently in the mandible, skull base, or maxilla (18). Most of the literature related to bone pain deals with bony metastasis. However, it is reasonable to assume that much of the pathophysiology underlying the pain due to bony metastasis is the same as that for direct bone invasion in the head and neck. Bone pain is also somewhat resistant to opioid medication alone, and the reasons for this appears to be related to the intermittent nature of the pain stimulated by motion as well as the cytokine-mediated inflammation and nociceptor activation (16,28,29). Decreasing the associated inflammation through the use of NSAIDs or corticosteroids may substantially reduce bone pain through a direct effect on the inflammation and other less well-defined central pathways (29). A spectrum of NSAIDs including the newer Cox-2 inhibitors is now available and should be liberally used in cases of bone pain. If one medication does not produce the desired effect, switching to another NSAIDs is recommended (29). In cases with obvious bone invasion, a bisphosphonate may be considered. These bone-stabilizing compounds have been shown to decrease the pain associated with bony metastasis by decreasing osteoclastic activity.

Along with the systematic approach to medication selection, a systematic approach to dose escalation is required. With mild pain, pain that is anticipated to be of short duration, or patients who have never had opioids, this type of intensive dose escalation regimen is generally not required. The approach outlined below is generally used for patients who have been on a suboptimal opioid regimen. This extremely useful method identifies an effective dose of opioid medication by establishing a 24-hour baseline dose using a short-acting opioid. The patient's current opioid regimen is converted to the oral morphine equivalent (another short-acting opioid and route of administration may be used as long as dosing is appropriate for the route and this stepwise approach is used) (Table 1). The total 24-hour dose is divided by six in order to establish a baseline q4-hour dose. If the patient's current pain control has been poor, this initial baseline dose may be increased by 30% to 50% depending on the level of current pain. This initial baseline dose is given as a fixed q4-hour dose for 24 hours. Breakthrough morphine is provided, which can be taken every one or two hours. The breakthrough dose is generally 10% to 15% of the total 24-hour baseline dose and should be used at a rate that keeps the pain rating below three or four. After 24 hours, the pain relief is quantified and the number of breakthrough doses required for adequate pain relief is counted. If more than three or four breakthrough doses were used during the 24-hour period, the amount of morphine used for breakthrough pain is added to the baseline 24-hour dose, and the process is repeated until an adequate baseline dose is found. After the satisfactory baseline

Table 1 Commonly Used Opioids in Palliative Care with Conversions Between IM/SC and Oral Dosing and Equianalgesic Doses

| Drug | Dose (mg) equianalgesic to 10 mg IM/SC morphine | | Half-life (hr) | Duration of action (hr) |
	IM/SC	PO		
Morphine	10	20–30	2–3.5	3–6
Codeine	130	200	2–3	2–4
Oxycodone	15	30	3–4	2–4
Hydromorphone	1.5	7.5	2–3	2–4
Methadone	10	20	15–120	4–8
Oxymorphone	1	10	2–3	3–4
Levorphanol	2	4	12–16	4–8
Fentanyl	0.1[a]	–	1–2[b]	1–3[b]
Tramadol	100	120	–	4–6
Buprenorphine	0.4	0.8	2–3	6–9

Continual infusion produces lipid accumulation and prolonged terminal excretion.
[a]Empirically, transdermal fentanyl 100 μg/hr = 2–4 mg/hr intravenous morphine.
[b]Single-dose data.
Abbreviations: IM, intramuscular; SC, subcutaneous; PO, by mouth.
Source: From Ref. 30.

dose is established, the short-acting opioid can be replaced with a long-acting opioid preparation or an appropriately sized fentanyl patch equivalent (30).

Using the systematic approach of the WHO and a structured dose escalation regimen, pain management in the majority of cases can be quickly brought under control, and the regimen "fine tuned" with various adjunctive medications. In approximately 5% of cases, control of pain in the HNC patient will not be possible with simple pharmocologic intervention. In this small group of terminal HNC patients, the use of a vast array of adjunctive medications to obtain the desired pain control is almost an art. In these circumstances, consultation with an expert in pain management is strongly encouraged.

In addition to the standard pharmacologic management of pain, a number of other specialized techniques are available, including epidural administration of opioid and other medications, pharmacologic, or surgical nerve block procedures, and adjunctive general anesthetic agents such as ketamine or nitrous oxide (31–38). These procedures and interventions are rare and are generally carried out by pain specialists in the fields of anesthesia and neurosurgery. Because these interventions are infrequently performed, few studies are available that objectively address the benefits and adverse effects. Most of the available literature consists of small case series with no control group. Physicians managing terminal HNC patients should be aware that these procedures are available. However, they should be reserved for resistant pain cases and undertaken through consultation with an expert in the field of pain management. Alternative or holistic techniques such as acupuncture or healing touch have many proponents within the field of palliative care. At centers in which experienced practitioners are available, many patients will find these techniques beneficial.

In the management of terminal HNC patients, particularly the elderly, several pitfalls to effective pain management should be kept in mind. Occasionally, a patient will express concern about addiction to strong opioids. Physical dependence on opioids when taken in large doses for a prolonged period of time is normal and patients should be aware of this. However, the psychological addiction to opioids that patients fear is very rare (16). In cases where the source of pain is no longer present, the overwhelming majority of cancer patients simply taper off and stop using the medication (22). In the overwhelming majority of HNC patients with terminal disease and severe pain, addiction should not be an issue. Many physicians are reluctant to administer opioids on a fixed dose schedule and use PRN dosing. As a general rule, with the exception of breakthrough dosing, the PRN administration of opioids has no useful role in severe cancer pain management. PRN dosing implies that the pain must be present in order for medication to be used. This is an extremely inefficient and ineffective method of chronic pain control (2,16,26). Dosage adjustments must be made when converting from IV, subcutaneous, or IM to oral medication, as is frequently done when a patient leaves the hospital. Table 1 gives the appropriate conversions. If this is not done, patients may be severely underdosed. The transdermal route of administration of fentanyl and sustained-release or long-acting opioids have become very popular in cancer pain management. These medications are very effective and convenient for many patients. However, during the initial titration of pain medication to find an effective baseline dose, the use of long-acting medications is very cumbersome because of the time required to attain a stable plasma concentration. It is much more efficient to determine the optimal dose of opioid with a short-acting drug and then convert to an equivalent long-acting preparation. All patients taking opioids on a regular basis should be on both a stimulant laxative (i.e., senna) and stool softener. The nausea associated with opioids in general does diminish with time and is rarely a significant problem after the first week. Antiemetics such as prochlorperazine can be very effective in the first few days of treatment at relieving this nausea. Sedation following the initiation of opioid medications is not uncommon. However, as with the nausea this generally diminishes substantially after two to three days (26,28).

The use of methadone for terminal HNC pain deserves mention. This medication has a very long half-life in comparison to its duration of action, and titration of methadone dose may be difficult due to this and the wide interindividual variability in analgesic effect and plasma half-life. Although Carroll et al. (19) have very successfully incorporated methadone into their four-drug regimen for HNC patients, the patients in that study were all managed very closely by pain specialists in the hospital for seven days to establish a baseline methadone dose. There are advantages offered by methadone, which include two to three times daily dosing, low cost, and no known active metabolites that are associated with the central nervous system (CNS) toxicity of some other opioids (primarily at very high dose in dehydrated patients). In addition, methadone may control some pain, which has proven resistant to other opioids (39). With the current availability of sustained-release preparations and transderm fentanyl, the convenience of BID or TID dosing is not a satisfactory reason to select methadone. However, it may be appropriate for some cases in which the use of other strong opioids has proven problematic. Consultation with a pain specialist is recommended if methadone is to be used for a HNC patient.

Airway

Death directly due to airway obstruction is a very frightening prospect for anyone. In palliative care, a peaceful death for the patient and family is a primary goal. Although it may occur in protracted cases of airway obstruction during which appropriate medications are used, few of us can envision a peaceful death as the result of airway obstruction. Patients and family members often voice a concern that the patient will suffocate. Due to the location of the tumors, patients with terminal HNC are at risk for airway compromise for a number of reasons. Uncontrolled cancer may directly invade the upper airway, lymphedema of the head and neck may result in laryngeal swelling, cranial neuropathies may result in pharyngeal laxity or vocal cord paralysis, an existing tracheostomy site may be locally invaded, reconstructive tissues may partially obstruct the airway, and infrequently the tracheal lumen may be compressed or invaded by disease in the upper mediastinum. These situations are characterized by anatomic obstruction of the airway. The respiratory compromise that results may be exacerbated by, but it is not caused by, end organ (lung) failure. This phenomenon is not respiratory insufficiency; it is airway obstruction. This distinction is important because a tracheostomy may not be an appropriate intervention for a terminal patient with end-stage lung disease or cardiac disease with respiratory insufficiency. However, tracheostomy is often very appropriate for an HNC patient whose primary symptom is upper airway obstruction.

It is difficult to identify the true incidence of airway obstruction in terminal HNC patients because approximately 50% of patients presenting for palliative care due to HNC have a tracheostomy (40). For HNC patients admitted to a hospice without a tracheostomy, airway problems will develop in approximately 20% (8,41). Unfortunately, by the time these terminal HNC patient are admitted to hospice, a tracheostomy that may have afforded palliation earlier in the natural history of the terminal illness is a significant undertaking and will likely not be performed.

There are a number of reasons to address the issue of airway obstruction or impending airway obstruction very early in the palliative care of HNC patients. Airway obstruction is a very frightening issue for the patient and family. Despite the possibility of a peaceful death due to gradual airway obstruction, the overwhelming majority of patients, if asked, do not want to face that situation. Many HNC patients and their families are very familiar with a tracheostomy, and many have previously had a tracheostomy. Many patients will communicate better with a small (#4 or #6) fenestrated metal tracheostomy than without a tracheostomy. The tracheostomy allows unobstructed inspiration, and in this regard, the tracheostomy actually facilitates communication. If the patient is able to take an oral diet, placement of a small metal tracheostomy is unlikely to alter that. It is also a very simple matter to plug the tracheostomy during the day to facilitate communication if the airway obstruction is partial, and again many HNC patients are familiar with doing this. The emotional upheaval for the patient, family, and caregivers associated with an emergent airway situation, and the difficulties attendant with an emergency tracheostomy are avoided by simply performing the tracheostomy when it becomes relatively certain that the airway is going to be compromised in the near future.

If the airway is currently adequate, and the patient would like to avoid tracheostomy for as long as possible, a reasonable follow-up schedule for airway checks should be set up. In these cases, the physician and patient will need to work together to identify the appropriate time for the tracheostomy. The key is to avoid having to perform the tracheostomy as an urgent or emergent procedure through the tumor or after the patient is physically unable to be intubated.

Unfortunately, a tracheostomy does not preclude problems with the airway, and problems due to tracheostomy blockage, local invasion of cancer at the tracheostomy site, or dislodging of the tracheostomy may occur. Forbes found that 5 of 34 patients admitted to hospice care had repeated tracheostomy problems. A plan of action for dealing with tracheostomy obstruction or severe bleeding at the tracheostomy site, which included administration of a short-acting anxiolytic medication, was discussed in advance with the tracheostomy patients (40).

Occasionally, a very difficult management situation may occur when tumor invades the tracheostomy site. In most of these cases with extensive tumor invasion, survival is a matter of days. In cases of extensive stomal invasion, the longest possible tracheostomy should be placed. Often an adjustable length, flexible tracheostomy works well (such as those offered by Portex). The tip of the tracheostomy may need to be at the carina to bypass extensive tumor. The tracheostomy tip should be positioned below the inferior extent of the tumor and confirmed with a flexible laryngoscope. If a tracheostomy tube is not available that will work, an endotracheal tube can be split to the appropriate length and substituted. The longest possible tube is inserted initially in order to avoid having to change the tube for the duration of the patient's life. If the majority of the tracheostomy tract is composed of friable cancer, changing the tube may be very difficult and often results in bleeding and acute airway obstruction. Unfortunately, many of the flexible tubes do not have an inner canulla. Therefore, meticulous cleaning and humidification are important in order to keep the tracheostomy patent. If the patient has an unsatisfactory tracheostomy and a change through tumor needs to be made, this can most safely be done over an endotracheal tube changer. Alternatively, the new tracheostomy can be placed over a flexible bronchoscope allowing direct visualization of the distal normal airway. The bronchoscope used must have a suction port. Both should be available when the tracheostomy is changed. In addition, a variety of endotracheal tubes, suction, an airway crash cart, and sedating medications should be immediately available. Lidocaine (4% topical) should be instilled in the existing tracheostomy to minimize coughing during the changeover. Often in an emergent situation with a bleeding stomal recurrence, an endotracheal tube is the easiest airway to insert due to the slightly beveled tip and flexible, curved contour of the tube.

Nutrition and Hydration

Many patients with terminal HNC and their families are very familiar with enteral feeding. Many of these patients will have had a nasogastric tube (NGT) or gastrostomy feeding tube following surgery or during radiation or chemoradiation. However, the issue of tube feeding for terminal patients in general engenders considerable debate (42–44). It is very important to clearly define the role of the feeding tube in terminal HNC patients and separate this from the use of feeding tubes in the general population of elderly, terminal patients.

There is clearly a case to be made against the routine use of feeding tubes in all terminal cancer patients. However, most of these arguments against feeding tubes do not apply to the terminal HNC patient. In the last weeks before death, it is natural for loss of appetite and thirst to occur, and it is tempting to think that enteral feeding will give the patient more energy and make the patient feel better and not be hungry. There is a tremendous cultural bias, which associates eating and weight gain with health. Unfortunately, for patients in the final phase of dying it is not true, and placement of a feeding tube in these circumstances is likely to cause the patient much more discomfort than symptom relief. There is substantial evidence to suggest that in the last month before death from chronic illness, hunger is very uncommon, and that death in a relative state of dehydration is much more pleasant than death in a normo- or hypervolemic state (45). Critics of tube feeding would also point out that there are no good data to suggest that a feeding tube actually improves the quality of life in terminal patients who are physically able to swallow but choose not to eat or are suffering from dementia. In addition, in this population acute and chronic complications associated with tube feeding are not uncommon (42–44). These scenarios, however, are very different from many cases of terminal HNC. Many terminal HNC patients are very coherent, are not in the final stages of death, and from a symptomatic standpoint would clearly benefit from enteral feeding. Most patients with terminal HNC are not able to eat due to neuroanatomic deficits in the upper aerodigestive tract, not terminal cachexia or dementia. As the terminal HNC patient enters the final stages of death, adjustments in tube feeding volume should be made.

In addition to nutrition, the feeding tube in many HNC patients is extremely useful as a route for delivery of medications. Many patients with terminal HNC are able to take nothing by mouth. This places severe limitations on the route of administering pain and other medications. Not all medications are appropriate for use through a feeding tube, and some medications will not be appropriate in combination with certain enteral feeding preparations. Consultation with a pharmacist and/or dietician may be helpful in preventing potential problems. Gilbar has published an excellent review on enteral drug administration in palliative care patients (46).

Aspiration is often a difficult issue with the terminal HNC patient and many other debilitated, elderly patients. Many patients have aspiration problems following intervention for HNC. In a number of patients a feeding tube is required because of aspiration. In many of these patients, there is a realistic expectation that swallowing will eventually improve and an oral diet resumed. In many others, the risk of fatal pneumonia substantially shortening life expectancy is the primary indication for the feeding tube. In the terminal cancer patient, it is unlikely that the clinical swallowing situation will change for the better, and the risk of fatal pneumonia must be weighed against the quality of life gained by being able to take some things by mouth. In these cases, an oropharyngeal swallow study may shed some light on the severity of aspiration and guide the clinician in counseling the patient about the risks of taking an oral diet. Often a speech pathologist can coach the patient on maneuvers that minimize aspiration, and in some cases prophylactic antibiotics would be appropriate. The final course of action should be left to the judgment of the patient with an understanding of the potential consequences of repeated aspiration.

Carotid Rupture

Despite the obvious potential for bleeding from the carotid artery or its major branches, death directly related to massive bleeding occurs in 1% or less of patients admitted to a palliative care program for terminal HNC (8,14,40,41). Over the past 20 years, substantial advances in the endovascular management of potential carotid rupture have been made. In addition to this, modern reconstructive procedures have afforded the carotid artery greater protection from pharyngocutaneous fistula contamination and overlying skin breakdown. Despite these advances, a number of patients will develop locally recurrent disease that puts the carotid artery at risk.

The current treatment paradigm for this problem is one of identifying the potential for vascular rupture and offering intervention early before a major carotid blowout with uncontrollable bleeding occurs. In the 1970s, endovascular occlusion of carotid-cavernous fistulas and intracranial aneurysms was developed, and in 1987 Zimmerman et al. (47) reported the use of detachable balloons to embolize the carotid artery in cases of impending rupture. The use of permanent detachable balloons to embolize the carotid was a significant advance over open surgical ligation. In many cases, surgical ligation of the carotid is extremely difficult because the involved carotid is not surgically accessible, the vessel walls are friable, or the vessel is encased in tumor (48). Unfortunately, endovascular carotid occlusion carries a risk of delayed cerebral ischemic complications in approximately 15% to 20% of cases, despite a satisfactory response to temporary test balloon occlusion. A further advance was reported by Lesley et al. (49) with the use of stents for endovascular reconstruction to bypass the compromised area of carotid in selected cases. This technique also allows for the endovascular management of patients who are deemed poor candidates for occlusion of the carotid artery due to an incomplete circle of Willis, occluded contralateral carotid, unstable clinical situation precluding balloon test occlusion, or failure of a test balloon occlusion study (49).

Most carotid blowouts do not occur without warning signs. Patients at highest risk include those who have had prior neck radiation and surgery with either a fistulous tract or recurrent cancer adjacent to the carotid. Sentinel bleeding from the oral cavity or neck is a late sign and indicates loss of vessel integrity. Of particular concern are active infection, necrotic tumor, and the absence of well-vascularized tissue within a wound through which the carotid artery passes. The potential for carotid rupture should be discussed with these patients. It may be very useful to obtain a computed tomography (CT) scan to clarify the potential risk. If there is a high level of concern due to necrotic tumor anatomically encroaching on the vascular space, prophylactic placement of a stent to bypass the compromised area or balloon occlusion should be offered to the patient. The decision to proceed with endovascular therapy will depend on the patient's anticipated survival. If the anticipated survival is weeks to months, endovascular management to prevent a vascular catastrophe should be strongly considered. In cases where death is very near, the patient is not going to be leaving the hospital, and the patient does not desire intervention unless a bleed is imminent, it is useful to have the patient meet with the interventional radiologist and discuss the procedure so that in the event a sentinel bleed occurs, they can be taken immediately to the angiography suite for management.

In cases where vascular rupture is not preventable and carotid rupture is a likely occurrence, family and caregivers should be educated about what to expect and counseled that death from carotid rupture is rapid and not painful. Most hospice programs have dark red or green bed sheets and towels that should be used with the patient. A short-acting benzodiazepine should be immediately available to administer if major bleeding occurs (40).

Tumor Hygiene

Local tumor ulceration, superinfection, and necrosis can be a significant detriment to the quality of life of the terminal HNC patient. Local infiltration with necrotic tumor is extremely disfiguring and may have a nearly unbearable odor. Localized surgery to decrease the size of or to remove surface lesions on the head and neck is rarely productive. If the lesion is a dermal metastasis, new metastatic lesions frequently appear before the excision site of the initial lesion is healed. If the lesion is due to skin involvement of an underlying tumor, complete excision is usually not possible. The resultant defect after partial excision is rarely much better than the original mass. If the area has not been previously treated with full-dose radiation therapy, occasionally a cone down field treated with a hypofractionated course may offer some benefit. This is not possible with large or deep lesions. One of the major problems with the larger lesions is that they become necrotic with surface ulceration that allows colonization with anaerobic bacteria, primarily *Bacteroides*. The odor emanating from these necrotic tumors is largely due to the volatile fatty acids released as a by-product of the anaerobic metabolism. In addition to routine debridement of necrotic tissues and dressing changes, systemic and topical metronidazole gel may have a very beneficial deodorizing effect (50,51). For painful lesions, opioids may be incorporated into the metronidazole gel preparation and, in some patients, additional pain relief obtained (52). The goal in these cases is to conceal the tumor, not the patient.

Terminal Care

Many patients with HNC remain mobile and prefer to be at home during the early period of terminal care. However, as we have discussed, many of these patients may have special needs (tracheostomy, enteral feedings, massive external cancers, significant comorbid illness, poor home support, and advanced age). When a patient is nearing death, becomes immobile, and enters the final phase of dying, adequate care for the patient may become difficult for home caregivers. In many circumstances, hospice home care is very satisfactory, and the hospice workers may be quite facile at managing the tracheostomy, feeding tubes, and external lesions. However, if the family is struggling, admission back to a head and neck oncology ward is often appropriate. The head and neck ward generally has familiar faces, the staff is comfortable with the peculiarities of HNC patients, and, as Meachen (9) has indicated, returning to the head and neck ward is, in a sense, returning to familiar ground for many of these patients. In some instances, the return may only be for several days. This gives the family a break and allows for a reevaluation of the medications, nutritional requirements, and status of any troubling symptoms. Having a terminal patient in an acute care hospital requires that they be protected from unnecessary interventions not appropriate in the terminal care of the patient. All staff managing the patient should be very clear on the management goals for the admission.

SUMMARY

Palliative care for HNC patients is often very challenging. The key to success lies in the identification of realistic patient-directed goals and the setting up of a systematic approach to address each goal individually.

In this chapter, we focused on the major physical issues faced by HNC patients. Many of these issues confront elderly patients without HNC who are at the end of life. The emphasis here has been a discussion of the physical problems. It is crucial to ensure that the emotional, social, and spiritual issues these patients have are addressed as well. There are a number of controversies in the palliative care of patients at the end of life. However, there is universal recognition that the management of these very complex, fragile patients and their families requires a multidisciplinary team.

CASE STUDIES

Case Study 1

A 57-year-old male presents to the otolaryngologist's office for evaluation of increasing dyspnea. The patient had a history of a T3 N0 M0 squamous cell carcinoma of the larynx treated with a chemoradiation protocol for organ preservation. He had done well for 1.5 years when he began developing difficulties with breathing on exertion. He was assessed by the local otolaryngologist and found to have edema and possible recurrence of his tumor. On endoscopy, a diagnosis of recurrent squamous cell carcinoma was made and a suggestion of laryngectomy for salvage was broached. As part of the preoperative work-up, metastatic disease throughout the pulmonary cavity was discovered. Bone pain precipitated a bone scan, which confirmed multiple bony metastasis. The patient presents for consideration of further treatment in management of his airway.

A laryngectomy was considered but, given the patient's prognosis with multiple bony and pulmonary metastasis, not felt to be warranted. Management of the patient's airway was felt to be of prime importance, and a tracheotomy was performed. The patient was taught the use of a Passy-Muir valve and is able to function well at home with his locally recurrent disease. Swallowing and pain control were not an issue, and he was entered into the hospice care program. His case demonstrates how management of end-stage HNC involving airway compromise can provide symptom relief of the upper aerodigestive tract and not compromise quality of life in terms of speech.

Case Study 2

A 74-year-old male presents for evaluation of his head and neck tumor. His history extended back four years when he was initially treated for a T1 carcinoma of the tongue. Surgical excision was performed and reconstruction performed with primary closure. He did well for one year and then developed a local recurrence. A formal hemiglossectomy with neck dissection was performed, and he was reconstructed with a radial forearm free flap. He received postoperative radiotherapy, which necessitated placement of a nasogastric feeding tube for a protracted period of time. Two months ago, he developed recurrence in the neck, as well as the primary site, and declined salvage surgery. He has had gradual loss of ability to maintain his weight by oral intake and had a nasogastric feeding tube placed by his family physician.

The gentleman is in the palliative care program and was referred for consideration of alternative feeding methodologies. On evaluation in the office, his recurrence in the oral cavity is obvious but does not compromise his airway. The neck recurrence is well contained and is not functionally or cosmetically debilitating.

Assessment by speech therapy is performed and confirms the slow transit time due to immobility and involvement of the entire tongue by tumor. There is evidence of aspiration and, while swallowing can be done safely with some modifications in head position and airway protection ensured with supraglottic swallow techniques, the feeling of the speech therapist in conjunction with the patient is that the time and effort required to take enough oral nutrition to maintain body weight is unlikely to be successful. The patient is very unhappy with his nasogastric feeding tube.

In this case, the patient's airway is stable and while the possibility of a tracheotomy was discussed with him, it is not something that requires placement at this point in time. Pain control is adequate, and there is no cosmetic or other functional debility from the tumor. The patient's main issues are oral supplementation and unhappiness with the nasogastric feeding tube. In these cases, consideration should be given to placement of a gastrostomy tube to enhance nutritional status, as well as facilitate oral medication administration. After an appropriate discussion between the patient and his family, a gastrostomy tube is placed by the General Surgery Service and the patient is discharged back to the hospice service.

Case Study 3

A 53-year-old male presents for management of his recurrent neck tumor. His history extends back approximately two years ago when he presented with a T2 N3 squamous cell carcinoma of the hypopharynx. He underwent total laryngectomy with partial pharyngectomy and radical neck dissection. Postoperative radiation therapy was given and after a long rehabilitation he was able to use his tracheoesophageal puncture for speech, as well as take enough oral nutrition to maintain his weight. Four months ago, he developed a recurrence in his neck. The neck tumor was wrapped around the carotid artery and invaded the prevertebral muscles. He was given one course of chemotherapy to which the tumor did not respond and referred to hospice. At this point in time, the tumor has eroded through the skin and is a fungating mass that is quite odorous. He also has many complaints concerning pain in the neck and area of the tumor.

On examination, he has a hard fixed mass fungating through the skin that is approximately 5×7 cm. It is ulcerative and quite necrotic. It is fixed to the muscles of the floor of the neck, and he has marked limitation of motion of the neck and head due to the tumor fixation.

This gentleman has two main issues. The first concerns the malodorous fungating neck mass. Metronidazole gel dressings are started and a short course of oral

Flagyl® is given. This results in some resolution of the malodor, and with good local wound care the cosmetic and social aspects of the recurrent tumor are managed.

Pain control is a more difficult issue. The patient was initially started on oxycodone but continued to have moderate pain at night. Hydromorphine was added along with an NSAID. This combination proved successful and alleviated his pain.

REFERENCES

1. Fox E. Predominance of the curative model on medical care a residual problem. JAMA 1997; 278:761–763.
2. World Health Organization report on cancer pain and palliative care. Technical report series No. 804. Geneva, Switzerland: World Health Organization—Marketing and Dissemination, 1990.
3. Hoffman HT, Karnell LHK, Funk G, et al. The National cancer data base report on cancer of the head and neck. Arch Otolaryngol Head Neck Surg 1998; 124:951–962.
4. Hodson DI, Bruera E, Eapen L, et al. The role of palliative radiotherapy in advanced head and neck cancer. Can J Oncol (suppl) 1996; 6(1):54–60.
5. Downing GM, Braithwaite DL, Wilde JM. Victoria BGY palliative care model—a new model for the 1990s. J Palliat Care 1993; 9:26–32.
6. Funk GF, Karnell LH, Dawson CJ, et al. Baseline and post-treatment assessment of the general health status of head and neck cancer patients compared to United States population norms. Head Neck 1997; 19:675–683.
7. Terrell JE, Nanavati K, Esclamado RM, et al. Health impact of head and neck cancer. Otolaryngol Head Neck Surg 1999; 120:852–859.
8. Aird DW, Bihari J, Smith C. Clinical problems in the continuing care of head and neck cancer patients. Ear Nose Throat J 1983; 62:10–30.
9. Meachen MA. Terminal care of a patient suffering from head and neck cancer. N Zealand Nurs J 1985; 78:8–9.
10. Kidder TM. Symptom management for incurable head and neck cancer. Wisconsin Med J 1997; 96:19–24.
11. Vecht CJ, Hoff AM, Kansen PJ, et al. Types and causes of pain in cancer of the head and neck. Cancer 1992; 70:178–184.
12. Olsen KD, Creagan ET. Pain management in advanced carcinoma of the head and neck. Am J Otolaryngol 1991; 12:154–160.
13. Talmi YP, Waller A, Bercovici M, et al. Pain experienced by patients with terminal head and neck carcinoma. Cancer 1997; 80:1117–1123.
14. Shedd DP, Carl A, Shedd C. Problems of terminal head and neck cancer patients. Head Neck Surg 1980; 2:476–482.
15. Kowalski LP, Carvalho AL. Natural history of untreated head and neck cancer. Eur J Cancer 2000; 36:1032–1037.
16. Emanuel LL, von Gunten CF, Ferris FD, eds. The Education in Palliative and End-of Life Care (EPEC) Curriculum: © The EPEC Project, 1999, 2003.
17. Foley KM. Pain assessment and cancer pain syndromes. In: Doyle D, Hanks GWC, Mac Donald N, eds. Oxford Textbook of Palliative Medicine. 2nd ed. New York, NY: Oxford University Press Inc., 1998:310–331.
18. Chua KSG, Reddy SK, Lee MC, Patt RB. Pain and loss of function in head and neck cancer survivors. J Pain Symptom Manage 1999; 18:193–202.
19. Carroll EN, Fine E, Ruff RL, Stepnick D. A four-drug regimen for head and neck cancers. Laryngoscope 1994; 104:694–700.
20. Shapshay SM, Scott RM, McCann CF, Stoelting I. Pain control in advanced and recurrent head and neck cancer. Otolaryngol Clin North Am 1980; 13:551–560.

21. Grond S, Zech D, Lehmann KA, et al. Transdermal fentanyl in the long-term treatment of cancer pain: a prospective study of 50 patients with advanced cancer of the gastrointestinal tract or the head and neck region. Pain 1997; 69:191–198.

22. Levy MH. Pharmacologic treatment of cancer pain. NEJM 1996; 335:1124–1132.

23. Zech DFJ, Grond S, Lynch J, et al. Validation of the World Health Organization guidelines for cancer pain relief: a 10-year prospective study. Pain 1995; 63:65–76.

24. Payne R, Gonzales GR. Pathophysiology of pain in cancer and other terminal diseases. In: Doyle D, Hanks GWC, Mac Donald N, eds. Oxford Textbook of Palliative Medicine. 2nd ed. New York, NY: Oxford University Press Inc., 1998:299–310.

25. Stanton-Hicks M, Janig W, Hassenbusch S, et al. Reflex sympathetic distrophy: changing concepts and taxonomy. Pain 1995; 63:127–133.

26. Storey P, Knight CF. American Academy of Hospice and Palliative Medicine, UNIPAC Three: assessment and treatment of pain in the terminally ill. Dubuque, Iowa: Kendall/ Hunt Publishing Co., 1997.

27. Grond S, Radbruch L, Meuser T, et al. Assessment and treatment of neuropathic cancer pain following WHO guidelines. Pain 1999; 70:15–20.

28. Ashburn MA, Lipman AG, Carr D, Rubingh C. Principles of analgesic use in the treatment of acute pain and cancer pain. 5th ed. Glenview, IL: American Pain Society, 2003.

29. Mercadante S. Malignant bone pain: pathophysiology and treatment. Pain 1997; 69:1–18.

30. Hanks G, Cherny N. Opioid analgesic therapy. In: Doyle D, Hanks GWC, Mac Donald N, eds. Oxford Textbook of Palliative Medicine. 2nd ed. New York, NY: Oxford University Press Inc., 1998:331–335.

31. Georgiou L, Louizos A, Sklavou C, et al. Cervical versus epidural morphine for the treatment of head and neck cancer pain. Ann Otol Rhinol Laryngol 2000; 109:676–678.

32. Varchese BT, Koshy RC. Endoscopic transnasal neurolytic sphenopalatine ganglion block for head and neck cancer pain. J Laryngol Otol 2001; 115:385–387.

33. Goto F, Ishizaki K, Yoshikawa D, et al. The long lasting effects of peripheral nerve blocks for trigeminal neuralgia using high concentration of tetrocaine dissolved in bupivicaine. Pain 1999; 79:101–103.

34. Varghese BT. Combined sphenopalatine ganglion and mandibular nerve, neurolytic block for pain due to advanced head and neck cancer. Palliat Med 2002; 16:447–448.

35. van Kleef M, Liem L, Lousberg R, et al. Radiofrequency lesion adjacent to the dorsal root ganglion for cervicobrachial pain: a prospective double blind randomized study. Neurosurgery 1996; 38:1127–1132.

36. Mullan S. Surgical management of pain in cancer of the head and neck. Surg Clin North Am 1973; 53:203–210.

37. Pagni CA. Maspes: problems in the surgical treatment of pain in malignancies of the head and neck. Current research in neurosciences. In: Wycis HT, ed. Topical Problems in Psychiatric Neurology. Vol. 10. Basel/New York: Karger, 1970:138–153.

38. Clark JL, Kalan GE. Effective treatment of severe cancer pain of the head using low-dose ketamine in an opioid-tolerant patient. J Pain Symp Manage 1995; 10:310–314.

39. Ripamonti C, Zecca E, Bruera E. An update on the clinical use of methadone for cancer pain. Pain 1977; 70:109–115.

40. Forbes K. Palliative care in patients with cancer of the head and neck. Clin Otolaryngol 1997; 22:117–122.

41. Talmi YP, Roth Y, Waller A, et al. Care of the terminal head and neck cancer patient in the hospice setting. Laryngoscope 1995; 105:315–318.

42. Campbell-Taylor I, Fisher RH. The clinical case against tube feeding in palliative care of the elderly. J Am Geriatr Soc 1987; 35:1100–1104.

43. Ciocon JO, Siverstone FA, Graver LM, Foley CJ. Tube feeding in elderly patients indications, benefits and complications. Arch Intern Med 1988; 148:429–433.

44. Rabeneck L, Wray NP, Peterson NJ. Long-term outcomes of patients receiving percutaneous endoscopic gastrostomy tubes. J Gen Intern Med 1996; 11:287–293.

45. Morrison RS, Morris J. When there is no cure: palliative care for the dying patient. Geriatrics 1995; 50:45–51.
46. Gilbar PJ. A guide to enteral drug administration in palliative care. J Pain Symp Manage 1999; 17:197–207.
47. Zimmerman MC, Mickel RA, Kessler DJ, et al. Treatment of impending carotid rupture with detachable balloon embolization. Arch Otolaryngol Head Neck Surg 1987; 113:1169–1175.
48. Chaloupka JC, Putman CM, Citardi MJ, et al. Endovascular therapy for the carotid blowout syndrome in head and neck surgical patients: diagnostic and managerial considerations. Am J Neuroradiol 1996; 17:843–852.
49. Lesley WS, Chaloupka JC, Weigele JB, et al. Preliminary experience with endovascular reconstruction for the management of carotid blowout syndrome. Am J Neuroradiol 2003; 24:975–981.
50. Anonymous. Management of smelly tumors. Lancet 1990; 335:141–142.
51. Dean MM. Metronidazole and fungating tumors. Can Med Assoc J 1990; 143:89–90.
52. Flock P, Gibbs L, Sykes N. Diamorphine-metronidazole gel effective for treatment of painful infected leg ulcers. J Pain Symp Manage 2000; 20:396–397.

ANNOTATED BIBLIOGRAPHY

Chua KSG, Reddy SK, Lee MC, Patt RB. Pain and loss of function in head and neck cancer survivors. J Pain Symptom Manage 1999; 18:193–202.

This article provides a detailed analysis of the types of pain encountered in all HNC patients and the difficulties that are encountered in managing them.

Forbes K. Palliative care in patients with cancer of the head and neck. Clin Otolaryngol 1997; 22:117–122.

This paper provides an excellent overall clinical picture of the HNC patient population admitted to hospice care and the problems encountered with this group of patients.

Gilbar PJ. A guide to enteral drug administration in palliative care. J Pain Symptom Manage 1999; 17:197–207.

This paper is extremely useful for anyone managing patients who are receiving medications and feeding through an enteral tube. A systematic evaluation of enteral medications is presented.

Levy MH. Pharmacologic treatment of cancer pain. NEJM 1996; 335:1124–1132.

This is a well-written and comprehensive review of the pharmacologic treatment of cancer pain.

Principles of analgesic use in the treatment of acute pain and cancer pain. 5th ed. Glenview, IL: American Pain Society, 2003.

This small pamphlet is available through the American Pain Society and is an excellent reference for all types of pain management. The tables of medications, doses, and conversions are very useful.

68

Hospice for the Otolaryngologist

Paul Bascom
*Palliative Medicine and Comfort Care Team, Division of General Internal Medicine,
Oregon Health and Science University, Portland, Oregon, U.S.A.*

HISTORICAL PERSPECTIVE

The term "hospice" originated in the middle ages. At its origin, a hospice was a shelter or lodging for travelers. Often, monastic orders developed hospices to serve pilgrims traveling from Europe to Jerusalem. In the 19th century, the word hospice became synonymous with a place where the dying received care. Religious orders established centers dedicated to the care of the dying, called hospices, in several European countries and subsequently in North America.

The rise of hospice as a place for terminal care dates to the establishment of St. Christopher's Hospice in London in 1967. St. Christopher's creation and much of the subsequent growth of hospice care around the world resulted largely from the efforts of one woman, Dame Cicely Saunders, MD. Dr. Saunders is credited with the inspiration that the medical, social, and spiritual needs of the dying be integrated in a place where the dying could receive comprehensive, holistic care.

Hospice in the United States developed with a distinctly American character. Connecticut Hospice was established in 1974 and modeled on St. Christopher's Hospice as a physical building where dying patients could come to spend their last days. However, the founders of Connecticut Hospice soon discovered that many Americans preferred to spend their last days at home and did not wish to enter a hospice facility. Thus was founded the unique American version of home-based hospice care. The initial home-based hospice programs in the United States emerged from community groups and not from established medical institutions. The programs sustained themselves on charitable funding, as there was not formal reimbursement for hospice services at the time. The focus of care centered less on the provision of technical medical services and more on the presence of lay volunteers providing presence and spiritual support for the dying.

The establishment of the Medicare hospice benefit in the 1980s provided financial stability that fueled the dramatic growth of hospice care over the next 20 years. Initial home hospice demonstration projects in the early 1980s demonstrated that hospice care was less expensive than traditional hospital-based care of the dying. This fact, that hospice care would save Medicare dollars, led to the enactment of the Medicare hospice benefit in 1982. From these humble origins, hospice care has grown to become the standard of care for dying patients. By 2000, 25% of the patients dying in the United States, more than 750,000 per year, received hospice care.

HOSPICE—A PHILOSOPHY OF CARE AND A PROGRAM OF SERVICES

Hospice care represents a philosophy of care that focuses on the physical, social, and spiritual needs of dying patients and their families. Hospice care is palliative rather than curative and seeks to maintain quality of life rather than to prolong life. In the United States, hospice became a program of services for those with terminal illness living in their own homes. Because of the historical roots, patients, families, and physicians may still often misidentify "hospice" as a physical place. Hospice care correctly refers to a program of services and a philosophy of care.

The Medicare Hospice Benefit

The particular features of the Medicare hospice benefit determine the eligibility criteria and scope of services available for hospice patients. Most geriatric patients with terminal illness are eligible for the Medicare hospice benefit. While the benefit does have many limitations, it is important to remember that it was also quite revolutionary for its time, in 1982. First, hospice care is fully capitated. Hospice programs receive a fixed daily reimbursement, around $100, for providing the totality of care the patients receive. Those who require minimal care offset the cost of providing care to complex, high-need patients. To that extent, hospice programs function in some ways like managed care organizations. Second, the family is the unit of care. Certain services such as bereavement and respite care are available for family members. Third, spiritual care, bereavement care, and volunteer services are required.

Scope of Services

Hospice care provides periodic home visits from nurses, social workers, chaplains, home health aides, volunteers, and others in support of family caregivers. These visits can range from daily to weekly depending on patient and family needs. Importantly, hospice does not provide 24-hour custodial care. Patients and families are responsible for the ongoing, daily care and other support that a patient may require. Family members often provide variable amounts of care. Options are available when the family is unavailable or incapable of providing needed custodial care. Some patients may move to, or may already reside in, nursing homes or assisted living facilities. Some families will choose to hire private caregivers.

Hospice provides coverage for all medications related to the terminal illness. Oxygen, supplies, and durable medical equipment, such as hospital beds, are also covered. Routine, long-term medications not related to the terminal condition remain the patient's responsibility.

While hospice care centers on the care of the individual in their own home, the hospice benefit allows hospitalization when symptoms persist despite optimal care in the home. The benefit also allows periodic five-day respite stays in a nursing home to relieve family caregivers. For patients who prefer not to be hospitalized and their families, hospice programs can provide a short-term continuous nursing presence in the home when symptoms remain uncontrolled despite periodic visits from hospice staff.

Eligibility Criteria

Enrollment in hospice requires the presence of an illness likely to cause death within six months. The caveat "expected course" reflects the difficulty of prognostication. Patients must be reevaluated periodically to ensure that they continue to meet the eligibility criteria of expected death within six months, even if their actual longevity exceeds six months. If their prognosis changes and patients no longer are expected to die within six months, then they can be discharged from hospice and reenroll at some future date when prognosis once again worsens.

Medicare patients who elect their hospice benefit waive traditional Medicare for all treatment related to their terminal condition. In essence, patients electing hospice choose to forgo expensive treatment designed to prolong life and instead elect hospice care with its expanded benefits. Patients may revoke their hospice benefit and reestablish traditional Medicare if they choose to pursue life-prolonging or curative treatment for their illness. Medicare continues to pay for all treatments not related to the terminal illness.

Limitations to the Medicare Hospice Benefit

The capitated structure of hospice reimbursement means that some patients with high cost treatments may not be eligible for hospice care. For example, some chemotherapy might be effective for a terminally ill patient but prohibitively costly for the hospice program as a whole. Large programs in urban areas can shoulder some expensive treatments, while small programs in rural areas cannot, since they have a limited number of low-cost patients on which to spread the burden of a single high-cost patient.

Definition of Palliative

Some confusion regarding eligibility for hospice originates around differing understandings of the word "palliative." Medicare rules require that hospice programs pay for "all palliative treatments related to the terminal illness." Some physicians contrast palliative treatments with curative treatments. Those treatments that cannot cure are considered palliative. These treatments usually have the primary goal of prolonging life without achieving cure. For hospice, the definition of palliative is more constrained. Palliative treatments are those whose primary goal is to alleviate symptoms, without the expectation of prolonging life.

DISCUSSING HOSPICE CARE WITH PATIENTS AND FAMILIES

Despite the impressive gains made by hospice in caring for the dying, many hospice patients receive hospice care very late in their illness. Fifty percent of patients are referred just weeks or even days prior to death; median lengths of stay under hospice care, or time to death after referral, for most hospice programs are 14 to 21 days.

Difficulty in Prognosis

The reasons for late referral are multifactorial and sometimes unavoidable. In certain acute, catastrophic illnesses, the time from development of a terminal condition to death may be quite brief. For example, a patient with an acute stroke, or a frail elderly patient with severe pneumonia may die just days after the illness begins. In these patients, the proximity of death could be predicted even the day prior to the onset of the terminal illness.

However, in many conditions common to otolaryngology, such as metastatic head and neck cancers or dysphagia with recurrent aspiration pneumonia, the inevitability and proximity of death can be predicted months prior to death. Yet physicians are remarkably inaccurate in their predictions of survival at the time of referral to hospice. In one study, the duration of the physician–patient relationship was inversely correlated with accuracy in physician prognosis. This may represent physician unwillingness to acknowledge a poor prognosis in a patient they care more deeply about, or may signify that the gradual changes that herald the proximity of death are less evident to those with a long, established relationship.

Providing Accurate Prognostic Information

Physicians have a responsibility to provide patients and families with accurate prognostic information, at least to the extent possible. When physicians refuse to provide an answer by saying "there is no crystal ball," they are abdicating this fundamental responsibility. As death nears, it becomes possible with increasing accuracy to predict survival. Patients with metastatic cancer who are rapidly losing functional capacity generally have weeks to a few months to live. When these same patients become bed-bound survival is measured by days to weeks, and when they are rarely awake they only have hours to days to live.

The familiar evasive answer of "you have less than six months to live" is also inadequate to meet patient and family needs. They may make plans as if they have exactly six months to live. They may also come to doubt the original diagnosis if they happen to live eight or nine months. No physician can accurately say that someone has "about six months to live." At that distance, it is possible only to estimate a range of possibilities, say, three to nine months, since the natural history of terminal illness varies substantially from patient to patient. However, physicians can advise patients and families that, as time progresses, the specific trajectory of their illness will become clearer. Those patients who at two months have declined significantly are likely to live only three months. Whereas those who at six months have shown no major change may indeed survive nine months or even longer.

Physicians often delay effective communication about prognosis. Two barriers to such effective communication include what have been called "the rescue fantasy" and "the conspiracy of silence."

The term "rescue fantasy" describes the illusion that repeated successful interventions for acute complications of an underlying condition somehow indicates that the underlying condition will not be ultimately fatal. For example, successful treatment of acute pneumonia in a patient with chronic recurrent aspiration may lead physicians to suggest that the patient can endure indefinitely. Instead, physicians should use these events to reinforce the understanding that the condition will ultimately cause the patient's death, even as they express gratitude of another successful intervention and a forestalling of death.

A related term, "the conspiracy of silence," reflects how physicians, patients, and families together conspire to ensure that no discussion of death ever occurs. This is understandable. Discussing a potentially terminal prognosis is always difficult for everyone involved. Thus, all parties have an interest in avoiding such conversations. Patients and families often wait for the doctor to raise the issue, while physicians may wait for patients to give some signal that they are ready to hear the news. However, all parties benefit when open and honest discussion of prognosis occurs.

Admittedly, a few patients may never acknowledge a terminal diagnosis and will resist any attempt to discuss the inevitability of death openly. In these rare cases, physicians should respect a patient's right to maintain their denial. It is helpful to ask a patient's permission to discuss their prognosis in a way that allows this denial to be maintained: for example, a physician might say, "I have some concerns about your illness. Is this something that we can discuss, or would you prefer not to discuss those possibilities?"

Effective Communication About Hospice Care

Some late referrals to hospice stem from ineffective communication with patients and families about prognosis and goals. When communication is not effective, physicians may present hospice inaccurately to patients and families. The false choice often mistakenly presented to patients and families is this: "Do you want to live, or do you want hospice?" All too often, hospice becomes the euphemism by which physicians inform their patients that they are dying. Physicians may say "you need hospice care" as a way of signaling to the patient that death is near and that no further treatment is likely to be of benefit. From the patient and family point of view, they may presume that by accepting hospice care, they are somehow "giving up" or forgoing other effective treatment. These patients and families may refuse hospice care upon these mistaken beliefs.

Effective communication about hospice care originates with clear discussions about prognosis and the risks and benefits of further treatment. To make an informed choice about hospice care, patients and families must understand that the illness is likely to cause death. They must also understand the risks and benefits of continuing aggressive treatment for their illness. For example, patients with metastatic head and neck cancer can be informed that further chemotherapy would not change inevitable death, but could provide the benefit of some prolongation of life, though at a risk of increased burden of symptoms, increased risk of hospitalization, and increased risk of uncontrolled hospital death with acute complications of therapy.

Hospice then becomes not a choice between living and dying, but a positive choice to embrace certain benefits at a cost of some modest risk. Hospice care offers the benefit of increased symptom control, improved support for family caregivers, decreased burden of treatment-related side effects, increased focus on living and maximizing quality of life, diminished focus on illness and its treatment, and increased chance for controlled death at home. The risk involves letting go of the small chance that further medical treatment might somehow prolong life in an unexpected way. When presented with the option of hospice in this way, as a positive choice to achieve certain goals in the face of inevitable death, most patients and families will gladly forgo the fleeting chance for increased life and will choose hospice and its focus on maximizing quality of life.

Hospice Means Living

Hospice has unfairly been cast as only a place to die, when it rightfully represents the possibility of living fully during terminal illness. As Dr. Cicely Saunders, the founder of modern-day hospice has said: "You matter to the last moment of your life, and we will do all we can, not only to help you die peacefully, but to live until you die."

Index